The New Mind-Body
Science of Depression

A Norton Professional Book

The New Mind-Body Science of Depression

Vladimir Maletic
Charles Raison

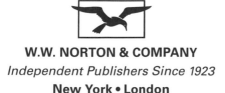

W.W. NORTON & COMPANY
Independent Publishers Since 1923
New York • London

Note to Readers: Standards of clinical practice and protocol change over time, and no technique or recommendation is guaranteed to be safe or effective in all circumstances. This volume is intended as a general information resource for professionals practicing in the field of psychotherapy and mental health; it is not a substitute for appropriate training, peer review, and/or clinical supervision. Neither the publisher nor the author(s) can guarantee the complete accuracy, efficacy, or appropriateness of any particular recommendation in every respect.

For information about permission to reproduce selections from this book, write to Permissions, W. W. Norton & Company, Inc., 500 Fifth Avenue, New York, NY 10110

For information about special discounts for bulk purchases, please contact W. W. Norton Special Sales at specialsales@wwnorton.com or 800-233-4830

Manufacturing by Maple Press
Production manager: Christine Critelli

Library of Congress Cataloging-in-Publication Data

Names: Maletic, Vladimir, author. | Raison, Charles L., author.
Title: The new mind-body science of depression / Vladimir Maletic, Charles Raison.
Description: New York : W. W Norton & Company, [2017] | Includes bibliographical references and index.
Identifiers: LCCN 2016039533 | ISBN 9780393706666 (hardcover)
Subjects: | MESH: Depressive Disorder, Major—psychology | Depressive Disorder, Major—physiopathology | Psychophysiology
Classification: LCC RC537 | NLM WM 207 | DDC 616.85/270651—dc23 LC record available at https://lccn.loc.gov/2016039533

ISBN: 978-0-393-70666-6

W. W. Norton & Company, Inc., 500 Fifth Avenue, New York, N.Y. 10110
www.wwnorton.com
W. W. Norton & Company Ltd., 15 Carlisle Street, London W1D 3BS

1 2 3 4 5 6 7 8 9 0

To my two primary teachers:

Edgar Michael Bravo and Andrew H. Miller

—C.R.

I dedicate this book to my wife Dr.Bernadette DeMuri-Maletic
and my son Stefan Maletic for their forbearance and
unconditional loving support.

—V.M.

Contents

Acknowledgments

This book would never have been possible without the wisdom, support, hard work and patience of many people at W.W. Norton & Company, especially Deborah Malmud, Mariah Eppes, Christine Critelli, Elizabeth Baird, Kevin Olsen, Julia Gardiner, and Natasha Senn. Thanks also to Sheryl Rowe for her sharp eye and hard work. We also wish to acknowledge and thank Roland Tuley and Fire and Rain productions, for their invaluable assistance with illustrations.

This book presents several clinical cases to illustrate general themes presented in previous chapters. All these cases are composites and do not represent the real life experiences of any single individuals.

The New Mind-Body
Science of Depression

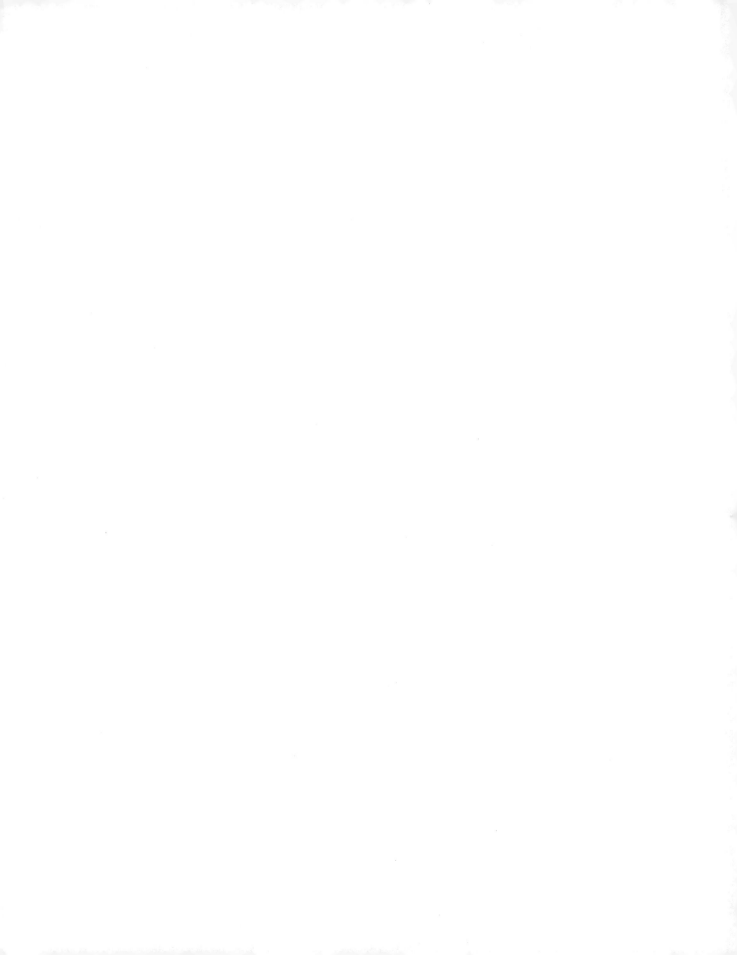

CHAPTER 1

Does Major Depression Exist?
Or, Why the Diagnostic Rule Book Is (Mostly) Wrong

There is increasing evidence that the very broad and heterogeneous Major Depressive Disorder (MDD) category, which has remained more or less unchanged since *DSM-III* has not led to advances in biological or treatment research. The MDD concept as it currently stands was created in *DSM-III* based on primarily political considerations, as documented in a recent history based on a reading of the minutes of the meeting of the *DSM-III* task force.

S. Nassir Ghaemi, personal communication, 2011

If we assume that the clinical syndromes based on subjective symptoms are unique and unitary disorders, we undercut the power of biology to identify illnesses linked to pathophysiology and we limit the development of more specific treatments.

Research Domain Criteria project description,
National Institute of Mental Health

The question of whether major depression exists must surely be one of the most rhetorical ones that ever started a book. If depression doesn't exist, we wouldn't be writing a book about it, and you never would have read the question in the first place. Moreover, people have been getting depressed since the beginning of recorded history.[1] Although it manifests a little differently in different cultures,[2] depression is found all over the world today[3,4] and tends to come about in similar situations everywhere.[4] Studies by anthropologists demonstrate that modern-day hunter-gather groups suffer from the same type of depressive symptoms as those in first-world societies, get depressed over the same types of issues, and have similar biological changes,[5,6] strongly suggesting that our hunter-gatherer ancestors probably also got depressed. So how can major depression not exist?

But as we hope you'll agree as you continue reading, we are asking this question in all earnestness, and we have an answer that might seem surprising, coming as it does from two psychiatrists. Shakespeare spoke of language providing things with a "local habitation and a name." Certainly major depression has a name, and in that way it exists. But just as certainly it has no local habitation. Compared with an entity that exists in the way a Rembrandt painting exists, or a blockage in a coronary artery exists, or a tumor exists, major depression is without existence.

Anyone who knows the full speech of Theseus in Shakespeare's *Midsummer Night's Dream* knows that the poet gives a local habitation and name to "airy nothings." Anyone who has ever suffered from depression or cared for someone with the condition will most emphatically assert that the disease is far from being an "airy nothing," and modern science couldn't agree more. When we say major depression doesn't exist, we mean that it doesn't exist as a separate, distinct disease state whose contours are exactly sketched by the diagnostic criteria one finds in that "bible" of psychiatry, the fifth edition of the *Diagnostic and Statistical Manual for Mental Disorders* (*DSM-5*).[7] In fact, as we shall see, overwhelming data show that depression is not a discrete illness at all but is, rather, a probabilistic tendency to exhibit any of a wide range of interrelated symptoms in response to many types of environmental adversity.

Many mental health clinicians might respond to this last statement with, "Say what?" For two generations we have been trained to see *DSM*-defined conditions as diseases like tuberculosis or cancer, with sharp boundaries that differentiate them from both health and other medical conditions. The idea of depression as a discrete illness has been enshrined, one might almost say entombed, in the official diagnostic schema of modern psychiatry for so long that many of us can't spontaneously see psychiatric conditions as anything other than hard little marbles of clear-cut pathology, each with its own "local habitation." Most of us have at least a vague sense that this doesn't quite fit our clinical experience or the findings of science, but when push comes to shove we can't let go of this way of looking at things.

The National Institute of Mental Health has been especially vocal about the problems with our same old way of doing psychiatric business.[8] One might think that if one of the major research bodies in the world believes that our current way of looking at conditions like depression is causing more harm than good in terms of promoting scientific discovery, the powers that be within psychiatry would make an urgent "all hands on deck" call for the profession to unite and figure out some better way of doing things. But as we shall see, scientific discoveries don't provide easy clues for how to supplant our current diagnostic system with a more accurate or more useful one. Still, the National Institute of Mental Health has taken a bold step in this regard with its efforts to draft a set of Research Domain Criteria that will supplement current *DSM*-based diagnoses with an organizational approach to mental disorders that is much closer to the perspective we espouse in this book.[8,9] But the government, in all its cautious wisdom, notes that this attempt to place psychiatric diagnoses on a scientific footing will only "be an early step in what is expected to be a long journey toward a new approach to classification."[9]

We aim in this book to cut that long journey short, at least regarding depression. It is our claim that scientific advances over the last 20 years provide answers to many of the issues regarding depression that matter most. We know why depression exists and what kind of illness it is. We know what causes it. We know the changes in brain and body that promote its development, and we know a lot about why treatment works—and doesn't work. We know why depression associates so closely with all other psychiatric and medical conditions, we know why it is typically a recurrent condition, and we are constantly learning more about why—and how—depression damages the brain and body over time. Moreover, we hope to demonstrate that many aspects of depression that are currently considered inexplicable, or are simply ignored despite their importance, can be explained by synthesizing already available information from neuroscience, cybernetics, anthropology, sociology, evolutionary biology, evolutionary psychology, neuroendocrinology, immunology, and yes, psychiatry—although the understanding of depression we espouse could not be derived from the mental health literature alone. Most important, a view of depression based on the new body-mind science generates clear—and testable—predictions to guide future scientific and clinical endeavors. Finally, while it is true that the full therapeutic implications of scientific findings will require significant time to come to full fruition, we feel strongly that viewing depression in ways consistent with our best current science already has some very novel and important treatment implications.

Before backing up these claims in the remainder of the book with all the evidence we can muster, we think it is important to give a quick accounting of how major depression came into existence as a discrete disease state and why subsequent science has snuffed it out. Mindful of George Santayana's dictum that "those who cannot remember the past are condemned to repeat it," we think that only by understanding at least the rudiments of how depression came to be misunderstood as a discrete illness can we be sure not to replace current conceptions with new ones that recapitulate the same old problems.

How Did Major Depression Come to Be?

Let's start by being clear by what we mean when we say *major depression*. In this book, when we write *major depression*, we mean nothing more or less than the current diagnostic criteria that describe—or, perhaps more accurately, create—the disorder, as expounded in the version of the *DSM* current at the time of this writing, the *DSM-5*. Table 1.1 lists diagnostic criteria, as well as relevant exclusionary

TABLE 1.1. Major Depressive Disorder Diagnostic Criteria[7]

A. Five (or more) of the following symptoms have been present during the same 2-week period and represent a change from previous functioning; at least one of the symptoms is either (1) depressed mood or (2) loss of interest of pleasure. **Note:** Do not include symptoms that are clearly attributable to another medical condition.
1. Depressed mood most of the day, nearly every day, as indicated by either subjective report (e.g., feels sad, empty, hopeless) or observation made by others (e.g., appears tearful). (**Note:** In children and adolescents, can be irritable mood.)
2. Markedly diminished interest of pleasure in all, or almost all, activities most of the day, nearly every day (as indicated by either subjective account or observation).
3. Significant weight loss when not dieting or weight gain (e.g., a change of more than 5% of body weight in a month), or decrease or increase in appetite nearly every day. (**Note:** In children, consider failure to make expected weight gain.)
4. Insomnia or hypersomnia nearly every day.
5. Psychomotor agitation or retardation nearly every day (observable by others, not merely subjective feelings of restlessness or being slowed down).
6. Fatigue or loss of energy nearly every day.
7. Feelings of worthlessness or excessive or inappropriate guilt (which may be delusional) nearly every day (not merely self-reproach or guilt about being sick).
8. Diminished ability to think or concentrate, or indecisiveness, nearly every day (either by subjective account or as observed by others).
9. Recurrent thoughts of death (not just fear of dying), recurrent suicidal ideation without a specific plan, or a suicide attempt or a specific plan for committing suicide.
B. The symptoms cause clinically significant distress or impairment in social, occupational, or other important areas of functioning.
C. The episode is not attributable to the physiological effects of a substance or to another medical condition. **Note:** Criteria A–C represent a major depressive episode. **Note:** Responses to a significant loss (e.g., bereavement, financial ruin, losses from a natural disaster, a serious medical illness or disability) may include the feelings of intense sadness, rumination about the loss, insomnia, poop appetite, and weight loss noted in Criterion A, which may resemble a depressive episode. Although such symptoms may be understandable or considered appropriate to the loss, the present of a major depressive episode in addition to the normal response to a significant loss should also be carefully considered. This decision inevitable require the exercise of clinical judgment based on the individual's history and the cultural norms for the expression of distress in the context of loss.
D. The occurrence of the major depressive episode is not better explained by schizoaffective disorder, schizophrenia, schizophreniform disorder, delusional disorder, or other specified and unspecified schizophrenia spectrum and other psychotic disorders.
E. There has never been a manic episode or a hypomanic episode. **Note:** This exclusion does not apply if all of the manic-like or hypomanic-like episodes are substance-induced or are attributable to the physiological effects of another medical condition.

criteria for a major depressive episode. From this point forward, we'll call these types of episodes, as well as the illness defined by them, *Major Depression* with capital M and D, to avoid confusion with the far larger, more biologically realistic, and fuzzier condition that most people diagnosed with Major Depression really have. To emphasize that depression as it exists in the real world is an inexact and heterogeneous condition, here we will refer to it simply as *depression*, with a lowercase d, to highlight that while therapeutically important it is not nearly as unique a condition—either symptomatically or biologically—as the *DSM* would have us believe.

As we noted above, people have almost certainly suffered from depression since the origin of our species. The roots of depressive symptoms are likely much more ancient still—how else would there be animal models for the disease, imperfect as they are? In this sense depression is a process, or vulnerability, somehow woven into the warp and woof of the human organism. As a recognized disease, depression is also old. Despite going by different names at different times, something recognizable as depression has been reported since antiquity. Consider the *melancholia* of Hippocrates (c. 460–377 BC), characterized by depressed/fearful mood, persistent sleeplessness, lack of appetite, a tendency toward social isolation, and aggressive behavior sometimes leading to suicide.[10]

In contrast, Major Depression is quite young, having been officially born in 1978 with the publication of a paper in the *Archives of General Psychiatry* titled "Research Diagnostic Criteria: Rationale and Reliability."[11] But Major Depression did not spring forth fully formed like Athena from the heads Robert Spitzer and the other authors of the paper; rather, it reflects a longer (but not much longer)— and very human—process that is worth recounting just to give the reader a sense of the profound contingency that underlies the entire modern psychiatric enterprise.[12]

To get a sense of how Major Depression became a discrete, billable illness that a person either had or didn't have, we've got to understand something of the intellectual and political situation in American psychiatry just prior to the disorder's birth. For good or bad, we can't tell this story without getting a bit personal because one of us (C. Raison) actually knew the men most responsible for creating Major Depression but knew so little about psychiatry at the time that this fact was lost on him until many years later. Our claim at the start of this chapter that Major Depression has no "local habitation" is true in terms of its status as a disease entity but needs revising regarding its history because, in fact, Major Depression, much like several styles of barbecued pork ribs, comes from St. Louis, Missouri.

After getting rejected by nearly every medical school to which he'd applied except the bottom-rated school in the country at the time, Chuck Raison was inexplicably admitted to Washington University School of Medicine in St. Louis. Then as now, the university was one of the top medical schools in the country, appended to a staggering city of medicine composed of giant hospitals and research buildings. Chuck went to medical school to be a psychiatrist. Having been enamored with the ideas of Freud while working on a PhD in English, he hoped to become a psychoanalyst. But he was pretty vague about all this at the time and so had not done any homework on the issue. Had he done so, he would have learned that he could not have possibly been relegated to a worse medical school in terms of his psychoanalytic aspirations. The faculty in psychiatry didn't just talk about their dislike of psychoanalysis; they had done something about it. In fact, more than any place in the country, they were responsible for psychoanalysis' long retreat from the scientific mainstream to the quiet (and profitable) backwaters in which it floats today.

To understand the radical transformation of psychiatry initiated at Wash U, we must try to imagine back to the generation that followed World War II, when psychoanalysis enjoyed near complete hegemony over academic and clinical psychiatry in the United States and was solely the province of medical doctors.[12–14] In direct opposition to the current *DSM* system, psychoanalysis disdained diagnosis in psychiatry for several very cogent reasons. First, it saw psychiatric disturbances as expressions of underlying, mostly concealed, intrapsychic conflicts. Symptoms were not to be taken on their own terms as problems to be treated but, rather, were understood as messages that required analytic decoding. From this perspective, psychiatric disorders were not an illness as we commonly understand the term but were, in the words of the famous American psychoanalyst Karl Menninger, "reducible to one basic psychosocial process: the failure of the suffering individual to adapt to his or her environment."[14] Unlike an illness, which we tend to think of as present or absent, adaptive failures run along a continuum. Again quoting Menninger, "Adaptive failure can range from minor (neurotic) to major (psychotic) severity, but the process is not discontinuous and the illnesses, therefore, are not discreet [*sic*]."[14]

The reader will see as we progress through this book that modern science does much to confirm this view, but for now we focus on two key points. First, psychoanalysis saw a continuum between normality and illness. Because everyone has trouble adapting to life's vicissitudes in one way or another, everyone can be seen as a little sick. On the other hand, because even the most deranged psychotic person can demonstrate remarkable strengths, even the most sick individual can be seen as somewhat well. Second, while recognizing various levels of pathological severity, the psychoanalytic perspective of those years tended to view mental disorders as one large process, more or less amenable to a single treatment, talk therapy.

Leaving aside the wisdom of these assumptions, they had very clear political and practical implications that in the end led to their undoing. Several excellent reviews are available that detail the concatenation of events and trends in the 1960s and 1970s that threatened the very existence of psychiatry as a medical specialty.[13,14] For present purposes, a couple of points are worth highlighting. First, although in the United States all psychoanalysts were MDs during these years, this treatment monopoly was being challenged on multiple fronts and by clinicians from other disciplines, such as psychologists and social workers, who saw no reason why they shouldn't be able to do therapy as effectively as a doctor, especially given that psychoanalysis contained nothing that required medical training to master. This put psychiatry in a rough spot. If it lost psychoanalysis to other professions that could do the same thing and at a fraction of the cost, what did it mean to be a psychiatrist? Second, psychiatry alone among medical specialties had no hard-and-fast disease states that could be their special province. Hot off the success of antibiotics for specific infectious disease states, doctors were venerated because they were able to diagnose disease and treat each of these diseases specifically. In contrast, psychiatrists had none of this special and powerful knowledge. Instead, a variety of power groups—including the government and private insurers, increasingly saw psychiatrists as catering to the worried well using a technique with no proven efficacy for therapeutic endpoints without standardization. By the mid-1970s the only even-remotely possible way out of this situation was clear: psychiatry would have to cede its monopoly of psychoanalysis to others and become a specialty that, like other nonsurgical disciplines, used medications to treat clearly defined disease states. From this realization, it was only a short step to the creation of the *DSM-III* and, with this document, the rebirth of psychiatry as a scientific discipline with a well-defined cadre of discrete disease states to call its own.

Well, that's more or less the official story, or at least one slightly jaded take on it.[14] But let's return now to Wash U in St. Louis in the mid-1980s, when as a third year medical student Raison did his first clinical psychiatry rotation. At that time the chairman of the department was Samuel Guze, MD, a personage of striking gravitas with ramrod-straight posture, slicked-back graying black hair, and a crisp, clean white doctor's coat that he always wore buttoned. When he lectured you knew you were in the presence of a great man, and a tough one, too. He was known for harshly reproving psychiatry interns and residents caught not wearing their white doctor's coats, even in hospital stairwells. In his hands psychiatry was an aggressively medical discipline, with diagnoses and treatments as tidy as a bed made with hospital corners.

Into this realm of antiseptic order would come a strange apparition whenever educational events were held within the department. Invariably, once everyone was seated, an older man would be brought in by wheelchair. In sharp contrast to all else in sight, this man looked anything but conservative, with his penchant for purple and pink suits and wild hats of similar colors. His contorted body was always akimbo in the wheel chair. He drooled a little. And he mumbled nearly inaudible and inarticulate bits of what seemed to Raison to be meaningless babble. When the man did manage understandable speech, it tended to be grossly inappropriate to the situation at hand. Remarkably, however, everyone who was anyone in the department would stop all activities and strain forward in an attempt to decipher the words, as if listening to some type of oracle from the ancient world.

This whole routine seemed so bizarre to Raison that—given his undergraduate training in anthropology—he wondered if underneath all the science the research psychiatrists at Wash U secretly believed in voodoo. What he didn't know at the time was the full extent to which the strange man in the wheelchair was responsible for creating Major Depression and many other important psychiatric disorders as they are diagnosed today. For the man in the chair was Eli Robins, previous chairman of the department and—quite arguably—the primary architect of modern psychiatry. It was under Robins's leadership that a group of clinicians and scientists with a profound antipathy toward psychoanalysis and a deep commitment toward "medicalizing" psychiatry gathered at Wash U just as psychotropic medications for schizophrenia and mood disorders were showing their initial promise.

For more than a decade Robins and his colleagues were the pariahs of their profession.[12] Their papers were routinely rejected for publication. They sat alone at national conferences—Raison can still remember seeing a picture of them huddled around a table at one such meeting. But all the while they were training their residents to see psychiatric disorders as genuine disease states, like any others, that could be reliably identified for purposes of treatment and accurate long-term prognostication. This process culminated in the 1972 publication of a paper popularly known as the "Feighner criteria,"[15] which provided specific inclusion and exclusion criteria for 14 psychiatric illnesses and became the primary source for the definitions of these disorders when they were incorporated into *DSM-III* in 1980.[11,12]

Had Robins not existed, it is almost certain that sociological and scientific pressures would have led to the establishment of some form of concrete psychiatric diagnoses. But as Kenneth Kendler suggests,[16] if we had a time machine and could run the historical process over again, it is unlikely that the same disorders would reemerge. We'd like to take this a step further and suggest that psychiatry might have looked very different if it had not been for Eli Robins's wheelchair. As a young man, Robins already suffered from inexplicable physical symptoms. Like the vast majority of psychiatrists of his time, he underwent psychoanalysis, which he found "silly."[12] More to the point, in good psychoanalytic fashion his physical symptoms were judged to be hysterical in nature, rather than the result of a medical illness,[17] which, as any psychiatrist truly believes in his or her heart of hearts—regardless of the official line on hysteria—means that they are more or less "made up." Misattributing Robins's developing multiple sclerosis to hysteria has been described as "perhaps the most fateful mistake of this type for the history of psychiatry,"[13] for at the least this experience must have infused all the energy of a personal vendetta into Robins's quest to replace psychoanalysis with what he considered to be evidence-based medicine.

How Could Anyone Believe That Major Depression Is a Single, Discrete, and Unitary Disease Entity?

Consider the following two people with major depression. Patient 1 is a 69-year-old Asian male who is experiencing his first episode of Major Depression. He complains of profoundly depressed mood, which he characterizes as a feeling of dejection and dread that is worst in the early morning but persists throughout his waking hours. He is able to fall asleep without much difficulty but awakens several hours later and then finds it impossible to fall back asleep, with the result that he is awake throughout the early morning hours, a time in which he normally is fast asleep. Despite his poor sleep he denies fatigue—if anything he says he feels "on edge," and his wife complains that his constant pacing during the day makes her nervous. His appetite has fallen off significantly, and he's lost 20 pounds in the last three months without trying to diet. He complains of difficulty concentrating and notes that he has been having trouble remembering things, a complaint that is reinforced by his wife's concern that he might be developing dementia. Finally, when you ask him if he has been bothered by anything he's done, after some hesitation he tells you that he is overwhelmed with guilt because he has failed his entire family by not making enough money in his life to make things "easier for his kids." When asked if he ever thinks of killing himself, he flatly denies this, saying "God would never forgive that kind of sin."

Patient 2 is a 23-year-old white female who tells you that her family thinks she's depressed. She admits to not really understanding why they think this, because she doesn't feel sad, down, or anything else that sounds like depression to her. All she notices is that she hasn't felt like doing anything for the last six months since her boyfriend "dumped her" for one of her best friends. When pressed, she acknowledges that many things she once found enjoyable now hold little interest. She denies changes in her sleep but complains of "waking up exhausted and feeling even more tired as the day drags on." She tells you she has struggled to stay thin since adolescence but has abandoned these efforts over the last half year, with the result that she has gained 50 pounds and is now obese. She complains of an uncomfortable feeling of heaviness in her arms and legs and says that she feels as if she is moving in Jell-O most of the time. On exam she is noted to move and speak slowly. Finally, despite denying feeling depressed per se, she freely admits that life seems so little worth living that she spends much of her time thinking about ways she could kill herself.

These clinical scenarios provide an most obvious challenge to the idea of Major Depression as a discrete, unitary illness, because they highlight the simple fact that—by definition from the *DSM-5*—two people with the disease need share no more than one symptom, because they need only five out of nine possible symptoms to qualify for the disorder. All that our two patients share is an alteration in eating pattern, and the alterations are opposite. Moreover, their life histories are profoundly different. Patient 1 spent the vast portion of his life depression-free, whereas Patient 2 is strikingly young to be so disabled. Would it make the situation any more discordant if we told you that upon further work-up neuroimaging revealed that Patient 1 had evidence of a fairly recent, albeit small, stroke in the anterior portion of his left anterior prefrontal cortex, an area notorious for causing depression when damaged?

What would the primary framers of the Feighner criteria say to all this? We'll never know for sure because they have all passed away, but taking their part for a moment and imaging ourselves back in the heady days of the early 1970s, when everything seemed much clearer—at least in St. Louis—than it does now, they might have responded by inviting us to imagine another two patients. Both are very sick. One is coughing up blood and complains of chest pain and difficulty breathing. The other has a cough but complains primarily of horrible pain that initially started in the left knee but has now spread to the lower back. On exam the left knee is hot and swollen.

As with our depressed patients, these two share only one symptom in common—coughing—and the second patient isn't coughing up blood. And yet upon further work-up they turn out to be suffering from the same illness, which in this case is tuberculosis (TB). Figure 1.1 depicts the fact that, on the one hand, the same pathophysiological factor can cause very different symptoms and, on the other, two different pathophysiological factors can cause the same symptom. Sensing their advantage, Robins and Guze would have pushed this example a little further. How does medical science successfully differentiate the quandary illustrated in the figure, and how might this apply to psychiatry? First, being self-professed followers of the great German psychiatrist Emil Kraepelin (1856–1926), they would invoke his postulates (a) that mental disorders are best understood as analogues with physical diseases; (b) that correct classification of mental disorders requires abandoning the types of untested etiological theories that form the bedrock of psychoanalysis and replacing them with careful observation of visible signs and symptoms as these manifest over the disease course; and (c) that in the future medical science will identify unambiguous organic causes for mental disorders.[14] To take the case of lung disease caused by TB versus heart failure (Figure 1.1B), Robins and Guze would point out that careful observation of signs and symptoms would go a long way toward demonstrating that they are separate disease states, even in the absence of any knowledge of either TB or cardiac function. TB tends to strike young people; heart disease afflicts the old. TB is almost always associated with fevers and night sweats; these are not part of heart failure unless a secondary infection develops. Both heart failure and TB patients cough, but

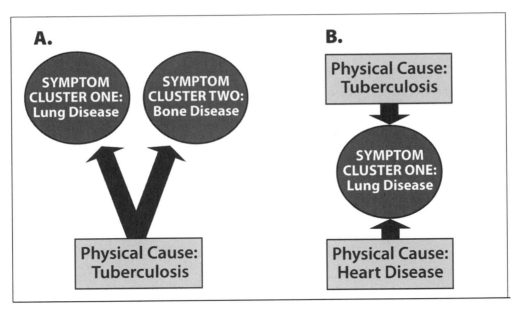

FIGURE 1.1. The same known physical cause can produce very different clusters of symptoms, such that if the specific cause was not known the symptom clusters would likely be considered different diseases (A). On the other hand, very different pathological mechanisms can produce similar symptom patterns (B). TB is well known for causing lung disease, but in the modern world more people develop cough and shortness of breath from heart failure than from TB. Without an ability to identify the different causal mechanisms producing these specific symptoms, it is likely that these very different disease states (i.e., pulmonary TB and heart failure) would be misidentified as belonging to one disease state.

heart failure doesn't typically lead to hemoptysis (coughing up blood). Many patients with TB recover; the vast majority of patients with heart failure will eventually die from their disease.

In fact, Robins, Guze, George Winokur, and others at Wash U took exactly this type of approach to establishing criteria for mental disorders. They recognized that the causes for these conditions were unknown, but because they were analogous to other medical illnesses, psychiatric conditions could be assumed to have clear physical causes awaiting discovery. In the meantime, just as close observation of medical illnesses can go a long way toward separating them into conditions with fairly homogeneous causes, similar close observation of psychiatric symptom patterns should do the same. It is only a short step from this assumption to the almost unspoken (but essential and essentialist) reification that the symptom patterns are themselves the disorder, or something very close to it. And if the initially proposed diseases turned out to have heterogeneous symptoms and outcomes over time, that only meant that more meaningful subtypes of the disorders or different arrangements of symptoms closer to the actual underlying patho-physiology would emerge from the iterative process of articulating and testing various symptom patterns.

Does the idea that Major Depression might be a discrete illness still seem so naïve? Indeed, if we could join Robins and Guze on the bow of 1972 and peer out into future seas, we might feel a sense of awe at the potential power of what these men had articulated. The problem with their ideas is not that they weren't great and not that they weren't in many ways useful and beneficial. The problem is that they were wrong.

Why Doesn't Major Depression Exist as a Discrete Illness?

HOW WOULD WE KNOW IF MAJOR DEPRESSION WAS A DISCRETE PATHOLOGICAL ENTITY?

Since we are in the midst of trying to see the world as it appeared in 1972 at the time the Feighner criteria were published, let us invoke Robins and Guze again regarding how psychiatric conditions might be shown to be the types of discrete illnesses that would allow them to be folded into the rest of medicine. In a land-mark paper published in 1970, Robins and Guze articulated five phases for establishing a condition as a genuine and unique psychiatric disease.[18] We have already discussed the first phase, which involves careful clinical description and extends beyond naming symptoms to considering other factors that might be relevant to the larger picture of the disease, such as typical age of onset, prevalence in different demographic/ethnic groups, and differential rates in men and women. If clinical researchers accomplished Phase 1 with sufficient rigor, the stage would be set for a second phase involving the development of laboratory tests that would tap into the underlying physical abnormalities causing the disorder in question.

Any clinical description of a disorder that had come close enough to "cleaving nature at the joints" to meet the other criteria enunciated by Robins and Guze would be expected to be associated with specific changes in specific biological tests that could be used to identify who did and did not really have the disorder in question. As an example from medicine, consider two patients with recurrent fevers, chest pain, shortness of breath, and hemoptysis. The doctor tests for TB. If the test is positive, the patient has TB. If negative, even though the patient has most of the cardinal symptoms of the disease, the search continues for other potential causes of the symptoms, such as cancer. Translated to psychiatry, one might imagine a world in which Major Depression was reliably characterized by specific results on a laboratory test, allowing the clinician to say with certainty that even though two patients were afflicted with negative feelings, anxiety, and sleep disturbance, one had "true" Major Depression and the other—despite appearances to the contrary—was not suffering from depression at all but, rather, from another disorder characterized by these types of symptoms, such as an anxiety condition. Sadly, and prophetically, Robins and Guze noted in their article that "consistent and reliable laboratory findings have not yet been demonstrated in the more common psychiatric disorders."[18]

Phase 3 is allotted only a brief paragraph in the original 1970 Robins and Guze paper, but it later became a cornerstone of psychiatric diagnosis as the disorders proposed in the Feighner criteria were melded by Robert Spitzer and colleagues first into the Research Diagnostic Criteria and then into *DSM-III*. Robins and Guze noted that, because similar clinical features and laboratory findings may be found in patients suffering from different disorders (like us, they invoked various lung diseases as examples), it is of great importance to establish exclusionary criteria so that patients with other conditions will not be included in the disorder at hand. This sounds well and good, but how do you exclude individuals who have the symptoms of your disorder when symptoms are all you have to go on?

There are a couple of ways to bootstrap oneself at least somewhat out of this tautology, one better than the other. Unfortunately, mainstream psychiatry elected what might be called a symptomatic approach, such that the cardinal symptoms of any given disorder were selected more for their supposed specificity to the disorder than for their prevalence within it. We'll discuss the evils this has produced in a moment. To their credit, Robins and Guze—echoing Kraepelin before them—generally appealed to (in our opinion) a more coherent approach, which forms the fourth phase of their validation process, which they labeled "Follow-up study." Kendler quotes Research Diagnostic Criteria coauthor Jean Endicott as saying Robins and Guze "were the first to tell us that we had to pay attention to more than the acute clinical picture. In defining disorders, we also had to be concerned with the course of illness and prognosis."[12] Half a century earlier Kraepelin had built an entire nosology (set of categories) around this same idea, believing that schizophrenia could be best differentiated from manic-depressive illness (now known as bipolar disorder) not by symptoms but by the fact that over time schizophrenics inevitably deteriorated, whereas manic-depressive patients maintained a cognitive/affective/functional baseline from which they deviated during times of illness but to which they returned upon recovery.[19] (Unfortunately we now know that even this cornerstone of Kraepelinian psychiatry is not true and that bipolar disorder is also typically characterized by deterioration over time in multiple domains of cognition, behavior, and psychosocial functioning.)[20]

If diseases with discrete causative processes breed true over time in terms of course and prognosis, it follows that they should also breed true when it comes time for breeding. Hence, the fifth and final phase of disorder validation proposed by Robins and Guze involved what they tersely referred to as "family study." The tendency for psychiatric disturbances to run in families had been noted since antiquity.[10] Robins and Guze elaborated upon this by noting that "the finding of an increased prevalence of the same disorder among the close relatives of the original patients strongly indicates that one is dealing with a valid entity."[18] As we'll see in a moment, Robins and Guze were right that their discrete psychiatric disease categories do indeed run in families, but they never could have guessed that this would do nothing to support their claims about valid entities.

PUTTING THE ROBINS AND GUZE CRITERIA TO THE TEST

Even with all the scientific advances the world has seen since Robins and Guze published their criteria for disease validity, there is probably no better way to show that Major Depression does not exist as a discrete, unique, specific disease state than to show that it violates each phase of the Robins and Guze criteria. Here we demonstrate this by taking each in turn.

Phase 1: Clinical Description of the Disorder

Our story of the two patients with Major Depression who share only a single symptom domain demonstrates in a straightforward manner that Major Depression, as codified in the *DSM*, runs the risk of being all things to all people. But ambiguities due to symptom counting within the *DSM-5* depressive criteria are minor compared with the challenges one faces when dealing with all the symptoms that are excluded from the official diagnosis. Because a person has to have either depressed mood or anhedonia (i.e., loss of interest in previously pleasurable activities) to meet criteria for major depression, it is not surprising that, taken together, these are the most common symptoms of the disorder. But other canonical symptoms, such as suicidal ideation, are less common in people with depression than are other symptoms that did not make the diagnostic cut.

Of particular relevance in this regard are physical aches and pains, irritability, and anxiety, which are frequent complaints in patients with major depressive disorder and are increasingly recognized as having profound, negative effects on treatment outcomes.[21–31] In this regard, these symptoms are probably more relevant to depression than are many of the official symptoms. But they are highly nonspecific. There are lots of reasons in life to be anxious, irritable, and in pain, so including them as diagnostic criteria would make the population of people with Major Depression even more diffuse than it is at present. Add to this dilemma the fact that, in addition to being common in depression, anxiety and pain also strongly predict the later development of Major Depression in initially nondepressed individuals.[32–34] Thus, their inclusion would swell the ranks of the officially depressed with many folk whose Major Depression developed secondary to a primary pain or anxiety condition.

What to do with the cloud of symptoms depressed people actually exhibit but are also frequently observed in other psychiatric or medical disorders? Or, more precisely, what have clinicians and researchers typically done over the last generation to cope with this type of problem? For the clinician the answer can be seen in the long list of additional psychiatric diagnoses that trail along behind many patients who are judged to suffer primarily with Major Depression. Indeed, our best epidemiological data suggest that comorbidity is the rule, not the exception, for most individuals with a diagnosable psychiatric disorder.[35] For researchers trying to understand the essential mechanisms underlying depression, the most typical strategy has been to exclude from study individuals with significant psychiatric or medical comorbidity, with the result that these populations bear little resemblance to the larger world of depressed individuals they are purported to represent.[36] Figure 1.2 graphs this larger symptomatic world of "real depres-

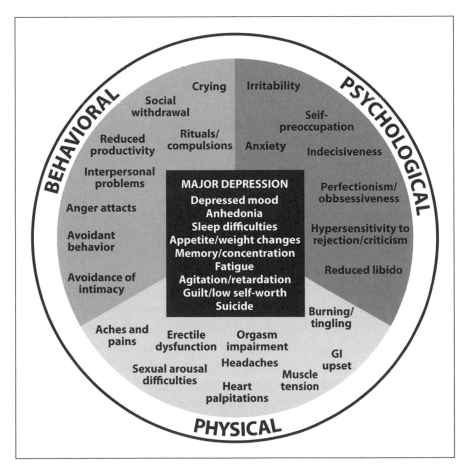

FIGURE 1.2. Major Depression, as diagnosed by the *DSM-IV-TR*, is a component of a larger group of symptoms that tend to co-occur. The currently recognized "official" symptoms of Major Depression are listed in the black box in the middle of the circle. The symptoms in the circle are also very common in depression, sometimes more so than the canonical symptoms in the box. Following Nierenberg et al.[37] we have divided these depression-related symptoms into psychological, behavioral, and physical.

sion" by showing both official diagnostic and nondiagnostic but frequent symptoms seen in Major Depression.[37]

A final problem with Major Depression can be seen even if we limit ourselves to the small cadre of "official" symptoms shown in the black box of Figure 1.2. Examination of a large cohort of twins is only one of the more recent demonstrations that *DSM-5*–specified depressive symptoms do not form an internally consistent entity.[38] Indeed, individual depressive symptoms differ significantly in their relationship with a wide range of factors relevant to clinical outcomes. These findings highlight the important point that symptoms composing Major Depression are more real and more clinically valuable than is the disorder itself.

In summary, then, the careful clinical description advocated by Robins and Guze as the surest way to build a foundation for the establishment of valid psychiatric diseases has not delivered the type of cut-and-dried depressive illness that would provide an optimal grounding for realizing their Phase 2, and one of psychiatry's greatest dreams—the identification of biological markers for diagnosing psychiatric illnesses.

Phase 2: Laboratory Studies

The fact that no biological diagnostic test for Major Depression has ever been discovered is widely used as evidence that we don't yet understand what causes the disorder. As we hope you'll agree by the end of this book, nothing could be further from the truth. In fact, we know a great deal about physical changes in the brain and body that tend to make people depressed, and we know even more about environmental risk factors for the disorder. Given this, we would suggest that it is far more plausible that the lack of a biological marker, or test, for Major Depression reflects not our lack of biological understanding but the fact that Major Depression is not a discrete, unitary disease entity that would be amenable to such marking.

In fact, we must digress at this point to emphasize that the very idea of a biomarker for Major Depression relies on unexamined and untenable assumptions that bedevil psychiatric thinking and that we will need to discard as we move forward. Let's begin this discarding process by exploring the biomarker issue with a thought experiment. Again, we consider two patients who present to your office, but this time they arrive in some golden future age when a biomarker for Major Depression has been identified.

The first patient breaks down sobbing when you begin inquiring into his emotional state. Upon further questioning he is found to have nine out of nine criteria for Major Depression. A call to his wife confirms that these symptoms have crippled every aspect of his life. Just to be sure that he does indeed have Major Depression, you obtain a little blood and send it off for the diagnostic lab test. Remarkably, the test comes back negative. What would you do? Would you tell the patient that he does not have Major Depression because the test is negative and that therefore you can't treat him? Or would you ignore the test and commence either psycho- or medicinal therapy?

In contrast to the first patient, the second patient presents to your office in a completely normal state of mind. He denies all depressive symptoms emphatically. A call to his wife confirms that the patient appears to be enjoying life fully and functioning at a near optimal level. If for no other reason than to protect yourself legally, you draw some blood and send it off for the diagnostic blood test. Amazingly, despite this patient's total lack of symptoms, his diagnostic test comes back as positive for Major Depression. Would you call him back and tell him he is sick with Major Depression but just doesn't know it? Would you start him on an antidepressant?

These examples expose several of the aforementioned unexamined assumptions, without which the very idea of a test for Major Depression becomes nonsensical. First, for such a test to be sensitive enough to pick up all true cases of Major Depression, it would have to tap into a pathway that was necessary to produce Major Depression. Said differently, Major Depression could not develop without the biological pathway identified by the marker becoming abnormal in a very specific way. Second, to really be of value, the diagnostic test would also have to be specific enough that if it was negative one could be sure that the individual could not have the symptoms of Major Depression. In other words, the abnormality indexed by the biomarker would have to be not only necessary for depression to develop but completely sufficient for its development. So, in essence, such a marker would have to identify the final causative factor that underlies all cases (or almost all cases of the disease), just as *Mycobacterium tuberculosis* underlies and is the final causal explanation for all cases of TB.

Put this way, you might protest that this is surely asking too much for Major Depression as a whole. But maybe biomarkers could be identified that would reliably tag more homogeneous subtypes of Major Depression. We acknowledge that this might be possible but also point out that this approach risks embarking on a potential infinite regress of more and more specific symptom patterns, until in the extreme case one is right back where psychoanalysis left off, with each individual demonstrating a unique constellation of symptoms produced by a unique causative factor. Note also that, infinite regresses aside, if a marker were found that identified a physiological abnormality that always produced the symptoms of Major Depression or some depressive subtype, then the symptoms would be just as accurate in predicting a positive diagnostic test as the test would be accurate in predicting the symptoms. In this circumstance the symptoms themselves would tell us all we need to know about the underlying pathophysiological disturbance without recourse to a needle stick. So the only circumstances that would allow for a useful biological diagnostic test for Major Depression would also make the test superfluous!

In fact, the two most reliable characteristics of biological changes associated with depression are that they are neither sensitive nor specific,[39] which is to say that no one has ever succeeded in identifying an abnormality that must be present in all people with Major Depression and that is only seen in the context of

Major Depression. All that has emerged from several decades of research are consistent tendencies for certain biological variables in the brain and body to differ between groups of depressed individuals and matched controls, but not to differ as consistently from groups of patients with other psychiatric disorders.[39] Here the word *group* is all important. Biological differences between people with and without Major Depression are only average differences. For any given individual, all one can say is something like, "For this biological variable the average person with depression is X percent more likely to have it than a person without depression."

But take a look at Figure 1.3, which compares a group of depressed individuals with a nondepressed control group on a biological variable that is abnormal in major depression. It is clear that the average level of the variable is higher in the depressed group (signified by the horizontal lines showing the mean values in

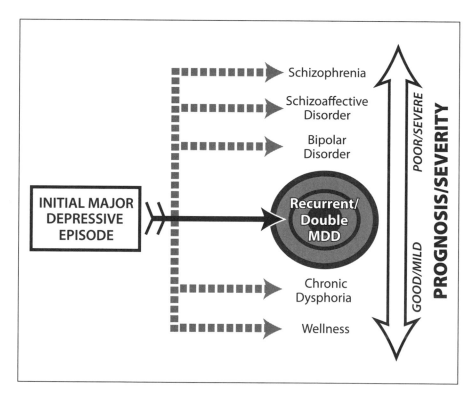

FIGURE 1.3. This figure demonstrates that symptoms that meet DSM-5 criteria for a major depressive episode do not always mean that a given patient will go on to have major depressive disorder (MDD) as a primary diagnosis across his or her lifetime. In some instances, an initial full depressive episode will occur just once in a person's life and he/she will go on to either experience normal moods or may develop various states of milder, but chronic dysphoria. Unfortunately, an initial major depressive episode, especially early in life may portend more severe and disabling psychiatric conditions, especially bipolar disorder, schizoaffective disorder and schizophrenia.

the two groups). But take a look at Subject 1. Even though she meets symptomatic criteria for major depression, she actually has low levels of the biological variable associated with Major Depression, lower in fact than the average value for the nondepressed group. Contrast this with Subject 2, who does not have major depression but has the highest levels of the biological variable of anyone in the study. This demonstrates that even though the biological variable is reliably associated with Major Depression, you can have Major Depression without an abnormality in this given biological variable, and you can have very abnormal levels of the variable and not be depressed. And note that this example is far from being merely theoretical but instead accurately reflects the distribution of many biological variables, such as cortisol and immune molecules, that have been linked to the pathophysiology of Major Depression.

It is a minor tragedy of psychiatric history that the quest for diagnostic biomarkers and other confirmations of our nosological system has blinded us as a profession to the true import of the numerous changes in the brain and body that have been reliably, although nonspecifically, associated with depression, and—as we hope to show in this book—to the fact that these changes are not random but coalesce to tell us a great deal about exactly the kind of disorder depression really is. Instead of interpreting our failure to discover clinically useful biomarkers as evidence that we don't understand the biology of depression, we suggest celebrating this fact for all it tells us about the pathophysiology of depression, as we shall see.

Phases 3 and 4: Delimitation From Other Disorders and Need for Follow-up Studies

Although Robins and Guze separate the need to delimit psychiatric conditions from the need for follow-up study, it is clear when we look at things with 20–20 hindsight that these two phases are really part of the same nosological effort, given that follow-up study played a major role in the Wash U's thinking regarding "how to cleave nature at the joints" in terms of psychiatric diseases. As Robins and Guze noted in their paper,[18] the challenge of accurately differentiating diseases from each other is not limited to psychiatry. They invoke the example of a patient with cough and blood in the sputum. These symptoms are common in lobar pneumonia and bronchiectasis, but also in lung cancer, and a standard chest X-ray cannot always differentiate pneumonia from a tumor.

What to do? This is where the analogy between these medical conditions and psychiatric disorders begins to break down, because the pulmonologist has multiple "next steps" at her disposal to resolve the diagnostic mystery, including her ability to simply go into the affected area in the lung, remove tissue, and see what is there. In the case of psychiatry all we have to guide us are symptoms, disease outcomes, and treatment responses. And with the development of medications, such as atypical antipsychotics, that are effective to some degree for all the major psychiatric conditions, treatment response isn't of much use anymore in this regard. This leaves only follow-up study as a means of differentiating symptomatically similar conditions.

This sounds straightforward enough, but there are a few sand traps dotting the terrain. Follow-up studies do show that Major Depression exists, if by this we mean that some people will spend their lives struggling with either chronic or recurrent symptoms that meet criteria for Major Depression and will not develop symptoms that qualify for other disease criteria. But much like Solon, who famously said, "Call no man happy till he dies,"[40] if we can only identify people who had pure (real?) Major Depression after they've died and no more possibilities are available to them, this is of no prognostic or diagnostic use whatsoever, although it might be of some scientific usefulness if the brains of these people were compared with the brains of people with less clean cases of depression and consistent differences were identified (which we doubt!).

These considerations point out a logical inconsistency in the criteria that launched modern psychiatric nosology—or perhaps a creative tension if we want to be more charitable. Clearly the extreme case of waiting until people have died to correctly classify them has no practical therapeutic use. On the other hand, if psychiatric symptoms do not map onto disorders in a simple one-to-one fashion (e.g., similar to cough and bloody sputum in relation to lung disease), how long do we need to watch people to be sure that the various underlying conditions that might be causing the symptoms have separated out from one another and demonstrated their true existence by "breeding true" over time? This is not a question that has ever been definitively answered, but such long-term data as are available suggest that *DSM-5* diagnoses tend to either congeal into larger entities or fracture into smaller pieces over time.[41]

In fact, one of the unspoken assumptions of our current diagnostic system is that if we look closely at symptom patterns and other factors that predict outcome for some period longer than an hour but less than forever, we should be able to predict from the symptom pattern what the disease is likely to be and hence what type of treatment is indicated and what type of outcome is most likely. Again we are back to an idea somewhat analogous to saying that if we just watch the cough and bloody sputum long enough and take important other factors into account, such as other symptoms, age, and disease course to date, we will be able to accurately determine whether the symptoms arise from pneumonia or cancer. Of course, as Robins and Guze presumed about psychiatric syndromes, if these cross-sectional variables don't disambiguate the various diagnostic possibilities for the patient with lung disease, watching the person long enough will usually do the trick. Left to their own devices, pneumonia patients either die fairly quickly or recover. On the other hand, almost all patients with lung cancer will gradually worsen and die.

Here again, several decades of investigation have shown that although many symptoms, biological measures, and psychosocial/demographic factors associated with depression do statistically predict long-term outcomes, these factors do not support the idea that Major Depression and other psychiatric diseases are discrete entities with unique underlying pathophysiologies.[9,39] Quite the contrary, as we shall show in the remainder of this book, data increasingly suggest that broad patterns of change in brain-body functioning underlie a wide range of psychiatric symptoms and outcomes and that associations between these patterns and any given symptom-based diagnostic category are probabilistic, not certain. Said another way, if you find a gene, or a neurotransmitter, or a pattern of brain activity that is associated with Major Depression, you would do well to immediately look for similar findings in psychiatric conditions that are either highly comorbid with depression (which is many of them) or that have depression as one of the components of the diagnosis (e.g., bipolar disorder).

Let's illustrate these ideas with a case history. Consider Susan, a 19-year-old white female experiencing her first full episode of Major Depression in the context of leaving home to attend college. When she presents to your office, you cannot believe the reports her mother provided by phone ahead of your meeting that Susan had been a high school cheerleader, class vice-president, and voted "Biggest Personality." In your office she moves and speaks slowly, never once making eye contact with you. She is disheveled, with greasy hair. She has the social smarts to apologize for her appearance but tells you that even the simplest tasks, like bathing, require so much effort that she can't bear to confront them. She tells you that her depression began when she and her roommate had a fight because her roommate is "a slob" who accused Susan of being an "impossible neat freak."

When the depression started she felt anxious and miserable and wanted to leave college, but as the weeks progressed these feelings were replaced by what Susan describes as "a dead, silent emotional desert inside me." She tells you her appetite is down but that she has gained "10 or 20 pounds," which she attributes to the fact that she spends much of the day in bed "staring at the ceiling." Sleep is her great escape, and she's been doing a lot of it, up to 18 hours a day. Nonetheless, she feels constantly exhausted. When asked if her concentration is reduced you get the one laugh of the entire interview. "I can't even follow the TV," she says. When you ask if she has suicidal thoughts, she tells you that she would love to kill herself but that planning "how to do it right" would require so much effort that she can't even begin to consider the idea. You ask if she has been hearing voices, seeing strange things, or having feelings that people are in some way talking about her behind her back or doing other strange things. She denies these symptoms, except for saying that she knows that people in her dorm must have talked widely about her condition because she notices people around campus staring at her on her few excursions out of her dorm room. You conclude the interview by asking about the possible presence of other psychiatric disorders. She assures you that prior to "the last month or so" she had no big troubles in her life. Specifically, she denies any history of generalized anxiety disorder, substance abuse, obsessive-compulsive disorder (OCD), eating disorder, or attention deficit hyperactivity disorder.

Susan is experiencing as classic a Major Depressive episode as anyone could ask for—and it is not complicated by any comorbid psychiatric diagnoses that might muddy the waters. You would think, therefore, that if there ever was a time for predicting that a person's psychiatric disorder will breed true, this should be it. In fact, nothing could be further from the truth, as any psychiatrist reading the case would tell you, because in females approximately 75 percent of cases of bipolar disorder start with just the type of depressive episode plaguing Susan. Knowing this, you gather additional information from Susan's mother and learn that, indeed, some type of psychotic condition that could be bipolar disorder has run in the family for generations. Does this mean that Susan has bipolar disorder? No. She may be at heightened risk for bipolarity, but, in fact, individuals with a family history of bipolar disorder are about twice as likely to suffer from a unipolar depressive disorder as a bipolar condition.

Susan's mother then tells you something else that causes even more worry. Although Susan did not confess to this, she had a bout of disabling OCD in her early teens that required treatment with therapy. OCD is frequently comorbid with bipolar disorder.[42–44] But it is also common for individuals eventually diagnosed with schizophrenia to have just this type of adolescent go-round with OCD as a prodromal state.[45–47] This gives you pause because you also know that schizophrenia can commence with symptom states that are difficult to differentiate from a major depressive episode.[48–51] On the other hand, although Susan is clearly at risk for a serious and potentially life-long psychiatric condition, she might also recover completely and never experience another full depressive episode. Or her depression might improve but not remit, leaving her with a chronic simmering dysphoria that becomes impossible to separate from her personality as the years pass and her misery takes over more and more of who she is.

Figure 1.4 summarizes what this case illustrates: an episode of Major Depression predicts trouble for a person's future but isn't very good at predicting what kind of trouble it will be. Even in large groups of people, we can make statistical predictions only about the likelihood of various outcomes resulting from an episode such as Susan's, and most of this predictive power comes not from the symptoms themselves but from other factors such as a person's age, family history, and premorbid functioning. Of course, as Robins and Guze surmised, it becomes easier and easier to delimit which diagnosis or group of diagnoses a person has the longer we watch the symptoms and behavior. But what they were silent on is the fact that this diagnostic delimitation becomes less and less useful as more time passes, until we reach the absolute limiting condition of the person's death, at which point our complete certainty is of no benefit to the patient whatsoever.

Moreover, a huge study from multiple cultures around the world powerfully demonstrates that even time is not the healer of diagnostic conundrums that Rob-

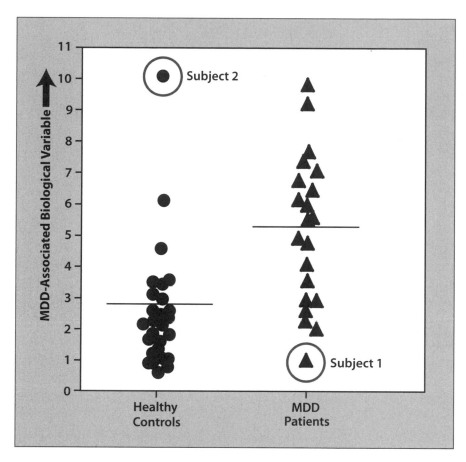

FIGURE 1.4. For the symptomatic presentation of Major Depression to qualify as a discrete, independent disease state, it should "breed true" over time, leading to a long-term condition dominated by the symptom patterns of the of the initial presentation, here represented as either recurrent or double major depressive disorder (MDD), with double depression signifying a disease course characterized by repeated full episodes of Major Depression superimposed on a baseline of chronic dysphoria. In fact, however, especially early in life, major depressive episodes can herald the onset of a number of psychiatric outcomes currently parsed as separate diagnostic conditions in *DSM-IV*, represented by the dashed arrows to a number of other psychiatric diseases. Alternately, a person can recover from the initial major depressive episode and have no further manifestations of psychiatric disease.

ins and Guze hoped it would be. With the caveat that having an internalizing disorder makes one somewhat more likely to subsequently develop another internalizing disorder rather than an externalizing disorder and vice versa, the really striking finding from a World Health Organization study is how having any one psychiatric condition strongly, but nonspecifically, predicts the later development of other disorders, and does so all around the world.[52] As noted by the study authors, these findings suggest that "common causal pathways account for most of the comorbidity among the [18 *DSM-IV*] disorders considered herein."

Seventy-two percent of patients with Major Depression will meet criteria for at least one additional *DSM*-based mental disorder (Figure 1.5).[53] Just as these high rates of comorbidity argue against the existence of Major Depression as an independent, discrete disease, an analogous situation pertains when one attempts to delineate Major Depression from the several milder forms of depression recognized in *DSM-5*, and in turn to delimit these conditions from normality. Given that the need to definitively separate psychiatric disease from normalcy was a prime motivator behind the creation of the modern psychiatric diagnostic system, it is remarkable that subsequent research has so thoroughly demolished all the diagnostic walls first suggested in the Feighner criteria and later constructed for *DSM-III*, most especially the wall between normal and depressed.

Let us think a bit more about how we decide that a set of symptoms reflects an underlying unitary disease state. First, and most crucial, we usually need recourse to some type of independent assessment that can locate a cause for the symptoms in any given patient, something sadly missing from psychiatry. But setting this aside for a moment, at the most basic level a disease is distinct and unitary if it can be shown that there are "zones of rarity" in key disease-related factors between people with the disease and both normal/healthy individuals and individuals with other diseases.[54,55] Said differently, it should be possible to identify a blank zone in any disease-related variable of interest between those with and without the illness, with this blank area serving as a natural boundary for the condition.[55]

Figure 1.6 illustrates this graphically by comparing individuals with human immunodeficiency virus (HIV) disease with individuals with chronic hepatitis C virus (HCV) infection and noninfected controls in terms of blood levels of the HIV virus, a measure known as *viral load*. You can see that noninfected control subjects have no HIV viral load and people with the disease have high viral loads. Between these groups is a blank area, a "zone of rarity" that separates the diseased from the normal.

Next, look at the group with HCV, which presents an interesting pattern of results. Most members of this group look like the noninfected group because, although they are infected with HCV, they are not HIV infected, so their HIV viral load is zero. But note that a small subgroup of the HCV population has HIV viral loads that overlap with the HIV group. This bimodal distribution separated by a zone of rarity suggests that some individuals must have both disease states and that, indeed, two separate disease processes are at work, which reflects true comorbidity.

If we apply this line of reasoning to depression, we would expect to see zones of rarity, or blank spaces, between people with and without Major Depression on any and all factors that are believed to be causative of, or even unique to, the dis-

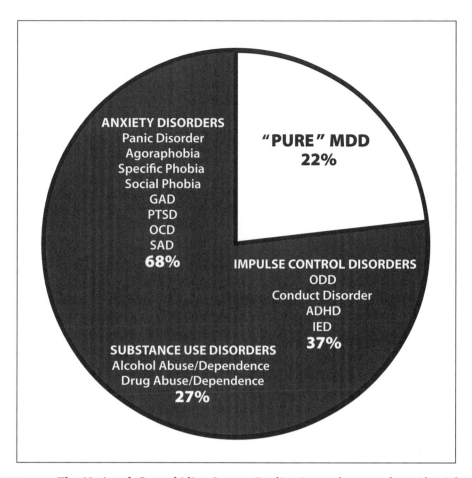

FIGURE 1.5. The National Comorbidity Survey Replication, a large-scale epidemiological study designed specifically to examine the prevalence of *DSM-IV* disorders as well as their patterns of comorbidity, found that 78 percent of individuals who met criteria for Major Depression in the prior 12 months also met criteria for at least one other comorbid *DSM-IV*–based mental disorder. Anxiety disorders were the most common comorbid class of disorders, followed by impulse control disorders and then by substance abuse disorders. Note that these comorbidity figures include only a subset of *DSM* disorders and do not include other common comorbidities, such as fibromyalgia, chronic fatigue syndrome, irritable bowel syndrome, and a host of other medical conditions such as heart disease, cancer, and metabolic syndrome. Abbreviations: GAD, generalized anxiety disorder; PTSD, posttraumatic stress disorder; OCD, obsessive compulsive disorder; SAD, separation anxiety disorder; ODD, oppositional defiant disorder; ADHD, attention deficit disorder; IED, intermittent explosive disorder.

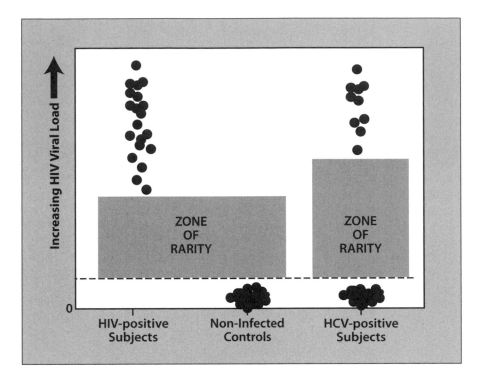

FIGURE 1.6. This figure illustrates that current many current ideas regarding disease work best for conditions that are either present or absent. These types of conditions demonstrate what we have termed a zone of rarity, meaning that there are no individuals who both have and do not have the condition. The figure demonstrates this in relation to human immunodeficiency virus (HIV) infection. Based on a reliable blood test, an individual will either have the virus or not. Within those with the virus the condition can be more mild or more severe, as measured by increasing viral load. This is true even in patients with hepatitis C virus (HCV) infection. In this population, some HCV-infected individuals will also be positive for the HIV virus, while others will be negative. But there will be individuals in the zone of rarity.

ease. Similar zones of rarity should be observed on depression-specific factors between Major Depression and other psychiatric conditions. This scenario is shown in Figure 1.7.

However, we know that for every biological, psychological, or symptom-based factor ever examined, depression is nothing like this. There are no zones of rarity anywhere to be found, only strong evidence for continuity between no depression and mild depression and between subsyndromal depression and Major Depression. Similarly, as we've already said, although Major Depression is reliably associated with patterns of changes in brain-body functioning, these patterns are no more specific for depression than are depressive symptoms (which are also observed in numerous other conditions), in relationship either to normalcy or to

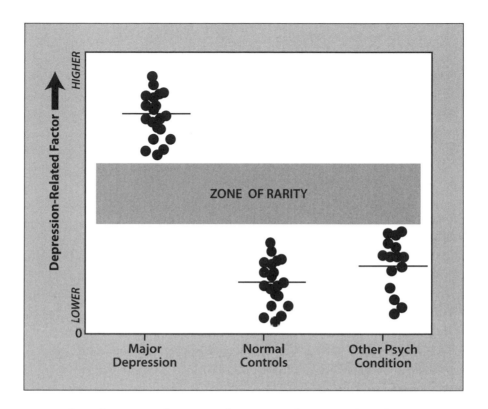

FIGURE 1.7. If psychiatric conditions, such as major depressive disorder (MDD) were discreet disease entities, as Robins and Guze initially envisioned, one would expect them to demonstrate zones of rarity, such as illustrated for human immunodeficiency virus (HIV) infection, as shown in Figure 1.6. Said differently, we should see that some individuals report very few, or no, depressive symptoms while others report many symptoms. Between these two groups should be an area of depressive symptomatology devoid of individuals. Similarly, if MDD was really a separate condition from other psychiatric disease, we might expect to see no depressive symptoms in these conditions. If an individual had both MDD and another psychiatric condition, we would still expect to see a zone of rarity in regard to depressive symptoms in these individuals, as we saw in relation to HIV infection in individuals also infected with hepatitis C virus (HCV) in Figure 1.6.

other psychiatric conditions. Another fact that is hard to square with Major Depression being some type of discrete unitary entity is the fact that for any physiological variable that has been reported as abnormal in the disorder, the range of values is wider in the depressed group than in the control group. That is, depressed people are typically less like one another in variables related to their illness than are people without depression, whose values tend to cluster closer together. This situation is depicted in Figure 1.8.

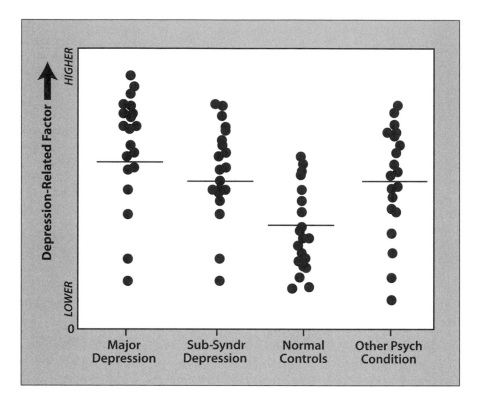

FIGURE 1.8. **Studies conclusively demonstrate that no zone of rarity exists for any psychiatric condition. Rather, major depressive disorder (MDD) is a spectrum condition with symptoms ranging from absent to profoundly severe. The imposition of MDD as a discrete disorder upon this continuous symptom spectrum produces an artificial construct that is useful for practical purposes, but that does not reflect the underlying biological bases of depression.**

Phase 5: Family Studies

Were Robins and Guze alive today they would likely be gratified by the extent to which the diagnoses they helped create have been subjected to family studies methodology, which comprises the fifth phase of their plan for validating the independent existence of psychiatric disorders as "natural types." However, we suspect that they would be equally disappointed by how consistently results of these studies have demonstrated that Major Depression does not meet criteria as a discrete disease state. Rather, like other psychiatric conditions, family studies suggest that Major Depression runs down through the generations in a pack with multiple other diagnoses.

Before turning to the data themselves, here we quickly review the various designs of family studies that have been used to examine the role of heritability of psychiatric disorders (Figure 1.9). Suppose you are just starting to study this issue. How should you commence? One good option would be to recruit a cohort

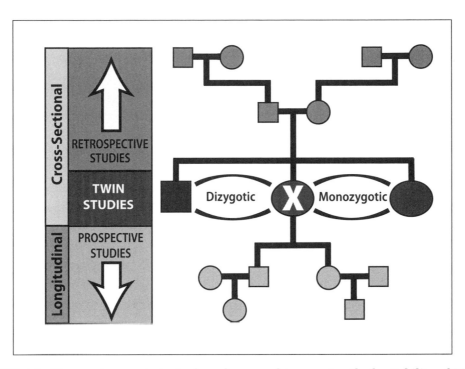

FIGURE 1.9. Three primary strategies have been used to examine the heritability of Major Depression within extended families. Two strategies, considered cross-sectional because they collect data at one point in time, are the use of *retrospective studies* and *twin studies*. Retrospective studies involve assessing the patterns of psychiatric disease in family members of an individual with the condition of interest, called the proband (marked with an "X" in the figure). Twin studies utilize differences in genetic closeness between monozygotic and dizygotic twins to examine the relative contributions of genes versus environment to the disease state and can be employed to examine the degree to which genetic and environmental factors promote specific *DSM*-based diseases versus other more or less inclusive constructs. *Prospective studies*, in contrast, use a longitudinal design: they assess people repeatedly as time moves forward. This is generally considered the strongest study design.

of people with Major Depression and ask them their opinions about the psychiatric conditions of their family members, and any ancestors they know enough about to discuss. Of course, this method has the obvious weakness that the subject might not really know the true histories of his or her family. So a better approach would be to go yourself and interview every family member you can find who would agree to be interviewed. In fact, this was the first strategy employed at the birth of diagnostic psychiatry. But this approach still suffers from a limitation inherent to all cross-sectional assessments: family members are asked to report on not just their present condition but their past. And as we know, memory can be remarkably fickle—with men in particular being likely to underestimate how depressed they were in the past.

A more reliable approach would be to recruit people with Major Depression, follow them until they have children, and then see what happens to these children in terms of mental illness as they grow up. This approach reduces recall bias impressively but is expensive and time-consuming in the extreme. Thankfully, Myrna Weissman and colleagues committed themselves to this type of Herculean effort in the early 1980s,[56] and as a result we now have these type of data added to an original study that first looked cross-sectionally at psychiatric illnesses in the families of the original probands (i.e., the subjects who were followed long enough to have kids).

A third type of family study design examines differences between monozygotic and dizygotic twins in terms of concordance for a given illness, as well as whether this concordance is specific to the illness in question or results from sharing some type of larger pathophysiological and/or symptom domain. Because monozygotic twins are assumed to be genetically equal (which isn't exactly true, we now know), whereas dizygotic twins share only half their genes, this design has been used extensively to explore the relative contributions of genes versus environment in disease pathogenesis. However, this design can also be employed to evaluate whether the genetic and environmental risk factors for a condition such as Major Depression code specifically for the disorder or for some type of larger disturbance of which Major Depression is a part.

The fact that Major Depression runs in families can be seen regardless of the type of family study methodology employed. Moreover, the younger depression strikes a person and the more anxiety symptoms he or she has, the more likely it is that the family will be loaded with Major Depression. Conversely, the more generations in one's family that have depression, the more likely it is that subsequent generations will continue the unfortunate trend. For example, by age 12, 60 percent of children with depressed parents and grandparents will have developed a psychiatric disorder.[57] But even taking all comers in terms of age of onset, Weissman and colleagues found that by the time children of depressed parents reached age 35, 65 percent of them had developed Major Depression and fully 80 percent had some type of mood disorder.[58]

So far so good for the status of Major Depression as a disease entity, but when we turn to the full picture of what runs in the families of probands with Major Depression, we see a mirror reflection of the extensive comorbidity that is apparent when we look specifically at depressed individuals themselves. People with Major Depression come from families that also have markedly elevated rates of bipolar disorder, a variety of anxiety disorders, attention deficit hyperactivity disorder, and substance abuse problems.[58,59] Using a twin-study methodology, Kenneth Kendler took these patterns of comorbidity a step further by demonstrating that within families Major Depression and generalized anxiety disorder run together so commonly because they share exactly the same genetic risk factors.[60] Even the finding that probands with early-onset Major Depression come from families with a higher prevalence of the disorder does not translate into genetic specificity, because these families also have strikingly increased rates of substance abuse and antisocial personality disorder compared with both the families of people who develop depression later in life and people with no personal or family history of Major Depression.[61] And invoking more homogeneous subtypes of Major Depression, based on symptom patterns, as a potential solution to this nonspecificity doesn't appear to help either, as these do not predict either familial loading for Major Depression or any specificity for this loading.[62]

Whether more genetically homogeneous brain-body abnormalities hypothesized to underlie, or form the building blocks for, depression (known as endophenotypes) will show more specificity of inheritance has yet to be seen. However, the plausibility of this possibility is strengthened by the finding that what appears to be passed down through families are not vulnerabilities to specific *DSM* disorders but more basic underlying patterns of maladaptive emotions/cognitions/behaviors most frequently labeled *internalizing* and *externalizing disorders*.[63] However, even here a caveat is in order, because families in which one of these apparently opposite behavioral clusters predominates are at greater risk than the general population to have members with disorders from the other category. Moreover, data show that these larger behavioral clusters are not stable across time and hence likely not to offer much promise as being more discrete than the *DSM-5* disorders they are hypothesized to underlie.[64]

Of course, narrowly defined psychiatric conditions are not the only comorbidities that bedevil the lives of people with Major Depression. Here again, when considering nonpsychiatric illnesses, the extensive comorbidities that we see within depressed individuals also play out across time in their families. For example, several studies have shown that families with Major Depression have markedly increased rates of fibromyalgia, chronic fatigue, and irritable bowel syndrome (and vice versa).[65,66] In all cases the data do not support the co-inheritance of separate disorders as an explanation for this comorbidity. Rather, the data are most consistent with the possibility that these disorders (i.e., Major Depression, fibromyalgia, irritable bowel syndrome) are different symptomatic expressions of the same underlying pathophysiological disturbances. Said differently, although these disorders are currently considered to be different disease syndromes, they all fall on the same spectrum, and it is the spectrum, not the disorders, that is passed down in families.

It is no longer big news that Major Depression is a risk factor for developing a host of medical illnesses, including heart disease, stroke, cancer, diabetes, and dementia, or that the development of Major Depression in the context of one of these other disease states (an all too common phenomenon) bodes poorly for one's health and survival. Bound as the mental health field has been to the vision of psychiatric disorders as discrete mental illnesses, we psychiatrists have made much of these patterns of comorbidity, because they help emphasize "how real" our emotional disorders are. But again, we have to ask ourselves, do these associations represent true comorbidity between separate disease processes, or do they reflect the fact that depressive symptoms are produced by physiological changes in the brain and body that also increase the risk of developing medical illnesses?

Family studies cannot resolve this issue definitively, but it is intriguing that, once again, associations between Major Depression and medical illness that exist within individuals also exist across families through time. For example, compared with children from families without depression, the children of parents with Major Depression are at significantly increased risk of developing a respiratory condition such as asthma in childhood and/or adolescence.[67] In fact, they are at greater risk of developing a respiratory condition during these years than they are of developing Major Depression.[58] And the relationship between a family history of Major Depression and childhood respiratory illness is independent of a number of factors that might account for it, such as any history of respiratory disease in the parents or whether they smoked or not. In the same study population, when these children were followed into early middle age they began to show evidence for an increased prevalence not just of respiratory conditions but of other medical illnesses, such as cardiovascular problems, which—even by the relatively youthful age of 35—were already five times more common in these individuals than in individuals from families without Major Depression.[58]

Back to Where We Started: Does Major Depression Exist?

Perhaps the simplest answer to this question is that Major Depression does not exist the way the field of psychiatry hoped it would back in the diagnosis-drunk days of the 1970s and 1980s, but to loosely quote the philosopher Daniel Dennett (as he said about free will),[68] it exists in all the ways worth wanting—or, we might add, that matter. What we hope to have shown in this chapter (and which is hardly a novel claim at this point in our history!) is that Major Depression does not exist as a natural kind, a discrete entity, or any type of condition that derives from some type of unified, essential, pathophysiological process. It is not like gold, for example, which provides an outstanding example of a natural kind, because all if its features (which we value so highly) derive from the exact makeup and arrangement of its constituent parts. Add one little proton and you've got mercury, which is nothing at all like gold. In contrast, you can add to and subtract all sorts of symptoms from Major Depression without appreciably changing its disease course, social/occupational impairment, or pathophysiological correlates. And, as we've shown with pain and anxiety, several of the symptoms most likely to affect the course and treatment response of Major Depression aren't even part of the official disorder.

Writing this chapter has reaffirmed our respect for the pioneers of diagnostic psychiatry, but it has also filled us with a haunting melancholy, especially for those who have passed away and so have no chance to respond to, or comment on, the ongoing collapse of their intellectual edifice. Would Eli Robins have remained entrenched in his hope that symptom patterns and disease course would identify "real" psychiatric diseases, or would he have risen from that wheelchair, waved his purple plumed hat in the air, and gotten with the times by eschewing his own handiwork? At any rate, a major thrust of this book is the attempt to demonstrate that we have lost nothing worth wanting, and stand to gain much, if we abandon our old, flawed certainties and look the truth of scientific discovery (imperfect as it is) straight in the face. Because it is time to rebuild the edifice of depression, we had first to bring in the wrecking ball to clear away what remains of the old structure, while saving some of the original foundation. Although this chapter has not been comprehensive in attempting this task (to do so would require a book all its own), we hope that it has been useful and persuasive.

References

1. Ebbell B. *The Papyrus Ebers: The Greatest Egyptian Medical Document*. London: Levin & Munksgaard; 1937.
2. Kleinman A. Culture and depression. *N Engl J Med*. 2004;351(10):951–953.
3. Simon GE, VonKorff M, Piccinelli M, Fullerton C, Ormel J. An international study of the relation between somatic symptoms and depression. *New Engl J Med*. 1999;341(18): 1329–1335.
4. Moussavi S, Chatterji S, Verdes E, Tandon A, Patel V, Ustun B. Depression, chronic diseases, and decrements in health: results from the World Health Surveys. *Lancet*. 2007;370(9590):851–858.
5. Stieglitz J, Schniter E, von Rueden C, Kaplan H, Gurven M. Functional disability and social conflict increase risk of depression in older adulthood among Bolivian forager-farmers. *J Gerontol B Psychol Sci Soc Sci*. 2015;70(6):948–956.
6. Stieglitz J, Trumble BC, Thompson ME, Blackwell AD, Kaplan H, Gurven M. Depression as sickness behavior? A test of the host defense hypothesis in a high pathogen population. *Brain Behav Immun*. 2015;49:130–139.
7. American Psychiatric Association. *Diagnostic and Statistical Manual of Mental Disorders, 5th Edition: DSM-5*. Arlington, VA: American Psychiatric Association; 2013.
8. Insel TR, Wang PS. Rethinking mental illness. *JAMA*. 2010;303(19):1970–1971.
9. Sanislow CA, Pine DS, Quinn KJ, et al. Developing constructs for psychopathology research: Research domain criteria. *J Abnorm Psychol*. 2010;119(4):631–639.
10. Solomon A. *The Noonday Demon: An Atlas of Depression*. New York: Scribner; 2001.
11. Spitzer RL, Endicott J, Robins E. Research diagnostic criteria: rationale and reliability. *Arch Gen Psychiatry*. 1978;35(6):773–782.
12. Kendler KS, Munoz RA, Murphy G. The development of the Feighner criteria: a historical perspective. *Am J Psychiatry*. 2010;167(2):134–142.
13. Galatzer-Levy IR, Galatzer-Levy RM. The revolution in psychiatric diagnosis: problems at the foundations. *Perspect Biol Med*. 2007;50(2):161–180.
14. Mayes R, Horwitz AV. *DSM-III* and the revolution in the classification of mental illness. *J Hist Behav Sci*. 2005;41(3):249–267.

15. Feighner JP, Woodruff RA, Winokur G, Munoz R, Robins E, Guze SB. Diagnostic criteria for use in psychiatric research. *Arch Gen Psychiatry.* 1972;26(1):57–63.

16. Kendler KS. An historical framework for psychiatric nosology. *Psychol Med.* 2009; 39(12):1935–1941.

17. Healy D. Samuel Guze: The neo-Kraepelinian revolution. In: Healy D, ed. *The Psychopharmacologists.* London: Arnold; 2000:395–415.

18. Robins E, Guze SB. Establishment of diagnostic validity in psychiatric illness: its application to schizophrenia. *Am J Psychiatry.* 1970;126(7):983–987.

19. Kraepelin E. *Manic-Depressive Insanity and Paranoia.* Edinburgh: Livingston; 1919.

20. Goodwin FK, Jamison KR. *Manic-Depressive Illness: Bipolar Disorders and Recurrent Depression.* 2nd ed. New York, NY: Oxford University Press; 2007.

21. Fava M, Rush AJ, Alpert JE, et al. Difference in treatment outcome in outpatients with anxious versus nonanxious depression: a STAR*D report. *Am J Psychiatry.* 2008;165(3): 342–351.

22. Geerlings SW, Twisk JW, Beekman AT, Deeg DJ, van Tilburg W. Longitudinal relationship between pain and depression in older adults: sex, age and physical disability. *Soc Psychiatry Psychiatr Epidemiol.* 2002;37(1):23–30.

23. Fava M, Mallinckrodt CH, Detke MJ, Watkin JG, Wohlreich MM. The effect of duloxetine on painful physical symptoms in depressed patients: do improvements in these symptoms result in higher remission rates? *J Clin Psychiatry.* 2004;65(4):521–530.

24. Huijbregts KM, van der Feltz-Cornelis CM, van Marwijk HW, de Jong FJ, van der Windt DA, Beekman AT. Negative association of concomitant physical symptoms with the course of major depressive disorder: a systematic review. *J Psychosom Res.* 2010;68(6): 511–519.

25. Mittal D, Fortney JC, Pyne JM, Edlund MJ, Wetherell JL. Impact of comorbid anxiety disorders on health-related quality of life among patients with major depressive disorder. *Psychiatr Serv.* 2006;57(12):1731–1737.

26. Kim JM, Kim SW, Stewart R, et al. Predictors of 12-week remission in a nationwide cohort of people with depressive disorders: the CRESCEND study. *Hum Psychopharmacol.* 2011;26(1):41–50.

27. Silverstein B, Patel P. Poor response to antidepressant medication of patients with depression accompanied by somatic symptomatology in the STAR*D study. *Psychiatry Res.* 2011;187:121–124.

28. Bair MJ, Robinson RL, Eckert GJ, Stang PE, Croghan TW, Kroenke K. Impact of pain on depression treatment response in primary care. *Psychosom Med.* 2004;66(1):17–22.

29. Ohayon MM, Schatzberg AF. Using chronic pain to predict depressive morbidity in the general population. *Arch Gen Psychiatry.* 2003;60(1):39–47.

30. Perlis RH, Fraguas R, Fava M, et al. Prevalence and clinical correlates of irritability in major depressive disorder: a preliminary report from the Sequenced Treatment Alternatives to Relieve Depression study. *J Clin Psychiatry.* 2005;66(2):159–166.

31. Fava M, Hwang I, Rush AJ, Sampson N, Walters EE, Kessler RC. The importance of irritability as a symptom of major depressive disorder: results from the National Comorbidity Survey Replication. *Mol Psychiatry.* 2010;15(8):856–867.

32. Barkow K, Heun R, Ustun TB, Maier W. Identification of items which predict later development of depression in primary health care. *Eur Arch Psychiatry Clin Neurosci.* 2001;251(suppl 2):II21–II26.

33. Garcia-Cebrian A, Gandhi P, Demyttenaere K, Peveler R. The association of depression and painful physical symptoms—a review of the European literature. *Eur Psychiatry.* 2006;21(6):379–388.

34. Stringaris A, Cohen P, Pine DS, Leibenluft E. Adult outcomes of youth irritability: a 20-year prospective community-based study. *Am J Psychiatry.* 2009;166(9):1048–1054.

35. Kessler RC, McGonagle KA, Zhao S, et al. Lifetime and 12-month prevalence of *DSM-III*-R psychiatric disorders in the United States: results from the National Comorbidity Survey. *Arch Gen Psychiatry.* 1994;51(1):8–19.

36. Zimmerman M, Mattia JI, Posternak MA. Are subjects in pharmacological treatment trials of depression representative of patients in routine clinical practice? *Am J Psychiatry.* 2002;159(3):469–473.

37. Nierenberg AA, Eidelman P, Wu Y, Joseph M. Depression: an update for the clinician. *Focus.* 2005;3(1):3–12.

38. Lux V, Kendler KS. Deconstructing major depression: a validation study of the *DSM-IV* symptomatic criteria. *Psychol Med.* 2010;40(10):1679–1690.

39. Hasler G, Drevets WC, Manji HK, Charney DS. Discovering endophenotypes for major depression. *Neuropsychopharmacology.* 2004;29(10):1765–1781.

40. Herodotus. *Herodotus, the Histories: New Translation, Selections, Backgrounds, Commentaries.* New York, NY: Norton; 1992.

41. Marneros A, Roettig S, Roettig D, Tscharntke A, Brieger P. The longitudinal polymorphism of bipolar I disorders and its theoretical implications. *J Affect Disord.* 2008; 107(1–3):117–126.

42. Adam Y, Meinlschmidt G, Gloster AT, Lieb R. Obsessive-compulsive disorder in the community: 12-month prevalence, comorbidity and impairment. *Soc Psychiatry Psychiatr Epidemiol.* 2012;47(3):339–349.

43. Dell'osso B, Buoli M, Bortolussi S, Camuri G, Vecchi V, Altamura AC. Patterns of Axis I comorbidity in relation to age in patients with bipolar disorder: a cross-sectional analysis. *J Affect Disord.* 2011;130(1–2):318–322.

44. Ruscio AM, Stein DJ, Chiu WT, Kessler RC. The epidemiology of obsessive-compulsive disorder in the National Comorbidity Survey Replication. *Mol Psychiatry.* 2010;15(1): 53–63.

45. Niendam TA, Berzak J, Cannon TD, Bearden CE. Obsessive compulsive symptoms in the psychosis prodrome: correlates of clinical and functional outcome. *Schizophr Res.* 2009;108(1–3):170–175.

46. Eisen JL, Beer DA, Pato MT, Venditto TA, Rasmussen SA. Obsessive-compulsive disorder in patients with schizophrenia or schizoaffective disorder. *Am J Psychiatry.* 1997;154(2):271–273.

47. Devulapalli KK, Welge JA, Nasrallah HA. Temporal sequence of clinical manifestation in schizophrenia with co-morbid OCD: review and meta-analysis. *Psychiatry Res.* 2008;161(1):105–108.

48. Bensi M, Armando M, Censi V, et al. [Early signs and symptoms before the psychotic onset: a study on the Duration of Untreated Illness (DUI) in a sample of patients with diagnosis of "non-affective psychotic disorders"]. *Clin Ter.* 2011;162(1):11–18.

49. Herz MI, Melville C. Relapse in schizophrenia. *Am J Psychiatry.* 1980;137(7):801–805.

50. Schothorst PF, Emck C, van Engeland H. Characteristics of early psychosis. *Compr Psychiatry.* 2006;47(6):438–442.

51. Hafner H, Maurer K, Trendler G, an der Heiden W, Schmidt M, Konnecke R. Schizophrenia and depression: challenging the paradigm of two separate diseases—a controlled study of schizophrenia, depression and healthy controls. *Schizophr Res.* 2005;77(1):11–24.

52. Kessler RC, Ormel J, Petukhova M, et al. Development of lifetime comorbidity in the World Health Organization world mental health surveys. *Arch Gen Psychiatry.* 2011; 68(1):90–100.

53. Kessler RC, Berglund P, Demler O, et al. The epidemiology of major depressive disorder: results from the National Comorbidity Survey Replication (NCS-R). *JAMA*. 2003;289(23): 3095–3105.

54. Regier DA, Narrow WE, Kuhl EA, Kupfer DJ. The conceptual development of *DSM-V*. *Am J Psychiatry*. 2009;166(6):645–650.

55. Kendell R, Jablensky A. Distinguishing between the validity and utility of psychiatric diagnoses. *Am J Psychiatry*. 2003;160(1):4–12.

56. Weissman MM. Depression. *Ann Epidemiol*. 2009;19(4):264–267.

57. Weissman MM, Wickramaratne P, Nomura Y, et al. Families at high and low risk for depression: a 3-generation study. *Arch Gen Psychiatry*. 2005;62(1):29–36.

58. Weissman MM, Wickramaratne P, Nomura Y, Warner V, Pilowsky D, Verdeli H. Offspring of depressed parents: 20 years later. *Am J Psychiatry*. 2006;163(6):1001–1008.

59. Faraone SV, Biederman J. Do attention deficit hyperactivity disorder and major depression share familial risk factors? *J Nerv Ment Dis*. 1997;185(9):533–541.

60. Kendler KS, Neale MC, Kessler RC, Heath AC, Eaves LJ. Major depression and generalized anxiety disorder: same genes, (partly) different environments? *Arch Gen Psychiatry*. 1992;49(9):716–722.

61. Rende R, Weissman M, Rutter M, Wickramaratne P, Harrington R, Pickles A. Psychiatric disorders in the relatives of depressed probands. II. Familial loading for comorbid nondepressive disorders based upon proband age of onset. *J Affect Disord*. 1997;42(1): 23–28.

62. Weissman MM, Merikangas KR, Wickramaratne P, et al. Understanding the clinical heterogeneity of major depression using family data. *Arch Gen Psychiatry*. 1986;43(5): 430–434.

63. Kendler KS, Davis CG, Kessler RC. The familial aggregation of common psychiatric and substance use disorders in the National Comorbidity Survey: a family history study. *Br J Psychiatry*. 1997;170:541–548.

64. Wittchen HU, Beesdo-Baum K, Gloster AT, et al. The structure of mental disorders reexamined: is it developmentally stable and robust against additions? *Int J Methods Psychiatr Res*. 2009;18(4):189–203.

65. Wojczynski MK, North KE, Pedersen NL, Sullivan PF. Irritable bowel syndrome: a co-twin control analysis. *Am J Gastroenterol*. 2007;102(10):2220–2229.

66. Raphael KG, Janal MN, Nayak S, Schwartz JE, Gallagher RM. Familial aggregation of depression in fibromyalgia: a community-based test of alternate hypotheses. *Pain*. 2004;110(1–2):449–460.

67. Goodwin RD, Wickramaratne P, Nomura Y, Weissman MM. Familial depression and respiratory illness in children. *Arch Pediatr Adolesc Med*. 2007;161(5):487–494.

68. Dennett DC. *Elbow Room: The Varieties of Free Will Worth Wanting*. Cambridge, MA: MIT Press; 1984.

CHAPTER 2

Building a New Phenomenology of Depression Where Genes and the Environment Meet

The fact that *DSM* mental disorders are distinct entities, felt to reside within an individual, having a threshold, such that they are either present or absent, makes the current categories "ontologically" suitable for underlying biological explanation. I think there was initial hope that the signs and symptoms of specific *DSM* disorders cluster together as they do because they share a specific biological etiology. Of course, this hope has been dashed by mounting evidence to the contrary. . . . Mental disorders may be so complex and multifactorial in origin that they will never rightly be understood in terms of simple and specific biological etiology.

Douglas Porter, "Consequences and the Normative Dimension," 2010

We propose that a diagnostic rubric may be said to possess utility if it provides nontrivial information about prognosis and likely treatment outcomes, and/or testable propositions about biological and social correlates.

Robert Kendell and Assen Jablensky, "Distinguishing Between the Validity and Utility of Psychiatric Diagnoses," 2003

Simply stated, descriptive psychiatric diagnosis does not now need and cannot support a paradigm shift. There can be no dramatic improvements in psychiatric diagnosis until we make a fundamental leap in our understanding of what causes mental disorders.

Allen Frances, "A Warning Sign on the Road to DSM-V: Beware of Its Unintended Consequences," 2009

A new edition of the *Diagnostic and Statistical Manual of Mental Disorders* (*DSM*) was released in 2013 to much controversy.[3,4] This hubbub resulted from strong disagreements about how best to cope with the failure of Robins's and Guze's vision that conditions like major depressive disorder would turn out, in the end, to be natural types amenable to cure via the reductionist discovery of their under-lying biological causes. On one side of the debate about how to incorporate this failure were those who feel that, because science should trump tradition and over-ride clinical practicality, the new edition should have been extensively revised to reflect the fact that all mental difficulties—depression included—are continuums and not clear-cut categories, in relation both to normality and to one another. On the other side of the debate were those who countered that we are so far from iden-tifying unambiguous causes for psychiatric disorders that radically transforming the current diagnostic categories would be no more scientifically sound than leav-ing the traditional ones in place. While the debate raged around the new version of the *DSM*, these proponents of diagnostic stasis eloquently described the hornet's nest of practical difficulties that would descend upon clinician, researcher, and patient alike if the well-established conventions of diagnostic psychiatry were overturned and an increasingly healthy segment of the population was recruited into the camp of the unwell. They asked for practical proof that any good that might emerge from the proposed changes would at least balance the clinical confu-sion and increased stigmatization that would also result. At the same time they pointed to evidence that going to a spectrum approach that would include increas-ingly normal people would expose these individuals to interventions they likely wouldn't need and from which they wouldn't benefit.

In the end caution trumped dreams of scientific grandeur, and the creators of *DSM-5* backed away from their initial grand visions of articulating a new psy-chiatry, producing a document that did little to change the basic diagnostic strat-egies and categories of biological psychiatry. However, the debate about how to conceptualize psychiatric conditions has, if anything, intensified. Although Thomas Insel, director of the National Institute of Mental Health (NIMH), backed off from his original strong condemnation of *DSM-5* and acknowledged its "clini-cal usefulness," the NIMH itself has largely abandoned funding studies that take current *DSM-5* disease states as their primary object of study.[1] Thus, in a very real sense, the NIMH has made a decision that takes us back to the question with which we started this book, which is whether depression exists. The NIMH says no in all the practical ways that matter to science.

Oddly, we find ourselves in sympathy with both sides of the diagnostic fray. On the one hand, there is no doubt that we are in deep trouble if we can't adjust the structure of our diagnostic system in light of scientific discovery, but on the other hand, it is not clear that making such diagnostic/nosological adjustments will make much difference in any of the ways that matter most. We suspect that a deep truth underlies our conflicted feelings, and this is that diagnoses—be they categorical or spectral—have done about all they can do and have little juice left to fuel the types of knowledge that would substantially enhance our scientific understanding or therapeutic efforts. Given this, it is ironic that Allen Frances, "father" of the *DSM-IV* and most outspoken opponent of diagnostic change in

DSM-5, has so clearly articulated our rationale not for maintaining a status quo, as he proposes, but for radically reconceptualizing depression as we present in this book. With him, we agree that we will understand what depression is only when we understand what causes it. Where we part company with Frances is in our sense that we do, in fact, have enough scientific evidence to make a reconceptualization of depression not just possible but of some practical use.

Something We Can All Agree on (in Our Different Ways): The Role of Gene-Environment Interactions in Depression

In different guises, the question of what causes depression reappears repeatedly in the pages that follow. Buried within the question's seemingly simplicity are hidden dimensions of how and why that require a good deal of thought. To fully slake our curiosity, we want to know what causes depression in at least two senses. First, we want to know *how*, in a mechanical way, biological and cognitive factors produce the condition. Second, we want to know what causes depression in a deeper sense, which boils down to the question of *why* depression exists in the first place.

Much space will be devoted in subsequent chapters to addressing these issues in depth. For now let's start our exploration of depressive causality from the broadest perspective possible, where—above the jumble of details—we discover a remarkable unanimity of evidence showing that depression results from genetic vulnerabilities interacting with environmental risk factors.[4–11] This is often expressed as a sort of balancing seesaw equation. As shown in Figure 2.1, the essence of the idea is that certain forms of genes (allelic variants) are more or less likely to produce depression in response to any given environment. Risk alleles are those that produce depression in response to even relatively mild conditions of environmental risk (Figure 2.1A), and protective alleles are those that allow significantly greater exposure to environmental risk without producing depression. Similarly, depression risk environments are those likely to produce depression in people with even mild levels of genetic risk (Figure 2.1B), and protective environments are those that promote depression only in those at most genetic risk. This all falls along a continuum. On one end of this hypothetical continuum are genes that never produce depression no matter how intense the environmental risk exposure, and on the other end are genes that promote depression in response to any degree of environmental risk at all. Because we each carry many risk and protective allelic variants, most of us fall somewhere between these two extremes in terms of our risk, which means that most of can withstand some degree of environmental risk without developing depression but will almost certainly develop at least some degree of depression if the environmental risk becomes great enough.

When the cause of depression is put at this level of abstraction, almost no one would disagree with it—which is really quite remarkable in light of the oft-

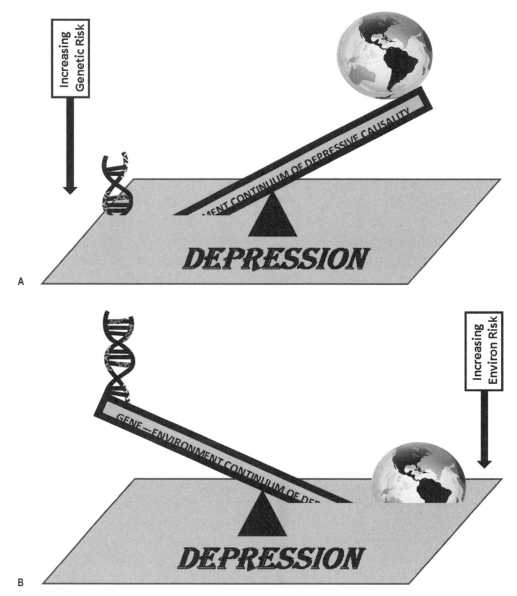

FIGURE 2.1. Panel A demonstrates depression developing almost exclusively as a result of significant genetic risk. In such cases, even minor environmental adversities are likely to produce depression. Panel B demonstrates the opposite situation in which depression occurs almost exclusively as a result of severe environmental adversities that overwhelm even genetic make-ups that are resilient to stress.

repeated assertion that we don't understand the causes of depression. In fact, we already know more about the cause(s) of depression than we generally acknowledge. Thus, we can say with confidence that gene–environment interactions are at the heart of depressive causality.

But this is where agreement ends and things quickly get complicated, because it turns out to be impossible to talk about the cause of depression without also asking about its location. Where, along the gene–environment continuum (GEC), can the cause of depression be said to most truly exist? Let's compare this question with an analogous one more in keeping with our everyday experience. Let's say we are trying to figure out who is to blame for a fight between a husband and wife. On some level we all know that it "takes two to tango" and that blame for marital hostilities is usually a function of the relationship itself. But if we really believed this in our guts, we wouldn't spend so much time gossiping about who did what in the most recent fight or who is "really to blame." The wife complains to her friends about what "he did," and even if the friends can see how she also contributed to the fray, they side with her and place the balance of blame on him. Same with the husband's friends. The human brain seems to crave one-to-one relationships between causes and outcomes, and this is as true for the causes of depression as it is for our hypothetical married couple. Much akin to blaming the husband or the wife, answers to the question of what really causes depression have been staked at all locations along the GEC, from the most inclusive environmental frame (e.g., the physical environment or whole societies) down to specific point mutations within the genes themselves. Indeed, entire research empires have been constructed at every conceivable spot along the continuum, each buttressed with data in support of the causal primacy of its particular patch of GEC turf.

While this variegated and sometimes contradictory welter of theoretical positions can give one the impression that as a field we know nothing definitive, when viewed from a high enough altitude the fact that each position along the GEC has powerful data to support itself is exactly what one would expect if the gene–environment interaction model is correct. In fact, if there was a section of the continuum without known causal efficacy, this would suggest that the model was wrong, or at the least in need of revision. For example, if data showed no effect of the physical environment or widespread social factors on the development of depression, we might rightly conclude that only certain levels of the environment are causally active—that depression is perhaps induced by environmental effects only at close range, such as within the family. Similarly, if no evidence existed suggesting that specific genes increase the risk of depression, one might conclude that depression was primarily environmental in its causation.

So let's launch our investigation by celebrating rather than cursing the fact that the causes of depression appear to be dispersed across systems that come in a wide range of sizes and complexity. In fact, in this regard there is nothing unusual about depression. Most complex phenomena in the world are similarly dispersed and lacking in single, point-like, causal fountainheads.[12] Indeed, the "smudge-like" nature of complex phenomena can be seen in the quantum structure of atoms, in the neural generation of consciousness, and in the definition of what qualify as species. Having said this, however, we are still left with the task of creating at least provisional categories through which the smudge-like entity of depression can be best understood—and by best understood we (being clinicians) mean how it can be conceptualized in ways that open up new methods for preventing and treating it. Moreover, even for smudge-like entities with complex, interactional risk/causative factors, one can often assign a ranking of these factors in terms of importance. So what is really most to blame for causing depression? Or, to rephrase the question with more of a geographic spin, where along the GEC are the causes of depression most truly located?

Let's begin our attempt to answer these questions by recognizing that like all scientific ideas the GEC is a metaphor standing in for an infinitely more complex underlying reality, and like all metaphors the GEC has its strengths and weaknesses. For example, it is natural to picture the GEC as a line anchored on one end by genes and on the other by the environment. But this prompts an immediate question: what is in the middle? Or consider another metaphor hidden within the GEC, which is that some things are on the inside and some things are on the outside. Depression happens when some entity meets conditions that trigger the disorder. The line between the entity and these conditions forms a boundary between things that are inside (i.e., that belong to the entity) and things that are outside (i.e., that belong to the larger environment). Most of the time we tacitly assume that point mutations (or single-nucleotide polymorphisms, SNPs) in genes are the smallest entities that can encounter conditions to produce depression. Thus, SNPs are as far "inside" as you can get. How far outside we can go depends on where we think the environment stops having relevant effects on depression: is it at the level of family, society, biosphere, visible universe? So the question of what causes depression is very closely aligned to the question of where the inside ends and the outside begins. In fact, this is very similar to asking what is in the middle of the GEC, because the line between inside and outside also marks the most relevant midpoint along the continuum.

As it turns out, the answer to what is inside or outside depends on where one is standing. If one wants to focus on the role of societal factors in depression, then all sorts of smaller things are on the inside, including families, individuals, biological pathways, and genes (Figure 2.2). But how would things look from a gene's perspective? Then almost everything in the world is outside and thereby qualifies as being "the environment." From the point of view of a single gene, in fact, the body that houses it is part of the environment. Even other genes are part of the environment, and extremely important parts at that, given increasing evidence that interactions between genes (known as epistasis) may be important in depression. This line of reasoning can be just as easily extended down to the level of SNPs within a gene. From this tiny vantage point, even other patterns of DNA base pairs within the same gene are part of the environment, are "outsiders" that can modulate the effect of the point mutation in ways that change its relevance to depression (Figure 2.3).

So in a very real sense our task of creating provisional categories along the GEC comes down to deciding the best spot for placing a line of demarcation

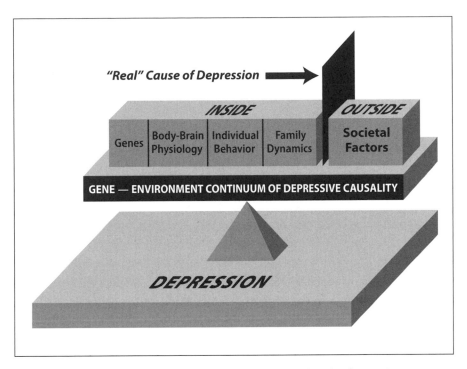

FIGURE 2.2. Given many studies showing that negative family dynamics are among the strongest risk factors for depression in adults and children, this figure demonstrates the fact that from the position of family systems theory the real cause of depression can be located between family systems and the larger societal environment in which the family is situated. From this perspective, everything from the family system down to genes is on the inside and the larger world beyond the family is on the outside.

between inside and outside. This task is of utmost importance because wherever the line is drawn also tends to become the spot that people see as the "real cause" of depression or, perhaps more often, as "the most important cause" of depression. Geneticists draw the line between genes and everything else; neuroscientists, between the brain and everything else; psychologists, between patterns of thought and emotion and everything else; systems theorists, between interaction patterns in the family or larger social groupings and everything else; and sociologists/anthropologists, between society or culture and all that is smaller.

An interesting fact about each of these strategies for demarcating inside from outside is that none of them includes much in the way of a middle zone between what's in and what's out. In fact, nothing but a thin lines separates in from out in most conceptualizations of the GEC. We think much mischief has been perpetuated as a result of this (mostly unexamined) thin-line approach to depressive causality. For while it fits easily enough with the GEC metaphor, it encourages us—without requiring conscious awareness on our part—to minimize the middle in favor of the edges, and it builds the equivalent of a Berlin Wall through the

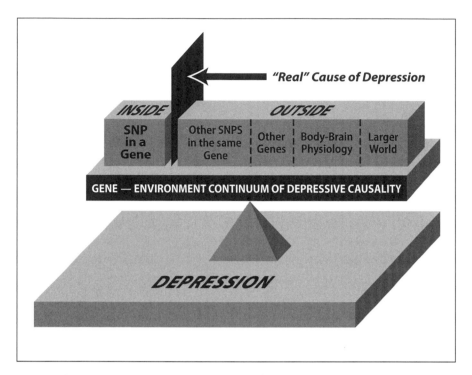

FIGURE 2.3. Although no single gene or single nucleotide polymorphism (SNP) within a gene has ever been definitively established as a risk factor for depression, it is clear that variations within genes contribute risk to the disorder. So from the perspective of one of these putative risk SNPs the real cause of depression lies between it and other genetic factors that can increase the gene's effects, or diminish them. Only the SNP is on the inside and even the rest of the genome is on the outside.

middle of the continuum, in the process forcing near neighbors into one extreme camp or the other, when in fact they have far more in common with one another than with either extreme. Let's expand the theoretical and practical implications of "fattening up the middle" by making use of a study and a metaphor inspired by summers backpacking in the high Sierra.

Of all gene–environment interactions relevant to depression, none has been more exhaustively examined than the tendency for the "short form" of the gene for the serotonin transporter to increase the risk for developing mood symptoms (including suicide) in response to environmental stress, especially when the stress occurs in childhood.[13] Serotonin is a neurotransmitter widely implicated in the development of depression, and most currently available antidepressants are believed to work, at least in part, by enhancing serotonin availability as a result of blocking the serotonin transporter. The short and long forms of the gene for this transporter are in an area of the gene called the promoter region, which— as the name suggests—plays a central role in determining how many serotonin transporter molecules are made. People with the short form of the allele make fewer transporters than do people with the long form.

With this background, consider a study that examined relationships between the short and long forms of the serotonin transporter gene and the risk for developing depression in response to a profound societal stressor.[14] In the early 1960s the eruption of war forced more than a million French citizens living in Algeria to flee the country and repatriate to France. These people typically lost their homes, most of their possessions, and an entire way of life. Many witnessed or suffered traumatic experiences. To make matters worse, upon arrival in France many of these displaced people faced harsh living conditions for the first time in their lives. Within the last several years approximately 900 of these people were genotyped to determine their status regarding the long/short polymorphism of the serotonin transporter (abbreviated here as 5HTTLPR). For purposes of comparison, 632 people of the same age, living in the same area in France, were also genotyped. In addition, all subjects were interviewed to determine how much depression they had suffered in their lives since 1962.

The results of this study reinforce several points we will make throughout the book. First, stress increases the risk for depression: people who lived through the Algerian war and were repatriated to France had more lifetime depression than did people born and raised in France, with the effect being especially strong for those who had suffered trauma in addition to relocation. Second, genes in themselves do not seem to directly cause or not cause depression. In the case of the study we are describing, the 5HTTLPR genotype had no effect on lifetime depression risk. On the other hand, an interaction between 5HTTLPR and stress history was apparent. In the long years following war and repatriation, individuals with two copies of the short 5HTTLPR allele experienced more depression than did people with one short and one long allele, who in turn experienced more depression than did people with two copies of the long allele. The more trauma people experienced, the stronger the effect.

These results (and many others like them) highlight the fact that the phrase *depression risk gene* is a misnomer of the first order. Based on studies to date, genes appear to have precious little ability to directly produce depressive symptoms. Rather, the best-studied "depression risk genes" appear not to cause depression but, rather, to increase a person's sensitivity to environmental conditions, for good or bad.[5,6] When conditions are bad, this sensitivity translates into an increased risk of developing depression. On the other hand, when conditions are good, these same genes may actually protect against depression.[6]

Now let's return to the GEC and note that the study of Algerian war survivors, and others like it, points to yet another metaphor hiding along the spectrum of depressive causality. The line labeled "'Real' Cause of Depression" in Figures 2.2 and 2.3 doesn't just demarcate the most potent causal point on the GEC or separate the inside from the outside. It also identifies a point of meeting, the place

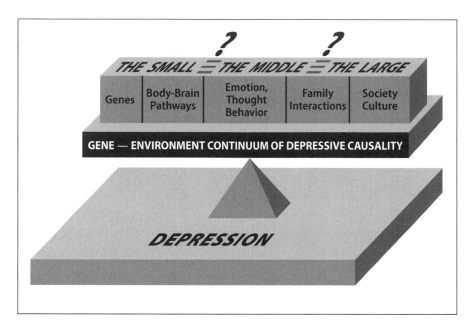

FIGURE 2.4. This figure splits the gene-environment continuum into three parcels without specifying the optimal location for bounding the middle region.

where the key depressogenic interactions between genes and environment occur. So where do genes and environments meet? Genes don't carry guns, retreat from war zones, or deal with petty government bureaucrats in their new homelands. Nor do wars enter the genome via specific transcription sites or use bullets to damage our DNA. So when we say that a certain form of a gene increases the risk of depression in response to war, we are ignoring an incredibly broad range of "middle men" who carry the message back and forth between the DNA and the trauma and its painful aftermath. And in contradistinction to the frequent claims of late-night advertisers, when it comes to the GEC there is no way to "skip the middleman," because genes can only survive by creating organisms, which in turn can only survive when placed in environments conducive to their survival. This interdependence of all zones of the GEC on one another—combined with the fact that each zone has unique functional patterns that differentially affect depressive causality—will turn out to be incredibly important for the way this book reenvisions depression. As it turns out, just as middle men make much of the money in three-party transactions, the middle men between genes and environment play no small role in making depression the kind of illness it is.

For now, the important point is that our inability to skip the middle man in gene–environment interactions is equivalent to saying that we need a far wider middle zone along the GEC if we are to optimally understand the causes of depression. Said differently, we suggest splitting the GEC into three pieces instead of two, so that in the middle of the GEC we have an inside area bounded by two

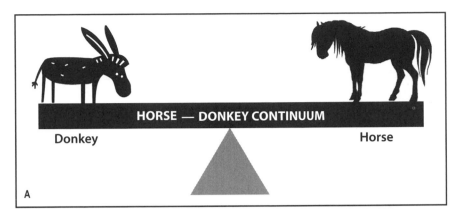

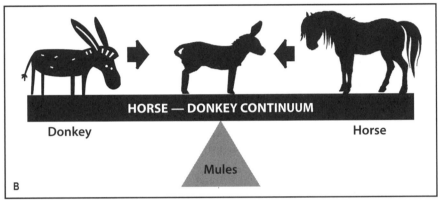

FIGURE 2.5. Panel A demonstrates donkeys and horses occupying either end of a potential continuum that is established in Panel B when horses and donkeys mate to produce mules.

outsides—with one of these being the "outside" of the small and the other the "outside" of the large (Figure 2.4). We are now left with the task of deciding where to place two borders instead of one. Where does the middle end in terms of the small, and where does it end in terms of the large?

Allow us to address this question by way of an admittedly unlikely metaphor. Instead of the gene–environment continuum, imagine a very different spectrum, one with horses at one end and donkeys at the other (Figure 2.5A). Somewhere in the middle of this continuum the horses and donkeys meet in sexual union, and from this meeting something is created: the mule (Figure 2.5B). Mules occupy a place on the horse–donkey continuum (HDC) that is remarkably analogous to our place as individuals along the GEC. Just as we are absolutely dependent for our existence upon genes and the larger suprapersonal environment, mules exist in absolute dependence on the prior existence of horses and donkeys, because mules are sterile and cannot reproduce themselves, any more than we could reproduce ourselves without either a genetic blueprint or a receptive larger environment. As befits their horse/donkey parentage, mules share many traits with both horses and donkeys and can in this way be seen as composites of the two far ends of the HDC. Just as mules are clearly composites of the horses and donkeys that created them, we are each composites of the interactions of genes with environment—although whether genes should be considered horses or donkeys in the analogy we leave to the reader.

To be complete, however, there is an important difference between mules and us, and therefore between the HDC and the GEC. Because mules are sterile, they have no effect on either donkeys or horses, both of which would continue existing just fine if the last mule on Earth perished. On the other hand, our relationship with the "far ends" of the GEC is far more complex, because both genes and the most depression-relevant parts of the suprapersonal environment are absolutely dependent on us for their existence. Suppose the last human being passed away alongside the last mule. Horses and donkeys go their merry way, but what happens to human genes if there are no humans to propagate them? Similarly, what happens to human social interactions—from the intimacies of the family to the formality of the state—without people around to enact these interactions?

With these limitations of the HDC firmly in mind, let's nonetheless put it to work as a thought experiment to compare "thin-line" and "fat-line" approaches to the middle of the GEC. Take a look at Figure 2.6A, which illustrates a thin-line approach splitting up a more realistic depiction of the HDC, complete with multiple horses, mules, and donkeys. We know that the important point of interaction between horses and donkeys is in the realm of the mules, so it makes sense to place the line of demarcation in their area of the HDC. But take a look what happens when we follow this up by dividing all the quadrupeds into two groups based on this thin-line split (Figure 2.6B). This nicely demonstrates what we described referred as a "Berlin Wall" effect. By separating mules from fellow mules, we are left with two heterogeneous groups and an empty middle. In addition, if we think a little more about why this thin-line split doesn't feel right, we'll recognize that although some mules more closely resemble horses and other more closely resemble donkeys, all mules more closely resemble one another than they do their parents. So even if we'd sent the horse-like mules with the horses and the donkey-like mules with the donkeys, we'd still be doing more damage to common sense than if we admitted the obvious and recognized that mules form a unique middle group—related to, but different from, either horses or donkeys.

Mules, in fact, are excellent examples of a category that maps closely onto what in philosophy is sometimes referred to as a natural type. For our purposes the important characteristics of a natural type are that (a) elements within the category are more closely related to one another than they are to any elements outside the category and (b) the category is bounded on all sides by an empty space, a discontinuity, or a "zone of rarity." In the case of mules, this means that there is a gap between mules and horses and between mules and donkeys. Using these two natural-type criteria, it is obvious that if we want to "cleave nature at

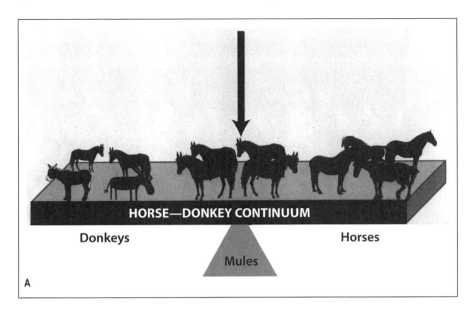

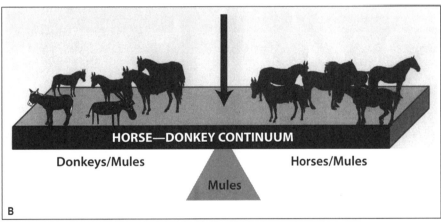

FIGURE 2.6. Panel A represents an effort to apply a thin line approach to splitting the middle regions of the continuum that exists between donkeys, mules and horses. Panel B shows that this approach produces to groups, both of which are heterogeneous because one group contains donkeys and mules and the other contains horses and mules.

the joints" along the HDC, we need two lines, one separating mules from horses and another separating mules from donkeys. With these lines in place (Figure 2.7), we can see that we have produced a rigorously defined middle zone within the HDC.

This tripartite division makes the HDC immediately more understandable than it was when perceived through the lens of a thin line and two groups, each a motley mixture of either horses and mules or donkeys and mules. Moreover, this enhanced understanding allows us to do practical work. We now know what each of the groups is good for. Mules are smarter than horses and can carry far

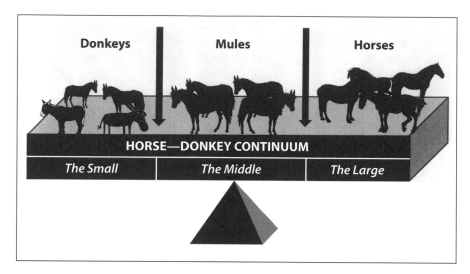

FIGURE 2.7. The figure demonstrates that creating three categories along the horse-donkey continuum produces a grouping that more closely reflects natural types and produces more homogeneous categories than did the two-category scheme shown in Figure 2.6.

more weight on their backs than can donkeys. They'll follow a pack horse anywhere, so they make great companions on an extended high-country expedition. But you wouldn't want to run one in the Kentucky Derby! This illustrates an important point. The more closely we can define entities by the natural-type criteria, the more we will understand about any complex phenomenon of which the entities are a part. (As an aside, it is because current psychiatric diagnoses do not meet these two criteria that our nosological system is in such a mess.)

We wouldn't have gone to such great lengths about donkeys and horses if we didn't think there was the equivalent of a mule munching grass somewhere in the middle of the GEC that drives major depressive disorder. To spot such a beast we can avail ourselves of the two natural-type criteria outlined above and search for an area between genes and the environment characterized by strong internal relationships among its elements and zones of discontinuity between itself and smaller and larger elements along the GEC. Let's start at the edges and work inward. Can we identify scientifically defensible borders where the middle abuts the large and small ends of the GEC?

For the border with the "large" we can use evolutionary theory and common-sense perceptions. In all deference to data showing that depression passes easily from one person to another and thus can be seen to a certain degree as a group affliction,[15–17] it is still the case that the thoughts, emotions, behaviors, and physiological changes that comprise—and by which we diagnose—the condition exist most powerfully within the skin of individual humans. That's common sense, but common sense buttressed by evolutionary biology, because, unlike the situation that pertains between individuals and their genes—where significant evidence suggests that genes are themselves as relevant to natural selection as the whole organisms they construct[18,19]—the border between individuals and their larger environments (typically defined by the skin/endothelial interface with the outside world) actually appears to represent a phase shift in the workings of evolution, the place where biological processes recognize a boundary between inner and outer. This can be shown in many ways, but it boils down to the fact that elements within individual bodies, because they live and die together, are far more tightly bound to one evolutionary fate than are elements shared between an individual body and its environment.

You can see this truth at work simply by noting the far greater amount of cooperation that occurs between bodily elements than between elements of any larger system. With the exception of the social insects, is there a social collective in the world that works together as seamlessly as do, for example, the cells of the immune system, even when it comes time for them to unceremoniously kill themselves to keep the body going? They do this, from an evolutionary point of view, because all the cells of a body (more or less) share the same genes, whereas—with the exception of identical twins—once you leave the boundary of the skin you won't find any connection between elements closer than the 50 percent genetic commonality seen between parents and children or between full siblings. Think of all the murders, mayhem, and general dysfunction that occur within families, and the significance of the skin boundary—with its immediate 50 percent or more reduction in shared genes—is disturbingly apparent.

Demarcating a lower boundary for the middle, or midrange, of the GEC is a more contingent exercise from the point of view of evolutionary biology, precisely because genes and the organisms they program are so enmeshed in terms of their overall fitness that it is hard to tell them apart in terms of natural selection.[20] After all, genes and organisms mutually specify each other biologically, such that genes produce bodies that then maintain and reproduce the genes. The difficulty of deciding where genes stop and their creations begin is reflected in many years of debate within evolutionary biology regarding the most potent unit for natural selection processes: the gene or the individual. So if evolutionary theory is less helpful than it might be in identifying an optimal boundary between the "middle" and the "small" along the GEC, perhaps another scientific discipline can come to our rescue?

Of course, we wouldn't raise the question if we didn't think the answer was yes. Indeed, let us suggest that computational science is admirably suited for the job, because by adopting its perspective we are able to reframe the question of where genes end and their biological creations begin as the question of what counts functionally as software versus hardware in the human organism.[18] If we do this, it is immediately apparent that genetic material—although obviously a physical part of the body—is uniquely information-rich in ways that separate it from other biological elements and systems. Indeed, if you think about it for a moment, you'll realize that when you use the word *gene* you are not referring to a physical object as much as to a parcel of information that produces predictable effects when embedded in the appropriate physical environment (a human body, in this case). When we say a gene is "millions of years old" we don't mean that the particular purine and pyramidine bases (A, C, T, G) in any given copy of that gene have existed that long, only that the information encoded in their patterning has existed for this period, and has done so in settings in which it affected the development and/or functioning of living organisms.

Contrast this with other configurations of matter within the body, such as the heart, brain, or liver, all of which can be seen as containing information, but none of which can be thought of in quite the same way as existing independently of their specific instantiations, and none of which are information-rich in a way that allows them to recreate themselves across time. That type of information, in fact, is in the genes—which is another way or demonstrating how, from a computational point of view, genes are very different from other configurations of matter within the body. So to return to our original metaphor, we might say that the difference between genetic material and all other bodily elements boils down to the fact that genes can be understood as software and the biological systems within which they operate as hardware.

So computational science helps us spot a discontinuity between genes and everything else in the body that is not readily apparent from the vantage point of evolutionary biology but that is of at least equal magnitude to the discontinuity between individual organisms and their surroundings. Thus, while fully recognizing the provisional nature of all categories, by employing both evolutionary and computational theory it is possible to set intellectually defensible upper and lower boundaries for the middle zone of the GEC. The middle zone begins where genes leave off and extends up to the skin/endothelial interface with the larger world and includes everything between, from chemical reactions to whole organism behavior. We propose calling this collection of midrange elements and processes the *body-brain complex*. Figure 2.8 shows the GEC parsed into three pieces with lines of demarcation set at the software/hardware and skin/world boundaries suggested by evolutionary theory and computer science. Representative elements within each domain, which are discussed in coming chapters, are also listed. Turning to the question of how a "tripartite" model of gene–environment interactions—complete with the body-brain midzone we have selected—helps clarify what we do and do not know about the causes of depression, all the while keeping in mind that it is only by understanding what causes depression that we will be able to more deeply understand what it is.

What We Do and Do Not Know About the Causes of Depression: Insights from a Tripartite Approach to the GEC

So don't be sad, two out of three ain't bad.

Meatloaf, "Two out of Three Ain't Bad"

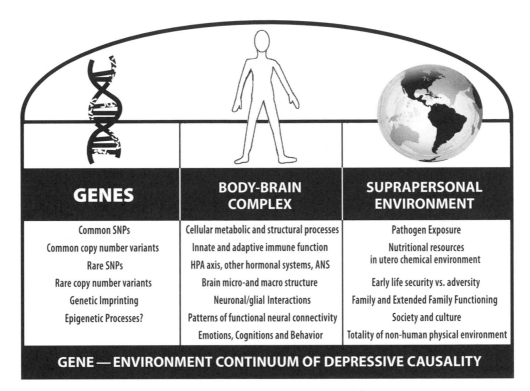

GENES	BODY-BRAIN COMPLEX	SUPRAPERSONAL ENVIRONMENT
Common SNPs	Cellular metabolic and structural processes	Pathogen Exposure
Common copy number variants	Innate and adaptive immune function	Nutritional resources in utero chemical environment
Rare SNPs	HPA axis, other hormonal systems, ANS	
Rare copy number variants	Brain micro-and macro structure	Early life security vs. adversity
Genetic Imprinting	Neuronal/glial Interactions	Family and Extended Family Functioning
Epigenetic Processes?	Patterns of functional neural connectivity	Society and culture
	Emotions, Cognitions and Behavior	Totality of non-human physical environment

GENE — ENVIRONMENT CONTINUUM OF DEPRESSIVE CAUSALITY

FIGURE 2.8. The figure demonstrates a conceptualization of the gene-environment continuum that inserts a middle Brain Body Complex.

Let's take a final look at the GEC, first from the perspective of genes interacting with environmental risk factors and then from a tripartite perspective in which genes and environment meet to give rise to a midrange entity (i.e., the "mule" of the GEC), the body-brain complex, which plays its own unique causal role in the development of depression. Figure 2.9 illustrates several standard assumptions of a gene–environment approach. Best estimates suggest that 60 percent or so of the risk for depression is environmental and approximately 40 percent is genetic. Reflecting this, the dark gray environment triangle in the figure occupies more of the GEC than does the light grey gene triangle. In the narrow zone where the triangles meet a line demarcates the spot of most relevance to the etiology of depression. If this line moves rightward, the influence of genes increases at the expense of the environmental influence, and vice versa if the line moves leftward. This figure illustrates how this type of approach promotes a tendency to highlight the contributions of the ends of the GEC at the expense of the middle. And, in fact, the history of psychiatric theorizing reflects the assumptions inherent in this view of the GEC, given the emphasis on environmental causation featured in most formulations of depression during the first half of the twentieth century and the primacy of place afforded to genes thereafter in accounting for all mental afflictions, depression included.

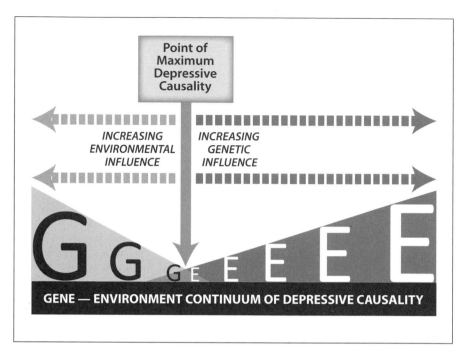

FIGURE 2.9. As the arrow moves rightward the genetic influence increases; as it moves left-ward the environmental triangle would grow and the environmental component would grow.

Contrast this with the implications of a tripartite perspective on the GEC (Figure 2.10). You might object that we are unfairly plugging our point of view by making this drawing so much fancier than the last figure. However, we would counter that this is exactly the point: all sorts of hugely important things exist between the genes and the skin (us, for one thing!), and they require special high-lighting if we are to give them their full due as agents of depressive causation. Note also that this figure introduces important changes in how genes and envi-ronment interact. Because the body-brain complex is "wide," meaning that it has complexity across time and space, it blurs gene–environment interactions, mak-ing any point-like approach impossible. And while it is true that the body-brain complex is in many ways constructed by gene–environment interactions, its whole is more than the sum of these parts, which means that we cannot under-stand gene–environment causality without also understanding patterns of body-brain functioning that promote depression.

Before providing an overview of how a tripartite perspective enhances our understanding of depressive causality (and, by extension, depression itself) we briefly double back and clarify our earlier comment that we were acting common-sensically when we placed the upper boundary of the "middle" of the GEC at the skin. In fact, this choice of an upper boundary is a radical departure from current vogues in the study of mental illness. Instead of assigning a central role to the

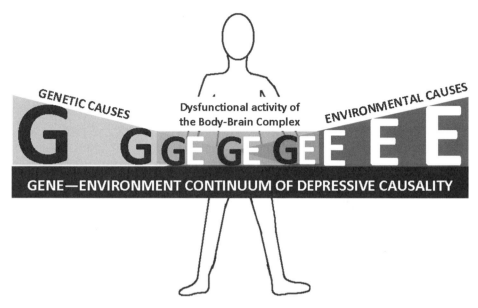

FIGURE 2.10. The figure presents a richer perspective on the importance of the middle zone of the gene-environment continuum, suggesting that this area, the brain-body complex, likely plays a pre-eminent role in the development and maintenance of depression in most people with the disorder.

body-brain complex in the etiology of depression, psychiatry seems at present intent upon casting its lot primarily with neuroscience by recognizing—again in the words of NIMH director Thomas Insel—that "mental disorders can be addressed as disorders of brain circuits."[21]

While no one in his or her right mind would argue against the centrality of the brain to mental disorders, an important part of our task moving forward will be to demonstrate that this "brain bias," while containing significant truths, is incomplete enough that it risks hampering efforts to optimally understand and treat depression, which—in a very irreducible sense—is a body-brain condition. By naming the skin/endothelium as an upper boundary of the GEC midzone we are in effect also militating for an advance of the research frontline from central nervous system circuitry to the totality of body-brain interactions. An important aim of this book is to examine how adopting a body-brain perspective helps resolve many ambiguities and contradictions in our current understandings of depression, while at the same time suggesting novel treatment strategies not readily apparent from a solely brain-based perspective.

But we are getting ahead of ourselves. For our purposes now, the great advantage of dividing the GEC into three segments instead of two is that this approach allows us to see far more clearly what we do and do not know about the causes of depression. Here is the big pay-off: our tripartite division makes immediately apparent a gradient of certainty regarding our knowledge of depressive causality. Ranked by decreasing certainty this gradient runs from the suprapersonal environment, through the body-brain complex to the genes. Indeed, we feel it is neither hubris nor an overstatement to say that we know what causes depression in the suprapersonal realm and have a pretty good idea of what causes it within the body-brain complex. What remains to be known is how genes cause depression. And as we shall see, current explanatory top contenders in the field of genetics lead to very different visions of depressive causality and, by extension, to what kind of illness depression is. Unfortunately, because genetic influences are so central to all biological functions, our lack of knowledge in this regard places a hard limit on what we can currently say about the status of depression as a disease entity and also constrains how far we can go in optimally treating the problem. But again to quote Meatloaf, "two out of three ain't bad," and we propose, as we move forward, to capitalize on this insight by showing how what we do know now might be translated into practical therapeutic advances that wouldn't be apparent without a methodology for clearly identifying and then honestly confronting our areas of ignorance.

So onward then into genes, body-brain physiology, and the suprapersonal environment, but not in that order. After going to such trouble to create a middle zone in the GEC, we need to ask now for a bit of forbearance, because we propose to set this midzone aside for a bit and turn our attention back to the GEC's two far ends: genes and the suprapersonal environment. We adopt this strategy because initially confronting the realms of our greatest certainty (the environment) and uncertainty (genes) will allow us to do two things at once. First, we'll be able to set into stark relief the two most likely scenarios for what kind of illness depression actually is and, by doing so, point to very different potential future scenarios for psychiatric nosology and treatment. Second, by approaching depressive causality from its two extreme ends we will be able to get a pincer grip on the middle, because as we shall see, the body-brain physiology that generates depression can be visualized as the meeting place of two great rivers, where the clear waters of environmental causality blend with, and then lose themselves in, the muddy currents flowing up from the genetic world of the very small.

References

1. Insel, TR, Lieberman, JA. DSM-5 and RDoC: Shared Interests. Retrieved from https://www.nimh.nih.gov/news/science-news/2013/dsm-5-and-rdoc-shared-interests.shtml?utm_source=rss_readers&utm_medium=rss&utm_campaign=rss_summary
2. Frances AJ, Widiger T. Psychiatric diagnosis: lessons from the *DSM-IV* past and cautions for the *DSM-5* future. *Annu Rev Clin Psychol.* 2012;8:109–130.
3. Suppes T, Frank E, DePaulo JR, et al. Letter to the editor in response to 2012 article by Frances and Jones. *Bipolar Disord.* 2014;16(2):214–215.
4. Caspi A, Hariri AR, Holmes A, Uher R, Moffitt TE. Genetic sensitivity to the environ-

ment: the case of the serotonin transporter gene and its implications for studying complex diseases and traits. *Am J Psychiatry.* 2010;167(5):509–527.

5. Homberg JR, Lesch KP. Looking on the bright side of serotonin transporter gene variation. *Biol Psychiatry.* 2011;69(6):513–519.

6. Dobbs D. Orchid children. *Atlantic.* 2009:50–60.

7. Uher R. The implications of gene-environment interactions in depression: will cause inform cure? *Mol Psychiatry.* 2008;13(12):1070–1078.

8. Karg K, Burmeister M, Shedden K, Sen S. The serotonin transporter promoter variant (5-HTTLPR), stress, and depression meta-analysis revisited: evidence of genetic moderation. *Arch Gen Psychiatry.* 2011;68(5):444–454.

9. Bradley RG, Binder EB, Epstein MP, et al. Influence of child abuse on adult depression: moderation by the corticotropin-releasing hormone receptor gene. *Arch Gen Psychiatry.* 2008;65(2):190–200.

10. Mitchell C, Notterman D, Brooks-Gunn J, et al. Role of mother's genes and environment in postpartum depression. *Proc Natl Acad Sci U S A.* 2011;108(20):8189–8193.

11. Mandelli L, Serretti A, Marino E, Pirovano A, Calati R, Colombo C. Interaction between serotonin transporter gene, catechol-*O*-methyltransferase gene and stressful life events in mood disorders. *Int J Neuropsychopharmacol.* 2007;10(4):437–447.

12. Gell-Mann M. *The Quark and the Jaguar: Adventures in the Simple and the Complex.* New York, NY: Freeman; 1994.

13. Sharpley CF, Palanisamy SK, Glyde NS, Dillingham PW, Agnew LL. An update on the interaction between the serotonin transporter promoter variant (5-HTTLPR), stress and depression, plus an exploration of non-confirming findings. *Behav Brain Res.* 2014;273: 89–105.

14. Artero S, Touchon J, Dupuy AM, Malafosse A, Ritchie K. War exposure, 5-HTTLPR genotype and lifetime risk of depression. *Br J Psychiatry.* 2011;199(1):43–48.

15. Pilowsky DJ, Wickramaratne P, Talati A, et al. Children of depressed mothers 1 year after the initiation of maternal treatment: findings from the STAR*D-Child Study. *Am J Psychiatry.* 2008;165(9):1136–1147.

16. Weissman MM, Pilowsky DJ, Wickramaratne PJ, et al. Remissions in maternal depression and child psychopathology: a STAR*D-child report. *JAMA.* 2006;295(12):1389–1398.

17. Fowler JH, Christakis NA. Dynamic spread of happiness in a large social network: longitudinal analysis over 20 years in the Framingham Heart Study. *BMJ.* 2008;337:a2338.

18. Dennett DD. *Darwin's Dangerous Idea: Evolution and the Meanings of Life.* New York, NY: Penguin Science; 1995.

19. Dawkins R. *The Blind Watchmaker: Why the Evidence of Evolution Reveals a Universe Without Design.* New York, NY: Norton; 1986.

20. Wilson DS. *Evolution for Everyone: How Darwin's Theory Can Change the Way We Think About Our Lives* New York, NY: Delacorte Press; 2007.

21. Insel T, Cuthbert B, Garvey M, et al. Research domain criteria (RDoC): toward a new classification framework for research on mental disorders. *Am J Psychiatry.* 2010;167(7): 748–751.

CHAPTER 3

Environmental Adversity, Loss of Evolutionary Fitness, and the Development of MDD

Generic low mood and related negative affect have been shaped to deal with unpropitious situations . . . [and] natural selection has partially differentiated several negative affects to deal with different kinds of unpropitious situations.

Randolph M. Nesse, "Is Depression an Adaptation?" 2000

Over? Did you say *over*? Nothing is over until we decide it is! Was it over when the Germans bombed Pearl Harbor? Hell no! And it ain't over now. 'Cause when the going gets tough . . . the tough . . . get going. Who's with me? Let's Go! Come on!

Bluto Blutarsky's response to college expulsion in *Animal House*

The contrast between our lack of knowledge regarding genetic causes and our certainty regarding environmental causes of major depressive disorder (MDD) could hardly be more striking. Given our ignorance in so many other areas, you would think that our firm grasp of environmental causality would have been widely trumpeted within the world of mental health research and a cause for much celebration. In fact, the opposite is true. Half a century's worth of consistent findings are usually given little more than a passing nod. Maybe it just seems so obvious to us now that stress causes depression that it hardly seems worth a comment. But nothing could be further from the truth. It is remarkable that stress causes depression for several reasons.

First, most of us use the word *stress* as shorthand for situations that challenge our well-being in one way or another. These situations are usually best handled with a clear head, an energetic body, and a calm heart. One would think, therefore, that evolutionary processes might have selected for genes that promote these types of responses to stress under the rubric of "survival of the fittest," rather than the responses we so often observe in humans. For every "take charge" Bluto

Blutarsky in *Animal House* there must be hundreds of real-life John Belushis (the actor who played Bluto), who respond to stress with fear, despair, paralysis, or various detrimental escape strategies, such as drugs and alcohol. Why should stress so reliably produce emotions, thoughts, and behaviors that seem so counterproductive? Consider an analogy: would you not find it odd if the heart responded to running for one's life by slowing down? The heart speeds up when you run because you need extra blood to supply extra oxygen. Why doesn't the brain respond to psychological stressors with a similarly reasonable, survival-promoting strategy?

We'll address these questions in Chapter 9. For now, let's consider another reason that it is remarkable that stress causes depression. Suppose that scientists discovered a gene that incontrovertibly caused depression. Anybody's first question would be, what does it do? We'd ask this because, of course, if we knew what the gene did we might be able to use the information to figure out at least one physiological cause for depression. We know that stress causes depression. Doesn't it make sense, therefore, that if we knew what stress does to the body-brain complex we should be able to use this information to identify physiological mechanisms that cause depression? We think so, and we take this approach as an entrée to our discussion of the pathophysiology of MDD in Chapters 5 and 6.

Everyone knows what stress is, but it turns out to be devilishly difficult to pin it down with a firm definition. Is stress what happens in the external world? Or is it how we perceive external happenings? Does it only cover bad things that happen? We all know good things can be stressful, too, but if we allow this, how do we separate stress from opportunity? The complications are endless. One way to sidestep these issues is to suggest, as many researchers have, that stress is anything that activates the body's stress system. We used to reject this definition on principle because it is a complete tautology, but as the years have passed we've never found one we liked better. And the idea that stress is anything that activates the stress system has a powerful advantage for our present purposes, because activation of the body's stress systems, especially when prolonged, is one of the most reliable physiological mechanisms by which depression is induced. Another advantage of this definition is that it allows us to expand our everyday ideas of stress to include all sorts of things in the world that we don't normally think of as stressors but that activate the stress system and also increase the risk for depression. For example, infections, cancers, metabolic disturbances, and tissue damage all strongly activate stress pathways and are all associated with high rates of MDD.[1,2]

So stress—as we commonly use the word—certainly is a risk factor for depression. But its connotations are too narrow to account for everything we are interested in. For this reason, we prefer the broader term *environmental adversity*, which comes much closer to encompassing the essence of how and when the world beyond ourselves promotes depression. The obvious next question is, what is it about environmental adversity that is depressogenic? Said differently, why do adversities increase the risk of depression? But before addressing this issue, let's review data showing that, indeed, all sorts of environmental adversities, from the very large to the very small, reliably increase the risk of developing depression.

Does Environmental Adversity Really Cause Depression?

AN OVERVIEW OF THE PROBLEM AND THE FINDINGS

No one likes air pollution, high pollen counts, lead poisoning (even when subtle), or second hand-smoke from cigarettes. We'd all agree that they are environmental adversities. They seem to have nothing to do with depression, but if the theory is correct that environmental adversities promote depression, these types of very impersonal features of the physical environment should be depressogenic. And, in fact, they are.[3-8] Even sunspots appear to increase the risk of depression.[8] On the other hand, environmental conditions with "built-in" antidepressant properties should protect against depression. Striking support for this possibility comes from studies showing that geographic regions with higher natural lithium concentrations in drinking water have reduced rates of attempted and completed suicide (lithium has antidepressant properties).[9]

The fact that these types of purely environmental and largely impersonal stressors promote or impede depression is a powerful argument for the depressogenic power of environmental adversity. But we all know from our personal experience that these types of problems pale in comparison to the things that really make us depressed: deaths, romantic breakups, fickle and wayward children, uncaring and harsh parents, financial reversals, uninspiring but stressful jobs, publicly embarrassing incidents, loss of status. And like the wag who said he drank to forget that he had a drinking problem, anyone who has been depressed knows that depression is a huge stressor in and of itself and, moreover, tends to either cause or worsen many of the problems listed above, further driving the depression in a vicious circle that can become impossible to break.

Many years' worth of research confirms that these are exactly the types of problems most likely to make people depressed.[10-14] And these everyday heartaches and disappointments also pose the biggest challenge to our argument that environmental adversity produces depression.[10] Before reading on, stop for a moment and see if you can hazard a guess as to why this is so.

A useful way to approach the issue is to follow the lead of most research in the field and make a crude distinction between independent and dependent stressors. If you become depressed after a spinal cord injury that resulted from a car wreck in which you—while stone sober—were hit by a drunk driver, we would all consider this cruel fate, or bad luck, and nothing more. That is, the stressor that set off the depression was independent of your habitual behavior, emotions, or way of looking at the world. Hurricanes, earthquakes, oil spills, and innumerable possibilities for being in the wrong place at the wrong time are all examples of independent stressors that have been associated with increased rates of depression.[15–21] On the other hand, there are many other painful experiences in life that are either caused or worsened by our own choices, thoughts, feelings, and actions. Take a look again at the list of stressors from two paragraphs ago. With the exception of death, they are all problems to which the suffering person contributes to some degree. That is, they are dependent stressors.

Because these stressors are to a large degree a hell of our own making, how do we know that they cause depression as opposed to being themselves caused by other underlying factors within ourselves that also cause depression? Or perhaps the deepest factors underlying depression (i.e., genes) do their dirty work by driving people to unconsciously make life choices guaranteed to make them miserable? It is clear, in fact, that both these scenarios are true. Studies in identical and fraternal twins have revealed a genetic link between the tendency to make stressful life choices and vulnerability to depression.[14] Said differently, people at genetic risk for depression seem wired to make choices that will make their lives more stressful, and this does indeed appear to be an important pathway whereby genes promote depression. Genes may also promote depression by contributing to personality styles, such as neuroticism, that create little whirlwinds of stress around the afflicted individual and his or her close associates.[22]

Just to complicate things further, everything we are saying about genetic risk factors is also true about early environmental experiences. Especially in the genetically vulnerable, adversity in childhood profoundly increases the risk of adult depression, and does so with equal potency in every culture examined to date.[23,24] Kids who are abused, neglected, or exposed to traumas such as loss of a parent are far more likely than others to suffer with MDD in adulthood, to commit suicide, and/or to develop a whole range of medical conditions for which MDD is a risk factor.[23,25–29] These children are also more likely to develop personality styles that increase the risk for interpersonal conflict.[30–33] As adults, they are more likely to make life choices that place them in inherently stressful situations.[34–37] So when survivors of early-life adversity become depressed as adults following a dependent-type stressor, did the stressor do the deed, or is it truer to say that the stressor and the depression are both reflections of the long-term effects of childhood trauma?

Of course, the strong association of early-life stress with later MDD provides one of the strongest possible arguments in support of the causative role of environmental adversity in producing depression. However, it also raises the possibility that environmental adversity has this true causative potency only when it occurs during certain developmental periods. Poets have pondered this possibility for centuries. William Wordsworth famously said that "the child is the father of the man," and the great German poet Rainer Maria Rilke warned, "Do not think that fate is more than the density of childhood." If so, early adversity, like genetic makeup, may program people to behave in ways likely to produce dependent stressors and subsequent depression, or it may be that early adversity more directly produces both a stressor-generating lifestyle and MDD.

TWO APPROACHES TO RESOLVING THE CAUSATION VERSUS ASSOCIATION ENIGMA

Let's examine two approaches that have been taken to disentangle these possibilities and see whether they support our claim that environmental adversity causes depression. The first approach utilizes a combination of a co-twin design and complex statistics. The second approach explores stressor–depression relationships not between individuals within a culture but among individuals across different cultures.

Twin Studies and Propensity Analyses

Championing the first approach is Kenneth Kendler, one of our great psychiatric research heroes, who as much as anyone else in the last half century has asked and tried to answer all the questions about genes and environment that matter most. (In fact, we often tell our students that if they want an intellectual feast they need do nothing more than enter "Kendler KS" in PubMed [a major biomedical search engine, available at http://www.ncbi.nlm.nih.gov/pubmed], and read the abstracts to his numerous articles.) Many of the answers he offers come from a huge registry of identical and fraternal twins he and his colleagues have assembled in Virginia. To understand how he has used this large study population to explore the question of whether dependent stressors actually cause (vs. being merely associated with) depression, it is worth describing one of his later studies in some detail,[10] although admittedly with some simplification.

Kendler's team began their work by assessing the occurrence of a list of 11 personal and 4 network-type stressful life events in each of approximately 5,000 male and female twins, determining by interview in each case the degree to which any and all of these stressors were likely the result of the individual's behavior. At the same time, the researchers evaluated the degree to which each individual demonstrated any or all of 18 factors associated with the development of MDD that are known to also increase the risk of experiencing a dependent stressful life event (dSLE). These factors (or covariates, as Kendler calls them) provide a type of doomsday list for MDD. They are worth perusing as a cautionary tale for what to avoid in life, if at all possible. As a final step in the assessment process, Kendler's team evaluated whether a depressive episode had occurred in the month of the dSLE or in the subsequent two months. With these data in hand, the analysis commenced.

To quote Kendler, "The critical question is whether the association between these risk factors [i.e., dSLEs] and MDD is causal or arises from covariates influencing both risk factors and disease. As articulated by the counterfactual/interventionist theories of causation, if the association is causal, reducing risk factor exposure will reduce rates of disease. If the association is non-causal, altering risk factor exposure will not affect illness rates."[10] Said differently, if dSLEs really cause depression, this effect should be seen in people who share the same genes and the same general risk factors for MDD and differ only in the fact of experiencing or not experiencing a dSLE. If the relationship between dSLEs and depression is not causal, then these life stressors should not increase the risk of subsequent depression in people who share the same genes and number of depressogenic covariates.

So what did Kendler find? First, and to our knowledge consistent with every other study that has examined the issue, people who experienced a dSLE were far more likely than people who did not experience such a stressor to subsequently experience an episode of MDD. Men were 455 percent and women were 585 percent more likely, to be exact. But people who experienced a dSLE were also far more likely to "test positive" for most of the risk factors for MDD that also increase the risk for dSLEs. To begin the process of disentangling things, the researchers first looked at fraternal and identical twins that differed in their exposure to a dSLE. Fraternal twins share 50 percent of their genes on average and usually share the same family environment in childhood. Identical twins, of course, share all their genes in common and are even more likely to experience very similar early environments. So if genes and early environment cause both a tendency toward dSLEs and depression, then no difference in rates of depression should be seen between identical twins discordant for a recent dSLE, because the dSLE did not cause the MDD but, rather, was caused by the same factors that caused the MDD. By the same logic, differences in rates of depression between fraternal twins discordant for a dSLE should be far lower than differences seen in the general population. To augment this examination in twins, the researchers also conducted a propensity score analysis, which matched each person in the study group who'd experienced a dSLE with a person matched as exactly as possible on the presence of the 18 depression-risk covariates. Even more than in the twins (who might be expected to vary somewhat on covariate number), this strategy allowed Kendler and his team to ask whether a dSLE leads to depression if most other conceivable causal possibilities are held constant.

The results of these analyses are a classic example of the glass being either half empty or half full, depending on one's theoretical biases. Consistent with his idea that underlying factors explain both the tendency to accumulate dSLEs and to develop depression, Kendler found that the association between a dSLE and subsequent depression weakened considerably in fraternal twins, weakened even further in identical twins, and weakened yet again in the propensity analysis.

Also consistent with the possibility that underlying factors explain away the apparent causal connection between dSLEs and depression, Kendler observed that fraternal twins discordant for experiencing a dSLE or an episode of depression tended to be far more similar in covariate exposure than were individuals discordant with a dSLE/MDD in the general population. The similarities were even stronger in identical twins. (The only difference between depressed and nondepressed identical twins was in the quality of their marriages—you can guess which one had the bad marriage!)

But to our eyes Kendler's findings also provide strong support for the contention that environmental adversity (even if of our own making) causes depression. Although weakened, the association between dSLEs and subsequent depression did not drop to zero in either fraternal or identical twins, or in the propensity analysis. Indeed, compared with their nonstressed twin sibling, male fraternal twins who experienced a dSLE were still 331 percent more likely and male identical twins were 219 percent more likely to experience an episode of MDD. The comparable numbers for female twin pairs discordant for a dSLE were 323 percent for fraternal twins and 229 percent for identical twins. The propensity analysis (which matched people on exposure to depressogenic covariates) found that men who experienced a dSLE were 79 percent more likely and women who experienced a dSLE were 66 percent more likely than their matched controls to develop an episode of MDD.

Kendler's perspective on these findings is well taken. If you just look at whether dSLEs predict subsequent depression, the effect is huge. But controlling for other potential causal explanations whittles much of this effect away. Seventy-nine percent and 66 percent are a long way down from 455 percent and 585 percent. But to keep things in perspective, the blockbuster diabetes medication Avandia (rosiglitazone) saw its sales collapse and was nearly pulled from the U.S. market for increasing the risk of cardiovascular death by 64 percent and risk of stroke by 27 percent.[38,39]

Cross-Cultural Studies of Environmental Adversity and Depression

Having evoked the old cliché about the glass being half empty or half full, permit us to start this section with another one: not being able to see the forest for the trees. We all know from our own experience that within any group some individuals appear to weather life's challenges far more easily than others. Stress may cause depression, but in addition to bringing stressful situations upon themselves, many people vulnerable to depression seem especially sensitive to life's buffeting. They also often appear to take a more negative view of things than most of us would consider warranted (unless we are struggling with depression ourselves). We'll return to these issues at some length as we progress, but for now, let's consider the possibility that these complexities may actually blind us to larger patterns of association between environmental adversity and depression. Kendler's work indicates as much: if you want to see truer associations between dependent stressors and depression than first meets the eye, you must be prepared to use natural experiments such as twin births or cutting-edge statistical/study design methodology.

We turn now to another, and in many ways more straightforward, approach to examining whether environmental adversity actually causes depression as opposed to being merely associated with it. This approach involves taking a step back from the particularities of individuals within a culture to focus on differences among cultures themselves. If environmental adversity causes depression, then rates of MDD within a culture or country should rise in lockstep with the average degree of adversity confronted by its people.

Among the many demonstrations of the truth of this hypothesis are several studies examining the prevalence of mental disorders in war-torn regions of the Middle East and Asia.[40–42] Perhaps the most chilling piece of statistics from this research is the report that in the war-ravaged tribal areas of northwest Pakistan 21 percent of men and 39 percent of women endorsed active suicidal ideation. By way of comparison, our best estimates for the prevalence of MDD over any 12-month period in the United States is 6.6 percent,[43] which is higher than the rate observed in most other Western nations and or in traditional cultures not beset by warfare or environmental catastrophe.

While certainly consistent with the idea that broad increases in environmental adversity increase rates of depression on a large scale, the argument that stress causes depression would be further strengthened (a) if rates of mean exposure to depressogenic life stressors within a society tracked with mean rates of depression within the society and (b) if societies with high rates of depression were also especially conducive to the types of stressors most likely to cause depression. The best evidence we know of in support of these ideas comes from the work of British psychologist George W. Brown. An early pioneer in the exploration of causal factors for depression, Brown and his colleagues spent many years administering detailed questionnaires about stressful life experiences while simultaneously assessing the prevalence of depression in widely divergent societies around the world. Because the assessment procedures were standardized, Brown was able to convincingly examine the degree to which stressor exposure accounted for different rates of depression around the world.

Across six widely divergent social groups, rates of depression during a given 12-month period increased in tandem with the likelihood that individuals within the society had previously experienced the severe, disruptive life events known from previous studies to be especially associated with the development of MDD.[12] The 12-month prevalence rate for depression among females in Harare, Zimbabwe, the group with the highest burden of stressful life events (87 percent), was 30 percent, more than 10 times higher than the rate of depression in the group with the lowest rate of severe life events (women in rural Basque society), who had a 12-month prevalence rate of depression of 2.5 percent and no incidence of severe, disruptive life stressors during the study period. Populations with intermediate levels of stressor exposure had intermediate levels of depression, suggesting a dose–response—and causal—relationship between environmental adversity and MDD.

What about the question of whether populations with high rates of depression are also characterized by high rates of the types of stressors most likely to cause depression? To answer this, we have to digress to examine what we know about which types of environmental adversity are especially depressogenic. We've already made the useful distinction between independent and dependent life stressors and noted that dependent events are the more depressogenic of the two. But as with most seemingly obvious distinctions, the one between dependent and independent stressors begins to fray when looked at more closely. As it turns out, when one shifts perspective from the personal to the population level, events that initially appeared to be independent suddenly seem dependent, and dependent events no longer appear to be so thoroughly the responsibility of the individuals involved.

When first making the distinction between independent and dependent stressors, we offered the example of being paralyzed after being hit by a drunk driver as an independent stressor likely to be depressogenic. Within a society this type of event may be largely random—a matter of bad luck rather than personal decision making. But imagine two societies, one in which drunkenness—and motor vehicles—are rampant, and another composed entirely of bike-riding tee-totalers. The risk of being hit by a drunk driver would obviously be far higher in the first society than in the second. So despite being independent from the point of view of members within a society, this stressful event is actually dependent when viewed at the level of the societies as a whole. Conversely, most of us would consider the legion of life stressors that follow in the wake of alcoholism to be entirely dependent events. But imagine identical twins born with a profound genetic vulnerability to alcoholism separated at birth and raised in either the first or second society described above. Alcohol is everywhere in one society, and its abuse is built into the warp and woof of the culture. In the other society, alcohol is essentially unavailable. The twin in the first society becomes a terrible alcoholic who drowns in his own vomit on a dingy street corner after a life of chronic stress and recurrent depression. The twin in the other society grows up to be a pillar of society who passes away in old age surrounded by his loving family. Would you blame the first twin for his miserable fate? He's the one who chose to drink. Is it his fault? But given the contribution of his society to his downfall, can we really say that the stressors he endured were completely dependent on his own behavior and choices?

With the dissolution of hard-and-fast distinctions between dependent and independent stressors, what are we left with in terms of how to conceptualize the properties of stressors that make them particularly depressogenic? Fortunately, many years' research provides a consistent answer. The most depressogenic stressors are severe, disruptive, and irregular, and they involve loss. *Severe* and *disruptive* are self-explanatory. *Irregular* means events that are not consistent with the expected tragedies of life. Death at 80 is regular, no matter how heart-rending. Death at 25—in the modern world—is highly irregular and so would qualify as a type of stressor especially likely to induce depression. When we hear the word *loss*, most of us think of death, or a romantic breakup, or being fired or perhaps one's house being destroyed by a fire, hurricane, or some other disaster. In fact, while all these are depressogenic, when it comes to depression the most powerful losses are more abstract. In a word, defeat is worse than death. And humiliation is worse than hurt. The most deeply depressogenic losses involve not heartbreak per se or deprivation of any particular thing or person but, rather, loss of social status, social options, and relationships upon which one's self-esteem depends, leading to humiliation, loss of hope, and despair. These types of losses are especially depressogenic when they are inescapable, or are seen as being such. A husband who drinks and beats the children would make anyone miserable. A conviction that one is stuck with this husband forever is a potent formula for converting misery to clinical depression. Add to this the humiliation of being the only one in the family to have made a bad marriage and the burden of depressive despair may be enough to prompt suicide.

With this background in place, we can reapproach the question of whether societies with high rates of stress and depression are also societies that promote these types of especially depressogenic dependent stressors characterized by defeat, loss, and entrapment. The answer is an unqualified yes. We think this is best seen by turning again to Brown's work comparing rates and types of stressors across very dissimilar Western and non-Western societies. Using in-depth standardized interviews, he and his colleagues demonstrated a 600 percent increased rate of humiliating and entrapping-type stressors in the population with the highest rate of depression in his study (females in Harare, Zimbabwe) compared with the population with the lowest prevalence of depression (females in the Outer Hebrides).[12] Across all populations examined, the rate of humiliation/entrapment stressors rose in a dose–response relationship with the prevalence of depression in each society. To quote Brown: "The key conclusion to be drawn . . . is that the severe events that differ most across populations and subpopulations are just those that aetiological research within populations have shown to be the most depressogenic."[12]

Although lacking in the rigorous cross-cultural design employed by Brown and colleagues, studies are consistent with the hypothesis that societies with very high rates of depression as a result of catastrophic events (i.e., Afghanistan, tribal regions of Pakistan, Palestine) are also fertile breeding grounds for humiliation/defeat/entrapment-type stressors. In fact, evidence suggests that society-wide adversities (e.g., chronic war) may produce depression to no small degree by increasing the likelihood that individuals will experience these more quotidian stressors, as either dependent or independent events.[40,41,44,45]

In summary, over and above the multiple complications we've discussed, findings from within and across societies do indeed support the notion that environmental adversities, especially those of a dependent, humiliating, defeating, socially rejecting, and entrapping nature, are causally related to depression.

What Is It About Environmental Adversity That Causes Depression?

Let's start with a thought experiment. Suppose you had worked hard all of your life and had risen to the top of your profession. As a result of your skills, dedication, and natural talent you had achieved a place of prominence in society that brought with it material comfort, great power, and easy access to all the interpersonal resources that makes life both secure and deeply pleasurable. Now suppose that in the midst of this success, an invading army ravaged your country, destroyed your culture, and sent you and a sizable portion of your compatriots into exile. After a miserable and dangerous trek across high, snow-bound mountains you arrived in a neighboring country that, while offering hospitality, was poor and lacked the resources and infrastructure to give you anything but the most meager of existences. You lost everything in the escape, and now you lose even more as you watch so many of your fellow displaced countrymen die from starvation and deadly diseases. From a position of high power and prestige you are reduced to the only available employment, which is hard labor for pennies a day on a road crew high in the very mountains across which you recently escaped.

By almost any reckoning this type of scenario would be powerfully depressogenic, given that it contains almost every type of loss known to induce MDD: loss of status, loss of homeland, loss of close friends and associates, loss of any hope for a future that will be anywhere near as satisfying as the past. But let's continue the thought experiment and imagine that a few years pass and conditions improve markedly for your exiled community. Not only are physical conditions better, but your society has reorganized itself in exile and established many of its old institutions, albeit in diminished form. In fact your old place of employment is up and running and ready for you to return to your old position of power and prestige. With this position will come a markedly improved lifestyle and a huge increase in personal safety and opportunity. Here is the thought experiment: would you leave the back-breaking, anonymous, and futureless work on the road crew and resume your old life of comfort and prestige?

If you said anything but "Of course!" you are an unusual human. But we've told this story for two reasons. First, it's true. Second, the gentleman whose story it is elected not to leave the road crew. Rather, he told his monastic colleagues that had come to rescue him from his earthly perdition that he had no desire to leave because he saw the rocks he was splitting as precious jewels and his road gang colleagues as enlightened Buddhas.

The tantric master's ability to radically reenvision reality serves here to highlight a key fact about the relationship between environmental adversity and depression. Adversity is in the eye of the beholder. It is the perception of environmental adversity—especially the sense that one has lost and/or been defeated, trapped, or shamed—and not the adversity itself that is depressogenic. The reason external adversities so reliably produce depression is because these events also reliably produce a perception of adversity in most people. From this perspective, environmental adversity causes depression because most people see the world with enough fidelity to recognize actual adversities as true signals that an internal felt sense of loss is appropriate.

If our tantric master is at one extreme of perceiving environmental adversities as opportunities rather than losses, depression is a condition strongly promoted by viewing and experiencing the world from the opposite extreme of seeing even neutral events as adversities. Environmental events and circumstances are almost always ambiguous and open to multiple interpretations. Moreover, the outcome of events often depends on our feelings and actions. Given these obvious truths, depression can be understood as a state of brain/body functioning that (a) promotes a perception of the self as being in a position of loss/defeat in relationship to the external world and (b) increases the likelihood that a person will make choices and behave in ways that make interpersonal loss and defeat more likely. Overwhelming evidence exists for each of these assertions. For example, in young adults, those who saw themselves in terms of failure, inadequacy, and worthlessness were 350 percent to almost 700 percent more likely than people with more positive views of themselves to develop depression over the ensuing two years,[46] and multiple studies by Kendler and colleagues[10,14] show that people with depression make more stressful life choices than do unaffected individuals. It is easy to see how these perceptual and behavioral components might be mutually reinforcing, which helps explain why many people with depression seemed doubly cursed, first by making choices and/or behaving in ways that increase actual environmental adversity and then by being overly sensitive to the adversity that ensues. This type of heightened sensitivity leads to further maladaptive choices, in an often inescapable cycle of misery.

Saying that it is the perception of adversity that provides the causal link between actual negative environmental events and depression is straightforward enough, but it immediately points to a deeper question: what is it within the perception of adversity that causes depression? Many lines of evidence provide a compelling answer. Just as data (and common sense) forced us to move beyond the occurrence of actual adverse events to their perception, now we need to move beyond the notion of adversity altogether to embrace a more abstract, but ultimately more satisfying, truth. We have to ask why adversity is so depressing. It's a tricky question because it seems so self-evident: adversity is depressing because adversity feels so terrible. But why does it feel so terrible?

We want to take what may seem like a conceptual leap and suggest that adversity feels horrible because it so reliably signals a risk to the deepest (and largely unconscious) mandate of our being, which is to maximize our Darwinian fitness. From this perspective we can say that depression results from the perception that events and circumstances have reduced, or threaten to reduce, one's Darwinian fitness. From this perspective, environmental adversities so potently promote depression because across evolutionary time they were true markers that an individual was about to suffer, or had already suffered, a reduction in overall personal fitness. (We highlight personal here to differentiate this level of selection from either inclusive or multilevel selection processes, both of which we discuss later.)

Although humans have created innumerable markers of—and surrogates for—overall personal evolutionary fitness, in the end it boils down to the likelihood that one's genes will be propagated into the next generation. For this to occur, two things must happen: an individual must survive long enough to reproduce, and he or she must reproduce. Because human infants are unique in their reliance upon extended nurturing and training for survival and later breeding success, it also likely that fitness was greatly enhanced across evolutionary time when individuals were able to survive long enough not just to reproduce but also to provide these advantages to their offspring. Following this line of reasoning, it has been suggested that humans live so much longer than other primates, at least in part, because our collaborative/cooperative lifestyle allowed older adults to continue contributing to their inclusive fitness (i.e., fitness related to success of relatives with whom one shares genes) by serving as grandparents.

A clear implication of these ideas, which together comprise a model we refer to as the threat to overall fitness (TOF) model of depressive pathogenesis, is that the most depressogenic adversities should be those that, across evolutionary time, were most likely to cause death prior to completion of child-rearing and/or those most likely to reduce one's access to high-quality sexual partners. By the same logic, people who for one reason or another perceive the world as especially dangerous or who view themselves as being more unworthy or unattractive than their peers should be especially prone to depression, regardless of their actual real-world circumstances. Putting it all together, we might formulate the following general two-part rule: (a) the perception of reduced overall personal evolutionary fitness should promote the development of MDD, and (b) the depressogenic potential of any environmental condition should be proportional to its average tendency to induce a perception of reduced overall personal evolutionary fitness.

Evolutionary Fitness I: Threats to Survival Should Induce Depression

DEPRESSION, INFLAMMATION, AND A SENSE OF EARLY DEATH

Nothing is more detrimental to one's evolutionary fitness than dying young, especially when death occurs prior to successful reproduction. Therefore, those things in the ancestral environment that most reliably signaled an increased risk of early-life mortality should have evolved to become especially potent inducers of depression. Like all evolutionary ideas, this one makes some surprising predictions. For example, if most humans in the ancestral environment died at the hands of carnivorous animals, one would expect, from a TOF perspective, that prolonged time spent in zoos should be a first-degree emotional bummer—don't even think about wildlife safaris! So, although predation was probably a bigger factor in human mortality than we tend to believe today,[47] by reverse engineering using the TOF model we might guess that it wasn't a prime concern. So what—or who—did kill young people back in the eons before modern hygiene and medicine changed everything? And does contact with, or perception of, these killers reliably induce depression, as would be predicted by TOF theory?

It is hard for those of us living in the industrialized world to grasp how many of our forebears perished from infectious causes and did so early enough in life to fall afoul of evolution's twin mandates to survive and reproduce. In fact, in most places and times, it is likely that 50 percent of all children born perished from infection in the first year of life, which may help account for the fact that certain tribal groups—the Hopi Indians, for example—didn't give their children names until their first birthdays (they were considered to be "on loan" until that time). It was certainly the case in ancestral environments, as in many parts of the Third World today, that deaths from infection decreased as childhood progressed and the immune system gained competency, but we need look no further than the nineteenth century to observe that death from infection remained more the rule than the exception throughout adolescence and early adulthood. For example, today it would be considered a national tragedy if three of a U.S. president's four children died before reaching age 21, but we make little note of this horrific aspect of Lincoln's life story. Charles Darwin, born the same day as Lincoln, fared better: only three of his ten children died in childhood from infection. And these were in the good times for people with significant societal resources. Among the poor and downtrodden, or during any of the innumerable plagues that ravaged human social groups at regular intervals, the death toll from infection led to scenarios unmatched by any Hollywood horror movie. Consider this eye witness account of the black death of 1348 as it ravaged Italy:

> At the beginning of October, in the year of the incarnation of the Son of God 1347, twelve Genoese galleys . . . entered the harbor of Messina. In their

bones they bore so virulent a disease that anyone who only spoke to them was seized by a mortal illness and in no manner could evade death. The infection spread to everyone who had any contact with the diseased. Those infected felt themselves penetrated by a pain throughout their whole bodies . . . then there developed on the thighs or upper arms a boil about the size of a lentil which the people called "burn boil." This infected the whole body, and penetrated it so that the patient violently vomited blood. This vomiting of blood continued without intermission for three days, there being no means of healing it, and then the patient expired. Not only all those who had speech with them died, but also those who had touched or used any of their things. Soon men hated each other so much that if a son was attacked by the disease his father would not tend him. If, in spite of all, he dared to approach him, he was immediately infected and was bound to die within three days. Nor was this all; all those dwelling in the same house with him, even the cats and other domestic animals, followed him in death.[48]

Because microorganisms and larger parasites such as worms have been the primary source of early-life mortality across human evolution, they have also been the greatest threats to the survival facet of overall personal evolutionary fitness. Therefore, TOF theory predicts that they should be powerful drivers of depression, as indeed they are. Unlike contact with predators, which typically produces a mixture of fear and awe in humans, contact with infectious agents does indeed promote depression, as shown from studies demonstrating that many infections, including the flu, produce decrements in mood that extend well beyond the period of sickness.[49–56] Usually these pathogen-instigated mood episodes are mild and self-contained, but occasionally they are long lasting and severe in vulnerable individuals and in response to microbes that are especially depressogenic, such as Epstein-Barr and SARS viruses. Moreover, we are exquisitely sensitive to signs of infection in other humans and tend to respond with disgust and shunning, both of which activate psychosocial processes that are depressive in their own right and are capable of further increasing the depressogenic potential of infection.

Earlier we said that it is the perception of adversity, rather than environmental adversity per se, that promotes depression. If this idea has merit, it should be as applicable to our struggles with pathogens as it is in our conflicts with fellow humans. So, does the perception of infection produce depression? The answer is a resounding yes. In fact, the perception of infection is probably the most reliable of all depressogenic stimuli, a fact which now requires us to turn our attention to the immune system and ask an obvious follow-up question: we use our eyes and ears to recognize social danger, so how do we perceive pathogen danger? If depression is produced by changes in brain functioning, how does the brain find out that the body is infected?

A Quick Primer on Inflammation as a Sense Organ

There are lots of ways of looking at the immune system. In a fanciful mood it can be envisioned as analogous to the army of ancient Troy, valiantly defending its bodily metropolis by keeping the hordes of invading pathogens outside the city gates in a battle it is destined to eventually lose. From another perspective, the immune system seems better conceptualized as a draconian police state replete with a vast contingent of cellular agents patrolling the body's highways and byways, checking everyone's ID cards and instantly executing anyone caught trespassing from a potentially hostile foreign state. Less fancifully, the immune system is like a brain in that it learns from experience and uses this knowledge to enhance its performance in the future.

These metaphors are all valid, and each touches upon a specific function of immunity. But first and foremost the immune system is the body's grandest sense organ, tasked with the overwhelming responsibility of identifying what belongs to the self and what is foreign. Once this basic sensory discrimination has been accomplished, the immune system must perform a second, equally daunting sensory function: it must determine whether any given foreign object is a friend (e.g., food in the gut), a foe (e.g., pneumococcal bacteria in the lung), or a neutral entity (e.g., pollen).

For now let's focus on what the immune system does when it recognizes an invading pathogen, as this is of most direct relevance to demonstrating that the perception of infection promotes depression. Let's start with a thought experiment based on our invocation of ancient Troy. Imagine you are given an army and charged with the task of protecting a walled city from a far larger invading force that is even now approaching across the horizon. What would you do first? Would you gather all your troops together and have them wait in the center of the city for the enemy? Probably not, given all the pillaging and plundering the invaders would inflict within the city on their way to meet you. Alternately, would you send your troops out onto the plain in an attempt to destroy the invaders before they reach the gates? Again, probably not, given that the invading army is so much larger. The smartest course of action would be to post sentries at all the cities most vulnerable spots—the walls, the gates, and such—and have these sentries call out immediately upon seeing the enemy. This strategy would both alert the entire army that battle is near and allow you to send most of your troops to the sites of potential invasion where they would be of most use.

By placing the equivalent of cellular sentries at the walls and gates of the body, the immune system adopts exactly the same strategy. Even if you knew nothing about the geography of the human body, you would be able to identify the body's "walls and gates" merely by asking yourself where most infections happen or come from. For every one infection of the muscles or the bones, we've all had any number of gastrointestinal, respiratory, and skin infections because these are the primary boundary zones—the walls and gates—between us and the larger world. Each of these areas is also chock full of macrophages, neutrophils, and dendritic cells, all of which serve as sentries for the immune system. These sentry cells have surfaces studded with receptors specialized in the recognition of foreign entities called, appropriately enough, pattern recognition receptors (PRRs). This recognition is possible because microbes of all stripes have molecules on their surfaces that are missing from our own cells. When combined with other complex signals from the local environment, these molecules provide pathogen-associated molecular patterns (PAMPs) that alert the immune sentry cells that a potentially dangerous invader is at the gates.

It is amazing how powerful a good metaphor can be for understanding complex physical realities, so back to our thought experiment about the walled city under approaching siege. Unfortunately, the metropolis you are charged with protecting has a huge array of enemies, each with very different invasion strategies, and any one of which could have dispatched the army that is now approaching the city gates. Fortunately, however, while small compared with the invaders, the force at your disposal is remarkably versatile in its fighting skills and so, if given enough time, can tailor its battle strategies to optimally defeat any given enemy. Given this, how would you want your sentries to proceed? Say an enemy regiment attacks a position on the city wall. Would you have the relevant sentry to wait to send any message of danger until he (or she) was completely sure of which enemy this was? Certainly not—such a strategy would be certain death. The sentry doesn't need to read the exact insignia on the uniforms of the advancing foe to know that the drawn swords and lances mean nothing good. First things first: you want a sentry who can recognize an enemy in a general sort of way and who can send a quick message that danger is afoot and to send reinforcements. Because there isn't time to figure out exactly who the enemy is before entering into battle, it is also essential that the message that the sentry sends be as general as possible, so that every possible weapon that can be quickly deployed is rushed to the site of potential invasion.

This is exactly how the immune system proceeds. The PRRs on the surfaces of sentry cells such as macrophages have evolved to act quickly and nonspecifically. They are able to do the equivalent of recognizing that the drawn swords and lances of a foreign invader mean a big dose of trouble that needs to be addressed as quickly as possible. And because they haven't had time to figure out exactly who the enemy is, they activate immune processes that are as widespread and nonselectively damaging as possible. These processes comprise the complicated biological response that is inflammation. And inflammation is the sense organ that tells the brain that the body has become infected.

Just to complete our brief sketch of how the immune system operates, we need to digress to complete our discussion of the sentry before returning to inflammation and depression. So back to the poor beleaguered sentry who is under attack on the walls of your city. While you certainly want this sentry to sound a major alarm immediately upon seeing the approaching enemy, it would also be profoundly useful if the sentry could provide information that would allow command central to ascertain the exact identity of the invader. This would allow you to begin training your troops for how to deal with this specific enemy, even while the pitched battle raged at the city walls. Again, this is exactly how the immune system operates. In addition to sending out a general call to arms when PRRs are stimulated, immune sentry cells capture invading pathogens, swallow them, digest them, and put pieces of the now-defunct microbes out on their cell surfaces for the purpose of presenting these bits of molecular information to T cells, which are the equivalent of command central for the mammalian immune response. Unlike the sentry cells, which can detect foreignness in only a general sort of way, T cells have the capacity to exactly identify specific pathogens and, having done this, to raise an army of other T and B cells all programmed to specifically attack and kill the particular microorganism that has invaded the body.

So immune sentry cells, when functioning properly, launch two very different types of immune responses to any given invading pathogen. By recognizing that a foreign invader is at hand and by immediately launching an all-out immune war, the sentry cells initiate what is variously referred to as innate, natural, or nonspecific immunity. By presenting pieces of the vanquished microbial foe to T cells (a process officially known as antigen presentation), these sentry cells also initiate a much slower and more costly, but ultimately more effective, type of immune functioning, known as adaptive or acquired immunity.

Turning again to our walled city analogy, we can imagine the innate immune system as citizen militia armed with spears, clubs, and shotguns. They are not well trained, but they are ready to attack anything or anybody that looks like a foreigner, and they are ready at the instant to rush pell-mell into battle wherever they are needed. The result is a lot of death by friendly fire and more than a little damage done to the walls of the city itself, but in the end the collateral damage is worth the cost if it keeps the invaders from destroying the city. The adaptive immune system, on the other hand, can be imagined as elite special forces, highly trained killers able to target an enemy very specifically with minimal collateral damage. These elite troops take time and resources to recruit and train, but when up and ready they can carry out complex missions far beyond the province of any innate immune militia. On the other hand, if the militia wasn't available to keep the invaders at bay, the city would be destroyed long before the special forces had the chance to be recruited, trained, and deployed.

How Does the Innate Immune System Alert the Brain to Infection?

A sentry might be brave and ready to die fighting mano a mano with each invader that scales the city walls, but he won't be much of a sentry unless he can also figure out a way to get the message out that the city is under attack and to broadcast this news as rapidly and widely as possible. Innate immune sentries, such as macrophages and dendritic cells, face the same challenge. They need to join the local fight in an attempt to stop invading pathogens at the site of bodily entry, but they also need to get an urgent danger message off to command central, which in this case is the brain and bodily immune tissues. To accomplish this, these cells—when activated by contact with a pathogen—produce a variety of chemicals called cytokines that are highly effective at commandeering both brain and body for the purpose of fighting infection. Cytokines come in all flavors, from highly proinflammatory to strongly anti-inflammatory. The most important proinflammatory cytokines are interleukin-1 (IL-1), tumor necrosis factor-alpha (TNF), and IL-6, all of which are produced in high quantities at sites of infection and all of which have powerful effects on the brain, even at very low concentrations.

Figure 3.1 provides an overview of pathways by which proinflammatory cytokines signal the brain. Multiple pathways provide both rapid and a more time-released type of signaling.[57] Infectious pathogens in the gut are especially likely to stimulate cytokines that interact directly with paraganglia of the vagus nerve to send a rapid-fire neural signal to the brain. Cytokines released in other bodily regions typically course through the blood at a slightly more leisurely pace but have a wider array of signaling options once they approach the central nervous system (CNS). It is only recently that we've appreciated yet another pathway by which inflammatory signals reach the brain. Despite being gospel for several generations that the brain is an "immune-privileged (i.e., wholly separate from) organ," it is now clear that this is a partial truth at best and that infectious signals from the periphery can be literally carried to the CNS by cells such as macro-

FIGURE 3.1. Although traditionally thought of as a psychological problem, psychosocial stress produces changes in the immune system that resemble those seen during infection and that produce changes in brain functioning that promote the development of depression and anxiety. Psychosocial stress activates the release of catecholamines (norepinephrine and epinephrine), which have multiple immune effects, including stimulating the production and release of monocytes from the bone marrow. These monocytes then enter circulatory systems within the body, where they encounter stress-induced danger-associated molecular patterns (DAMPs) and bacteria and bacterial products such as microbial associated molecular patterns (MAMPs) leaked from the gut in response to stress. These DAMPs and MAMPs subsequently activate inflammatory signaling pathways such as nuclear factor-kappa beta (NFκB) and the nod-like receptor protein-3 (NALP3) inflammasome. Stimulation of NLRP3 in turn activates caspase 1, which leads to the production of mature interleukin-1 (IL-1) and IL-18, while also inactivating the glucocorticoid receptor (GR), which contributes to glucocorticoid resistance. Activation of NFκB stimulates the release of other proinflammatory cytokines, including tumor necrosis factor (TNF) and IL-6, which together with IL-1β and IL-18 can access the

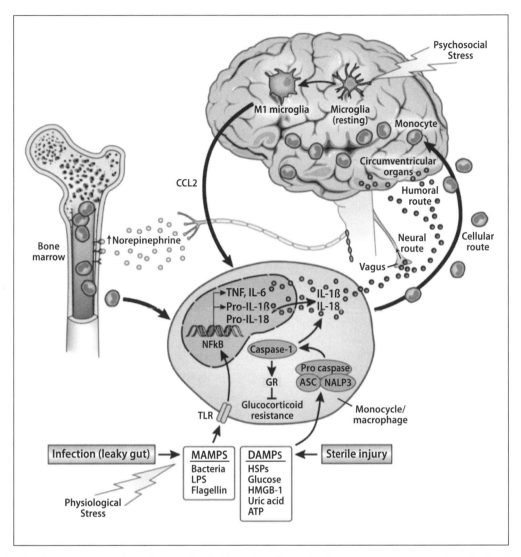

brain through several pathways, including signaling via the vagus nerve, entering the brain through leaky regions in the blood–brain barrier and signaling across the humoral and neural routes. Another important cellular route has also been identified by which peripheral monocytic and T cells traverse from the body either to the brain parenchyma or to the meninges, where they influence central nervous system functioning. It is believed that this cellular route is engaged via activation of microglia to a M1 proinflammatory phenotype which releases chemokine (C-C motif) ligand 2 (CCL2) that in turn attracts activated myeloid cells to the brain. Once in the brain, activated macrophages can perpetuate central inflammatory responses. ASC, apoptosis-associated speck-like protein containing a C-terminal caspase-recruitment domain; ATP, adenosine triphosphate; HMGB-1, high-mobility group box 1; HSPs, heat-shock proteins; LPS, lipopolysaccharide; NALP3, NACHT, LRR, and PYD domains–containing protein 3; TLR, toll-like receptor.

phages and T cells that cross the blood–brain barrier to enter brain tissue.[58] In terms of our walled city analogy, this would be equivalent to a sentry that had engaged the enemy leaving the site of battle to run back himself to command central, all bloodied up and desperate, to carry the bad tidings of trouble to his leaders in person.

Several facts of immune–brain communication highlight its centrality to optimal functioning. First, the very multiplicity and redundancy of pathways by which inflammatory signals can reach the CNS testify to the extreme importance of cytokine signaling for survival across evolutionary time (think key operating systems on a space ship, which have huge redundancy for the same reason). Second, even miniscule concentrations of cytokines far below the levels needed to induce full-on sickness powerfully affect how an animal (or human) behaves. Indeed, the interchange of inflammatory information appears to be so critical that cytokine activation in the body causes de novo production of cytokines in the CNS, and vice versa. This is really quite remarkable—not only does an infection in the body cause the brain to make inflammatory cytokines, but an infection in the brain causes even an organ as far distant as the liver to begin cranking up its production of cytokines. One can only conclude from this that a localized infection anywhere within an organism is so great a risk for subsequent widespread contagion that the body-brain complex hedges its bets and fires up inflammatory readiness everywhere.

Regardless of the path a particular inflammatory signal takes to reach the CNS from the periphery of the body, once there it encounters a rich cytokine network within the brain itself. Neurons have receptors for proinflammatory cytokines and can even synthesize them under inflammatory stimulation. But by far the biggest source of "homegrown" inflammation in the CNS are microglial cells, which are often characterized as the "macrophages of the brain." (We say a good deal more about these cells in Chapter 7.) As you might predict, not all brain areas are equally endowed with the ability to create and/or receive cytokine messages. In fact, the brain areas most sensitive to proinflammatory cytokines are exactly those areas (hypothalamus and various limbic and paralimbic areas) that are known to produce the behavioral patterns and physical symptoms that we recognize as sickness.

INFLAMMATION, PERCEPTION OF INFECTION, AND THE DEVELOPMENT OF DEPRESSION

If inflammation serves as the body's "eyes and ears" for perceiving infection, and if it is the perception of infection that drives depression, then inflammatory molecules should cause depression, even when administered in the absence of an actual pathogen. In fact, inflammatory molecules, or anything that activates them, are among the most potent inducers of depression known to science. If you enter "lipopolysaccharide" and "behavior" into PubMed, almost 2,000 references immediately pop up. Most of these references report that administration of lipopolysaccharide (LPS) to various types of animals reliably produces behavioral patterns widely considered to be equivalents of human depression and anxiety, that is, patterns of behavior that are also produced when animals are stressed and that can be blocked by antidepressant treatment. LPS is an important component of the cell walls of many bacteria and is a PAMP recognized by PRRs on cells of the innate immune system. When detected anywhere in the body by the PRRs of innate immune cells, LPS powerfully stimulates the production and release of proinflammatory cytokines, especially TNF, IL-1, and IL-6, and induces all the symptoms of sickness seen during an actual infection. However, LPS still has a tie to the pathogens from which it derives. An even more powerful demonstration that inflammation itself induces depression comes from the many studies showing that proinflammatory cytokines not only produce all the symptoms of sickness observed following LPS administration but also induce classic depression- and anxiety-like behavior in various animal models.[59] A particularly vivid example of this phenomenon comes from the work of Steven Maier's group at the University of Colorado. They have shown that mice, when stressed with social isolation, develop cognitive difficulties and changes in brain chemicals similar to those seen in MDD.[60–62] Social isolation also potently increases secretion of the proinflammatory cytokine IL-1β in the hippocampus (a brain area central to depressive pathology) of these mice. Remarkably, when the scientists administered an antagonist of IL-1β into the brain prior to the social isolation, the negative effects of the stressor on both behavior and brain chemistry were completely abolished.

Consistent with animal data, studies in humans show that even small doses of a proinflammatory stimulus produce depressive symptoms in most individuals. For example, a dose of LPS too small to produce obvious sickness nonetheless induced feelings of depression and anxiety and impaired memory in healthy volunteers. The more proinflammatory cytokines increased in response to the LPS, the more depressed and anxious the volunteers became.[63] A separate study demonstrated that pretreating people with the selective serotonin reuptake inhibitor citalopram (but not the noradrenergic agent bupropion) prior to LPS exposure blocked the depressogenic effects of the inflammatory stimulus.[64,65] Short-term decrements in mood and cognitive ability have also been reported following typhoid vaccination.[66] Of course, as anyone who has had the flu knows, inflammatory activation may induce depression, but it produces many other feelings as well. For example, ever been in the throes of the flu and felt an irresistible desire to go out to a party and be really social? Assuming you said no, the reason for this is because, in addition to making you sick, proinflammatory cytokines inhibit our ability to take pleasure in things and make us feel socially disconnected. As it turns out, even mild immune stimuli—LPS in this case—produce powerful feelings of social disconnection, and these feelings play an important role in generating depressive emotions.[67]

If inflammatory stimuli such as LPS or a typhoid vaccine induce depression even in the absence of an actual infection, one would predict that these stimuli should also induce changes in brain function similar to those seen in depression. In fact, this is exactly what studies show. Typhoid vaccine has been reported to acutely increase activity in the subgenual region of the anterior cingulate cortex (sgACC), which is a very common finding in people with MDD.[66] The more the vaccine increased activity in the sgACC, the more depressed people became. Interestingly, the same study observed that typhoid vaccine also impaired the ability of many mood-relevant brain areas (e.g., sgACC, amygdala, medial prefrontal cortex, and nucleus accumbens) to work together, a process technically known as functional connectivity. Similar patterns of reduced functional connectivity have been repeatedly observed in patients with MDD. Strongly supporting a direct role for inflammation in this process, people who produced more IL-6 in response to the typhoid vaccine also showed greater impairments in CNS functional connectivity. In a separate study done at UCLA, Naomi Eisenberger and her colleagues observed that the short-term depression induced by LPS was also associated with changes in an area deep in the brain known as the ventral striatum.[68] This brain region activates in response to novel stimuli, especially pleasurable ones, and has been repeatedly identified as a primary site of action for all drugs of abuse, including alcohol. It is also a primary brain region implicated in the pathogenesis of MDD. As you might guess LPS, reduced activity in this brain region in response to a pleasurable/exciting stimulus (winning money!), and the more LPS reduced activity in this region, the more depressed people became.[68]

Is Chronic Inflammation More Depressogenic Than Acute Inflammation?

Taken together, studies examining the mood effects of acute inflammatory stimuli provide compelling evidence that, as with psychosocial stress, it is the perception of infection (measured as cytokine activity), rather than infection itself, that promotes depression. But now we need to extend this line of reasoning and ask a follow-up question. One of the most striking features of the association between psychosocial adversity and depression is the fact that stressors become more and more depressogenic the longer they last. We all know this from personal experience: one negative event is bad; a string of them is hellish. This makes sense from a TOF perspective because chronic and/or inescapable stressors almost always signal a greater risk to survival and reproduction than do single bad events that don't outright kill you. So from a TOF perspective, chronic inflammation should be more depressogenic than the types of acute inflammatory stimuli we've discussed thus far. Is this true?

In fact one of us (C.R.) spent more than a decade conducting studies that directly address this question. This work was made possible by the fact that one inflammatory cytokine, interferon-alpha (IFN-α), enjoyed many years of wide use for treating a number of disorders for which enhanced immune functioning is thought to be of benefit, including several cancers and chronic infection with the hepatitis C virus (HCV). While not very powerful for treating cancer, IFN-α was often almost a miracle cure for HCV infection (it has been replaced by even more effective and less burdensome treatments in recent years). It is also a potent inflammatory stimulus, which allowed us to use it as a model for the effects of chronic inflammation on brain, body, and behavior. There is nothing subtle about IFN-α's ability to induce depression when administered over periods of weeks to months. Depending on the dosage used and the average level of pretreatment risk factors in any given study, rates of clinical depression during IFN-α treatment have been reported to range from a low of around 20 percent to a high of high of 82 percent.[69–71] Importantly, although sickness symptoms develop within hours of receiving a first injection/infusion of IFN-α, depressive symptoms emerge to a significant degree only after weeks to months of treatment, clearly establishing that chronic inflammation is more depressogenic than is acute inflammatory exposure (although acute sickness in response to IFN-α initiation strongly predicts the later development of depression).

Several lines of evidence demonstrate that IFN-α–induced depression is a "real" depression. Our colleague Andrew H. Miller at Emory University has provided the key data. Working with Lucile Capuron, he compared patients who met *DSM-IV* criteria for major depression as a result of ongoing IFN-α treatment with medically healthy people suffering from "regular" idiopathic MDD in terms of the number and type of depressive symptoms they demonstrated.[72] Their symptom profiles were remarkably similar. Patients on IFN-α tended to be more psychomotor retarded (i.e., they moved and responded to things more slowly) and less guilty and suicidal than people with idiopathic MDD, but otherwise the groups were essentially identical. Miller and his colleagues provided even more powerful evidence for the equivalence of cytokine-induced and idiopathic MDD in a study in which patients receiving high-dose IFN-α therapy for malignant melanoma were randomized in double-blind fashion to treatment with either the selective serotonin reuptake inhibitor paroxetine or a placebo prior to and during their cytokine therapy.[73] Although all subjects were depression-free prior to commencing IFN-α, at the end of three months of treatment almost 50 percent of patients in the placebo group had experienced MDD, compared with only 9 percent in patients receiving adjunctive paroxetine. A final line of evidence that inflammation produces "real" depression comes from a series of studies done by us and others showing that chronic IFN-α exposure produces many of the pathophysiological changes associated with MDD, including glucocorticoid resistance, flattening of the diurnal cortisol rhythm, disruptions in sleep continuity and reduced slow wave sleep, decreased peripheral serotonin availability, increased CNS concentrations of quinolinic acid (a powerful excitotoxin and stimulator of glutamatergic *N*-methyl-D-aspartate receptors), and changes in the activity of several depression-relevant brain regions, including the anterior cingulate cortex and basal ganglia.[74–89] In general, the more a given patient shows these changes, the more likely he or she is to develop clinically significant depression during IFN-α therapy.

With all these physiological changes afoot, it is a fair question to ask whether evidence supports a direct link between increased inflammation and the development of depression during IFN-α treatment. In other words, how do we know that IFN-α makes people depressed because it increases inflammation rather than via some other more general mechanism? Again, our work with Andy Miller provides a likely answer.

To help make this work intelligible, we need to digress and provide a bit more background information on the physiology of inflammation. We've already described about how PRRs on immune cells are able to identify PAMPs on the external walls of infectious pathogens, with the result that these immune cells become activated and commence secreting proinflammatory cytokines. But how does the message get from the receptor on the immune cell surface down into the nucleus, where most changes in cellular function are initiated and regulated? This feat is accomplished by a variety of mechanisms, alternately referred to as second-messenger or intracellular signaling cascades. To visualize these cascades, imagine a group of people racing to fill sandbags to save their city from flooding, who would typically line themselves up in a sort of transfer chain. At one end people fill sand bags, which they hand to the next person, who hands it to the next and the next until the bag reaches someone at the site where it will be placed. In this analogy, the people filling the bags are like cell-surface receptors, the people placing the bags onto the growing flood-control wall are like the cellular nucleus, and all the people handing the bags along the chain are like an intracellular, second-messenger signaling cascade. The analogy breaks down at this point because typically the people passing along the sandbags make no decisions regarding which bags go where or when they get there. But we might imagine a scenario more consistent with actual second-messenger behavior in which the sand bag transfer line had various branch points, allowing bags to be diverted to any of a number of vulnerable locations along the flood-control wall. This scenario begins to approach the complexity of second-messenger signaling, in which different pathways regulate one another and in which activation of individual pathways can result in very different biological effects depending on local conditions within the cell.

Intracellular signaling cascades form a warren of complexity that would do the center of any medieval city proud. Indeed, there is a second-messenger pathway for every aspect of cellular functioning. For present purposes, let's focus on two pathways: nuclear factor kappa-beta (NFκB) and p38 mitogen-activated pro-tein kinase. These pathways live at the crossroads of cellular function and so contribute to almost every process necessary for life. Because of this, we cannot assign an overriding, unitary function to either NFκB or p38. Nonetheless, at the risk of oversimplifying, it is clear that both these pathways are essential for acti-vating inflammation in response to a wide variety of infectious signals, including LPS and proinflammatory cytokines. When activated, these pathways stimulate coordinated activity throughout the cell to release stored proinflammatory medi-ators and to stimulate gene expression to create new inflammatory molecules. Conversely, agents that block either NFκB or p38 are powerfully anti-inflammatory and as such are being actively explored as therapeutic agents for a range of inflam-matory conditions, including cancer, heart disease, and depression.

With these details in mind, let's return to the question of whether IFN-α pro-duces depression by directly activating inflammation. As part of an elaborate evaluation of the effects of IFN-α on the body, brain, and behavior, we admitted patients to a special research unit in the Emory University Hospital and drew their blood on an hourly basis before and immediately after they received their very first dose of IFN-α. We did this to see if we could identify immediate physio-logical responses to the acute immune challenge that might predict later develop-ment of depression during chronic IFN-α treatment. Even though we hypothesized that the body's initial inflammatory response to IFN-α would predict the later development of depression, we were astonished to see how powerfully one key inflammatory pathway actually did this: that of p38. The amount of increase in p38 in the hours following a first IFN-α shot almost perfectly predicted how much depressive symptoms would go up over the succeeding month of IFN-α therapy.[90] This means that we could have told people their depression score a month in the future armed only with their current score and their p38 response in the hours following that first IFN-α shot, and we would never have been off by more than a point or two.

These findings provide the strongest demonstration we know of that IFN-α induces depression first and foremost by activating inflammation. But there are other lines of evidence as well. We and others have shown that the development of depression during IFN-α is highly correlated with the degree of inflammation engendered by the medication. For example, Francis Lotrich and his colleagues demonstrated that IL-6 responses to IFN-α both were associated with depression scores cross-sectionally during treatment and, more important, predicted depres-sion scores at subsequent time points.[88] Similarly, we found that the more TNF signaling increased over the first three months of IFN-α treatment, the more depressed people became over the same time period.[78] Absolute confirmation that the body's inflammatory system must be activated for IFN-α to produce depres-sion would require demonstrating that blocking the production/activity of pro-inflammatory cytokines prevents depression during treatment. Sadly from the point of view of science (but fortunately for the treatment of HCV), IFN-α essentially vanished as a treatment before these studies could be conducted.

INFLAMMATION AS A UNIVERSAL DEPRESSOGEN

The argument we have been making is straightforward. TOF theory suggests that environmental conditions indicating an increased risk for early mortality should be powerfully depressogenic because dying young is a certain way to reduce one's overall fitness. More specifically, it is the perception of increased risk for early mortality that is depressogenic. And because infection has been the primary cause of early mortality across human evolution, it is not surprising that the perception of infection, accomplished via activation of the body's inflammatory response system, is one of the most powerful of depressogenic stimuli.

A more surprising, but very logical, extension of this line of thought is that anything that increases inflammation should be depressogenic, not necessarily because it actually poses an actual threat to overall fitness but because the brain has evolved to perceive inflammation in this way. Conversely, anything that reduces inflammation, regardless of whether it actually improves overall fitness, should have antidepressant properties in people with elevated inflammation for the simple reason that it reduces the brain's hard-wired perception of impending doom. So what sorts of things increase inflammation, and are they reliably depressogenic?

Inflammation as a Link Between Medical Illness and Depression

Let's start with the most obvious of proinflammatory conditions: medical illness. Although most people in the modern world no longer die young from infection, we eventually succumb to any one of a host of diseases that have inflammatory activation at their core. Indeed, inflammation is the sine qua non of all the major modern medical maladies, from cardiovascular disease, stroke, and cancer to diabetes and dementia. These conditions vary widely in their average inflammatory burden, and wide ranges of inflammation are seen across individuals with each disease. However, despite this, medical illnesses are all characterized by levels of inflammatory activity known to predict the development of depression, even in people who are apparently medically healthy.

Most of us rightly associate the development of depression with psychosocial stressors, but in fact medical illness is at least as powerful an inducer of depression as any psychosocial factor, and maybe more so. Although estimates of the prevalence of MDD in various illnesses vary widely, we've never seen a study that didn't find that sick folks have higher rates of depression than do medically healthy individuals. The most definitive study conducted to date examined the association of depression with a number of common chronic medical conditions in 60 countries around the world. In a sample of nearly 250,000 adults, having one chronic medical condition increased the risk of also having depression by

300 to 600 percent.[1] Having two medical conditions increased the depression risk by almost 800 percent.

Of course, anyone who has had a serious medical disorder knows that these diseases can be very powerful psychosocial stressors in and of themselves. So how do we know that medical illness produces depression via increased inflammation as opposed to via the more mundane fact that "you'd be depressed too if you were seriously sick"? In fact, the stress associated with illness is highly depressogenic. So perhaps it is more appropriate to reframe the question and ask after evidence that inflammation contributes to depression during medical illness over and above the effects of chronic stress. A first line of evidence comes from studies showing that diseases with higher levels of inflammation also tend to produce more depression than less inflammatory conditions.[91] A second line of evidence comes from the fact that, with any given medical condition, patients with higher levels of inflammation tend also to be more depressed.[92] Finally, blocking inflammatory signaling pathways, TNF in particular, has been shown to reduce depression in the context of several autoimmune conditions, including psoriasis and Crohn's disease.[93–95]

Exploding a False Dichotomy

Before turning from medical illness to other sources of inflammation, we have to set aside a false dichotomy between sickness and psychosocial stress that we've thus far indulged. When we say that sickness causes depression in part because it is a significant stressor, this in no way marginalizes the role of inflammatory processes, because psychosocial stressors themselves robustly activate inflammatory pathways in the brain and body.[96] Stress is proinflammatory. A huge literature reports that people under stress, whether young or old, have higher levels of circulating inflammatory biomarkers (e.g., IL-6 or C-reactive protein) than do their less stressed compatriots. Supplementing these cross-sectional findings are multiple studies demonstrating that even mild stressors reliably increase inflammatory markers in humans. (For a good review of this literature, see Steptoe et al.[97]) An important early demonstration of this effect came from the finding that exposure to a public speaking and mental arithmetic stressor (known as the Trier Social Stress Test) significantly increased activity of the fundamental inflammatory transcription factor NFκB in peripheral blood mononuclear cells compared with individuals who were spectators of the task, but not participants.[98] We and many others have shown that the Trier Social Stress Test also increases plasma concentrations of inflammatory cytokines, especially IL-6, and does so more in people with a history of early-life adversity than in others.[99,100]

Is Everything That Causes Depression Proinflammatory?

Depending on how much one knows about the role of the immune system in the pathogenesis of depression, this question might sound either rhetorical or preposterous—it's neither. It's not preposterous because, in fact, many factors known to

TABLE 3.1. **Risk Factors for Depression That Also Increase Inflammation**

Medical illness	Female sex
Psychosocial stress	Low socioeconomic status
Sedentary lifestyle	Smoking and second-hand smoke exposure
Obesity	Air pollution
Diminished sleep	Change of seasons (e.g., winter in those with
Social isolation	seasonal affective disorder)
Diet (e.g., low ratio of omega-3 to omega-6 fatty acids, high-fructose sugars)	

promote depression are also proinflammatory.[101] Nor is the question rhetorical, because not every known depressogen has been carefully examined in terms of immune effects, and as we describe in Chapter 9, if a powerful depression risk factor turned out not to increase inflammatory activity, this would pose a challenge to many ideas central to this book. Table 3.1 lists important risk factors for depression that are also known to be proinflammatory.[1–8,43,97–99,102–129] Many of these are unique to the modern world, such as obesity and the consumption of processed food. As we discuss in Chapter 9, the proliferation of these types of inflammatory factors may help account for the dramatic increase in MDD that has occurred over the last 50 years. Other noninfectious promoters of inflammation have been around for at least millennia (i.e., psychosocial stress), and some have been around since the beginning of life (i.e., change of seasons), suggesting that our depressive responses to them may serve adaptive purposes.

Evolutionary Fitness II: Circumstances That Threaten Both Survival and Reproduction Should Be the Most Depressogenic of All

> And those whose names were never called, when choosing sides for basketball.
>
> Janice Ian, "At Seventeen"

Years ago one of us had an experience with a medical psychiatry service that we've never forgotten. As the attending physician with the service, we listened during daily rounds to a young resident who told us about an elderly man he'd just seen who would soon be dead from cancer. The old gentlemen had developed a profound depression. Our young resident physician colleague was of a philosophical bent, so he concluded his case presentation with an extended discussion of how the old fellow was likely depressed as a result of the existential misery inherent in facing certain and imminent death. It seemed reasonable. But then, with the whole team in tow, we went to evaluate the patient. The resident had been dutiful in asking all the questions on the depression criteria list and had correctly established that the elderly gentleman was clear-headed and not delirious. What he'd failed to do was ask the old man why he was so damn miserable. We did this and were immediately regaled with a long story of how his brother-in-law was screwing him out of an important business deal because he was stuck in a hospital bed. We asked directly about the patient's understanding of his current medical condition. He shrugged and said, "I'll be dead in a couple of weeks. That just makes me angrier that this guy is taking advantage of me." Based on this interview, we instructed the resident to call a family meeting to address the patient's business dealings. The meeting was held, and the errant brother-in-law was called on the carpet by other family members. An agreement was struck, and the patient died three weeks later completely depression-free.

We tell this story to highlight an aspect of the human world that is so obvious that we typically fail to grasp its strangeness and profundity. People are remarkably good at denying the certainty of their upcoming death but will die and kill others for even minor threats to their honor, status, or control of material resources. We easily ignore the true life-and-death aspects of our existence (i.e., we are alive now, and will soon—in the grand scheme of things—be dead) and behave as if all sorts of minor slights, affronts, and conflicts are of life-and-death importance, even when they are clearly not. Overwhelming evidence documents the high price we pay for this pattern of misperception, in costs both to real-world resources (think wars, divorces, failed business deals) and to our health (think of the correlations between anger/hostility and medical illnesses in particular and early death in general).[130,131] Moreover, we know from many studies that people who are able to keep their cool and not overreact to these multiple, but minor, threats to well-being have heightened overall fitness as a result of enhanced social success and better health compared with their more short-sighted and short-tempered peers. So why has natural selection programmed us to be so unrealistically hotheaded about all the relatively unimportant social challenges that make up the warp and woof of our daily lives?

The peacock's tail posed a similar challenge to the theory of evolution in the mid-nineteenth century, leading Darwin to famously say, "The sight of a feather in a peacock's tail, whenever I gaze at it, makes me sick." Darwin had seen enough vain male peacocks get taken down by small-time predators to know how great a survival liability those big, glorious tails were. So why hadn't the tails been clipped by natural selection? His eventual answer presaged all of twentieth-century biology. He realized that traits such as the peacock's tail could undergo positive selection, even at risk to life and limb, if they made an individual more effective in passing along his or her genes to the next generation.[132] This is the evolutionary equivalent of the Madison Avenue truth that "sex sells," and it points to a biological reality that was only fully understood nearly a century after Darwin's death: evolutionary change is driven not by the survival of individuals but by the survival of their genes. From this perspective, individual life forms, including humans, are like missiles loaded with genes and pointing toward to the future. The missile is not important for its own sake. It is only the delivery of the payload that matters, and if the genetic payload doesn't make a direct strike on the next generation, the game of life is finished.

In the case of peacocks, Darwin theorized—correctly, as it turned out—that the grandiose tail might have sexual benefits that outweighed any costs to individual survival. This insight has been greatly expanded in recent years as sexual selection theory, once considered Darwin's great mistake, has experienced a Renaissance in the world of evolutionary biology.[132] The essence of natural selection is that any genetically determined trait that increases the odds of an organism surviving to reproductive age is likely to increase in prevalence over time because organisms with the trait are more likely to contribute the trait (and underlying gene) to the next generation. Similarly, the essence of sexual selection is that any genetically determined trait that increases the odds of an organism successfully reproducing will likely spread throughout a population simply because it produces more offspring in the next generation that have inherited the trait (and the gene).

At first blush you would expect these two great selection forces to cooperate, because it is obvious that any trait that enhances both fitness by natural and sexual selection is a complete winner. Some traits do indeed follow this pattern; for example, good health both increases survival and is sexually attractive. But much of the resurgent interest in sexual selection has been fueled by our growing appreciation that the forces of natural and sexual selection can—and often do—actually compete with each other.[132] This notion comes to its most extreme and logical conclusion with costly signaling theory, first articulated in the 1970s by Amotz Zahavi as the handicap principle.[132] The idea here is that sexual ornaments in animals (e.g., the peacock's tail) evolved precisely because they signal to members of the opposite sex that the possessor of the ornament is fit enough to sacrifice energies needed for survival to produce the ornament. These ornaments, therefore, are costly and difficult to fake and for this reason send a reliable message to a potential mate regarding the genetic quality of the suitor. Many studies have demonstrated that the egregiousness these types of sexual displays can take is limited only by the unflinching demand of natural selection that the organism survive long enough to procreate.

A clear implication of TOF theory is that anything that negatively impacts either natural or sexual selection should promote depression. And the most depressing environmental adversities should be those that at one and the same time reduce both aspects of fitness, survival, and reproduction. To examine this assertion, let's return for a bit to inflammation before turning our focus to the question of whether the most depressogenic psychosocial adversities are indeed those most likely to reduce both survival and reproductive opportunity.

INFLAMMATION AND DEPRESSION BEFORE AND AFTER
THE AGE OF REPRODUCTION

From the point of view of your genes, once you've raised your children you've served your purpose and are now more or less superfluous (we write "more or less" in deference to theorizing regarding the importance of grandparents in human evolution). On the other hand, your death prior to reproduction is a catastrophe of the first order. Thus, early death meets the criteria par excellence of being an environmental adversity that reduces both aspects of overall fitness, survival and reproduction, in a way that death later in life does not. If inflammation serves as a "sixth sense" for detecting infectious danger, and if infection has been the primary cause of early death across hominid evolution, then TOF theory predicts that inflammatory conditions should be more depressogenic when they occur prior the end of the age of reproduction and/or successful child-rearing than when they occur later in life. Said differently, inflammation may be depressogenic at any point in life because it is a reliable indicator of reduced fitness secondary to reduced survival, but inflammation early in life also runs afoul of sexual selection. It does this in two ways: first by indicating that one is not likely to survive to reproduce, and second, by making people less sexually attractive. In regards to this second mechanism, many studies have shown that all around the world people are able to both consciously and unconsciously recognize people who are infected and tend to shun them.[133] Sickness, far from being sexy, triggers disgust.

Several lines of evidence support the notion that inflammation is more depressogenic before versus after the end of the age of reproduction. People instinctively feel that death early in life is more tragic than death in old age. Without questioning why, we say, "Young people have so much more to lose." This is incontrovertible and no doubt plays a large role in the repeated finding that medical illnesses are more likely to produce depression in younger versus older individuals.[134–140] But TOF theory provides a complementary perspective to these findings, because the illnesses that demonstrate a depressogenic age gradient are also states of increased inflammation, raising the possibility that inflammation itself might be might be more powerfully depressogenic when experienced prior to the age of reproduction/successful child-rearing.

On this point, the jury is still out. But a tantalizing clue supports this prediction of TOF theory. In the early 2000s we made the curious observation that younger people were more likely than older individuals to develop clinically significant depression during chronic cytokine exposure resulting from use of IFN-α to treat HCV infection.[141] None of the ideas we are discussing here had formed in our minds in those days, and we were far more interested in other more powerful predictors of developing IFN-α–induced depression, so we never reported the strange age finding when we published the study. But other research groups have reported age as a risk factor for developing IFN-α–induced depression. The findings are not consistent, but the bulk of available data point to younger age as a likely risk factor for IFN-α–induced depression.[142,143] But none of these studies (including ours) has tested the clear implication of TOF theory that the association between age and depression during inflammation should be not linear but discrete, with cut points based on average ages of reproduction and completion of child-rearing in ancestral human environments. Said differently, no one has tested the idea that people below the average ages of successful reproduction or successful child-rearing are more likely than people past these ages to develop depression during chronic cytokine exposure. Interestingly, we saw the strongest effect of age when we split our IFN-α population between those younger and older than 40 years, which is a credible age for completion of child-rearing in ancestral environments. But confirmation of these ideas awaits more definitive studies.

DO THE MOST DEPRESSOGENIC PSYCHOSOCIAL ADVERSITIES REALLY THREATEN BOTH SURVIVAL AND REPRODUCTIVE SUCCESS?

Psychosocial Messages of Danger, Disappointment, and Despair From Ancient Environments

Why are people so much more afraid of flying on commercial jets than they are of driving their cars around town, when flying is several hundred times less likely to kill you than is driving, on a mile-per-mile basis? From an evolutionary perspective the answer is simple: people evolved in a world with heights, and heights have posed a risk to life and limb since time immemorial. Genes that promoted fear of heights prevented death by falling often enough to have undergone positive selection. That this fear is now instinctual (i.e., in our genes) can be seen in experiments showing that babies show fear when encouraged to crawl over a clear surface stretched over a height. On the other hand, until the nineteenth century no one ever traveled faster than 10–15 miles an hour (except those unlucky enough to fall from a high place!), so we never had a reason to evolve a fear of high speeds on land. Few people have absolutely no fear of flying, and few people are truly terrified of driving speeds on land, testifying to the astounding power that the realities of the ancestral environment continue to wield on our modern existences.

We provide the example of flying versus driving to emphasize that we cannot answer the question of whether the most depressogenic stressors are really those that threaten survival *and* reproduction without first attempting to identify the events and circumstances that were most likely to pose these dual threats in the ancestral environment, often referred to as the environment of evolutionary adaptedness (EEA). From an evolutionary perspective, it should be these ancient threats to survival and reproduction, and not their modern counterparts, that most reliably produce depression. This, of course, begs the question of what these ancient threats actually were. But before examining this, let's pause for a moment to examine how this "ancient terrors perspective," as it might be called, helps explain an apparent challenge to TOF theory.

If threats to overall fitness are really the most powerful risk factors for depression, why don't modern young Americans become overwhelmed with despair whenever they contemplate taking a drive or working with power tools, and why don't the various available birth control methods come with an FDA black box warning about their risk for producing profound depression? In modern America unintentional injury is the leading cause of death through early middle age, and more reproductive fitness has been lost to birth control than to any other factor in our lives. You can see that the answer to this question is similar to the answer for why driving doesn't frighten us as much as it should. In our emotional life, no less than in much of our thinking, we shadowbox with long-gone environments that no longer pertain but that drive much of our behavior.

This truth provides a possible explanation for another odd fact about the circumstances most likely to depress us. While we all understand depression in response to the death of a child or loss of a long-time spouse, we've also all had the experience of wondering why our friends and loved ones are so devastated by circumstances and/or occurrences that don't seem worth all the misery. Sure, he was an OK guy, but is the world really over because he broke up with you? Yes, that job promotion would have helped your bottom line, but you've still got a job and a family that loves you—is it really worth considering suicide? And so on. TOF theory suggests that although these types of adversities no longer deeply threaten either survival or reproduction, they must be tapping into archetypal dangers to overall fitness in the EEA.

Does the Link Between Early Adversity and Depression Reflect Ancient Truths?

We've already invoked the EEA in our discussion of inflammation as an evolved signal of increased risk of death from infection. Inflammation still depresses us in the modern world, regardless of its real danger in any given situation, as would be predicted by TOF theory. In extending the discussion from the immunological to the psychosocial adversities that reduced overall fitness in the EEA, we would do well to start with childhood, because an "ancient adversities" perspective helps clarify an observation that is so well established and so seemingly commonsensical that it no longer puzzles us, although it should. All over the world maltreatment and/or neglect from parents produces depression, not just in childhood but throughout adulthood, long after those childhood adversities pose any danger to daily life.[144] Death of a parent (especially a mother) in childhood has a similar long-lasting proclivity to produce depression in adulthood,[145] again, long after any practical need for the parent's presence has passed. Why? The last decade has seen huge strides in our understanding of *how* childhood adversity programs the brain and body in ways that promote depression, but we've thought less often about the more obvious question: why does early-life adversity do this? Why does early adversity set an entire lifetime upon an arc of depression?

We suggest an adaptive answer to this question in Chapter 9, but for now let's train TOF theory upon the question. From this perspective, the types of early adversity that produce depression in today's world must have been powerful signals of reduced overall fitness in the EEA. In fact, this is likely true. Of all animals, humans are most dependent upon parental nurturance for survival to reproductive age. Because of this, traits that enhance a child's ability to bond with his or her caregivers have undergone tremendous positive selection across evolutionary time in humans. One such trait is a heightened ability to recognize and react to any parental behavior that signals disruption in the nurturance required for survival. In the modern world, psychologically healthy parents find these abilities/gestures on the part of their children lovable. In earlier times, these abilities were often a matter of life and death.

In all deference to the current widespread romanticization of our hunter-gatherer origins, children in ancestral environments likely had much to fear from their parents, and much to fear from the loss of their parents. Although the types of abusive/neglectful behavior that are sadly rife in the modern world appear to be rare in social groupings that more closely approximate the human EEA (i.e., hunter-gatherers), parents in these societies routinely make very hard choices that directly affect which of their children survive and prosper and which do not. The implications of Sarah Hrdy's work on infanticide in primates scandalized the academic world several decades ago but turned out to be prescient in relation to humans, given increasing evidence of the widespread use of infanticide and other types of more subtle (but equally lethal) parental abandonment in hunter-gatherer groups, as well as other types of traditional human societies.[146]

The specifics of how and why these devastating choices are made varies from one type of society to another and from one type of environmental condition to another, but the overarching message is clear. Across human evolution: violence and rejection on the part of parents toward a child were tantamount to a death sentence. Similarly, the death of a parent in hunter-gatherer societies not infrequently signals a significantly increased likelihood of death for the children, from either infanticide or abandonment. In fact, it appears that Paleolithic hunter-gatherer groups may be more likely than societies that evolved later, such as agriculturists, to practice infanticide or abandonment of children in general, and likely orphans in particular.[147] So from a TOF perspective, parental abuse, neglect, and death are so depressogenic now because these types of behavior were a true signal for reduced probability of a child's actual physical survival in the EEA. (Of course, it is still true that abused/neglected children die younger—either in childhood or as adults—than do appropriately cared for children.)[144]

A parental decision to end a child's life—via either infanticide or abandonment—is the ultimate threat to overall fitness. In this regard it is remarkably similar to the effects of early-life infection. Perhaps it is no surprise, then, that these two types of adversities are among the most depressogenic known, or that they produce similar changes in the body-brain complex, as we discuss in Chapters 5 and 6. Evidence suggests that females are generally at greater risk for infanticide in hunter-gatherer societies, and thus presumably in the EEA, which may help explain the consistent finding that females in the modern world are significantly more likely than males to develop MDD as a result of early adversity.[148] Early adversity in the form of parental violence/neglect may be more depressogenic for females because in the EEA it was a truer signal of increased risk of early mortality.

But infanticide and abandonment are only the far extremes of a long continuum in parental decision making regarding how many resources to invest in any given child, and studies suggest that even minor discrepancies in parental behavior likely had long-term health consequences for children in the EEA. Still, these more subtle types of parental favoritism would not often have killed their offspring outright. So why are even relatively minor levels of parental violence/neglect so profoundly depressogenic in today's world? A TOF perspective suggests that the "missing misery" might be found in the realm of sexual selection. That is, TOF theory suggests that the degree to which any negative parental behavior produces depression should be proportional not just to its effect on survival but also to its effects on the ability of the affected offspring to reproduce. A simple way to test this idea would be to examine in hunter-gatherer societies whether differences in parental behavior toward their offspring predicted the number of grandchildren that were born from each of these children. Children who received more support/resources/affection from their parents should in turn have more children themselves, if this idea is correct. We know of no such study; however, a similar investigation has been conducted in Hungary. In that country, the Gypsy population favors female offspring, whereas the general Hungarian (i.e., non-Gypsy) population favors male offspring (as assessed by a variety of metrics). Consistent with an effect of parental investment on reproductive success, and hence sexual selection, Gypsy females have higher reproductive success than do Gypsy males, and the exact opposite pattern is observed among the general Hungarian population.[149,150]

Before Turning to Adulthood, TOF Theory Offers Novel Explanations for Known Childhood Depressive Risk Factors

TOF theory provides a simple and unifying perspective on why childhood adversity so powerfully promotes the development of depression. In the EEA, even minor gradations in the provision of parental resources likely had significant effects on both survival and reproductive success and hence on overall evolutionary fitness. Moreover, because reproduction is an adult activity, it is perhaps not surprising that the full depressogenic effects of childhood maltreatment often do not manifest until adulthood, when this second "hit" to overall fitness is fully realized. In fact, from this perspective, the fact that childhood adversity so commonly causes depression years after the survival dangers have largely passed is strong circumstantial evidence for the power of sexual selection in this process.

As a field, psychiatry has held to the commonsense notion that early-life abuse and neglect are so depressing . . . because they are so depressing. They are obviously horrible, so why shouldn't they cause depression? TOF theory provides an escape from this tautology by suggesting that early-life abuse and neglect are only extreme cases of the larger phenomenon of reduced parental investment. As true signals of drastic reductions in parental investment, abuse and neglect powerfully predict reduced overall fitness. And that is why they are depressing. Now let's consider an obvious extension of these ideas. If parental investment, rather than abuse or neglect, is the core issue, then anything that reduces parental investment in the EEA should still cause depression today. Many such factors present themselves, but we'll focus on two: limited resources and the presence of siblings

Children are less likely to get resources if there are fewer resources to be had, so, on average, environmental conditions with limited or unpredictable resources should be depressogenic. Of most relevance to ancestral hunter-gatherer societies in which food procurement is the primary live-or-die resource, longitudinal studies demonstrate that malnutrition in early childhood predicts the development of depression in adulthood, even if the nutritional deficits are time limited and fully corrected.[151,152] Drawing on animal data, explanations offered to date for this phenomenon have pointed to the fact that neonatal malnutrition selectively disrupts the development of brain regions most implicated in the pathogenesis of MDD. (Specifically, it deranges glial and dendritic development in prefrontal cortex and hippocampus.)

TOF theory offers the complementary perspective that early malnutrition may promote depression because it signals a reduction in parental investment (even if involuntary) and hence of overall evolutionary fitness. To test this idea, one would want to separate the direct physical effects of malnutrition from the effect any involved maternal behavior—be it behavior that caused the malnutrition or behavioral responses to the fact that such malnutrition is inescapable. TOF theory predicts that if malnutrition produces depression at least in part because it is a true signal of reduced parental investment, then the parental behavior associated with malnutrition should itself produce depression in the affected offspring, independently of any direct effect of the food shortage.

Whether this is true for humans is unknown (at least as far as we know), but a series of studies by Jeremy Copland and colleagues in nonhuman primates provide very strong support for this TOF prediction. They have shown that macaque mothers react to experimental environments with difficult-to-find and unpredictable food sources in ways that program their offspring to demonstrate depressive behavior as adults, as a result of multiple changes in brain-body functioning that are similar to those seen in human depression.[153,154] Importantly, the variable foraging demand (VFD) paradigm does not result in infant macaques receiving less nutrition than infants raised in environments in which food is reliably present. This rules out the possibility that the long-term behavioral changes observed in response to VFD result directly from the physical effects of malnutrition. Rather, from a TOF perspective VFD produces depression-like behavior and physiology in affected offspring because the difficulties of food finding reduce the investment in time, attention, and care that mothers can provide to their infants.

Ethnographic analyses support the validity of VFD as a model for inducing depression because, like the female macaques in Copland's studies, human mothers invest fewer resources in their offspring under environmental conditions of uncertainty or danger, such as pertain during periods of war, famine, or pestilence.[155] Findings from Afghanistan tragically demonstrate that this withdrawal of parental investment is as likely to produce depression in humans as it is in monkeys. As we noted previously, researchers from the Centers for Disease Control and Prevention have observed sky-high rates of depression in Afghanistan as a result of the ongoing horrific violence, societal collapse, and political schisms afflicting that war-torn country.[42] However, when researchers turned to examining emotional distress in Afghani children and adolescents, they found something surprising. The primary driver of depression and anxiety in these young people was not the generalized environmental hell in which they lived but, rather, the effect that this generalized environmental adversity had on the behavior and mental health of their parents.[45,156] As predicted from the ethnographic literature,[155] under the unpredictable and dangerous circumstances in Afghanistan parents behave in ways that signal a withdrawal of resource investment in their children, and it is this parental behavior (including engaging in violent/abusive behavior) that is the strongest depressogenic risk factor for Afghani children and teens.

Brothers and sisters are not typically mentioned in the same breath as war and famine. But from a TOF perspective they pose similar dangers in terms of depriving one of parental investment. The potential seriousness of this danger is well illustrated by the fact that in many species of birds and mammals, stronger siblings either directly kill their weaker brethren or do things to assure that weaker brothers and sisters won't survive. Similar behavior has been the norm even in humans under exceptional circumstances, such as among the multiple sons of Ottoman sultans, only one of whom would inherit the throne.

Generally, however, sibling rivalries are mellower among human children. Nonetheless, anyone raised with a sibling knows that, even in our world of plenty, competition for parental attention and affection can at times be brutal. From an evolutionary point of view the explanation for this is obvious. Although we share half our genes with our siblings and so are biologically programmed to care for them via kin selection, we share all our genes with ourselves so are even more likely to favor self-interests when they matter most. And nowhere do they matter more than in the procurement of parental resources in early childhood, especially in the EEA when such resources were literally a matter of life and death.

Given the complexities of self versus kin selection that are inherent in all familial dynamics, we should expect complicated associations between the presence of siblings and risk for depression. Nonetheless, TOF theory would assert that, good, bad, or ugly, siblings should have some type of impact on one's risk of developing depression, precisely because siblings pose a primary challenge to obtaining limited parental resources.

A study published in 2007 provides strong support for this possibility.[157] The study recruited 268 male college sophomores in the period 1939–1942 who were judged to demonstrate exceptional mental and physical well-being. At the initial assessment, interviews were conducted with the subjects as well as with family members and parents to assess myriad psychosocial factors thought to contribute to well-being. The subjects were then followed up regularly over the next 30 years. Using this very powerful design, researchers found that the quality of subjects' youthful relationships with their siblings more powerfully predicted the subsequent development of adult depression than did any measure of the quality of the relationship subjects had with their parents when growing up. Said differently, bad relationships with one's brothers and sisters were much more depressogenic than a bad relationship with one's parents.

Lacking a TOF perspective at the time, when we first saw these results we found them impossible to believe. That siblings would be more depressogenic than parents seemed to fly in the face of everything we were learning about the centrality of parent–child bonds for adult emotional functioning. But from a TOF perspective the findings make perfect sense. Sibling relationship quality is likely a surrogate for families in which parental investment was sufficient for each child that siblings did not have to fight one another to get their "fair share." In this way, it may have been a truer measure of parental investment in each subject than were reports of parent–child relationships, which we now know are frequently cast in an overly optimistic light (especially by parents, who are notorious for not acknowledging practicing favoritism with their children).[158,159] Importantly, parental reports of favoritism do not appear to be associated with depression in their adult offspring, whereas the perceptions of favoritism by the offspring themselves do associate with depression. It is favoritism in general, and not toward a particular child, that predicts increased offspring depression,[159] consistent with the idea that favoritism activates ancient associations with resource scarcity, and hence with danger and—consistent with TOF predictions—with depression.

Back to the Question of Why People Don't Get Depressed Over the Things That Really Matter: Proximate Versus Ultimate Mechanisms of Reproductive Success

If, as TOF theory predicts, the most depressogenic adversities should be those that signal a reduction in the likelihood of both survival and reproduction, why is it that people don't reliably get depressed over the fact that they can't live and produce children for 200 years? Why do people in retirement communities tend to get more depressed over the death of a spouse (despite the spouse no longer producing or caring for your offspring), or bad finances, or failing health (long after an age where their personal survival matters to their reproductive success), or for that matter being snubbed on the golf course or at the bridge table, rather than in response to the fact that their children have decided not to have children? If reproductive success is truly what matters, there should be a linear relationship in older age between the number of grandchildren one has and one's risk for MDD. Although we are not aware of anyone studying this, we can assure you from many years clinical experience that, as with the our story of the dying gentleman angry at his brother-in-law, reproductive failure, while sometimes depressogenic, is hardly the major cause of MDD that one would predict from a TOF perspective.

In our scientific work we've discovered that it is often helpful to answer one question by asking others. For example, why do most people—men and women—daydream more about sex and/or sexual relationships than they do about having children? Why do sea turtles like to eat plastic bags even though doing so is usually lethal? Why will birds get off a perfectly good egg and abandon it to die while they pointlessly care for a perfectly smooth, round ball?

The answer to all these questions highlights a key distinction in evolutionary thinking between proximate and ultimate explanations. People daydream about sex and seek sexual relationships because sex feels (or should feel) intensely pleasurable. In fact, it feels so good, and seems so desirable in and of itself, that people often do it when they shouldn't. That is a proximate explanation. On the other hand, an ultimate explanation for sex, and one that invokes evolutionary theory, would be that people have sex because sexual intercourse effectively gets one's genes into the next generation and, because one's genes are mixed with those of another, does it in a way that enhances the likelihood that any resulting offspring will be able to more effectively fight off rapidly evolving infectious agents. Similarly, a proximate explanation for why people invest huge amounts of time and effort to look good in front of other people—doing everything from good deeds to amassing significant amounts of power and material resources in this pursuit—is because it feels so good to have people's respect and to feel the security that comes from knowing you have a valued place in the world. An ultimate explanation for the universal human need to belong and to do so with enough status to be able to affect other people's thoughts and behaviors would point to two facts: first, that group belonging has long been essential not just for reproductive access but for survival itself; and second, that enhanced status within any given social group has been shown repeatedly to translate into enhanced survival and reproduction (and hence improved overall reproductive fitness) across a wide range of current and historical societies, even those that most closely approximate likely social conditions that would have been normative in the EEA (i.e., within hunter-gatherer groups).[132]

As these examples suggest, the key to understanding why reproductive success, as such, is not as strongly associated with depression as are any number of other circumstances is to recognize that in many instances the most successful evolutionary strategy for achieving ultimate reproductive goals is for organisms to pursue proximate goals for their own sakes. Said more simply, evolution seems to "understand" that people (and probably all other life forms) are more likely to do something because they want to rather than because they have to. One factor that may have contributed to the evolution of proximate goals being pursued for their own pleasurable rewards is the fact that reproduction in many species comes at a cost to the individual. No more spectacular example of this exists than spider species in which the female devours the male while he copulates with her.[132] In this case he literally pays for the opportunity to contribute genes to the next generation with his life. One can only imagine that if these male spiders feel anything while they mate, they must be experiencing one of the world's ultimate emotional highs, given that only such an immediate reward would propel an organism to partake in such foolishness simply to have some kids.

Although far subtler, a similar effect has been observed in humans. Significant data suggest that people who reproduce pay a survival price compared with those who don't. Especially in environments with limited resources (which would have been commonplace in the EEA), people who have children are not as healthy and do not live as long as those who don't. So although reproduction is essential for accomplishing evolution's primary mandate, it also sets up a genetic conflict that must be resolved. If I maximize my own life, I protect all my genes. If I have a child, I pass on only half these genes and with no guarantee that the child will survive (especially in ancestral environments where, based on data from hunter-gatherer populations, 50 percent of children may have died by age 15). And simply having more children doesn't solve this genetic conflict. While having more children means passing along more of one's genes, each child comes at an additional cost to parental fitness, with this cost increasing the more closely spaced the subsequent offspring. A trace of this phenomenon can be seen even today in studies showing an increased risk for depression in mothers who have twins or who space their children too closely, as well as in studies suggesting that—in America, at least—people who are married but do not have children lead happier lives, overall, than people who do.[160] Given the metabolic costs of prolonged lactation and the high rates of childbirth-related mortality in traditional societies (and hence almost certainly in the EEA), the cost of each additional child would have been spectacularly higher, especially for women.

We might call the evolutionary strategy of accomplishing costly ultimate goals by making the means to these goals important, and/or pleasurable, in themselves the Mary Poppins principle, in recognition of the lyrics to her song in the Disney movie: "Just a spoonful of sugar makes the medicine go down." Given its ubiquity, the Mary Poppins Principle represents an evolutionarily stable strategy, meaning that it works so well that no alternative approach to getting organisms to maximize their reproduction has been able to evolve to outcompete and replace it. But this doesn't mean that it works perfectly by any means. Like all evolutionarily stable strategies, the Mary Poppins principle is reliable as long as conditions don't change radically or rapidly in ways that disconnect the previously reliable connection between the proximate aim and the ultimate result. The sea turtle proximate strategy of swallowing anything that looks like a jellyfish works perfectly well as long as only jellyfish look like jellyfish but becomes a death sentence as our oceans fill with plastic bags that look like jellyfish. Similarly, the avian proximate mechanism of "if you see something small, smooth, and round that looks like an egg, sit on it" works well unless you tempt the bird away with a man-made object that possesses these qualities to an even higher degree than does the poor abandoned egg.

When environmental changes lead to a disconnection between proximate goals and the ultimate reproductive outcomes they evolved to serve, a condition of evolutionary mismatch ensues. As one might guess from the profound and rapid changes humans have inflicted on themselves and the rest of the world, our lives are replete with examples of evolutionary mismatch in which we pursue proximate goals for their own sakes even if they clearly no longer benefit our reproductive fitness. The widespread use of contraception is a fairly benign example, given that it doesn't damage us as individuals. But other examples are more catastrophic. For example, using pleasure as a guide that one is on the right reproductive track is fine until society invents paths to pleasure that are powerful and that actually threaten survival and reproduction. Drugs and alcohol, which directly stimulate the brain's pleasure centers, are the most striking example of an evolutionary novelty for which people will sacrifice their evolutionary fitness.

In addition to explaining much craziness in the modern world, evolutionary mismatch provides a parsimonious explanation for our earlier observation that people don't get depressed over cars, birth control pills, or other facets of the modern world that actually most threaten reproductive fitness now. Evolutionary forces have not been able to keep up with our pace of innovation. Because of this, novel aspects of the modern threaten or thrill us only to the degree that they tap into mechanisms that reliably enhanced reproductive fitness in the EEA. And even in the EEA these mechanisms were pursued not always to explicitly enhance reproductive fitness but because they were perceived as pleasurable and/or important in their own right. Combining these two insights, we are now in a position to make an important refinement to the threat to overall survival, or TOF, theory of depression. Environmental circumstances should be depressogenic to the degree that they reliably induce a perception that one is blocked from access to, or successful utilization of, proximate mechanisms that, while consciously desired for their own sake, enhanced overall evolutionary fitness in ancestral environments by promoting individual survival, personal reproductive success, and the success of one's genes in related individuals.

Depression and the Remembrance Things Past

With this prediction in place, all that remains is to examine whether, in fact, current conditions that tap into proximate mechanisms of reproductive success from ancestral environments are indeed especially depressogenic today. One approach to this addressing this question, based on an excellent summary of evolutionary social psychology by Neuberg, Kenrick, and Schaller,[161] points to a convergence of data showing that humans, like all other species, have evolved specific adaptations to solve the primary problems posed by their existence. Some of these problems, such as self-protection, disease avoidance, and mate attraction, are universal, or nearly universal, in all vertebrate species. Other problems, such as mate retention, are less common, given that fewer species have engaged in prolonged pair bonding. Other problems, such as issues around coalitional cooperation, while present to some degree in other primates, are largely unique to humans. For present purposes, the striking point is that failure to adequately address any of these problems, or challenges, is strongly associated with the development of depression and, in the case of threat to self-protection, also with the closely related condition of posttraumatic stress disorder. We've already discussed at some length the strong association between disease and depression. We all know from our own experience how much effort most of us have invested in attracting and retaining a mate (or mates, as the case may be), and the scientific literature is replete with evidence that failure in either activities domain is powerfully depressogenic, especially for women.[162]

"Coalitional collaboration" sounds bland, as scientific jargon often does, but in many ways it subsumes all the other basic social challenges humans have confronted across evolutionary time. We are the beings we are, and live the lives we do, because evolution hit upon the fact that (for beings like us) belonging to a group and having status within that group were two of the most powerful ways to avoid and/or survive threats to our survival, reduce disease risk, and attract and retain a high-quality mate. To employ a bit of scientific jargon ourselves, we might say that humans evolved as a primary proximate mechanism for reproductive success a strong cognitive and emotional drive to seek affiliation with a group and, once so affiliated, to enhance one's agency within that group. Across human evolution this drive became a self-fulfilling prophecy of sorts, such that individuals with strong group affiliations and higher status within their groups (however measured in any given group/society) were more likely to survive and reproduce. This assured that forms of genes that promoted these outcomes underwent positive selection and became more prevalent with the passing of time, with the result that the drive and need of humans for affiliation and status also increased over time. We can see plenty of evidence for this phenomenon in the modern world. There is not a society on Earth in which people don't pursue status-enhancing goals with the utmost determination, nor is there a society (as far as we know) in which high status is not associated with better health and a longer life-span. As one would predict from this line of reasoning, reproductive success, as measured by number of children who survive to reproductive age, is universally associated with increasing social status in societies in which the link between sexual opportunity and conception has not been severed by birth control.

We have been using the word *status*, but we like the word *agency* better because it comes closer to connoting the full range of social effects that most humans crave. *Agency*, in relationship to a group, suggests power, the ability to get people to listen to and agree with one's point of view, the ability to do things, to get things done, and to get things done in ways that will benefit oneself and the people one loves. In the modern world, agency is usually pursued through an accumulation of some combination of wealth, power, and fame. It is no surprise, then, that poverty, powerlessness, and anonymity (i.e., social isolation) are all hugely depressing. But to fully see how enmeshed the drive for affiliation and agency is with depression, we have to ask ourselves how affiliation and agency manifested in the small, kin-based coalitional groups that were the norm for most of our existence as a species.

To get a flavor for this, let's engage in a brief thought experiment. Imagine that, after roaming through the skies for a bit, a tornado touches down in your city exactly on top of your house. The results are disastrous. Although you and your family escape with your lives, your home is completely destroyed and with it all your earthly possessions. Standing amid the wreckage. you realize that you foolishly allowed your home and homeowners insurance to lapse. You cast your eyes farther afield and see that, remarkably, yours is the only home that has been damaged by the tornado. Where would you rate this scenario on a 1-to-10 depressogenic scale, with 10 being the most depressing situation you can imagine? We'd put it at 6, maybe 7.

But now imagine that word of your disaster spreads immediately through your small city. Neighbors immediately take you and your family in. In fact, you hear them arguing among themselves over who should have the privilege of hosting you. Being unable to decide, they finally flip a coin. The neighbor who wins puts you and your family up in their finest quarters, insisting they will have it no other way when you protest. The man of the house makes a surprising statement. He tells you that his heart is broken over your loss, but if there is a silver lining to the tragedy it is that at last he will be able to make some small gesture to repay you for the wisdom and generosity you have shown him and his family over the years. The next morning you awake to the sound of heavy machinery next door on your ruined property. You go out to inspect the situation only to discover that news of your catastrophe has spread to the architectural and construction concerns of the city, which have come to first clear your property and then rebuild a house for you. You are about to protest that this is all too much when you notice the bulldozer operator silently weeping as he surveys your damage. You put your arm around him to offer comfort and decide to let him continue with his work. Stories like this are repeated endlessly over the next several weeks, as the entire citizenry rallies to your aid, all the while assuring you that it is the least they can do given all you've done for them. In fact, your near demise has driven home to everyone how precious you and your family are to the life of the city. A long-planned bust of you is hurried to completion and placed in city hall, but not before a formal dinner is held in your honor.

OK, now where would you place this scenario on the 1-to-10 depressogenic scale. If you're like us you might want to put it somewhere less than zero, because almost anyone would be profoundly cheered up by these types of events, even if your house had been destroyed. In fact, if this story was typical of tornado victims, these horrible storms might be celebrated as boons to human well-being. Why? Why would the events of this story make almost anyone feel as good as a human can feel?

We suggest that the answer to this question is apparent once we understand how affiliation and agency manifested in the EEA. For most of our existence as a species we lived in small, kin-based groups that rarely numbered more than 50–100 people. By modern or historical standards, these groups were remarkably egalitarian, with few material possessions. Rather than pursuing status by accumulating goods as we do, data from hunter-gatherers suggest that status in the EEA was more closely associated with one's power to give essential resources such as food away to others. In addition to engendering a sense of indebtedness that might yield much needed material returns in times of personal need, the ability to obtain and share valuable resources was a primary source of building reputation, and with reputation all the reproductive benefits that still accrue to those highly admired by others.

Thus, in a way hard for us to understand today, life, death, and reproductive success in the EEA depended upon one's ability to belong to a group and to behave in ways that fostered collaborative ties and gave one influence over the minds and emotions of others. The reason our tornado story turns from tragedy to triumph is that it highlights how strongly feeling good or bad still depends upon our perception of where we stand in the minds and hearts of those with whom we live. Under the noise, complexity, and confusion of our modern lives, those things that made us feel good or bad 100,000 years ago remain firmly entrenched in the deepest recesses of our emotional lives and are prime determinants of our risk for developing depression.

In today's world success usually involves flouting the egalitarian and sharing mores of our distant ancestors to one degree or other, but it is interesting to note that rates of depression are lower and rates of happiness are higher the more egalitarian a society is—that is, the more equally resources of all types are shared.[163] But in the EEA failure to develop valuable skills and resources or to be equitable with them once they were acquired put one at risk for being stigmatized and in extreme cases ostracized. While a source of much misery, by ensuring that those who violated the rules of fair exchange or had nothing to give were excluded or punished, these behaviors also likely made possible the development of all the forms of cooperation that characterize human groups.[164] Although much has been written about these closely related human tendencies to reject and shun those seen by the larger group as dangerous, derelict, or in some way deficient or different, little attempt has been made to connect these universal human tendencies to major depression (but see Allen and Badcock[165]). And yet, once one looks, surprising links become obvious. For one thing, social isolation, exclusion, and rejection are among the most powerful of depressogenic stimuli. For another, people with MDD often feel and behave as though they have been stigmatized, even if no objective evidence for this exists. In fact, depression can almost be viewed as an internal state of perceived stigmatization, given how common it is for depressed people to feel different, rejected, outcast, isolated, inadequate, and generally shameful to themselves.[166]

When one examines potential adaptive reasons for the evolution of stigmatization, the link between social exclusion and MDD becomes even more elemental.[165] Theorizing suggests that stigmatization proved adaptive by limiting the range of human cooperative behavior to those people most likely to benefit cooperative individuals, while assuring the exclusion of those with whom cooperative behavior was likely to consistently incur more costs than benefits.[164] Without such protective measures, genes that promoted cooperation would be outcompeted by those that encouraged the development of individuals who would benefit from cooperative people while making no sacrifices on their own part. This strategy would spread through cooperative groups, replacing cooperative people with manipulators and their socially manipulative genes. To stop this from happening, cooperative groups had to be perpetually on guard against three types of people: those who engage in unfair trading of any and all sorts (i.e., cheaters), those perceived as requiring far more investment than they are likely to be able to return (i.e., those with little to give), and those harboring parasites and other infectious agents that might spread through a group of humans in close contact with one another.

Considerable data demonstrate that, even today, people are fast to stigmatize and shun just these types of people. Being known as a cheater is one of the surest ways to be excluded from the company of good people, especially in modern domains that are especially close to ancient arenas for displaying fitness, such as sports and entertainment, where cheating is the ultimate sin. We are less likely to acknowledge our tendency to think poorly of or avoid people we perceive as having little to give, but once one becomes aware of this phenomenon one sees it everywhere. It is especially noticeable when one enters any highly competitive, high-stakes social grouping where people are sacrificing much of their lives to accumulate the modern equivalents of ancient status markers, such as fame or beauty. Most of us in the modern world don't encounter much in the way of highly dangerous infectious illness, so we might not be aware of how powerfully infection can engender stigmatization. But in fact, many studies show that even subtle signs of infection, often perceived below the level of consciousness, affect brain function in the observer and produce feelings of disgust and withdrawal.[133] Moreover, anyone old enough to remember the beginnings of the AIDS epidemic can remember, now with embarrassment for our culture, how the early victims of the infection were often treated like social pariahs.

If being stigmatized and/or ostracized was a sure way to reduce overall evolutionary fitness in ancestral environments, then clear-cut links should be apparent between the primary causes of stigmatization in those long lost worlds and depression in our lives today. We've already discussed at some length the fact that stressors that contain the elements of exclusion, rejection, shame, and failure are the most depressogenic of all social adversities, consistent with the idea that depression is a response to ancient threats to reproductive fitness. But there is another very powerful—and to our knowledge never noted—connection between stigmatization and depression. Not only do depressed people often feel and behave as if they've been stigmatized, but the three primary ancient causes for stigmatization (cheating, lack of worth, infection) manifest very powerfully in the symptom structure of depression itself.

To examine this, let's ask ourselves how normal people feel when caught cheating, found to be inadequate, or are overcome by infection. Cheating, broadly construed as breaking the rules and/or trying to obviously get more than we give, is at the heart of much that we do that is wrong. How do we feel when we've been caught in these types of activities? Guilty and ashamed. The strength of these feelings, as well as their profoundly aversive nature, is amply attested to by the lengths most of us will go to fool ourselves and others regarding our actions and motives when we do things that even begin to border on cheating. It is notable, then, that guilt is one of the cardinal cognitive/emotional symptoms of depression. And although not an official depressive symptom, guilt's close associate shame is also commonplace in depression. Moreover, being disgraced—which usually occurs after one has been caught cheating in one way or other—is powerfully depressogenic. Similarly, the perception of being inadequate or without value to others is strongly associated with depression, both as a symptom and as a risk factor for the condition.[167] Indeed, worthlessness, like guilt, is a cardinal cognitive/emotional symptom of the disorder. From this perspective, depression can be seen as a state characterized by a profound feeling that one has somehow (and often inexplicably) run afoul of the perceptions of others in a way that, in ancestral environments, at best would have reduced one's hopes of successfully reproducing, and at worst would have greatly increased one's chances of early mortality, either through direct physical attacks from others or from restricted access to group-controlled resources (i.e., food) or from outright ostracism.

However, many people with depression experience feelings of guilt and worthlessness that are out of proportion to anything they have done or any realistic estimate of their value to others. This strongly suggests that abnormalities in brain systems that evolved to promote these feelings may contribute to the pathogenesis of depression. Said differently, perhaps depression can be conceptualized as a condition in which the brain's stigmatization alarm system is either hypersensitive (like a smoke alarm that goes off in a house when someone smokes a cigarette) or flat out broken, stuck in the on position. Strong support for this possibility comes from many years' worth of neuroimaging studies showing that a midline brain structure called the anterior cingulate is activated whenever feelings of guilt are induced in healthy volunteers.[168] An intriguing study suggests that different brain networks are activated when someone feels guilt over violating internal principles of right or wrong versus when someone contemplates doing something specifically unfair to others.[169] However, both types of guilt strongly activate the anterior cingulate. If depression results from functional abnormalities of brain regions that evolved, at least in part, to produce feelings of guilt and/or worthlessness as a signal of impending stigmatization/ostracism in ancient environments, one would predict that the anterior cingulate should be involved in depression. As we discuss more fully in Chapter 8, innumerable studies support this prediction by showing that MDD is reliably associated with abnormalities in both the structure and function of this brain area.[170]

So if depression often appears to be a kind of free-wheeling version of what normal people feel when caught doing things that make them feel guilty or less than adequate, might it also be the case that the disorder is a free-wheeling version of what normal people feel when they are infected? Said differently, if being infected was a powerful risk factor for being stigmatized or ostracized in ancestral environments, following the logic of our argument, infection should promote depression, and depressed people should behave as if they are infected, even if they are otherwise perfectly healthy. We've already presented evidence for the first. Do depressed people behave as if they are infected?

Suppose you saw a friend for the first time in six months. You know nothing of what's happened to her, but you immediately know something is wrong. Her eyes are downcast when you find her huddled on the couch. She speaks slowly and softly. When she gets off the couch she moves slowly. You ask if she wants to go out with you to see some mutual friends and she declines, explaining that she doesn't feel like seeing anyone she knows or doing anything other than sitting on the couch. You ask a little more about this, and she tells you that nothing is giving her much pleasure. In fact, just getting through the day is a struggle. She has lost her appetite, and her sleep has become abnormal. She tells you that she is exhausted. Even minor tasks feel overwhelming. She complains of being in a mental fog, barely able to concentrate on one simple thing at a time and completely unable to cope with anything that might tax her brain. Worried, you take her temperature and note that she is running a low-grade fever.

If you hazarded a guess that your friend was sick, you'd be wrong. She is, in fact, depressed. If you object that she has a fever, you might be surprised to learn that depression has been repeatedly shown to be a febrile condition,[171] as we discuss at greater length in Chapter 11. What we didn't mention were symptoms that might be characterized as "self-evaluative," in other words, the terribly painful symptoms we've already mentioned: guilt, shame, worthlessness, feelings of being overwhelmed and inadequate, all those horrible feelings of internal condemnation and failure that are so integral a part of most serious depressive episodes. Anyone who has ever been really depressed at one juncture and really sick at another would likely tell you that this is how one can tell which is which. When you're sick, you feel down, nothing much brings pleasure, you are exhausted, and your sleep and appetite are disrupted, but you don't typically feel guilty for getting the flu or feel like being sick has somehow reduced who you are as a person or is a cause for mortifying shame. Lacking these feelings, being sick doesn't make most of us contemplate suicide the way a good case of depression is wont to do.

As already mentioned, a study from Emory University provides strong support for this felt sense of difference between depression and sickness. Andrew Miller and colleagues got the ingenious idea of comparing people receiving the cytokine IFN-α with medically healthy individuals suffering from MDD to see whether chronic cytokine exposure produces a set of symptoms different from those seen in what we might call "regular" or idiopathic depression.[172] The most noticeable finding was that people who received IFN-α and didn't develop Major Depression looked much different from either people with IFN-α–induced depression or those with idiopathic depression. In contrast, people who developed MDD on IFN-α showed a remarkable symptom overlap with those with idiopathic MDD. Only two differences emerged: patients on IFN-α were more likely to be physically slowed down, and people with idiopathic MDD were more likely to feel guilty and worthless and to think about killing themselves. Other studies paint a similar picture: inflammation makes everyone feel sick, and many people feel depressed. Sometimes it produces feelings of despair, guilt, and self-loathing that match the best that social stressors can do, but this is less common. More often, people who become depressed in response to inflammatory stimuli have a condition that is heavy on apathy, irritability, anxiety, exhaustion, poor sleep and appetite, and a variety of cognitive complaints ranging from mental fog to profound impairments in memory and reasoning. Indeed, a study demonstrates that in medically healthy individuals with Major Depression, increased inflammation correlates more strongly with physical symptoms shared with sickness than with emotional symptoms that are more specific to depression.[173]

Is this semispecificity of symptoms unique to the infectious basis for stigmatization, or might depressions that develop as a result of guilt-producing situations show, on average, symptoms different from those that arise as a result of situations suggesting that one is inadequate and/or devalued by others? To our knowledge the question has never been asked in quite this way, but Matthew Keller and Randolph Nesse came close when they conducted a study to test the idea that different types of adverse situations should produce different clusters of symptoms that might have some adaptive value in helping people cope with those situations (more about that in Chapter 9).[174] As with all psychiatric phenomena, the results were messy, but not so messy that a pattern could not be discerned. In fact, people were more likely to report guilt, ruminations, fatigue, and pessimism following a failed effort and were more likely to report crying, sadness, and desire for social support following a social loss. Keller replicated and extended these findings in a far larger longitudinal study. Although some of the details differed, as is always the case when psychiatric studies are replicated, the hypothesis that different types of life adversities produce different depressive symptom patterns was upheld.[175]

A Final Objection to the Possibility That Stress Causes Depression: Stress Causes Everything

The question of what legitimately qualifies as a cause for something else has a distinguished history in philosophical systems of both the East and the West and has bedeviled thinkers of both ancient and modern times. Setting aside the generally held conclusion that the philosopher David Hume forever destroyed any hope for iron-clad demonstrations of cause and effect, let's take a standard pragmatic approach and distinguish between necessary, sufficient, and contributory causes. When a cause is *necessary*, you will never see the effect without also seeing the cause. When a cause is *sufficient*, its effect will always be found whenever the cause is present, but the effect itself may have other causes. A cause is judged to be *contributory* if occurs before an effect and if altering the cause changes the effect, but not everyone with the cause will experience the effect and not everyone with the effect will have experienced the particular contributory cause.

It is clear from this description that stress cannot be either a necessary or a sufficient cause for depression for the simple reason that plenty of stressed people do not develop depression and at least some people appear to develop depression without a clearly preceding stressor (although this is less clear because very minor stressors may be depressogenic in very vulnerable individuals). This means that stress must be a contributory-type cause for the disorder. Based on everything we've discussed thus far, we know that environmental adversities are powerfully depressogenic, but we have yet to address a final challenge to the notion that environmental adversity (or, more properly, its perception) is an important contributory cause to depression, and this relates to its specificity as a risk.

Let's start with a *reductio ad absurdum* thought example: breathing is an important cause for depression; in fact it is a necessary cause for depression, given that whenever a person is depressed (the effect) he or she will always be found to be breathing (the cause). Although no everyone who breathes is depressed (so it is not a sufficient cause), you will never find a depressed person who isn't breathing.

Why doesn't this causal explanation for depression satisfy, given that it is obviously true? The answer lies in the fact that that it is too general. Yes, you've got to be breathing to be depressed, but you've got to be breathing to do or think anything else in the world, too. Exactly the same challenge, on a slightly truncated scale, faces stress as a risk for depression. Stress isn't just a risk factor for depression; it is also a risk factor for developing bipolar disorder, schizophrenia, and addiction and is a major risk factor for relapse in addicted individuals who have managed to achieve abstinence. Stress is a risk for all sorts of health problems, including insomnia, obesity, fibromyalgia, chronic fatigue syndrome, diabetes, heart disease, dementia, and maybe cancer, just to name a few. And the malignant effects of stress aren't restricted to individual health. Stress also increases the risk for divorce, child abuse, and poor job performance. Perhaps stress is like breathing when it comes to illness: it is somehow conducive to everything without being specifically involved in the pathogenesis of anything. Said more formally, it is permissive but not causative.

Before suggesting two reasons that we do not believe this, let's take a moment to acknowledge an obvious implication of the association between stress and so wide an array of troubles. Stress, or its perception, must very rarely cause any type of illness directly, or there would be one condition that would be so much more common an outcome of stress than any other that it would be obvious and we would call it something like "stress disease." This suggests that stress must interact with other things to cause specific diseases. This line of reasoning suggests that under stress individuals with vulnerability in their coronary arteries develop cardiac disease, people with metabolic vulnerabilities develop diabetes, people with vulnerability to sadness, hopelessness, and pessimism develop depression, and so on. It is in this way that stress is permissive: it allows vulnerabilities to be translated into disease in instances in which they might not have otherwise done so. But which disease is permitted by stress depends on each individual's vulnerabilities.

With this said, let's discuss the two reasons that stress is merely permissive when it comes to depression. The first reason can be best explained as illustrated in Figure 3.2. Without questioning it, most of us would view the relationship between stress and disease as it is presented in Figure 3.2A: stress is an amorphous, generalized risk factor for a wide array of very solid and distinct disease states. But we think that scientific evidence increasingly turns this view on its head, as shown in Figure 3.2B. Here the human stress response is seen as a stereotyped physiological phenomenon with crisp boundaries, and it is the disease states that have become fuzzy and intermingled. Obviously cardiac disease is not the same thing as depression, or everybody with depression would have heart disease and vice versa. But on the other hand, neither are they totally separate. They are highly comorbid and share environmental and genetic risk factors.[176] And they seem to cause each other, or at least to be caused by some shared third factor, given that young people with depression are at increased risk of cardiac disease as they age, and people with cardiac disease and no prior depression history are nonetheless at a hugely increased risk of eventually developing depres-

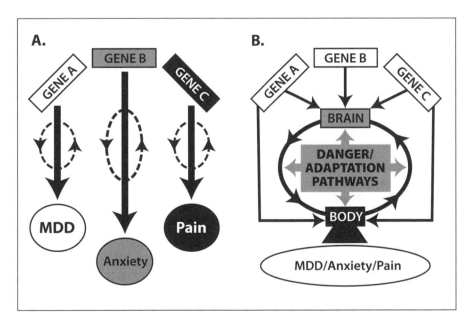

FIGURE 3.2. Panel A shows stress (pictured as the dotted line circles) as contributing along with genes to very specific disease states. In this model, stress is non-specific and the disease states are specific. Panel B presents the model we prefer in which stress is biologically specific but the disease states to which it contribute are amorphous and overlapping.

sion compared with the general population. The same relationships hold between depression and all the other conditions shown in Figure 3.2: they are not the same as depression, of course, but neither are they fully separate. This perspective suggests that stress may directly cause disease, but the disease it directly causes is currently spread across, or through, a variety of illnesses that we currently consider separate conditions. Stress may cause one lifelong health condition that manifests in different ways at different ages and in different people depending on their other vulnerabilities.

In seeking to explain this intermingled state of affairs, we come to our second reason for believing that stress causes a larger condition of ill health, of which depression is an integral part. Although the modern diseases of aging and metabolism to which most people in the developed world eventually succumb have multiple causes, they all share many common patterns of dysregulation in the body's primary stress response systems. This pattern is especially prominent in depression, which may help explain why, if there were a condition that could qualify as "stress disease," depression might be it. This pattern of stress and immune system activity, and the role of abnormalities in these systems in the pathogenesis of depression, is discussed at some length in Chapters 5 and 6.

References

1. Moussavi S, Chatterji S, Verdes E, Tandon A, Patel V, Ustun B. Depression, chronic diseases, and decrements in health: results from the World Health Surveys. *Lancet.* 2007;370(9590):851–858.

2. Evans DL, Charney DS, Lewis L, et al. Mood disorders in the medically ill: scientific review and recommendations. *Biol Psychiatry.* 2005;58(3):175–189.

3. Bouchard MF, Bellinger DC, Weuve J, et al. Blood lead levels and major depressive disorder, panic disorder, and generalized anxiety disorder in US young adults. *Arch Gen Psychiatry.* 2009;66(12):1313–1319.

4. Hamer M, Stamatakis E, Batty GD. Objectively assessed secondhand smoke exposure and mental health in adults: cross-sectional and prospective evidence from the Scottish Health Survey. *Arch Gen Psychiatry.* 2010;67(8):850–855.

5. Bandiera FC, Arheart KL, Caban-Martinez AJ, et al. Secondhand smoke exposure and depressive symptoms. *Psychosom Med.* 2010;72(1):68–72.

6. Postolache TT, Stiller JW, Herrell R, et al. Tree pollen peaks are associated with increased nonviolent suicide in women. *Mol Psychiatry.* 2005;10(3):232–235.

7. Szyszkowicz M, Tremblay N. Case-crossover design: air pollution and health outcomes. *Int J Occup Med Environ Health.* 2011;24(3):249–255.

8. Yang AC, Tsai SJ, Huang NE. Decomposing the association of completed suicide with air pollution, weather, and unemployment data at different time scales. *J Affect Disord.* 2011;129(1–3):275–281.

9. Kapusta ND, Mossaheb N, Etzersdorfer E, et al. Lithium in drinking water and suicide mortality. *Br J Psychiatry.* 2011;198(5):346–350.

10. Kendler KS, Gardner CO. Dependent stressful life events and prior depressive episodes

in the prediction of major depression: the problem of causal inference in psychiatric epidemiology. *Arch Gen Psychiatry.* 2010;67(11):1120–1127.

11. Skarsater I, Agren H, Dencker K. Subjective lack of social support and presence of dependent stressful life events characterize patients suffering from major depression compared with healthy volunteers. *J Psychiatr Ment Health Nurs.* 2001;8(2):107–114.

12. Brown GW. Genetic and population perspectives on life events and depression. *Soc Psychiatry Psychiatr Epidemiol.* 1998;33(8):363–372.

13. Taylor PJ, Gooding P, Wood AM, Tarrier N. The role of defeat and entrapment in depression, anxiety, and suicide. *Psychol Bull.* 2011;137(3):391–420.

14. Kendler KS, Karkowski LM, Prescott CA. Causal relationship between stressful life events and the onset of major depression. *Am J Psychiatry.* 1999;156(6):837–841.

15. Amstadter AB, Acierno R, Richardson LK, et al. Posttyphoon prevalence of posttraumatic stress disorder, major depressive disorder, panic disorder, and generalized anxiety disorder in a Vietnamese sample. *J Trauma Stress.* 2009;22(3):180–188.

16. Kim SC, Plumb R, Gredig QN, Rankin L, Taylor B. Medium-term post-Katrina health sequelae among New Orleans residents: predictors of poor mental and physical health. *J Clin Nurs.* 2008;17(17):2335–2342.

17. Kilpatrick DG, Koenen KC, Ruggiero KJ, et al. The serotonin transporter genotype and social support and moderation of posttraumatic stress disorder and depression in hurricane-exposed adults. *Am J Psychiatry.* 2007;164(11):1693–1699.

18. McLeish AC, Del Ben KS. Symptoms of depression and posttraumatic stress disorder in an outpatient population before and after Hurricane Katrina. *Depress Anxiety.* 2008;25(5):416–421.

19. Chadda RK, Malhotra A, Kaw N, Singh J, Sethi H. Mental health problems following the 2005 earthquake in Kashmir: findings of community-run clinics. *Prehosp Disaster Med.* 2007;22(6):541–546.

20. Onder E, Tural U, Aker T, Kilic C, Erdogan S. Prevalence of psychiatric disorders three years after the 1999 earthquake in Turkey: Marmara Earthquake Survey (MES). *Soc Psychiatry Psychiatr Epidemiol.* 2006;41(11):868–874.

21. Palinkas LA, Petterson JS, Russell J, Downs MA. Community patterns of psychiatric disorders after the *Exxon Valdez* oil spill. *Am J Psychiatry.* 1993;150(10):1517–1523.

22. Kendler KS, Myers J. The genetic and environmental relationship between major depression and the five-factor model of personality. *Psychol Med.* 2010;40(5):801–806.

23. Nanni V, Uher R, Danese A. Childhood maltreatment predicts unfavorable course of illness and treatment outcome in depression: a meta-analysis. *Am J Psychiatry.* 2011; 169(2):141–151.

24. Cong E, Li Y, Shao C, et al. Childhood sexual abuse and the risk for recurrent major depression in Chinese women. *Psychol Med.* 2012;42:409–417.

25. Danese A, Moffitt TE, Harrington H, et al. Adverse childhood experiences and adult risk factors for age-related disease: depression, inflammation, and clustering of metabolic risk markers. *Arch Pediatr Adolesc Med.* 2009;163(12):1135–1143.

26. Danese A, Moffitt TE, Pariante CM, Ambler A, Poulton R, Caspi A. Elevated inflammation levels in depressed adults with a history of childhood maltreatment. *Arch Gen Psychiatry.* 2008;65(4):409–415.

27. Danese A, Pariante CM, Caspi A, Taylor A, Poulton R. Childhood maltreatment predicts adult inflammation in a life-course study. *Proc Natl Acad Sci U S A.* 2007;104(4): 1319–1324.

28. Wegman HL, Stetler C. A meta-analytic review of the effects of childhood abuse on medical outcomes in adulthood. *Psychosom Med.* 2009;71(8):805–812.

29. Pickles A, Aglan A, Collishaw S, Messer J, Rutter M, Maughan B. Predictors of suicidality across the life span: the Isle of Wight study. *Psychol Med.* 2010;40(9):1453–1466.

30. Moran P, Coffey C, Chanen A, Mann A, Carlin JB, Patton GC. Childhood sexual abuse and abnormal personality: a population-based study. *Psychol Med.* 2011;41(6):1311–1318.

31. Fergusson DM, Horwood LJ, Lynskey MT. Childhood sexual abuse and psychiatric disorder in young adulthood: II. Psychiatric outcomes of childhood sexual abuse. *J Am Acad Child Adolesc Psychiatry.* 1996;35(10):1365–1374.

32. Allen B, Lauterbach D. Personality characteristics of adult survivors of childhood trauma. *J Trauma Stress.* 2007;20(4):587–595.

33. Golier JA, Yehuda R, Bierer LM, et al. The relationship of borderline personality disorder to posttraumatic stress disorder and traumatic events. *Am J Psychiatry.* 2003;160(11):2018–2024.

34. Magnusson A, Lundholm C, Goransson M, Copeland W, Heilig M, Pedersen NL. Familial influence and childhood trauma in female alcoholism. *Psychol Med.* 2012;42:381–389.

35. Hodgins DC, Schopflocher DP, el-Guebaly N, et al. The association between childhood maltreatment and gambling problems in a community sample of adult men and women. *Psychol Addict Behav.* 2010;24(3):548–554.

36. Vaddiparti K, Bogetto J, Callahan C, Abdallah AB, Spitznagel EL, Cottler LB. The effects of childhood trauma on sex trading in substance using women. *Arch Sex Behav.* 2006;35(4):451–459.

37. Lang AJ, Stein MB, Kennedy CM, Foy DW. Adult psychopathology and intimate partner violence among survivors of childhood maltreatment. *J Interpers Violence.* 2004;19(10):1102–1118.

38. Nissen SE, Wolski K. Effect of rosiglitazone on the risk of myocardial infarction and death from cardiovascular causes. *N Engl J Med.* 2007;356(24):2457–2471.

39. Graham DJ, Ouellet-Hellstrom R, MaCurdy TE, et al. Risk of acute myocardial infarction, stroke, heart failure, and death in elderly Medicare patients treated with rosiglitazone or pioglitazone. *JAMA.* 2010;304(4):411–418.

40. Canetti D, Galea S, Hall BJ, Johnson RJ, Palmieri PA, Hobfoll SE. Exposure to prolonged socio-political conflict and the risk of PTSD and depression among Palestinians. *Psychiatry.* 2010;73(3):219–231.

41. Husain N, Chaudhry IB, Afridi MA, Tomenson B, Creed F. Life stress and depression in a tribal area of Pakistan. *Br J Psychiatry.* 2007;190:36–41.

42. Cardozo BL, Bilukha OO, Crawford CA, et al. Mental health, social functioning, and disability in postwar Afghanistan. *JAMA.* 2004;292(5):575–584.

43. Kessler RC, Berglund P, Demler O, et al. The epidemiology of major depressive disorder: results from the National Comorbidity Survey Replication (NCS-R). *JAMA.* 2003;289(23):3095–3105.

44. Catani C, Jacob N, Schauer E, Kohila M, Neuner F. Family violence, war, and natural disasters: a study of the effect of extreme stress on children's mental health in Sri Lanka. *BMC Psychiatry.* 2008;8:33.

45. Panter-Brick C, Goodman A, Tol W, Eggerman M. Mental health and childhood adversities: a longitudinal study in Kabul, Afghanistan. *J Am Acad Child Adolesc Psychiatry.* 2011;50(4):349–363.

46. Alloy LB, Abramson LY, Whitehouse WG, Hogan ME, Panzarella C, Rose DT. Prospec-

tive incidence of first onsets and recurrences of depression in individuals at high and low cognitive risk for depression. *J Abnorm Psychol.* 2006;115(1):145–156.

47. Hart D, Sussman RW. *Man the Hunted: Primates, Predators, and Human Evolution.* Boulder, CO: Westview Press; 2009.

48. Nohl J. *The Black Death.* London: Allen and Unwin; 1926.

49. Meijer A, Zakay-Rones Z, Morag A. Post-influenzal psychiatric disorder in adolescents. *Acta Psychiatr Scand.* 1988;78(2):176–181.

50. Okusaga O, Yolken RH, Langenberg P, et al. Association of seropositivity for influenza and coronaviruses with history of mood disorders and suicide attempts. *J Affect Disord.* 2011;130(1–2):220–225.

51. Morag M, Yirmiya R, Lerer B, Morag A. Influence of socioeconomic status on behavioral, emotional and cognitive effects of rubella vaccination: a prospective, double blind study. *Psychoneuroendocrinology.* 1998;23(4):337–351.

52. Lee AM, Wong JG, McAlonan GM, et al. Stress and psychological distress among SARS survivors 1 year after the outbreak. *Can J Psychiatry.* 2007;52(4):233–240.

53. Mak IW, Chu CM, Pan PC, Yiu MG, Chan VL. Long-term psychiatric morbidities among SARS survivors. *Gen Hosp Psychiatry.* 2009;31(4):318–326.

54. Morroy G, Peters JB, van Nieuwenhof M, et al. The health status of Q-fever patients after long-term follow-up. *BMC Infect Dis.* 2011;11:97.

55. Petersen I, Thomas JM, Hamilton WT, White PD. Risk and predictors of fatigue after infectious mononucleosis in a large primary-care cohort. *QJM.* 2006;99(1):49–55.

56. White PD, Thomas JM, Amess J, et al. Incidence, risk and prognosis of acute and chronic fatigue syndromes and psychiatric disorders after glandular fever. *Br J Psychiatry.* 1998; 173:475–481.

57. Miller AH, Raison CL. The role of inflammation in depression: from evolutionary imperative to modern treatment target. *Nat Rev Immunol.* 2015;16(1):22–34.

58. Louveau A, Harris TH, Kipnis J. Revisiting the mechanisms of CNS immune privilege. *Trends Immunol.* 2015;36(10):569–577.

59. Dantzer R, O'Connor JC, Freund GG, Johnson RW, Kelley KW. From inflammation to sickness and depression: when the immune system subjugates the brain. *Nat Rev Neurosci.* 2008;9(1):46–56.

60. Barrientos RM, Sprunger DB, Campeau S, et al. Brain-derived neurotrophic factor mRNA downregulation produced by social isolation is blocked by intrahippocampal interleukin-1 receptor antagonist. *Neuroscience.* 2003;121(4):847–853.

61. Barrientos RM, Higgins EA, Sprunger DB, Watkins LR, Rudy JW, Maier SF. Memory for context is impaired by a post context exposure injection of interleukin-1 beta into dorsal hippocampus. *Behav Brain Res.* 2002;134(1–2):291–298.

62. Pugh CR, Nguyen KT, Gonyea JL, et al. Role of interleukin-1 beta in impairment of contextual fear conditioning caused by social isolation. *Behav Brain Res.* 1999;106(1–2): 109–118.

63. Reichenberg A, Yirmiya R, Schuld A, et al. Cytokine-associated emotional and cognitive disturbances in humans. *Arch Gen Psychiatry.* 2001;58(5):445–452.

64. Hannestad J, DellaGioia N, Bloch M. The effect of antidepressant medication treatment on serum levels of inflammatory cytokines: a meta-analysis. *Neuropsychopharmacology.* 2011;36(12):2452–2459.

65. DellaGioia N, Devine L, Pittman B, Hannestad J. Bupropion pre-treatment of endotoxin-induced depressive symptoms. *Brain Behav Immun.* 2013;31:197–204.

66. Harrison NA, Brydon L, Walker C, Gray MA, Steptoe A, Critchley HD. Inflammation

causes mood changes through alterations in subgenual cingulate activity and mesolimbic connectivity. *Biol Psychiatry.* 2009;66(5):407–414.

67. Eisenberger NI, Inagaki TK, Mashal NM, Irwin MR. Inflammation and social experience: an inflammatory challenge induces feelings of social disconnection in addition to depressed mood. *Brain Behav Immun.* 2010;24(4):558–563.

68. Eisenberger NI, Berkman ET, Inagaki TK, Rameson LT, Mashal NM, Irwin MR. Inflammation-induced anhedonia: endotoxin reduces ventral striatum responses to reward. *Biol Psychiatry.* 2010;68(8):748–754.

69. Raison CL, Borisov AS, Broadwell SD, et al. Depression during pegylated interferon-alpha plus ribavirin therapy: prevalence and prediction. *J Clin Psychiatry.* 2005;66(1): 41–48.

70. Raison CL, Demetrashvili M, Capuron L, Miller AH. Neuropsychiatric adverse effects of interferon-alpha: recognition and management. *CNS Drugs.* 2005;19(2):105–123.

71. Raison CL, Borisov AS, Woolwine BJ, Massung B, Vogt G, Miller AH. Interferon-alpha effects on diurnal hypothalamic-pituitary-adrenal axis activity: relationship with pro-inflammatory cytokines and behavior. *Mol Psychiatry.* 2008;15(5):535–547.

72. Capuron L, Fornwalt FB, Knight BT, Harvey PD, Ninan PT, Miller AH. Does cytokine-induced depression differ from idiopathic major depression in medically healthy individuals? *J Affect Disord.* 2009;119(1–3):181–185.

73. Musselman DL, Lawson DH, Gumnick JF, et al. Paroxetine for the prevention of depression induced by high-dose interferon alfa. *New Engl J Med.* 2001;344(13):961–966.

74. Felger JC, Li L, Marvar PJ, et al. Tyrosine metabolism during interferon-alpha administration: association with fatigue and CSF dopamine concentrations. *Brain Behav Immun.* 2012;31:153–160.

75. Felger JC, Cole SW, Pace TW, et al. Molecular signatures of peripheral blood mononuclear cells during chronic interferon-alpha treatment: relationship with depression and fatigue. *Psychol Med.* 2012;42(8):1591–1603.

76. Raison CL, Rye DB, Woolwine BJ, et al. Chronic interferon-alpha administration disrupts sleep continuity and depth in patients with hepatitis C: association with fatigue, motor slowing, and increased evening cortisol. *Biol Psychiatry.* 2010;68(10):942–949.

77. Raison CL, Dantzer R, Kelley KW, et al. CSF concentrations of brain tryptophan and kynurenines during immune stimulation with IFN-alpha: relationship to CNS immune responses and depression. *Mol Psychiatry.* 2010;15(4):393–403.

78. Raison CL, Borisov AS, Woolwine BJ, Massung B, Vogt G, Miller AH. Interferon-alpha effects on diurnal hypothalamic-pituitary-adrenal axis activity: relationship with pro-inflammatory cytokines and behavior. *Mol Psychiatry.* 2010;15(5):535–547.

79. Raison CL, Borisov AS, Majer M, et al. Activation of central nervous system inflammatory pathways by interferon-alpha: relationship to monoamines and depression. *Biol Psychiatry.* 2009;65(4):296–303.

80. Kenis G, Prickaerts J, van Os J, et al. Depressive symptoms following interferon-alpha therapy: mediated by immune-induced reductions in brain-derived neurotrophic factor? *Int J Neuropsychopharmacol.* 2011;14(2):247–253.

81. Wichers MC, Koek GH, Robaeys G, Verkerk R, Scharpe S, Maes M. IDO and interferon-alpha-induced depressive symptoms: a shift in hypothesis from tryptophan depletion to neurotoxicity. *Mol Psychiatry.* 2005;10(6):538–544.

82. Wichers MC, Kenis G, Leue C, Koek G, Robaeys G, Maes M. Baseline immune activation as a risk factor for the onset of depression during interferon-alpha treatment. *Biol Psychiatry.* 2006;60(1):77–79.

83. Robaeys G, De Bie J, Wichers MC, et al. Early prediction of major depression in chronic hepatitis C patients during peg-interferon alpha-2b treatment by assessment of vegetative-depressive symptoms after four weeks. *World J Gastroenterol.* 2007;13(43): 5736–5740.

84. Wichers MC, Kenis G, Koek GH, Robaeys G, Nicolson NA, Maes M. Interferon-alpha-induced depressive symptoms are related to changes in the cytokine network but not to cortisol. *J Psychosom Res.* 2007;62(2):207–214.

85. Capuron L, Pagnoni G, Demetrashvili M, et al. Anterior cingulate activation and error processing during interferon-alpha treatment. *Biol Psychiatry.* 2005;58(3):190–196.

86. Capuron L, Pagnoni G, Demetrashvili MF, et al. Basal ganglia hypermetabolism and symptoms of fatigue during interferon-alpha therapy. *Neuropsychopharmacology.* 2007; 32(11):2384–2392.

87. Lotrich FE. Major depression during interferon-alpha treatment: vulnerability and prevention. *Dialogues Clin Neurosci.* 2009;11(4):417–425.

88. Prather AA, Rabinovitz M, Pollock BG, Lotrich FE. Cytokine-induced depression during IFN-alpha treatment: the role of IL-6 and sleep quality. *Brain Behav Immun.* 2009; 23(8):1109–1116.

89. Franzen PL, Buysse DJ, Rabinovitz M, Pollock BG, Lotrich FE. Poor sleep quality predicts onset of either major depression or subsyndromal depression with irritability during interferon-alpha treatment. *Psychiatry Res.* 2010;177(1–2):240–245.

90. Felger JC, Alagbe O, Pace TW, et al. Early activation of p38 mitogen activated protein kinase is associated with interferon-alpha-induced depression and fatigue. *Brain Behav Immun.* 2011;25(6):1094–1098.

91. Raison CL, Miller AH. The neuroimmunology of stress and depression. *Semin Clin Neuropsychiatry.* 2001;6(4):277–294.

92. Musselman D, Pisell T, Lewison B, et al. Interleukin-6 plasma concentrations in cancer patients with depression. Paper presented at: Annual Meeting of the Society for Neuroscience; 1997; New Orleans, LA.

93. Tyring S, Gottlieb A, Papp K, et al. Etanercept and clinical outcomes, fatigue, and depression in psoriasis: double-blind placebo-controlled randomised phase III trial. *Lancet.* 2006;367(9504):29–35.

94. Persoons P, Vermeire S, Demyttenaere K, et al. The impact of major depressive disorder on the short- and long-term outcome of Crohn's disease treatment with infliximab. *Aliment Pharmacol Ther.* 2005;22(2):101–110.

95. Abbott R, Whear R, Nikolaou V, et al. Tumour necrosis factor-alpha inhibitor therapy in chronic physical illness: a systematic review and meta-analysis of the effect on depression and anxiety. *J Psychosom Res.* 2015;79(3):175–184.

96. Haroon E, Raison CL, Miller AH. Psychoneuroimmunology meets neuropsychopharmacology: translational implications of the impact of inflammation on behavior. *Neuropsychopharmacology.* 2012;37(1):137–162.

97. Steptoe A, Hamer M, Chida Y. The effect of acute psychological stress on circulating inflammatory factors in humans: a review and meta-analysis. *Brain Behav Immun.* 2007;7:901–912.

98. Bierhaus A, Wolf J, Andrassy M, et al. A mechanism converting psychosocial stress into mononuclear cell activation. *Proc Natl Acad Sci U S A.* 2003;100(4):1920–1925.

99. Pace TW, Mletzko TC, Alagbe O, Musselman DL, Nemeroff CB, Miller AH. Increased stress-induced inflammatory responses in male patients with major depression and increased early life stress. *Am J Psychiatry.* 2006;163(9):1630–1633.

100. Carpenter LL, Gawuga CE, Tyrka AR, Lee JK, Anderson GM, Price LH. Association between plasma IL-6 response to acute stress and early-life adversity in healthy adults. *Neuropsychopharmacology.* 2010;35(13):2617–2623.

101. Raison CL, Lowry CA, Rook GA. Inflammation, sanitation, and consternation: loss of contact with coevolved, tolerogenic microorganisms and the pathophysiology and treatment of major depression. *Arch Gen Psychiatry.* 2010;67(12):1211–1224.

102. Simon GE, Von Korff M, Saunders K, et al. Association between obesity and psychiatric disorders in the US adult population. *Arch Gen Psychiatry.* 2006;63(7):824–830.

103. Miller GE, Freedland KE, Carney RM, Stetler CA, Banks WA. Pathways linking depression, adiposity, and inflammatory markers in healthy young adults. *Brain Behav Immun.* 2003;17(4):276–285.

104. Suarez EC. C-reactive protein is associated with psychological risk factors of cardiovascular disease in apparently healthy adults. *Psychosom Med.* 2004;66(5):684–691.

105. Tanskanen A, Hibbeln JR, Tuomilehto J, et al. Fish consumption and depressive symptoms in the general population in Finland. *Psychiatr Serv.* 2001;52(4):529–531.

106. Dai J, Miller AH, Bremner JD, et al. Adherence to the Mediterranean diet is inversely associated with circulating interleukin-6 among middle-aged men: a twin study. *Circulation.* 2008;117(2):169–175.

107. Lee O, Bruce WR, Dong Q, Bruce J, Mehta R, O'Brien PJ. Fructose and carbonyl metabolites as endogenous toxins. *Chem Biol Interact.* 2009;178(1–3):332–339.

108. Kiecolt-Glaser JK, Preacher KJ, MacCallum RC, Atkinson C, Malarkey WB, Glaser R. Chronic stress and age-related increases in the proinflammatory cytokine IL-6. *Proc Natl Acad Sci U S A.* 2003;100(15):9090–9095.

109. Miller GE, Rohleder N, Cole SW. Chronic interpersonal stress predicts activation of pro- and anti-inflammatory signaling pathways 6 months later. *Psychosom Med.* 2009;71(1):57–62.

110. Miller GE, Chen E, Sze J, et al. A functional genomic fingerprint of chronic stress in humans: blunted glucocorticoid and increased NF-kappaB signaling. *Biol Psychiatry.* 2008;64(4):266–272.

111. Fuligni AJ, Telzer EH, Bower J, Cole SW, Kiang L, Irwin MR. A preliminary study of daily interpersonal stress and C-reactive protein levels among adolescents from Latin American and European backgrounds. *Psychosom Med.* 2009;71(3):329–333.

112. Vieira VJ, Valentine RJ, McAuley E, Evans E, Woods JA. Independent relationship between heart rate recovery and C-reactive protein in older adults. *J Am Geriatr Soc.* 2007;55(5):747–751.

113. Moyna NM, Bodnar JD, Goldberg HR, Shurin MS, Robertson RJ, Rabin BS. Relation between aerobic fitness level and stress induced alterations in neuroendocrine and immune function. *Int J Sports Med.* 1999;20(2):136–141.

114. Anton SD, Newton RL Jr, Sothern M, Martin CK, Stewart TM, Williamson DA. Association of depression with body mass index, sedentary behavior, and maladaptive eating attitudes and behaviors in 11 to 13-year old children. *Eat Weight Disord.* 2006; 11(3):e102–e108.

115. O'Connor MF, Bower JE, Cho HJ, et al. To assess, to control, to exclude: effects of biobehavioral factors on circulating inflammatory markers. *Brain Behav Immun.* 2009;23(7): 887–897.

116. Breslau N, Roth T, Rosenthal L, Andreski P. Sleep disturbance and psychiatric disorders: a longitudinal epidemiological study of young adults. *Biol Psychiatry.* 1996; 39(6):411–418.

117. Irwin MR, Wang M, Ribeiro D, et al. Sleep loss activates cellular inflammatory signaling. *Biol Psychiatry.* 2008;64(6):538–540.

118. Irwin MR, Wang M, Campomayor CO, Collado-Hidalgo A, Cole S. Sleep deprivation and activation of morning levels of cellular and genomic markers of inflammation. *Arch Int Med.* 2006;166(16):1756–1762.

119. Vgontzas AN, Zoumakis M, Papanicolaou DA, et al. Chronic insomnia is associated with a shift of interleukin-6 and tumor necrosis factor secretion from nighttime to daytime. *Metab Clin Exp.* 2002;51(7):887–892.

120. Steptoe A, Owen N, Kunz-Ebrecht SR, Brydon L. Loneliness and neuroendocrine, cardiovascular, and inflammatory stress responses in middle-aged men and women. *Psychoneuroendocrinology.* 2004;29(5):593–611.

121. Cacioppo JT, Hawkley LC. Social isolation and health, with an emphasis on underlying mechanisms. *Perspect Biol Med.* 2003;46(3 suppl):S39–S52.

122. McDade TW, Hawkley LC, Cacioppo JT. Psychosocial and behavioral predictors of inflammation in middle-aged and older adults: the Chicago health, aging, and social relations study. *Psychosom Med.* 2006;68(3):376–381.

123. Cole SW, Hawkley LC, Arevalo JM, Sung CY, Rose RM, Cacioppo JT. Social regulation of gene expression in human leukocytes. *Genome Biol.* 2007;8(9):R189.

124. Alley DE, Seeman TE, Ki Kim J, Karlamangla A, Hu P, Crimmins EM. Socioeconomic status and C-reactive protein levels in the US population: NHANES IV. *Brain Behavior Immun.* 2006;20(5):498–504.

125. Howren MB, Lamkin DM, Suls J. Associations of depression with C-reactive protein, IL-1, and IL-6: a meta-analysis. *Psychosom Med.* 2009;71(2):171–186.

126. Wolf JM, Miller GE, Chen E. Parent psychological states predict changes in inflammatory markers in children with asthma and healthy children. *Brain Behav Immun.* 2008;22(4):433–441.

127. Elenkov IJ, Iezzoni DG, Daly A, Harris AG, Chrousos GP. Cytokine dysregulation, inflammation and well-being. *Neuroimmunomodulation.* 2005;12(5):255–269.

128. Miller GE, Chen E, Fok AK, et al. Low early-life social class leaves a biological residue manifested by decreased glucocorticoid and increased proinflammatory signaling. *Proc Natl Acad Sci U S A.* 2009;106(34):14716–14721.

129. Saules KK, Pomerleau CS, Snedecor SM, et al. Relationship of onset of cigarette smoking during college to alcohol use, dieting concerns, and depressed mood: results from the Young Women's Health Survey. *Addict Behav.* 2004;29(5):893–899.

130. Miller TQ, Smith TW, Turner CW, Guijarro ML, Hallet AJ. A meta-analytic review of research on hostility and physical health. *Psychol Bull.* 1996;119(2):322–348.

131. Appleton KM, Woodside JV, Arveiler D, et al. A role for behavior in the relationships between depression and hostility and cardiovascular disease incidence, mortality, and all-cause mortality: the prime study. *Ann Behav Med.* 2016;50(4):582–591.

132. Miller G. *The Mating Mind: How Sexual Choice Shaped the Evolution of Human Nature.* New York, NY: Anchor Books; 2000.

133. Schaller M. The behavioural immune system and the psychology of human sociality. *Philos Trans R Soc Lond B Biol Sci.* 2011;366(1583):3418–3426.

134. Lo C, Zimmermann C, Rydall A, et al. Longitudinal study of depressive symptoms in patients with metastatic gastrointestinal and lung cancer. *J Clin Oncol.* 2010;28(18):3084–3089.

135. Jones JM, Cheng T, Jackman M, Rodin G, Walton T, Catton P. Self-efficacy, perceived preparedness, and psychological distress in women completing primary treatment for breast cancer. *J Psychosoc Oncol.* 2010;28(3):269–290.

136. Rodin G, Lo C, Mikulincer M, Donner A, Gagliese L, Zimmermann C. Pathways to distress: the multiple determinants of depression, hopelessness, and the desire for hastened death in metastatic cancer patients. *Soc Sci Med.* 2009;68(3):562–569.

137. Schane RE, Walter LC, Dinno A, Covinsky KE, Woodruff PG. Prevalence and risk factors for depressive symptoms in persons with chronic obstructive pulmonary disease. *J Gen Intern Med.* 2008;23(11):1757–1762.

138. Arden-Close E, Gidron Y, Moss-Morris R. Psychological distress and its correlates in ovarian cancer: a systematic review. *Psychooncology.* 2008;17(11):1061–1072.

139. Mehnert A, Koch U. Psychological comorbidity and health-related quality of life and its association with awareness, utilization, and need for psychosocial support in a cancer register-based sample of long-term breast cancer survivors. *J Psychosom Res.* 2008;64(4):383–391.

140. Julian LJ, Tonner C, Yelin E, et al. Cardiovascular and disease-related predictors of depression in systemic lupus erythematosus. *Arthritis Care Res (Hoboken).* 2011;63(4):542–549.

141. Raison CL, Borisov AS, Broadwell SD, et al. Depression during pegylated interferon-alpha plus ribavirin therapy: prevalence and prediction. *J Clin Psychiatry.* 2005;66(1):41–48.

142. Evon DM, Ramcharran D, Belle SH, et al. Prospective analysis of depression during peginterferon and ribavirin therapy of chronic hepatitis C: results of the Virahep-C study. *Am J Gastroenterol.* 2009;104(12):2949–2958.

143. Smith KJ, Norris S, O'Farrelly C, O'Mara SM. Risk factors for the development of depression in patients with hepatitis C taking interferon-alpha. *Neuropsychiatr Dis Treat.* 2011;7:275–292.

144. Heim C, Binder EB. Current research trends in early life stress and depression: review of human studies on sensitive periods, gene-environment interactions, and epigenetics. *Exp Neurol.* 2012;233(1):102–111.

145. Crook T, Eliot J. Parental death during childhood and adult depression: a critical review of the literature. *Psychol Bull.* 1980;87(2):252–259.

146. Konner M. *The Evolution of Childhood.* Cambridge, MA: Belknap Press; 2010.

147. Milner L. *Hardness of Hearth/Hardness of Life: The Stain of Human Infanticide.* New York, NY: University Press of America; 2000.

148. MacMillan HL, Fleming JE, Streiner DL, et al. Childhood abuse and lifetime psychopathology in a community sample. *Am J Psychiatry.* 2001;158(11):1878–1883.

149. Bereczkei T, Dunbar R. Helping-at-the-nest and reproduction in a Hungarian Gypsy population. *Curr Anthropol.* 2002;43:804–809.

150. Bereczkei T, Dunbar R. Female-biased reproductive strategies in a Hungarian Gypsy population. *Proc R Soc B Biol Sci.* 1997;264:17–22.

151. Galler JR, Bryce CP, Waber D, et al. Early childhood malnutrition predicts depressive symptoms at ages 11–17. *J Child Psychol Psychiatry.* 2010;51(7):789–798.

152. Waber DP, Eaglesfield D, Fitzmaurice GM, Bryce C, Harrison RH, Galler JR. Cognitive impairment as a mediator in the developmental pathway from infant malnutrition to adolescent depressive symptoms in Barbadian youth. *J Dev Behav Pediatr.* 2011;32(3):225–232.

153. Coplan JD, Smith EL, Altemus M, et al. Maternal-infant response to variable foraging demand in nonhuman primates: effects of timing of stressor on cerebrospinal fluid corticotropin-releasing factor and circulating glucocorticoid concentrations. *Ann N Y Acad Sci.* 2006;1071:525–533.

154. Coplan JD, Smith EL, Altemus M, et al. Variable foraging demand rearing: sustained elevations in cisternal cerebrospinal fluid corticotropin-releasing factor concentrations in adult primates. *Biol Psychiatry.* 2001;50(3):200–204.

155. Quinlan RJ. Human parental effort and environmental risk. *Proc Biol Sci.* 2007; 274(1606):121–125.

156. Panter-Brick C, Eggerman M, Gonzalez V, Safdar S. Violence, suffering, and mental health in Afghanistan: a school-based survey. *Lancet.* 2009;374(9692):807–816.

157. Waldinger RJ, Vaillant GE, Orav EJ. Childhood sibling relationships as a predictor of major depression in adulthood: a 30-year prospective study. *Am J Psychiatry.* 2007; 164(6):949–954.

158. Kendler KS, Sham PC, MacLean CJ. The determinants of parenting: an epidemiological, multi-informant, retrospective study. *Psychol Med.* 1997;27(3):549–563.

159. Pillemer K, Suitor JJ, Pardo S, Henderson C Jr. Mothers' differentiation and depressive symptoms among adult children. *J Marriage Fam.* 2010;72(2):333–345.

160. Baumeister RF. *Meanings of Life.* New York, NY: Guilford; 1991.

161. Neuberg SL, Kenrick DT, Schaller M. Human threat management systems: self-protection and disease avoidance. *Neurosci Biobehav Rev.* 2011;35(4):1042–1051.

162. Kendler KS, Gardner CO. Sex differences in the pathways to major depression: a study of opposite-sex twin pairs. *Am J Psychiatry.* 2014;171(4):426–435.

163. Wilkinson R, Pickett K. *The Spirit Level: Why Greater Equality Makes Societies Stronger.* London: Allen Lane; 2009.

164. Kurzban R, Leary MR. Evolutionary origins of stigmatization: the functions of social exclusion. *Psychol Bull.* 2001;127(2):187–208.

165. Allen NB, Badcock PB. Darwinian models of depression: a review of evolutionary accounts of mood and mood disorders. *Prog Neuropsychopharmacol Biol Psychiatry.* 2006;30(5):815–826.

166. Sloman L, Gilbert P, Hasey G. Evolved mechanisms in depression: the role and interaction of attachment and social rank in depression. *J Affect Disord.* 2003;74(2):107–121.

167. Gilbert P, McEwan K, Bellew R, Mills A, Gale C. The dark side of competition: how competitive behaviour and striving to avoid inferiority are linked to depression, anxiety, stress and self-harm. *Psychol Psychother.* 2009;82(pt 2):123–136.

168. Muller-Pinzler L, Krach S, Kramer UM, Paulus FM. The social neuroscience of interpersonal emotions. *Curr Top Behav Neurosci.* 2016. doi: 10.1007/7854_2016_437.

169. Basile B, Mancini F, Macaluso E, Caltagirone C, Frackowiak RS, Bozzali M. Deontological and altruistic guilt: evidence for distinct neurobiological substrates. *Hum Brain Mapp.* 2011;32(2):229–239.

170. Hamilton JP, Etkin A, Furman DJ, Lemus MG, Johnson RF, Gotlib IH. Functional neuroimaging of major depressive disorder: a meta-analysis and new integration of base line activation and neural response data. *Am J Psychiatry.* 2012;169(7):693–703.

171. Raison CL, Hale MW, Williams LE, Wager TD, Lowry CA. Somatic influences on subjective well-being and affective disorders: the convergence of thermosensory and central serotonergic systems. *Front Cognit.* 2015;5:1580.

172. Capuron L, Fornwalt FB, Knight BT, Harvey PD, Ninan PT, Miller AH. Does cytokine-induced depression differ from idiopathic major depression in medically healthy individuals? *J Affect Disord.* 2009;119(1–3):181–185.

173. Jokela M, Virtanen M, Batty GD, Kivimaki M. Inflammation and specific symptoms of depression. *JAMA Psychiatry.* 2016;73(1):87–88.

174. Keller MC, Nesse RM. The evolutionary significance of depressive symptoms: different adverse situations lead to different depressive symptom patterns. *J Pers Soc Psychol.* 2006;91(2):316–330.

175. Keller MC, Neale MC, Kendler KS. Association of different adverse life events with distinct patterns of depressive symptoms. *Am J Psychiatry.* 2007;164(10):1521–1529.

176. Musselman DL, Evans DL, Nemeroff CB. The relationship of depression to cardiovascular disease: epidemiology, biology, and treatment. *Arch Gen Psychiatry.* 1998;55(7): 580–592.

CHAPTER 4

The Genetics of
Major Depressive Disorder

Several genetic epidemiological studies estimate heritability of major depressive disorder (MDD) to be in the moderate range of 31–42 percent.[1] Before we proceed with the discussion of the genetic origins of MDD, it would be only fair to warn the reader of the inexorable train of evidence. The largest mega-analysis of genome-wide association studies (GWAS), which included approximately 19,000 subjects in the MDD discovery phase, 57,000 subjects in the replication phase, and 32,000 subjects in the cross-disorder analysis of MDD and bipolar disorder, has failed to provide robust and replicable proof of specific gene involvement in the etiology of MDD.[2] Unfortunately, findings of this study mirror the conclusions of several other previous attempts to identify genes responsible for depression. There may be several explanations for this striking absence of identifiable genetic contributors.

For one thing, we may not be looking in the right places. MDD is currently a descriptive diagnosis without a precise reference to a common underlying pathophysiology. Certain forms of depression, such as early-onset depression, familial depression, and clinically established recurrent depression, may have higher heritability (48–75 percent)[3] and could provide a better opportunity for identification of responsible genes. On the other hand, it is not inconceivable that in some instances genetic factors may play a negligible role. Most of the GWAS start their search from a broad base of relatively common "suspect" genes. It is conceivable that some of the important but rare "culprit" genes have been omitted from the search base.[2] Sheer numbers make the task even more daunting—70 percent of all our genes are expressed in the brain, creating an overwhelming diversity of candidates.[4]

In addition, our premise about the origin of depression may be spurious. Etiology of MDD may include an interaction of several factors, none of which is sufficient to explain it on its own. At any given time the risk of developing depression could be a product of interactions among genetic epistasis, polymorphisms of multiple genes (each with small to moderate effect), potential copy number variants, epigenetic modulation, and chemical correlates of environmental adversity.

Copy number variants (CNVs) would have a more robust effect than more commonly occurring genetic polymorphisms but are unlikely to explain most of the occurrences of depression. Rare, spontaneously occurring mutations and CNVs tend to be associated with earlier disease onset and a greater frequency with advanced paternal age. Rare mutations and CNVs are more likely to be relevant in etiopathogenesis of autism and schizophrenia, both of which are influenced by paternal age, unlike MDD, where it does not appear to play a significant role.[5]

Timetable is also important. Because certain genes and their products have a greater role in earlier developmental stages (e.g., genes involved in regulation of neurogenesis, neuronal migration, and synaptic differentiation), other genes may have a more pronounced effect in the middle and later phases of etiopathogenesis, like the ones controlling neurotransmitter signaling, endocrine, and immune responses. Therefore, the genes that predispose may be a different set from the genes that contribute to initiation and the maintenance of the depressive process.

Epigenetic processes entail heritable changes in gene expression that are not encoded by the DNA sequence and are therefore of no influence in GWAS.[6] Early-life adversity may alter subsequent gene expression in an enduring way by silencing selected genes via DNA methylation.[6] Numerous studies have established connections between early-life adversity and subsequent risk of developing MDD, earlier disease onset, chronic course, inadequate response to antidepressant treatment, greater morbidity, and more frequent comorbidities.[3] Later stressful life events, such as the death of loved ones, disruptions of major relationships, serious and disabling medical illness, and extreme financial distress, can leave their epigenetic imprint by regulating the histone code. Information-rich DNA is wrapped around histone proteins in a spool-like manner. Acetylation and methylation work like on and off switches, allowing or denying transcription factors access to the DNA strand. Methylation of histone converts it into its heterochromatic off state, while acetylation produces euchromatin, which switches transcription on (epigenetic modulation is discussed in greater detail elsewhere in this chapter).[6] Unlike the alterations in the histone code, which can occur in a matter of minutes, early-life adversity, by impacting a developmentally sensitive period, may produce DNA methylation with long-lasting effects. Later in life, aging-related processes are interwoven with the epigenetic consequences of early and later adversity, providing an influential backdrop that actively shapes the expression of depressive symptoms.[7]

MDD does not appear to be a monolithic biological entity. Clinical symptoms of depression are most likely an expression of the activity in the final common pathophysiological pathways. Biological markers, such as neurotrophic factors, inflammatory cytokines and chemokines, monoamine transmitter turnover, sympathetic tone, and levels of hypothalamic-pituitary-adrenal (HPA) mediators, as well as imaging findings and clinical characteristics seem to be unevenly distributed in the population of depressed patients. Some depressed patients will manifest these biological markers to a greater or a lesser degree; in some they will be completely absent. Likewise, the relationship between genetic/epigenetic underpinning and clinical characteristics of this biologically heterogeneous diagnostic entity, which we identify as Major Depression, is most likely probabilistic in nature.

Pursuant our previous discussion, it may appear unavailing to review the studies exploring the relationship between single-nucleotide polymorphisms (SNPs) of the candidate genes and MDD. Paradoxically, we believe that our insight into the pathophysiology of MDD can profit from examining how the interface between common genetic variants and environmental adversity translates into clinical manifestations of depression. Polymorphisms of the genes that regulate various aspects of monoamine signaling, such as synthetic and catabolic enzymes, transporters (uptake pumps), and pre- and postsynaptic receptors, have most consistently been implicated in the etiopathogenesis of MDD. Numerous studies have investigated the relationship between the serotonin (5HT) transporter promoter locus (5HTTLPR), the 5HT2A and 5HT1A serotonin receptors, catechol-*O*-methyltransferase (COMT), monoamine oxidase (MAO), and predilection for depression, especially in adverse circumstances (see Table 4.1 for a list of gene and receptor abbreviations used in this chapter). Genes regulating the synthesis and/or activity of corticotropin-releasing factor (CRF) and its receptors have also been implicated.[8] In addition, genetic studies have established a link between genes coding for elements of glutamate and gamma-aminobutyric acid (GABA) signaling cascades, as well as neuroplasticity regulators, such as brain-derived neurotrophic factor (BDNF) and glial-derived neurotrophic factor, and the risk of developing depression. An exciting development in the field of psychiatric genetics is the recognition that genes are more likely to code for "endophenotypical traits" that increase the risk of psychiatric morbidity, rather than coding directly for any specific psychiatric diagnosis.[9] For mood disorders these endophenotypical indicators primarily center on the circuitry essential for regulation of emotions and arousal, cognition, and risk/benefit appraisal, as well as modulation of stress and immune activity. But here we focus primarily on the GWAS examining the relationship between common genetic polymorphisms and various elements of the MDD, especially pertaining to the interactions with environmental adversity.

Genes Involved in Regulation of Serotonergic Function

As noted above, "depression genes" frequently do not contribute directly to the development of the disorder but, rather, confer vulnerability to developing depres-

TABLE 4.1. **Gene, receptor, and transporter abbreviations used in this chapter**

5HIAA	5-hydroxyindoleacetic acid
5HT1A, 5HT2A	serotonin receptors
5HT	serotonin
5HTT	serotonin transporter
5HTTLPR	serotonin-transporter-linked promoter region
5MTHF	5-methyltetrahydrofolate
BDNF	brain-derived neurotrophic factor
BH2	7,8-dihydrobiopterine
BH4	tetrahydrobiopterin
CACNA1C	a gene that codes for the a1C subunit of LTCC
cAMP	cyclical adenosine monophosphate
cGMP	cyclical guanosine monophosphate
CNVs	copy number variants
COMT	catechol-*O*-methyltransferase
CREB1	cAMP response element binding protein-1
CRF	corticotropin-releasing factor
CRH	corticotropin-releasing hormone
CRHR1	corticotropin-releasing hormone receptor 1
DA	dopamine
DAT	DA transporters
FKBP5	a regulator of glucocorticoid receptor complex
GABA	gamma-aminobutyric acid
GR	glucocorticoid receptor
GRIA-1 to -4	four units composing the alpha-amino-3-hydroxy-5-methyl-4-isoxazolepropionic acid (AMPA) glutamate receptor
GRIK-4	kainite glutamatergic receptor
GRM-1 to -7	genes involved in glutamatergic synaptic transmission
GSK-3b	glycogen synthase 3-beta
GWAS	genome-wide association studies
IL-6	interleukin-6
KA	kainite
LTCC	Cav1.2 voltage-dependent L-type calcium channel
MAO	monoamine oxidase
MAOA	monoamine oxidase A
MR	mineralocorticoid receptor
MTHFR	methylenetetrahydrofolate reductase
NE	norepinephrine
NET	NE transporter
NMDA	*N*-methyl-D-aspartate
NPY	neuropeptide Y
PDE	phosphodiesterase
SLC6A4	solute carrier family 6 member 4
SNPs	single-nucleotide polymorphisms
TPH	tryptophan hydroxylase
TrkB	tropomyosin receptor kinase-B

sion in response to environmental calamity. Direct association between common genetic variants and common disorders is implausible.[5] An allele that would reduce reproductive fitness by as little as 0.003 percent would be removed from the population by natural selection.[5] Alternatively, if gene–environment interaction is a more prominent etiological factor, one would anticipate significant regional epidemiological differences. Indeed, cross-national epidemiological studies found a greater then 10-fold difference in lifetime Major Depression rates between Taiwan and Beirut.[10]

We start our review of specific candidate genes associated with depression with the 5HT-transporter-linked promoter region (5HTTLPR), by far the most researched allele with the presumptive ties to MDD etiology. Review of the role of the 5HT transporter (5HTT) polymorphism in MDD will be more detailed, as it will also serve as an illustration of the multilayered nature of the genetic influence. Gene coding for transcription of serotonin transporter (5HTT), also known as SERT, is referred to as SLC6A4 (see table 4.1). In proximity of SLC6A4 is 5HTTLPR, a promoter region, involved in regulating its transcription. Within this promoter or immediately adjacent to it are two SNPs, rs25531 and rs25532, both located upstream from the transcription site, jointly contribute to modulation of SLC6A4 transcription.[11] There are two basic variations of 5HTTLPR, a short version (S), comprised of 14 repeats and a long version (L), which has 16 repeats. "S" allele is associated with reduced SLC6A4 transcription and therefore diminished 5HT uptake, and consequently disrupted 5HT signaling. An embedded A/G substitution of rs25531, commonly labeled Lg, is functionally similar and most often grouped with the S-allele.[12] This minor Lg allele tends to be coupled with the L-allele of 5HTTLPR, thereby attenuating its function. Thus, there are three different functional alleles: La (highest expressing) and Lg and S (both low-expressing). Only a few of the most recent studies distinguish between Lg and La, most of the literature does not. A minor allele of rs25532 can also reduce gene expression levels by 15–80 percent depending on other background 5HTTLPR alleles.[13] A combination of the frequent and less common variants may thus act in a synergistic manner, resulting in 20-fold higher expression and function of the 5HTT in the higher-expressing variants compared with lower-expressing alleles.[11] This dramatic genetically determined difference in 5HT uptake capacity has a direct impact on 5HT levels in various brain and bodily areas. Indeed, an imaging study using a radiolabeled ligand of 5HTT demonstrated significantly reduced binding in the medial prefrontal cortex (mPFC) of homozygous short allele depressed carriers, compared with all other alleles (see Table 4.2 for a list of brain area abbreviations used in this chapter).[14] 5HTT is expressed not only in brain and bowel but also in the heart, vasculature, platelets, and pancreas, despite the absence of significant serotonergic innervation in these organs and tissues.[11] 5HT also has a prominent role in neuroendocrine regulation: it is involved in modulation of HPA axis activity and in oxytocin and prolactin signaling.[11] At this point

TABLE 4.2. Brain region abbreviations used in this chapter

ACC	anterior cingulate cortex
CSF	cerebrospinal fluid
dlPFC	dorsolateral prefrontal cortex
DMN	default mode network
EN	executive network
HPA axis	hypothalamic-pituitary-adrenal axis
mPFC	medial prefrontal cortex
PFC	prefrontal cortex
rACC	rostral anterior cingulate cortex
SN	salience network
vlPFC	ventrolateral prefrontal cortex
vmPFC	ventromedial prefrontal cortex

it is important that we remind ourselves that 5HTTLPR does not alter the function or composition of the transporter itself; it just influences its transcriptional efficiency.[15] Despite reports of decreased transcriptional efficiency in vitro of *SS* and *SL* alleles compared with *LL*, short allele does not appear to influence the availability of transporter in mature organisms in the resting state.[11,15] However, decreased 5HTT availability and elevated 5HT levels in response to adversity in the earlier developmental stages may result in downregulation and desensitization of the presynaptic 5HT1A/B and postsynaptic 5HT2A receptors, with subsequent epigenetic reprogramming of the stress response system, manifesting as trait anxiety and maladaptive response to stress later in life.[16]

Insufficient 5HT signaling in the depressed individuals is further reflected in elevated 5HT turnover and increased cerebrospinal fluid (CSF) concentration of the principal 5HT metabolite, 5-hydroxyindoleacetic acid (5HIAA), in depressed *SS* subjects compared with *LL* carriers. Dysfunctional 5HT neurotransmission is akin to trying to communicate during a loud sporting event. We find ourselves shouting in order to be heard. Elevated 5HT levels, and therefore its metabolites, in some depressed individuals may be an attempt to be "heard" above the elevated background noise, due to insufficient 5HT transmission. Impaired 5HT signaling may spread downstream to influence dopamine (DA) neurons in the ventral tegmental area of the brain, which are usually modulated by 5HT. Empirical evidence supports less efficient DA signaling in *SS* individuals affected by MDD, relative to *LL* patients, as evidenced by higher homovanillic acid levels in CSF.[17] One can speculate that this disturbance in DA transmission, caused by inadequate serotonergic modulation in *SS* patients, may be the neural basis for anhedonia, one of the cardinal features of MDD.[16]

A number of psychological traits and functions have been associated with 5HTTLPR polymorphism. Several, but not all, studies have reported an association between the short form of 5HTTLPR and a psychological trait labeled neuroticism. Individuals endowed with this trait have a greater than average propensity to react to environmental change with negative emotional states such as anxiety, depression, hopelessness, somatization, interpersonal sensitivity, obsessive-compulsive symptoms, anger, guilt, and hostility.[18–20] Some authors believe that it is precisely this psychological trait, neuroticism, that mediates the relationship between 5HTTLPR polymorphism and Major Depression.[20] Furthermore, in one study individuals who carried a less-expressing 5HTTLPR allele, compared with the rest of the 220 college student group, were more likely to report negative affect, a core feature of neuroticism.[21]

Could it be that negative emotions, associated with 5HTTLPR polymorphism, are driven by a perceptual bias? Some evidence points exactly in that direction. Different groups of researchers have noted that carriers of low-expressing 5HTTLPR genotype, compared with those carrying intermediate or high-efficacy genotypes, displayed attentional bias toward negatively valenced stimuli.[22,23] It is even possible that negative perceptual bias related to 5HTTLPR is active in utero: a Dutch group found an association between maternal anxiety during pregnancy and negative emotionality at six months of age in infants carrying one or more copies of the short allele but not in those homozygous for the long allele. There was no difference between the genotypes if maternal anxiety was low.[24]

Given the relationship between emotions and cognition, would 5HTTLPR polymorphism influence aspects of cognitive functioning? One study found a tendency for negative information processing in short-allele-carrying children following a negative mood prime. After viewing a sad video clip, children were presented with a list of 18 positive and 18 negative adjectives. Children with short allele recalled more negative adjectives than did children with other genotypes.[25] Since 5HTTLPR polymorphism has a considerable impact on function and structure of several components of neural networks involved in empathy, imitative learning, and communication (see text bellow), would it have a role in social cognition[26]? An interesting body of work suggests that collectivism may have developed and persisted in populations with a high proportion of putative social sensitivity alleles, such as the low-expressing 5HTTLPR allele, because it was more compatible with such groups. The relative proportion of "sensitivity alleles" was correlated with the lifetime prevalence of Major Depression across nations. The relationship between allele frequency and depression was in part influenced by individualism–collectivism trait, raising the question of whether lower levels of depression in populations with a high proportion of social sensitivity alleles are due to greater collectivism.[27]

Researchers have had difficulty establishing and consistently reproducing an association between 5HTTLPR polymorphism and complex psychological traits. It has been proposed that upward of 100 gene polymorphisms may contribute to shaping of the complex continuously distributed traits; thus, the effects of individual genes would be modest, and barely distinguishable, at best.[26] Even the hypothetical role of the interaction between 5HTT alleles and stressful life events in the etiology of depression remains controversial.[28] An alternative route would recommend pursuing imaging research into the influence of 5HTT alleles on neural structure and function, arguing that the impact of genetic polymorphism may be more straightforward and therefore easier to detect.

The S-allele of the 5HTTLPR gene has been associated with a number of alterations in brain function and morphology. One of the more prominent and reproduced findings in subjects bearing 5HTTLPR S-alleles involves compromised functional and structural integrity of amygdala–anterior cingulate cortex (ACC) circuitry engaged in regulation of emotional, behavioral, and endocrine response to stress, as well as in processing of the pain signals.[29–33] The short allele has also been linked with reduced ACC, amygdala, and hippocampal volumes in healthy individuals.[30] Additionally, healthy carriers of at least one copy of the 5HTTLPR short allele (SS and SL) were noted to have smaller superior temporal gyrus and areas of the PFC—ventrolateral (vlPFC), ventromedial (vmPFC), and dorsolateral (dlPFC)—compared with individuals with the LL genotype.[12,30,34] Furthermore, diffusion tensor imaging, a sophisticated technique to evaluate white matter tract integrity, has revealed abnormalities in the healthy S-allele carriers. Individuals endowed with at least one copy of the low-expressing 5HTTLPR S-allele, compared with ones with LL-alleles, had altered white matter microstructure in the tracts connecting the amygdala with the vmPFC and vlPFC.[35] Moreover, the same group of authors established that vlPFC morphology was inversely associated with sustained attention for positive and negative stimuli, but only among 5HTTLPR short-allele carriers. Similar associations between the attention and morphology did not exist for the vmPFC or the amygdala.

These study results strongly imply that brain regions involved in cognitive emotional control are also associated with attentional biases for emotional stimuli among 5HTTLPR short-allele carriers.[36] An intriguing elaboration of this report comes from primate research. The S-allele of the rhesus macaque analogue of human 5HTTLPR broadly affected cognitive and emotional choices in context of several learning and attentional tasks. Another study linked the brain structure and function with S-allele. Elderly individuals who were S carriers, compared with those of other genotypes, had increased morning cortisol, decreased hippocampal volume, and diminished delayed recall.[37] Could it be that 5HTTLPR polymorphism actively shapes our early emotional experiences, attentional bias, and learning by influencing function and structure of the key corticolimbic circuits? Is it possible that these genetically influenced neural propensities, embedded in our temperamental traits and personality, set the stage for subsequent encounters with life's adversities and potential risk for depression?

Primate studies clearly point in that direction. The observed differences in complex choice-making behavior were related to 5HTTLPR alleles and brain morphology but not to 5HTT or 5HT1A concentrations in vivo, suggesting that the complex behaviors were more influenced by the past dynamic interactions between genotype/neural function and structure and the environment rather than by static, cross-sectional determinants of 5HT signaling.[38] Findings of this study provide basis for an interesting speculation: the effect of 5HTTLPR polymorphism may be substantially mediated by its influence on early neural development rather than the subsequent change in serotonergic transmission.

The influence of 5HTTLPR polymorphisms on the brain structures differentially affects neural morphology in healthy individuals versus MDD patients. Thomas Frodl and his colleagues in Munich have provided us with some interesting insights. Their first study produced a completely unexpected outcome: MDD patients with the LL genotype had significantly smaller hippocampal gray and white matter than healthy controls, yet L is the more efficient allele. There were no differences in hippocampal volume between MDD patients and healthy controls if they carried one of the S-alleles.[39] Their subsequent study replicated this finding: contrary to healthy controls, where the 5HTTLPR S-allele was associated with a smaller hippocampal volume, the situation in MDD patients was reversed: LL homozygous individuals had reduced hippocampal volume. The authors speculated that the "corrosive" impact of the disease state might be more pronounced in LL carriers who had a larger hippocampal volume to start with, compared with SS or SL individuals.[34] Frodl et al. further argued that the change in the hippocampal volume in LL depressed individuals may be related to an interaction between diminished serotonergic transmission (due to excessive 5HT uptake) and consequent reduction in BDNF signaling.

A later study by the same group appeared to "restore the order." Depressed patients who were S-allele carriers with a history of emotional neglect before age 18 had smaller hippocampal volumes than did the patients who had only one risk factor (either S-allele or neglect without the S-allele). Consistent with the previous finding, hippocampal white matter reduction in S carriers correlated with intensity of the early emotional neglect.[40] Similar to the observations made by Frodl and colleagues, Taylor et al. found an association between the S-allele and smaller hippocampal volume in early-onset depression (before age 50), while in late-onset depression L/L carriers had smaller hippocampi.[41]

One can speculate that early-life adversity may hasten the onset of depression[42] and also interact with the S-allele to produce smaller hippocampal volumes, while L alleles may provide a protective effect against stress and adversity, sparing the hippocampal volume and delaying the onset of depression. On the other hand, patients with the La allele of 5HTTLPR-rs25331 suffered the greatest gray matter reduction once the disease process became active (having a greater volume to start with provided them with a greater opportunity for the gray matter loss).

The apparent controversy between these findings illustrates the complexity of the factors that influence the association between 5HTTLPR alleles and brain morphology in depressed patients, and indicates why the research outcomes can be so discrepant. Other studies have also described an association between the

S-allele and a smaller hippocampal volume in medication free depressed patients (mean age 33.6 ± 9.5 years);[43] greater microstructural white matter abnormalities in dorsal anterior cingulate cortex, rostral ACC (rACC), dlPFC, mPFC, posterior cingulate cortex, and the thalamus volume in elderly patients;[44] and smaller caudate nucleus and enlarged thalamic pulvinar volume and elevated neuronal numbers in a postmortem study.[45] Review of morphological differences associated with 5HTTLPR allows several inferences: (a) the affected areas are crucial components of the three major functional networks (salience, executive, and default-mode networks; see below) implicated in pathophysiology of depression, (b) some of the structural changes may be independent of the impact of 5HTTLPR alleles on serotonergic transmission, (c) the influence of 5HTTLPR on neural structure is modified by interaction with early adversity and the time of disease onset, and (d) alterations in neural structure are most often associated with a change in function.

Previously described structural changes associated with 5HTTLPR polymorphisms may in turn result in aberrant connectivity between the amygdala and the subgenual ACC (studies often include the adjacent vmPFC). Resulting disturbances in these key components of the corticolimbic circuitry are believed to interfere with emotional homeostasis and appropriate modulation of stress response.[30,31,46] Moreover, it appears that the S-allele may have a more extensive influence on several components of the salience network (SN). When a group of children experienced a period of transient sadness, induced by viewing sorrowful film excerpts, they responded with a dissimilar pattern of limbic activity, influenced by the difference in 5HTTLPR alleles. Children who had an S-allele, compared with the LL homozygous group, had significantly elevated ACC, insula, putamen, and caudate activation during functional MRI scanning while viewing sad movie excerpts.[47] It appears that increased SN activation may be accompanied by increased cortical excitability and compromised inhibitory processes in S-allele carriers, relative to carriers of other polymorphisms.[48] In view of these findings, one might be concerned about the double handicap in S carriers: exaggerated automatic limbic response to aversive stimuli, coupled with inadequate cortical "top-down" modulation. Fortunately, despite increased limbic (especially amygdala)/SN activation in response to aversive stimuli in S carriers, imaging studies suggest that the top-down, volitional regulation of the emotion is still partially intact in these individuals.[49,50] Another study extended these findings, reporting increased propensity toward rumination in response to a negative stimulus, coupled with the impaired automatic amygdala–ACC regulation in S carriers compared with the LL homozygous group.[50] Lower-expressing, 5HTTLPR S-allele carriers have also been noted to have increased bilateral PFC activity while performing a working memory task. Despite elevated PFC activity, most likely to compensate for inefficient neural processing, women with an S-allele had inferior cognitive performance compared with the ones with the LL genotype.[51] Thus, inadequately regulated limbic activity in lower-expressing 5HTTLPR allele carriers may be coupled with cognitive deficiencies.

Interestingly, one study found evidence that greater amygdala response to positive stimuli, such as looking at the photo of a favorite person, may have a beneficial effect. Healthy individuals with S/S genotype had both higher amygdala activity in response to looking at their favorite person and elevated natural killer cell mobilization. Natural killer cell activation in context of S/S polymorphism provides a significant evolutionary benefit because these cells form an important defense against the spread of tumor cells, as well as viral and bacterial infections.[52]

Given that negative emotions usually signal an environmental threat or loss, it might be interesting to know if 5HTTLPR polymorphisms also influence somatic responses to adversity. Indeed, Gotlib and colleagues have proposed relationships between the 5HTT S-allele, responses to stress, HPA reactivity, and susceptibility to MDD. They have substantiated this hypothesis by finding that girls homozygous for the S-allele reacted to stress with a prolonged elevation of cortisol, compared with ones with at least one L-allele, indicating greater reactivity to stress and possible increased susceptibility toward depression.[53] Furthermore, individuals homozygous for the 5HTTLPR S-allele, relative to other polymorphisms, exhibited exaggerated sympathetic response to a stress task, manifesting as blood pressure elevation and epinephrine secretion,[54] as well as an increased inflammatory response.[55]

Functional changes associated with 5HTTLPR polymorphism in MDD parallel the findings in healthy individuals. Patients with the lower-expressing 5HTTLPR S-allele have exhibited enhanced amygdala reactivity, in some instances associated with greater depression chronicity.[56,57] Other researchers have noted an association between the 5HTTLPR S-allele and recurrence and early onset of depression.[58] In addition to increased amygdala reactivity, depressed S-allele carriers also manifest elevated mPFC and vlPFC activity, possibly reflecting compromised automatic and volitional emotional regulation.[59] The 5HTTLPR S-allele has also been associated with elevation of morning cortisol and increased recurrence risk in depressed adolescents[60] and greater depressive symptoms in presence of elevated interleukin-6 (IL-6) plasma levels.[61]

Now that we have a better understanding of the impact of 5HTTLPR polymorphism on neural structure and function, both in healthy and in depressed individuals, let us try to elucidate the dynamic between the genes influencing the 5HTT function and the environmental forces. GWAS and meta-analyses have left us with equivocal evidence of association between 5HTTLPR and depression. While some large GWAS studies, including over 1,500 depressed patients and 2,500 controls, found significant associations between 5HTTLPR polymorphism and depression,[62] other large meta-analyses have failed to confirm this relationship.[63]

Could it be that the presence of the less-expressing 5HTTLPR allele has bearing on the etiology of depression in only a specific set of circumstances? Indeed, the 5HTT S-allele is more likely to be associated with depression when interacting with environmental stress. For example, a study by Caspi et al.[64] demonstrated that the inconsistently observed association between depression and the 5HTTLPR S-allele may in part be explained by intervening variables. A study of a nonclinical population found associations among the S-allele, life adversity, and somatization, depression, anxiety, paranoid ideation, and global symptom severity. No such association was noted in S-allele-carrying subjects who have not faced past life adversity.[64] Another study noted a connection between the less functional 5HTTLPR allele and increased risk of developing both depression and suicidal ideation, but only in individuals exposed to life stressors, unlike the ones spared the environmental adversity.[65]

Findings of gene–environment interactions involving 5HTTLPR polymorphism as a putative etiological factor of MDD have been replicated several times. There even appears to be a sort of dose–response relationship, whereby S-allele carriers have a greater likelihood of developing depression in face of multiple stressful, threatening, and adverse events; environmental calamity, financial crisis, disruption in intimate relationship, illness, injury, and death.[66–68] Interaction between stressful life events and the S-allele has also been associated with the severity of depression.[69,70] Moreover, Kendler et al.[71] observed an interactions between the 5HTTLPR S-allele, stressful life events, and the risk of developing MDD involving a gender effect: women with the 5HTTLPR S-allele were especially likely to develop depression in response to stress (odds ratio of 7 compared with males with the L-allele). Furthermore, the National Longitudinal Study of Adolescent Health reported an association between perceived stress and stable depressive symptomatology, moderated by homozygous SS-genotype in girls, but not in boys.[72]

It is important to mention that there are some contradictory findings. An Australian group reported an association between higher-expressing LL genotype and melancholy depression in females, with an odds ratio of 1.7, or 70% greater odds than in males (95 percent confidence interval, 1.1–2.6), the same was true for women with La/La genotype, with an odds ratio of 2.1 (95 percent confidence interval, 1.1–4.1). No such relationship was observed in the male group. However, although this study focused on the relationship between 5HTTLPR genotype and the subtypes of depression (melancholy vs. atypical), it did not evaluate an interaction with stressful events.[73] Another study established the relationship between the S-allele, combined with caregiving stress or low socioeconomic status, and higher depression scores in women, compared with participants with L-allele without stress. Perhaps, paradoxically, it was the stress combined with L-allele in males that showed an association with depression severity, relative to men who had an S-allele and reported no stressors.[74] Beyond the role of gender, there may be additional methodological explanations for the reported lack of association between MDD and the 5HTTLPR–environment interaction in some of the meta-analyses.[28,75] Most of the negative findings referenced in the meta-analyses are derived from the studies that relied on brief, retrospective self-reports of stress. On the other hand, studies that utilized objective evidence and detailed interviews to collect the information about adversity are almost invariably positive.[76–78]

The timing of the interaction between the adversity and 5HTTLPR polymorphism, as well as the type and duration of stress, appears to be quite relevant. Childhood maltreatment in individuals with the less efficient forms of 5HTTLPR seems to be particularly depressogenic.[79] Substance abuse and suicidal behavior have also been associated with interaction between the 5HTTLPR S-allele and childhood trauma.[80] A retrospective study has linked childhood sexual abuse and physical neglect, in combination with the S-allele, with the subsequent recurrent MDD.[81] The interaction between 5HTTLPR S-alleles and childhood maltreatment has also been associated with the chronic and persistent forms of depression.[82,83] Furthermore, chronic family stress predicted depressive symptomatology in a group of prospectively studied adolescents if they were S-allele carriers. If they lacked the S-allele or were exposed only to episodic stress, no such relationship was noted.[84]

If this 5HTTLPR polymorphism leads to a greater likelihood, chronicity, and recurrence of depression when interacting with early-life adversity, how is this association mediated, and does it also influence the role of later life stress in the etiology of depression? Two-stage models have attempted to answer this question. In brief, these models propose that early-life trauma interacts with this 5HTTLPR polymorphism and other genes causing changes in neuroplasticity and epigenetic programming, with consequent alterations in neural structure and function, HPA, and immune modulation, jointly contributing to a maladaptive stress response. In face of repetitive adult-life stress, already vulnerable stress-response systems breaks down, precipitating a second wave of structural and functional changes that give rise to symptoms of depression.[3,16,85]

Emerging evidence provides additional hypothetical pathophysiological explanations for the relationship between 5HTTLPR and depression. Recent stress appears to have a "generalizing" effect, by increasing the likelihood of ruminations in S-allele carriers, even in the circumstances in which the self-referential process is uncalled for.[50] In Chapter 8 we describe neurobiological processes underlying ruminations and their link with core MDD symptomatology.[86] It has been posited that ruminations in physiological circumstances act as a form of rehearsal, allowing stress-related information to be properly processed and stored in the memory. In context of MDD, ruminations are maladaptive, as they interfere with working memory and executive function and diminish hedonic drive.[86]

Another important point concerning the role of 5HTTLPR polymorphisms in etiopathogenesis of depression bears a more careful examination. Is the low-expressing 5HTTLPR allele a vulnerability or a sensitivity allele? Some very intriguing studies have explored this issue. Taylor and colleagues found an expected relationship between the short allele, stressful early family environment, and more intense depressive symptomatology. Interestingly, they also reported that S/S carriers in context of a supportive family environment or recent positive experience manifested significantly fewer depressive symptoms than did S/L or L/L carriers.[87] Extending these findings, a group of German researchers reported increased expression of anxiety and negative affect in 18-month infants who had an S/S variant of 5HTTLPR and insecure attachment to their mothers. By contrast, infants with the same genotype who were securely attached expressed less negative emotion in response to a strange situation than the ones with L/S or even the L/L genotype.[88] Therefore, the presence of social support moderated the interaction between 5HTT polymorphism and maltreatment in children, and environmental disaster in adults. Low-expressing gene carriers who benefited from good social support had attenuated response to adversity and were less likely to develop depressive symptomatology, compared with those who lacked such support.[89,90]

A human study focusing on the epigenetic modification of 5HTT-related gene (5HTTLPR) noted that complete or partial methylation of the corresponding histone substantially reduced the 5HTT activity.[91] This is of particular interest since alleles of 5HTTLPR, a 5HTT-linked polymorphic region, have been associated with a number of different neuropsychiatric conditions, including depression, bipolar and anxiety disorders, chronic pain, fibromyalgia, attention-deficit/hyperactivity disorder, insomnia, and substance abuse. Therefore, the genetic influence on 5HTT expression can be modified by the epigenetic alterations in response to life circumstances.

Another study assessed depressed mood in a group of women during the second and third trimesters of pregnancy, using the Edinburgh Postnatal Depression Scale and the Hamilton Depression Rating Scale (HAMD-RS). The methylation status of 5HTTLPR and BDNF-related genes was assessed in third-trimester maternal peripheral leukocytes and in umbilical cord leukocytes collected from their infants at birth. A gene regulating methylenetetrahydrofolate reductase (MTHFR), an enzyme with a key role in the synthesis of methyl group donors (and therefore influential in epigenetic methylation), was also studied. Future mothers with the MTHFR 677T (less functional) allele had greater second-trimester depressed mood, which was associated with decreased maternal and infant 5HTT promoter methylation.[92] The less-functional genetic variant of the 5HTT promoter was inadequately silenced. These findings suggest that maternal depression via altered epigenetic processes may contribute to developmental programming of infant behavior in utero.

In a separate study, adoptees, now in their late thirties, experienced a greater sense of loss and trauma if their less functional 5HTTLPR "S" allele was lightly methylated or, conversely, if their high-functioning L/L allele was silenced by heavy methylation.[93] Cumulatively, this research broadens our focus from purely gene–environment interactions to include a very significant role that environmentally driven epigenetic modulation may play in the etiology of depression

A number of studies have examined the relationship between 5HTTLPR polymorphisms and antidepressant response, with equivocal results. A large meta-analysis of 28 studies with 5,408 participants found no significant relationship between individuals with S/S genotype and those with S/L or L/L genotypes in antidepressant response or remission from MDD.[94] Other meta-analyses have offered conflicting conclusions. One reported a significant association of the 5HTTLPR S/S allele and lower remission rate. Additionally patients with S/S and S/L genotypes also had reduced response rates.[95] Furthermore, an earlier study reported threefold greater risk of reaching nonremission after 12 weeks of antidepressant treatment in patients with homozygous S/S genotype compared with all other genotypes.[96] Moreover, "core" and somatic anxiety symptoms in patients with the s/s genotype have had slower response to selective 5HT reuptake inhibitor (SSRI) treatment than do those with L/L and S/L genotypes.[97] The relationship between an antidepressant response and 5HTTLPR genotype can be further influenced by other factors. Huezo-Diaz and colleagues reported that depressed males who were L/L carriers, compared with those with different genetic variants, had significantly greater improvement in response to SSRI treatment.[98] A large randomized longitudinal study noted an intriguing interplay among preceding stressful life events, 5HTTLPR polymorphism, and differential response to an SSRI versus a predominantly noradrenergic antidepressant (nortriptyline). In general, a recent stressful event predicted a better response to escitalopram (an SSRI), while response to nortriptyline was unaffected by the presence of stress. Paradoxically, if depressed patients who have experienced a stressful event are homozygous for S-allele, they will actually have a reduced response to the SSRI, compared with those with other genotypes, while the response to nortriptyline will remain unineffected.[99] So potential reason for the discrepant findings may be the lack of control of relevant variables, such as gender or the precipitating effect of stress on depressive episodes.

Additionally, a study of predominantly persistently depressed patients, found the highest CSF levels of the metabolites for serotonin (5HIAA) and DA (homovanillic acid) in patients who were S/S carriers and the lowest in L/L group.[17] Several studies have found elevation of CSF monoamine metabolites in depressed patients, which most often normalized after several weeks of antidepressant treatment.[100–102] A most likely explanation for this phenomenon would suggest that the state of depression is accompanied by inefficient monoamine signaling (reflected in the high transmitter turnover and thus elevated metabolite levels), which may be ameliorated with successful antidepressant therapy. Patients with S/S genotype compared with L/L patients also experienced 9.5 times higher incidence of agitation and 3.5 times higher frequency of insomnia in the context of SSRI treatment but no difference in the incidence of other side effects.[11]

In conclusion, 5HTTLPR polymorphisms have been associated with alterations in 5HT signaling and, consequently, the sensitivity of 5HT receptors. Due to interactions of 5HT with other neurotransmitter systems, metabolic rates of other monoamines are also influenced. As we know, neural activity in the neural pathway is the key regulator of neurotrophic activity. Therefore it is not surprising that several limbic and paralimbic areas, such as amygdala, hippocampus, ACC, vmPFC, posterior cingulate cortex, dlPFC, and thalamus, have altered structure and function influenced by 5HTTLPR polymorphisms. Since these areas are involved in regulation of mood and stress response, it is no surprise that interaction with stress and early-life adversity increases the likelihood of depression in individuals with the less functional 5HTTLPR allele. Behaviorally, 5HTTLPR polymorphisms have been associated with greater harm avoidance, neuroticism, and propensity toward rumination. Some data suggest that the lower-functioning S-allele may be linked with a propensity toward collectivism, which may prove to be advantageous in nurturing and supportive environments. The same allele is also associated with more readily activated inflammatory response, another feature that may have provided evolutionary benefits in the historical context. Finally, 5HTTLPR polymorphisms may influence antidepressant response and incidence of adverse reactions to medications in some depressed patients.

Polymorphism of Genes Regulating MAO

A very intricate and carefully designed study examined the relationship between monoamine oxidase A (MAOA) and temperamental traits in healthy volunteers. Researchers reported that carriers of the low-expressing allele (MAO-L) had deficient regulation in the rACC–amygdala circuit. To compensate for faulty communication between amygdala and rACC, the vmPFC becomes involved and "overconnected" with the amygdala. These are the brain areas that have a prominent role in social cognition, including theory of mind (being able to see things from someone else's perspective), empathy, moral reasoning, and social decision making. Men (there was a genetic dimorphism) who were MAO-L carriers showed a correlation between amygdala and vmPFC connectivity, as well as a greater sensitivity to threat cues and lower sensitivity to cues that promote prosocial behavior.[103] Interestingly, the impact of MAOA polymorphism on the vmPFC–rACC–amygdala circuit is a relatively specific functional "fingerprint," as it has not been observed in conjunction with COMT polymorphisms, for example.

An important interaction between the low-expressing MAO-L allele and early adversity has also been repeatedly reported in the literature. One study found that polymorphisms of the MAOA gene interacted with maltreatment with adverse impact on children's mental health, especially in males.[104] Another study reported a greater risk for antisocial personality disorder and alcoholism in a group of sexually abused women who are homozygous for MAO-L allele, compared with those who had the MAO-H allele. Furthermore, other women who were homozygous for MAOA-L but had no prior history of sexual abuse showed no increase in psychopathology.[105]

Unlike the previously prescribed psychopathology, which is a product of interaction of adversity with the MAO-L allele, MDD has been associated with the MAO-H allele. Depressed MAO-H carriers tend to have compromised amygdala–PFC (dlPFC, dorsal anterior cingulate, vlPFC) connectivity and a greater illness duration and severity.[106]

COMT Gene Polymorphisms

There are several variables that introduce significant complexity into interpretation of influence of COMT (see table 4.1) polymorphisms on neural structure and function. COMT is a catabolic enzyme involved in degradation of dopamine (DA), epinephrine, and norepinephrine (NE). A common SNP of the COMT gene, Val-158Met is by far the best studied. The Val/Val COMT allele is associated with approximately 35–50 percent greater enzyme activity compared with the Met/Met allele,[107] and therefore lower DA, as well as (most likely compensatory) increased Dopamine-1 cortical receptor density.[108] The Val and Met alleles are almost evenly distributed in the general population in Europe and North America. There is an important gender difference in COMT activity due to interaction with estrogen. At least in the periphery of the body, estrogen diminishes COMT activity by approximately 30 percent.[109] Women are reported to have a higher tonic (basal, sustained firing rate) and lower phasic (altered firing rate in response to a specific stimulus) DA levels. Striatal DA is higher in females, along with diminished Dopamine-2 receptor activity (most likely compensatory).[110] It is questionable if estrogen's influence on COMT activity is sufficient to explain the gender difference. Despite the putative hormonal influence on enzyme activity, there are no gender-related differences in COMT protein levels. Furthermore, differences in the COMT activity were noted in the periphery of the body but not in the central nervous system (CNS). Moreover, there is an age-related increase in COMT activity in men between the third and fifth decade of life.[110] There are also important regional differences in the COMT impact on DA levels. Unlike striatum, cortex is virtually devoid of DA transporters (DAT), so COMT-mediated catabolism is the primary mechanism of DA removal from the synapses. As we would anticipate, COMT is responsible for 60 percent of DA metabolism in the PFC, as opposed to 15 percent in the striatum.[109]

The COMT Val158Met polymorphism has a significant impact on hippocampal and prefrontal gray matter volume.[111] Replicated studies have reported larger hippocampal gray matter volume in Met carriers compared with Val genotypes and, conversely, greater dlPFC and PFC volumes in individuals with the Val/Val genotype.[111–113] Several lines of evidence suggest that there is an inverted-U relationship between DA levels in the PFC and cognitive performance. Both inadequate and excessive DA levels are associated with suboptimal cognitive function.

Additionally, stress is known to increase PFC DA levels. Gender and stress most likely interact in modulating the cognitive performance. Men, but not women, have been reported to perform better in mildly stressful situations, such as the ones involved in routine cognitive tasks.[109] Not surprisingly, studies have noted better cognitive performance in Met/Met (higher PFC DA) males and Val/Val (lower PFC DA) females.[109] Met carriers, as we have already mentioned, have a higher tonic and lower phasic DA activity that translates into greater executive function and working memory but, at the same time, decreased neural network flexibility.[114] Paradoxically, Val carriers manifest greater PFC activity compared with Met carriers during a simple working memory task, most likely due to the low-DA-related cortical inefficiency.[115] Additionally, the Met allele has been associated with an increased limbic (hippocampus, amygdala, and thalamus) and cortical (vlPFC and dlPFC) reactivity to unpleasant stimuli and altered connectivity between the amygdala and the PFC.[116] Anxiety, increased parahippocampal response to fearful faces, cortisol response to social stress, and ventral striatal and anterior temporal cortical response to reward stimuli have all been associated with the Met (higher DA) relative to the Val allele.[9,107,113,117] Given that stress increases DA and that women have a lower COMT activity (translating into higher DA), will there be a gender effect in activation of limbic areas caused by negative stimuli? The answer is yes: women who are Val carriers manifest a "dose-related" (greater with the higher number of Val alleles) increase in amygdala and temporal pole activity in response to fearful and angry faces.[118,119]

How do these genetically influenced neurophysiological tendencies translate into predilection for depression? Although a lot of information is still missing, there are some interesting, and at first glance mutually opposing, indications stemming from relevant research. One study reported the relationship between the Val/Val genotype in males (very active COMT, thus lower synaptic DA levels) and increased negative/decreased positive emotionality compared with the Met/Met genotype. Surprisingly, an opposite but nonsignificant trend was observed in women (women have less COMT activity, thus relatively higher DA levels).[120] Another study found an interaction between the COMT polymorphism and genes influencing the DA transporter (DAT1) in shaping the positive emotionality. Subjects with Val/Val COMT genotype who were 9-repeat homozygous (9R/9R) for DAT1 (associated with lesser transcriptional efficacy) manifested greater positive emotionality and externalizing tendencies, compared with the other variances of these genes.[121]

How do we reconcile these ostensibly conflicting reports? We have to remind ourselves of the regional differences in the regulation of DA transmission. As we have previously mentioned, COMT has the greatest impact in the PFC, where there are relatively few DA uptake sites (DAT). In contrast, the greatest abundance of DAT is in the striatum and midbrain. While the Val/Val COMT genotype may lead to the more rapid metabolism, and therefore less synaptic DA, decreased

DAT density (less uptake) may compensate by increasing the transmitter availability. This is an exciting example of genetic epistasis (interaction between the two polymorphisms) that may produce an adaptive regional DA balance.

Now that we have reviewed the evidence of the COMT polymorphism influence on transmission, neural structure and function, let's examine its potential role in etiology of MDD. As you may already expect, genetic data concerning the role of COMT polymorphisms in MDD are complex and conflicting. Several studies have reported an association between the Val COMT allele and depression, especially in the interaction with the early adversity and male gender.[122–124] Other researchers have noted an increased frequency of Met/Met and Met/Val genotypes in depressed population, especially in context of childhood problems,[125] as well as a relationship between the Met COMT allele, subjective experience of stress, and increased epinephrine and cortisol in response to stress in healthy controls but not in depressed patients![126] Another study described a relationship between maternal depression and early-life adversity and subsequent depression in the probands, but no influence of the COMT polymorphism.[127] Several studies have reported a relationship between Val/Val COMT genotypes and significantly reduced response to a variety to antidepressants, including SSRIs, 5HT-NE reuptake inhibitors (SNRIs), tricyclic antidepressants, and mirtazapine, compared with other COMT genotypes.[123,128,129]

In conclusion, COMT polymorphisms most likely have a complex and varied relationship with MDD etiology and treatment response, moderated by age, gender, genetic epistasis, stress level, and interaction with the early-life adversity.

Other Genes Involved in Regulating Monoamine Transmission

Multiple studies have associated enhanced 5HT2A frontolimbic binding with neuroticism and the vulnerability for developing depression in healthy adults.[130] Despite these results, a lack of clarity remains regarding the role of 5HT2A alleles in the risk of depression. Several studies have associated C/C alleles with a greater risk, although some researchers have also noted an increased risk in T/T carriers, while others still have found no association between 5HT2A polymorphisms and the risk of depression.[131] Could it be that complex gene–gene and gene–environment interactions determine the influence of 5HT2A polymorphisms on the risk of developing depression? A large Finnish study reported an increased risk of depressive symptoms in urban C-homozygous individuals; conversely, the T allele conveyed a greater risk in the rural setting but not in suburban or urban environments.[132] Is it possible that T-allele carriers derive benefit from the greater population density in urban setting by availing themselves of social supports? Interestingly, a separate study by the same group noted that the same 5HT2A T/T allele, in the presence of high maternal nurturance was associated with lower depressive symptoms compared with the C/C genotype, consistent with the notion that "vulnerability" genes may have been maintained in the human gene pool because they are "opportunity" genes, given the proper environmental exposure.[131] Future genetic studies would likely have more consistent findings if they accounted for gene–gene interactions and environmental variables, such as urbanicity, gender, and nurturance. Polymorphisms of the 5HT2A gene have also been associated with antidepressant response, especially in patients who have experienced childhood trauma.[133,134] Variation in 5HT2A receptor gene also interacts with race and ethnicity in determining the antidepressant response.[135,136]

5HT1A receptors are densely distributed in nuclei raphae (principal serotonergic nuclei) and in cortical and limbic structures. While the receptors in nuclei raphae have a presynaptic location and act as autoreceptors, impeding 5HT release, the ones in limbic and cortical areas are postsynaptic[137,] and regulate GABA, glutamate and cholinergic signaling in the corticolimbic circuits. An rs6295 C/G variant of the 5HT1A gene promoter region HTR1A has been found to significantly influence receptor expression and function. Presence of the 5HT1A G-allele has been associated with a greater expression of the presynaptic receptors and hence reduced serotonergic transmission.[137] Polymorphisms of the 5HT1A gene have additionally been linked with increased amygdala activation in functional MRI studies, a feature that has been previously connected with predilection for MDD.[138] Furthermore, 5HT1A expression as measured by receptor binding potential negatively correlated with stressed plasma cortisol levels and inflammatory response (reflected by IL-6 levels) in MDD patients.[139] Extant literature suggests that G-allele carriers, compared with carriers of other 5HT1A variants, have a greater risk of developing depression and a poorer response to antidepressants.[140] While some studies reported a direct association between the 5HT1A G-allele and MDD, others have found no such relationship.[140,141]

Perhaps surprisingly, a report indicated a gene × gene × environment interaction, whereby individuals with high-expressing the 5HTTLPR LL genotype (usually associated with lower risk of MDD) and 5HT1A GG genotype had an approximately fourfold greater risk of developing depression when facing a prominent negative life event relative to those carrying the 5HTTLPR SS genotype and 5HT1A CC genotype.[142] This may be an example of genetic epistasis, whereby interaction of 5HTTLPR and 5HT1A genotypes resulting in diminished serotonergic transmission predisposes individuals toward developing depression in stressful circumstances, when serotonergic regulation of corticolimbic circuits is required. In addition to a direct influence of 5HT1A polymorphisms on the risk of developing MDD, interaction between the 5HT1A GG genotype and BDNF Met variant has also been associated with the risk of treatment-resistant depression.[140] Other studies have reported a relationship between the 5HT1A GG genotype and diminished response and remission rates following SSRI and SNRI antidepressant treatment.[137]

The tryptophan hydroxylase (TPH) gene(s) has also been implicated in the etiology of MDD. A TPH2 gene variant expresses an enzyme with compromised catalytic activity, resulting in impaired 5HT synthesis and reduced 5HT levels in the adult brain.[143,144] While several studies identified an association between the less efficient TPH2 allele and the amygdala reactivity,[145] MDD, and suicidality,[143,146] others have found no such relationship.[147,148] It appears that the low-expressing TPH2 allele may also modulate response to SSRIs, especially in the presence of early adversity or childhood trauma. Hypothetically, the less-functioning TPH2 allele, and consequent diminished 5HT signaling, may negatively influence early neural development, making individuals more susceptible to the harmful effects of early trauma and less responsive to subsequent SSRI treatment.[144,149,150]

Genes regulating the NE transporter (NET) and DAT and their roles in susceptibility toward MDD and treatment response to antidepressants have also received some attention. While a few studies have detected a direct association between NET polymorphism and MDD, others have not.[151] A GG genotype for the NET G1287A polymorphism has been associated with more robust NE turnover and elevated CSF levels of the principal NE metabolite, 3-methoxy-4-hydroxyph enylglycol, possibly reflecting less efficient NE signaling in the healthy individuals homozygous for this allele.[152] The same genotype was also linked with a higher depression risk in females living in a rural environment in China, especially if they have encountered recent stressful events.[151] Interestingly, the same study related NET AA and AG genotypes with increased risk of depression in urban women. The depressed NET GG homozygotes were also more likely to respond to SNRI antidepressants than to SSRIs. Furthermore, GG homozygous patients suffering from treatment-resistant depression had a more robust response to the combination of olanzapine and fluoxetine (believed to enhance all three monoamines: 5HT, NE, and DA), compared with individuals bearing other genetic variants.[153,154] Conversely, depressed NET AA-homozygous carriers had a lesser response to milnicipran (a predominantly noradrenergic antidepressant) relative to those with other genotypes.[155] Emerging evidence also supports a role of DAT polymorphisms in determining the response to several different antidepressant agents.[155,156]

The Role of Genes Regulating Neurotrophic Factors

Psychiatric literature abounds with analogies comparing the functions and structure of the brain to a computer. Anatomical structures, including their white matter "wiring," are often likened to the hardware, while our psychological processes and temperamental tendencies are commonly compared to software. Unfortunately, these analogies are in some respects woefully inadequate. In the human brain hardware and software are inextricably intertwined. Persistently elevated activity in a neural pathway triggers the mechanism that regulates neuroplasticity, thereby transforming the participating neural components in the service of facilitating future information processing.[157] Therefore, a functional change has precipitated an adaptive structural modification, which further elaborates and extends the initial change in the signaling pattern.

BDNF, one of the most important regulators of neuroplasticity, is in the center of these transformations. In addition to its role in regulating the neuroplastic processes, BDNF also acts as a resilience factor, assists the maturation and differentiation of the nerve cell progenitors,[158] and even acts as an immunomodulator in the periphery of the body.[159] BDNF is released from neurons in two forms: pro-BDNF and its chemically abbreviated version, mature BDNF. Pro-BDNF and mature BDNF act as yin and yang, participating in opposing functions: pro-BDNF binds to the p75 receptor, initiating apoptosis, or shriveling of the neurons, while mature BDNF has primary affinity for the tropomyosin receptor kinase-B (TrkB) receptor, which mediates neuroplasticity and resilience.[157,160] The gene regulating BDNF synthesis has two different alleles, depending on the valine-to-methionine substitution at position 66 of the pro-domain, leading three different genotypes: Val/Val, Val/Met, and Met/Met. Met variants are accompanied by decreased BDNF distribution in the dendrites and impairment in regulated secretion.[160] Therefore, BDNF genotype also likely plays an important role in the etiopathogenesis of MDD.[161,162]

Given the role of BDNF in neuroplasticity and early development, one would anticipate structural differences in the Met-allele carriers. Indeed, the Met allele has been associated with structural brain changes common both in healthy controls and in patients with MDD. These include reduced gray matter volume in dlPFC, lateral orbital PFC, amygdala, and hippocampus.[163–166] The Met BDNF allele predicted not only change in hippocampal structure in healthy subjects but also function. The Met-allele carriers had impaired performance on the hippocampal-related memory tasks, as well as more pronounced age-related decline in the reasoning skills.[167–169] Hippocampal volume is more affected by the Met allele in depressed patients than in healthy controls, indicating an interaction between genotype and the disease process.[170] Furthermore, the larger hippocampal volume in depressed homozygous Val/Val individuals has been associated with a shorter time to reach remission, reflecting a relationship between genotype, hippocampal size, and treatment outcome.[171] The overlap between the brain areas that have the highest concentration of BDNF mRNA, and therefore suffer the most pronounced structural reductions, associated with the BDNF Met allele and the structural abnormalities most often implicated in the pathophysiology of MDD by the imaging studies is striking.[160,172,173]

The hippocampus is also one of the major hubs in the brain involved with HPA axis regulation. It is therefore not surprising that depressed patients with two Met alleles were more likely to have a disturbed HPA feedback control and a greater incidence of cortisol nonsuppression during the dexamethasone/corticotropin-releasing hormone test than the Val carriers.[174] Furthermore, the BDNF Met allele may have an impact on the connectivity of the major brain networks.

The salience network (SN), comprising the thalamus, basal ganglia, limbic structures (amygdala, ventral striatum), and paralimbic areas (ACC and insula), provides information about important changes in the internal and external environment, encoded into the flow of emotions. The default mode network (DMN), anchored by posterior cingulate, vmPFC and dorsomedial PFC, participates in self-reflection, accessing autobiographical memories, social interactions, and future planning. Posterior parietal cortex, dlPFC, and vlPFC are the main components of the executive network (EN), which is involved with prioritization, problem solving, working memory, effortful sustained attention, and monitoring the outcomes of our adaptive behaviors.[175,176] In physiological circumstances or the absence of a pathological state, influx of emotions from the SN structures, signaling an important change in the environment, should put DMN deliberations on hold and engage EN-related problem-solving faculties.

However, in the context of MDD a different scenario takes place. SN and DMN are "short-circuited," presumably generating melancholy ruminations, in addition to the absence of effective EN-mediated coping.[175,176] The BDNF Met-allele carriers (Met/Met and Met/Val), compared with Val/Val homozygotes, had lower functional connectivity in the EN and DMN brain structures. Moreover, Met-allele carriers showed increased interconnectedness between the limbic and paralimbic SN areas, coupled with diminished connections with the EN cortical areas, relative to Val/Val individuals.[177] Interestingly, even the propensity to ruminate in the stressful circumstances, one of the key clinical characteristics of MDD,[86,178] involving aberrant connectivity between the SN and DMN, may be under genetic control. Even healthy individuals possessing BDNF Met alleles and 5HTTLPR S-alleles (both implicated in conferring susceptibility toward MDD), under conditions of life stress, respond with ruminations, which are proportionate in magnitude with the number of risk alleles.[179] It is therefore more likely that individuals bearing BDNF Met alleles, due to less adaptive connectedness and altered structure and function of the principal limbic and executive cortical regions, may be more vulnerable to developing depression in the face of adversity. These suspicions are unfortunately confirmed by epidemiological and treatment studies, which report higher incidence of depression and compromised response to antidepressants in individuals with BDNF Met alleles.[180,181]

The impact of BDNF genes can also be observed at the cellular and molecular levels. BDNF has been shown to influence monoamine synthesis, metabolism, and the release. One study reported that several BDNF gene polymorphisms were associated with higher CSF concentrations of the principal NE metabolite, 3-met hoxy-4-hydroxyphenylglycol, reflecting inefficient NE transmission, also a common feature of MDD.[182] Dwivedi et al. reported altered genetic expression of BDNF and its TrkB receptor in the hippocampus and PFC of depressed suicide victims.[183] Moreover, a large-scale GWAS with 706 adult participants has linked a gene responsible for coding for one of the BDNF receptors, neurotrophic tyrosine kinase receptor type 2, with increasing suicidal ideation during a course of anti-depressant treatment.[184] Further extending these findings, two separate research teams have found an association between polymorphisms of the pro-BDNF receptor p75 gene and suicide attempts in the depressed population, especially in individuals with early disease onset.[185,186]

In summary, it appears that BDNF genes impact neural function and structure at both macro- and microscopic levels, resulting in aberrant neural network communication and information processing, as well as compromised neurotransmission and neurotrophic signaling. In the face of adversity, anomalous genetic control of BDNF synthesis and release may compromise neuroplasticity and the complex interface between function and structure, resulting in an increased risk of depression.

The Role of Genes Regulating the HPA Axis in MDD

Dysregulation of the HPA axis is one of the central pathophysiological features of several stress-related disorders, including MDD, posttraumatic stress disorder, and various anxiety disorders.[187] Genetic variations of several regulatory components of the HPA axis have been implicated in the etiology of MDD, including receptor(s) for CRF, NR3C1 (the gene regulating neuron-specific corticosteroid receptor synthesis), FKBP5 (a regulator of glucocorticoid receptor complex), CRF-binding protein, and arginine-vasopressin receptor-1 (a potentiator of CRF signaling). Four peptide transmitters act on CRF receptors. CRF and urocortin 1 are agonists at CRF-1, while urocortin 1, 2, and 3, but not CRF, bind to the CRF-2 receptor.[187] The activity of CRF, and all of the urocortins, is restricted by their binding to CRF-binding protein. This binding protein is readily available in circulation and is expressed in several tissues, including brain (especially in pituitary, and in proximity to CRF pathways), heart, and lungs. CRF plays a regulatory role in both central and peripheral stress response systems. In addition to innervating the limbic areas, and its involvement in the emotional- and stress-response regulation, CRF neurons also project to the locus ceruleus (the cerebral NE hub). Furthermore, the CRF system exerts a local stimulatory influence on the adrenal gland, promoting corticosteroid synthesis and medullary catecholamine release.[187] Peripheral corticosteroids diminish CRF expression by providing a negative feedback via hippocampal and hypothalamic glucocorticoid receptors (GRs). Paradoxically, glucocorticoid activity in limbic areas, particularly the amygdala, enhances CRF signaling.[187] Another, short regulatory loop involves FKBP5. GR activation increases FKBP5 transcription. Greater quantities of FKBP5 desensitize GRs by decreasing ligand binding and translocation of the receptor complex to the cell nucleus. In other words, excessive glucocorticoids are capable of rapidly buffering their own signaling by muting the receptor response via the FKBP5 involvement.[188]

Cumulative genetic, epigenetic, and biochemical evidence suggests that there are several levels of disruption in the HPA regulation in MDD. Here we track the sequence of HPA disruptions and then discuss them individually. The initial phase of the stress response is associated with intense CRF signaling. Several studies have reported (a) elevation of CRF mRNA in the brains of depressed individuals, (b) greater CRF expression in the limbic areas, (c) increased CSF concentration of CRF, (d) an association between corticotropin-releasing hormone (CRH) receptor 1 (CRHR1) alleles and haplotypes and MDD, (e) an interaction between early-life adversity and CRHR1 polymorphisms, and (f) an influence of CRHR1 on the antidepressant response.[187,189,190] Furthermore, greater CRHR1-mediated signaling is associated with increased DA signaling in the amygdala (via D1 and Dopamine-5 receptors), with consequent elevation in glutamate input to mPFC, an area critically involved in the stress response and emotional regulation (described above). Additionally, CRHR1 signaling participates in regulation of NE and 5HT transmission, via CRF input to locus ceruleus (LC) and dorsal nuclei raphae (DNR), respectively.[189] Extending these findings, researchers reported an increased expression of arginine-vasopressin receptor-1 genes, potentially facilitating CRF transmission, combined with diminished expression of androgen receptors (mediating inhibition of CRF signaling), in the brains of depressed patients.[190] CRF elevation precipitates adrenocorticotropic hormone release from the pituitary gland, and eventually increased cortisol production in the cortex of adrenal gland. Cortisol elevation in the bloodstream provides a feedback to hippocampus and hypothalamus via GRs and mineralocorticoid receptors (MRs). Gene expression studies have noted increased expression of the MR gene in depressed patients. A change in MR/GR balance may contribute to the altered CRF transcription rate in MDD.[190] Multiple studies have provided evidence of the epigenetic modulation of the human neural GR gene (NR3C1) promoter, related to maternal depression,[191] childhood adversity (parental loss, maltreatment, and poor parental care),[192] childhood abuse,[193] and phosphorylation of the leukocyte GR in patients currently suffering from a depressive episode.[194] An interaction between polymorphisms of the FKBP5 gene (a regulator of GR sensitivity) and childhood adversity has also been implicated in the etiology of MDD.[195] Individuals homozygous for the FKBP5 T-allele are reported to have aberrant HPA regulation, a past history of more depressive episode recurrences, and more rapid response to antidepressants.[196] Moreover, an epigenetic × genetic × childhood trauma interaction involving FKBP5 has been reported. This complex interaction may predispose individuals toward a host of stress-related psychiatric disorders, including MDD and posttraumatic stress disorder.[188]

Numerous studies have established an association between CRHR1 polymorphisms and MDD and treatment response. Unmedicated depressed patients who are homozygous for the CRHR1 G-allele were reported to have an exaggerated subgenual ACC response to negative verbal stimuli relative to the individuals with other genotypes.[197] Abnormal subgenual ACC function, resulting in impaired emotional response to stress, is regarded as one of the central imaging correlates of MDD. Studies have provided evidence of direct association between a combination of CRHR1 alleles, GGT haplotype, and MDD.[198] A haplotype is a combination of three adjacent or jointly expressed SNPs, in this case composed of Guanine Guanine Thymine set. This set of genetic polymorphisms is typically inherited together from a single parent. Presence of CRHR1 A-allele was found to be protective from developing MDD in males with a history of childhood trauma,[199] TAT (thymine-adenine-thymine) haplotype was reported to be protective from developing MDD in two community cohorts of women reporting childhood maltreatment,[200] while a protective CRHR1 haplotype was associated with lesser depressive symptoms in a clinical sample of individuals who have experienced childhood abuse.[8] Furthermore, an epistatic interaction between CRHR1 TCA haplotype and the S-allele of the 5HTTLPR gene in individuals who have suffered childhood trauma predicted current depressive scores.[201]

Antidepressant response has also been linked to CRHR1 polymorphisms. Depressed Chinese patients with G/G genotype and homozygous GAG haplotype of the three SNPs had a better response to six weeks of fluoxetine therapy than did other genotypes. This was particularly true in MDD patients who experienced high anxiety.[202] Interestingly, researchers in the Sequenced Treatment Alternatives to Relieve Depression (STAR*D) study also reported lower remission rates and less reduction in depressive symptoms in response to citalopram therapy in CRH-binding protein T-allele carriers, effects that were also more pronounced in the patients suffering from anxious depression.[203] Carriers of the CRH-binding protein T-allele have diminished binding protein expression, which was associated with higher plasma CRF levels and greater GR resistance, both commonly accompanying MDD.

Childhood trauma, a known risk factor for stress-related disorders and Major Depression, has also been associated with allele-specific FKBP5 DNA demethylation. This epigenetic modification contributed to a greater FKBP5 transcription and elevated concentration, consequently producing GR resistance. Evidence suggests that these enduring epigenetic changes may occur only during the sensitive developmental period, as DNA methylation typically does not accompany adult trauma or recent life stress.[188] Thus, it is truly a gene × childhood trauma × epigenetic interaction that results in disease-predisposing HPA abnormalities, rather than a simpler gene × environment interaction to which disease risk was previously attributed.[188]

In conclusion, CRHR1 and FKBP5 polymorphisms have been directly associated with a direct risk of developing depression (even more pronounced in individuals exposed to childhood trauma), suicidal ideation in depressed patients, depression severity in males, age of onset and the seasonal pattern in females, and treatment response to antidepressants, especially in anxious depression.[189,204] Despite less then impressive evidence stemming from GWAS and linkage studies, candidate gene approaches have firmly established genes involved in HPA axis regulation as important etiological factors and major determinants of treatment response in Major Depression.[187]

Polymorphisms of Genes Involved in the Regulation of Inflammation and MDD

Recent years have witnessed burgeoning research into the role of inflammation as one of the key pathophysiological mechanism for a significant number of depressed patients. Inflammation is an integral component of the stress response, which is a known precipitant of depression. Additionally, proinflammatory cytokines have a profound impact on mood, HPA axis regulation, monoamine signaling, and regulation of neurotrophic factors and neuroplasticity.[205] Multiple lines of evidence support this notion: depressed patients tend to have higher levels of cytokines in their plasma and CSF; therapeutically administered interferon-alpha promotes symptoms that are indistinguishable from depression; and peripheral levels of stimulated inflammatory cytokines closely correlate with all of the cardinal depressive symptoms.[206,207] Furthermore, high levels of peripheral inflammatory molecules are associated with poorer response to antidepressant agents, possibly due to altered monoamine transporter function and less efficient monoamine signaling; conversely, successful antidepressant therapy tends to lower peripheral inflammatory modulators.[208] Further extending these findings, a postmortem study has found increased expression of a number of genes regulating inflammatory and anti-inflammatory cytokine signaling in the PFC of deceased depressed patients, relative to matched controls.[206] Additionally, polymorphisms of inflammation-related genes have been reported to confer susceptibility toward Major Depression and to effect antidepressant response.[209–211]

A high-expressing tumor necrosis factor-alpha (TNF) 308A allele, associated with elevation in levels of one of the principal inflammatory cytokines, was much more frequently identified in depressed patients than in healthy controls.[212] The same TNF allele has been linked with (a) diminished expression of the 5HTT, (b) compromised HPA regulation,[212] (c) impaired attention and cognitive processes in the healthy individuals,[213] (d) reversible depression-like behaviors caused by dim light in preclinical models,[214] (e) CNS inflammatory disorders,[215] and (f) incidence of depression in physically ill elderly patients.[216] Perhaps the strongest evidence linking TNF polymorphism with the risk of MDD comes from GWAS. The association between TNF and MDD was the only one in a large meta-analysis that remained significant, surviving all the corrections for multiple testing.[217] Conversely, the low-expressing TNF 308G allele, along with high-expressing IL-10 1082G allele (IL-10 is one of the main anti-inflammatory cytokines), has been associated with longevity.[218] A study that compared a sample of depressed patients and matched healthy controls found lower frequency of high-expressing IL-10 1082G allele and greater frequency of low-expressing A-allele in the depressed group.[219] In summary, preliminary evidence points to a potential role of genes regulating the synthesis of inflammatory mediators in etiopathogenesis of MDD and treatment response to antidepressants. Involvement of inflammatory genes does not appear to be specific to depression, as they have also been implicated in the etiology of bipolar disorder, CNS inflammatory conditions, and pain disorders.[173,219]

The Role of Glutamate and GABA Transmission-Related Genes in MDD

Glutamate and GABA represent the principal excitatory and inhibitory neurotransmitters in the CNS. Their presence in the brain is virtually ubiquitous. Although depression literature places a heavy emphasis on the role of monoamines in the etiology and treatment of this condition, it may be an opportune time to remind ourselves that glutamate- and GABA-operated neuronal circuits are indeed the primary targets of monoamine projections.[220] Emerging research suggests that we would be remiss not to include glial cells in our conversation about the role of glutamate and GABA in depression. Astroglia, the most numerous cell population in the brain, have the capacity to signal by releasing either glutamate or GABA. They also have a key role in restoring and maintaining the GABA/glutamate balance,[221] in part through utilization of the transporters capable of removing these transmitters from the synapse.[222,223] The glia–synaptic junction is an exchange space, where a rich "conversation" mediated by GABA, glutamate, and immune molecules takes place,[173,224] fundamentally influencing neural plasticity and resilience.[223] Interations between glutamate and inflammatory cytokines appear to be bidirectional, whereby inflammatory signals have the capacity to modulate glutamatergic signaling and vice versa.[225–227] One of the key transcription factors involved in GABA–glutamate–immune interaction,[223] nuclear factor kappa-beta, is also implicated in the regulation of glutamate uptake,[228] glutamate-mediated inflammatory signaling,[225] endocrine response,[229] neuroplasticity,[230] and neurogenesis.[231] It is therefore no surprise that we have a great interest in genetic regulation of GABA and glutamate and its role in etiopathogenesis of MDD.

Several postmortem studies have reported altered expression of GABA and glutamate transmission-related genes in depressed individuals and those who ended their life with suicide. Candidate genes implicated in the etiology of MDD —such as the ones regulating glutamate synthetase; high-affinity glial glutamate transporter; neuronal glutamate transporter; vesicular glutamate transporter; ionotropic glutamate receptors like N-methyl-D-aspartate (NMDA) (GRIN-1), α-amino-3-hydroxy-5-methyl-4-isoxazole propionic acid receptor (GRIA-1 and GRIA-3), and kainite (KA) (GRIK-1); and metabotropic glutamate receptors (GRM-1 and GRM-5)—have all shown altered expression in the brains of deceased depressed individuals.[232–234] One of these, GRIA-3, has also been implicated in antidepressant-associated suicidal tendencies.[232]

A meta-analysis of three large GWAS data sets, which comprised 4,346 cases and 4,430 matched controls, found a significant association between genes involved in glutamatergic synaptic transmission (especially GRM-7, the gene coding for metabotropic glutamate receptor 7) and MDD.[235] Genes coding for all four units composing the α-amino-3-hydroxy-5-methyl-4-isoxazole propionic acid receptor glutamate receptor (GRIA-1 to -4) have been associated with the risk of developing depression.[236,237] More specifically, GRIA-2 may be marginally associated with the age of onset of MDD, while GRIA-3 polymorphism may mediate the risk of developing depression in women who sleep less than eight hours a night.[236,237] A gene regulating synthesis of one of the subunits of the KA glutamatergic receptor (GRIK-4), and therefore presynaptic KA-mediated inhibition of glutamate release, has been reported to modulate hippocampal response to processing emotional facial expressions.[238] Given that GRIK-4 is highly expressed in the hippocampus, one of the brain formations most often implicated in pathophysiology of MDD,[239] but also in predicting treatment response, we would suppose that GRIK-4 polymorphisms may also be relevant in predicting the outcome of antidepressant therapy. Indeed, STAR*D study has reported an association between the marker alleles of the genes GRIK-4 and HTR2A (coding for the 5HT2A receptor) and a response to a 14-week course of the SSRI citalopram. Carriers of marker alleles of these two genes were 23 percent less likely to respond to SSRI treatment than participants who were endowed with other alleles.[133]

Similar to the studies that have found altered expression of glutamate-related genes in the brains of deceased depressed individuals, several studies have reported an association between the misexpression of the genes coding for that GABA-A receptor and GABA transporter, often accompanied by altered expression of the genes regulating astrocyte and oligodendrocyte function, in multiple brain areas of MDD patients.[221,232,233,240] Studies have also reported a relationship between polymorphisms of the genes coding for the subunits of the GABA-A receptor (alpha-1, -3, and -6 and gamma-2) and depression, especially in the female patients.[241,242] Another report has linked a polymorphism of the gene that transcribes for glutamic acid decarboxylase-67, an enzyme that regulates GABA synthesis from glutamine in neurons and astrocytes,[223] with Major Depression, anxiety disorders, and neuroticism.[243]

In summary, genes that regulate glutamate and GABA synthetic enzymes and receptor subunits have been linked with the risk of developing depression. Furthermore, GABA- and glutamate-regulating genes most likely have a substantial impact on neuroplasticity, neurogenesis, and immune and endocrine regulation in the context of MDD.

Other Candidate Genes Implicated in Etiology of MDD

The role of cannabinoid system in the etiology has also attracted some attention, given its role in the regulation of emotions and stress response. A cannabinoid receptor-1 gene polymorphism has been reported to predict neuroticism and depressive symptoms following recent negative life events and child abuse.[244,245]

Neuropeptide Y (NPY) is widely distributed in the brain. It is coreleased with a variety of other neurotransmitters, including GABA, in the cerebral cortex. Preclinical models have attributed anxiolytic properties to stress-associated release of NPY in the amygdala. Low-expressing NPY genotypes were reported with greater frequency in depressed individuals relative to other genetic variations.[246] Interestingly enough, this NPY polymorphism is one of the few that can claim a GWAS-established relationship with MDD.[217]

Several genes that regulate intracellular signaling cascades have also been linked with the risk of MDD. After monoamine neurotransmitters engage the cell-surface receptors, a sequence of events takes place. Many of the monoamine receptors belong to the G-protein-coupled receptor family. Binding of a ligand to the G-protein-coupled receptors commonly triggers activation of second messengers. Cyclical adenosine and guanosine monophosphate (cAMP and cGMP) are second messengers activated by hormones, growth factors, and neurotransmitters. Typically the role of the second messengers is to regulate transcription factors, one of which is cAMP response element binding protein 1 (CREB1). After they have accomplished their goal, and the signal is delivered to the genome, second messengers are broken down by catalytic enzymes. Phosphodiesterases (PDEs) are a family of 11 enzymes charged with responsibility of interrupting the cAMP- and cGMP-mediated signaling and therefore regulating the gene transcription initiated by extracellular signals.[247] Two genes regulating PDE-9A and PDE-11A have been associated with propagating susceptibility to MDD, while PDE-1A and PDE-11A also influence antidepressant response. Preclinical studies point to the role of CREB in cognition, long-term memory, and neuroplasticity. Downstream gene targets of this transcription factor are involved with regulation of emotions, circadian rhythms, HPA activity, and cell survival and repair.[248] Polymorphisms of CREB1 gene have been directly associated with the risk of depression (especially in women), expression of anger in MDD, early disease onset, and greater recurrence of depressive episodes.[248–250]

Conversion of dietary folate or dihydrofolate (a form of vitamin B) into the active metabolite of folate, 5-methyltetrahydrofolate (5MTHF, a.k.a. L-methylfolate) is to a significant extent regulated by the enzyme methyltetrahydrofolate reductase (MTHFR). 5MTHF is a predominant form of folate capable of crossing the blood–brain barrier and entering the CNS, where it participates in remethylation of the amino acid metabolite homocysteine, creating methionine. A downstream metabolite of methionine, S-adenosylmethionine, is involved in a number of biochemical methyl donation reactions, including the ones leading to monoamine neurotransmitter synthesis. In the context of an inadequate supply of 5MTHF, CSF levels of S-adenosylmethionine may be decreased, subsequently interfering with monoamine transmission, thus adding to the disease process of depression.[251]

The presence of adequate MTHFR activity and 5MTHF concentrations in the CNS seems to be particularly important in the circumstances of heightened inflammation and oxidative metabolism often encountered in the context of MDD. In such conditions, tetrahydrobiopterin (BH4), an essential enzyme cofactor for the synthesis of DA, NE, 5HT, and subsequently melatonin, but also highly labile and sensitive to nonenzymatic oxidation, becomes irreversibly converted to 7,8-dihydroxanthopterin or reversibly to BH2 (7,8-dihydrobiopterine).[252,253] Furthermore, a study that examined patients treated with an 11-week course of interferon-alpha, which is notoriously associated with onset of depression and anxiety, reported significant increases in the CSF BH2 concentrations in patients relative to healthy controls. In the same group of patients, elevation in inflammatory IL-6, strongly correlated with the declining BH4 levels in the CSF, while decreased DA levels were associated with the intensity of fatigue.[254] In further support of these findings, postmortem studies have documented reduced BH4 concentration in the brains of depressed patients, albeit not consistently.[255]

The proper function of MTHFR, and thus availability of 5MTHF, is particularly important in the setting of elevated oxidative stress and inflammation, necessitating that BH4 be reconstituted from BH2.[252–254] Not surprisingly, the role of the two polymorphisms of MTHFR gene (C677T and A1298C) in depression has received considerable attention. Whole-genome linkage scans and meta-analyses have found evidence of association of the 677T-homozygous MTHFR variant and recurrent depression, especially in females.[256,257] Large meta-analyses have also reported that the 677T-homozygous MTHFR variant may be a genetic vulnerability shared among schizophrenia, bipolar disorder, and MDD.[258] While the largest study found a link between MTHFR 677T-homozygous status and MDD, two smaller studies did not, possibly because they were underpowered.[258,259] Other research has reported a link between the MTHFR C677T polymorphism and loneliness, but not depression, in elderly males[260] and association between white matter intensities, cognitive decline and depression in elderly patients.[261] Furthermore, the presence of MTHFR and 5HTTLPR polymorphisms has also been reported to moderate the link between depression and the general health status in a population of elderly patients.[262] Relationship between MTHFR polymorphism and antidepressant response is as equivocal as its direct relationship with the disease state. While an open-label study found no relationship between MTHFR polymorphism and response to fluoxetine,[263] a larger randomized trial reported an association between MTHFR A-C haplotype and antidepressant response, particularly in males treated with SNRIs.[264] A-C haplotype is a set of two jointly inherited SNPs—adenine and cytosine are the bases involved.

A GWAS has identified CACNA1C, a gene that codes for the a1C subunit of the Cav1.2 voltage-dependent L-type calcium channel (LTCC), as a shared risk locus for depression, schizophrenia, autism spectrum disorders, bipolar disorder, and attention deficit hyperactivity disorder.[265] Additionally. both preclinical and human studies have identified SNPs in the CACNA1C gene as mediators of interaction between sex and genotype in the pathophysiology of mood disorders. Furthermore, CACNA1C may influence the relationship between affective disorders and migraines in women,[266] as well as (a) the difference in the mean gray matter volume, (b) verbal fluency,[267] (c) increased hippocampal and amygdala activity during emotional processing,[268] and (d) increased prefrontal activity during working memory tasks (indicative of inefficient function) in subjects who have no diagnosable psychiatric illness.[269] Genetically regulated decreases in Cav1.2 function may have a protective role in the development of mood disorders. Moreover, relevant to the interaction of CACNA1C and gender, physiological levels of estrogen potentiate LTCCs in vitro.

In some instances neuroprotective effects of estrogen on glutamate-induced excitotoxicity and cell death have been linked to L-type calcium channels.[267] The L-type calcium channels integrate and couple local calcium increases to cyclic CREB-dependent gene transcription via activation of intracellular signaling cascades. Thus, genetic regulation of LTCCs may be implicated in the modulation of synaptic transmission. Additionally, calcium influx through LTCCs, combined with calcium influx through NMDA receptors, controls BDNF synthesis. More specifically, calcium flow through LTCCs preferentially activates BDNF promoter I, while BDNF promoter III is equally driven by LTCCs and NMDA receptors.[268] Interestingly enough, CACNA1C is also involved in regulation of immune function, a finding particularly relevant in view of immune dysregulation that often accompanies MDD.[270]

In summary, evidence suggests that selected genes may influence the risk of MDD by acting sequentially. For example, CACNA1C genes responsible for regulating calcium influx may interact downstream with the ones that control cAMP, PDE, and CREB, thereby jointly influencing cerebral function and structure, possibly by mediating synaptic function and neuroplasticity. Other links may be less obvious. Obesity, CACNA1C, other genes regulating immune response, and MTHFR polymorphisms may combine forces in modulating monoamine neurotransmission in the key brain networks involved in the regulation of mood and stress response. Future research may provide us with insights into the interactions of gene networks and their role in the etiology of depression. In the meantime, we have to deal with vexing variability in associations of genes influencing intracellular signaling and neurotransmission with MDD. The elusive relationship between the genes and depression may be influenced by the study design, power, epigenetic modulation, genetic epistasis, and interactions with environmental factors.

Genetic Epistasis

It would be ludicrous to assume that the structural and functional consequences of a specific genotype can be observed in isolation. Genes and their products engage in myriad complex interactions, called epistasis. Our brief review of the role of genetic epistasis in etiology of MDD is not meant to be exhaustive or comprehensive. On the contrary, we aim to provide only a modest "tasting menu" of the types of consequences related to the genetic epistasis that may be germane to our discussion of the MDD etiopathogenesis. We provide only a few of the illustrative examples. Several reports have addressed the epistasis between the BDNF alleles and 5HTTLPR alleles, which influence their respective synthesis and the efficiency of the related signaling systems. In a seminal study, Kaufman et al. reported that the S-allele of 5HTTLPR, associated with deficient 5HT signaling, and the BDNF Met-allele of the Val66Met SNP act in a synergetic fashion by increasing the risk of developing depression in a group of children exposed to early-life adversity.[271] The additive effect of the two risk polymorphisms was mitigated by supportive environment, resulting in lower depression scores.[271] Two other studies have replicated these findings, reporting higher depressive symptoms in adults with lower-functioning BDNF and 5HTTLPR genes who have also suffered childhood adversity.[272,273]

On the other hand, Pezawas and colleagues reported an epistatic interaction between the 5HTTLPR S-allele and the BDNF Met allele pointing in a very different direction. In a volumetric MRI study of 111 healthy, nondepressed, individuals, they found that, contrary to expectations, the BDNF Met allele (which commonly increases depression risk) provided protection to circuitry linking amygdala and rACC. As noted above, this circuitry, which is involved in emotional modulation and stress responses, tends to function suboptimally and be reduced in volume in 5HTTLPR S-allele carriers. However, these abnormalities are significantly muted in 5HTTLPR Se carriers who also carry the BDNF Met allele, because this allele made amygdala–rACC circuitry relatively insensitive to 5HT signaling, therefore protecting these individuals from the rACC gray matter volume loss.[274] This finding may potentially have significant clinical implications, given that the rACC also plays a role in pain signaling and predicts treatment response to antidepressants.[275] Other epigenetic interactions influencing limbic activity and treatment response have been reported. For example, the combination of the 5HTTLPR S-allele with a functionally less competent allele of the 5HT1A receptor gene has been associated with exaggerated amygdala reactivity in medicated MDD patients.[276] These apparently contradictory findings, caution us to consider the consequences of genetic epistasis in a wider context, not only as gene × gene interactions, but also as potentially gene × gene × environment × gender × ethnicity × age interactions, maybe even including other social modifiers, such as urbanicity.

Studies have also reported that 5HTT, COMT, and MAOA polymorphisms have a convergent effect and interact with gender, exerting an influence on the HPA axis response to psychological stress and endocrine challenges.[277] Individuals with less functional 5HTT, COMT, and MAOA alleles had blunted baseline adrenocorticotropic hormone and cortisol responses to dexamethasone/corticotropin challenge, reflective of potential susceptibility toward MDD. This study also implies that monoamines play an important role in neuroendocrine homeostasis and maintenance of health.[277] An counterintuitive interplay between 5HTTLPR and COMT polymorphisms and chronically stressful family environment has been reported. Combination of 5HTTLPR LL genotype with COMT VV genotype (previously considered as a risk for developing MDD) was found to be protective from developing depression by the age 20 in individuals who at age 15 reported high family stress in their interview and in a response to the structured questionnaire.[278] However, in the presence of a single COMT Met allele, all 5HTTLPR genotype groups were susceptible to developing depression if exposed to chronic family stress. Studies of this type may shed some light on the inconsistent reports about the relationship between 5HTTLPR polymorphism and early-life adversity. Unless one accounts for epistatic interactions, we may easily arrive to spurious conclusions.

Another important interaction between BDNF polymorphisms and the genes regulating glycogen synthase 3-beta (GSK-3b) has been reported. GSK-3b is one of the more prominent cell-survival proteins, involved with a complex regulation of transcription factors and, ultimately, cell apoptosis.[279] BDNF, via an intricate intracellular signaling cascade, is one of the major regulators of GSK-3b. It comes as no surprise that carriers of combined at-risk polymorphisms of BDNF and GSK-3b genes tended to suffer from MDD four times as often relative to individuals endowed with other generic variants.[280] In addition to just described interaction between BDNF and GSK-3b, BDNF also modulates CREB activity by means of an intracellular cascade initiated by its binding to the TrkB receptor.

The BDNF/TrkB/CREB signaling cascade has a central role in activity-driven neuroplasticity and therefore in learning and memory processes. As one might anticipate, based on the previously described association between minor BDNF and 5HTTLPR alleles and depression in the face of adversity,[271] minor BDNF, neurotrophic tyrosine kinase receptor type 2 (a gene coding for TrkB receptor), and CREB1 allele carriers who were also exposed to childhood adversity were at a higher lifetime risk for developing depression. Perhaps paradoxically, genetic epistasis between BDNF and CREB1 major alleles was significantly associated with ruminations and current depressive symptoms but with not lifetime depression in this community-based sample.[281] If we conceive of rumination as a process associated with exaggerated retrieval of negative memories and congruent autobiographical reminiscence, which additionally taxes cognitive resources, it would make sense that these processes might be facilitated in individuals with genes that enhance cognitive processes. Thus, increased rumination would likely lead to depressive symptoms.[281]

As we have previously mentioned, genetic epistasis also plays a role in shaping antidepressant response. A complex gene × gene × gene × gender interaction, involving polymorphisms of the genes regulating 5HT receptors HTR1B, HTR3A, and HTR5A, predicted antidepressant response in women. Additionally, interactions between HTR1B and recent stress, and TPH2 and childhood trauma, also significantly influenced antidepressant response. Replicating previous findings, polymorphisms of 5HT1B and TPH2 genes also demonstrated a direct influence on antidepressant efficacy.[279] Despite these findings, genetic prediction of antidepressant response continues to be an elusive goal. A meta-analysis of the two large European and U.S. GWAS, which included over 2,000 patients treated with antidepressants for two weeks, concluded that a weak polygenetic signal, distributed over many polymorphisms, accounted for approximately 1.2 percent of the variance.[282]

Conclusion

In summary, GWAS and linkage studies have offered meager and inconsistent evidence of the role that individual genes may play in the etiology and treatment of MDD. When there are positive findings, they indicate a very small contribution by individual genes and point to a polygenetic pattern of inheritance and significant disease heterogeneity. Candidate gene research proved to be somewhat more fruitful. Several genes regulating monoamine receptors, transporters, and enzymes involved in their metabolism all seem to contribute toward MDD vulnerability,[146] as well as treatment response. Additionally, studies focused on genes involved in glutamate and GABA signaling have established their relationship with depression. These genes combined with the ones regulating corticosteroid, neurotrophic, and inflammatory signaling influence structural integrity and functional connectivity in the brain areas involved in mood regulation and adaptation to stress.[162,283,284] Moreover, a review suggests that genes associated with depression may act in unison by accelerating sensitization to stress.[285] Work elucidating the role of genes regulating intracellular signaling cascade in etiopathogenesis of MDD is also showing promise. However, the proof of direct relationship between any of the candidate genes and depression remains tenuous and equivocal. It appears that the influence of genes is moderated by social variables, gender, and environmental adversity. As a matter of fact, early-life adversity seems to have a more profound and enduring effect than stressful events in later life, possibly because it is more likely to produce the epigenetic modulation of DNA itself rather than change in histone structure. "Two-hit" theories, proposing that early-life adversity combined with genetic epistasis and subsequent epigenetic modulation may alter the neural function and substrate in a manner that renders individuals more susceptible to later-life stress, are gaining support. Studies aimed at identifying the resilience genes and clarifying their role in the etiology of MDD have added a new dimension to our understanding of this phenomenon.

It is unlikely that future research will provide us with simple answers about the genetic origins of depression. More likely, we will gain further appreciation of the genetic and biological diversity of MDD. Gender, early and late adversity, availability or absence of social supports, urbanicity, developmental phase, and resilience factors all interact in a dynamic fashion, with multiple genes and epigenetic modifications, to generate a panoply of phonotypical manifestations, yet all of these are similar enough to be included under the same diagnostic umbrella. So what do we have to show in the end, for all this painstaking and laborious genetic research? Maybe a far more advanced understanding of the intricate and dynamic factors participating in the etiopathogenesis of MDD. At some point in the future, this knowledge may be transformed into more effective diagnostic and treatment strategies.

References

1. Sullivan PF, Neale MC, Kendler KS. Genetic epidemiology of major depression: review and meta-analysis. *Am J Psychiatry.* 2000;157:1552–1562.
2. Major Depressive Disorder Working Group of the Psychiatric GWAS Consortium. A mega-analysis of genome-wide association studies for major depressive disorder. *Mol Psychiatry.* 2013;18(4):497–511.
3. Uher R. Genes, environment, and individual differences in responding to treatment for depression. *Harv Rev Psychiatry.* 2011;19:109–124.
4. Hasler G, Drevets WC, Manji HK, Charney DS. Discovering endophenotypes for major depression. *Neuropsychopharmacology.* 2004;29:1765–1781.
5. Uher R. The role of genetic variation in the causation of mental illness: an evolution-informed framework. *Mol Psychiatry.* 2009;14:1072–1082.
6. Schroeder M, Hillemacher T, Bleich S, Frieling H. The epigenetic code in depression: implications for treatment. *Clin Pharmacol Ther.* 2012;91:310–314.
7. Maletic V. Neurobiological aspects of late-life mood disorders. In: Ellison JM, Kyomen HA, Verma S, eds. *Mood Disorders in Later Life.* 2nd ed. New York: Informa Healthcare; 2009: 133–149.
8. Bradley RG, Binder EB, Epstein MP, et al. Influence of child abuse on adult depression: moderation by the corticotropin-releasing hormone receptor gene. *Arch Gen Psychiatry.* 2008;65:190–200.
9. Dreher JC, Kohn P, Kolachana B, Weinberger DR, Berman KF. Variation in dopamine genes influences responsivity of the human reward system. *Proc Natl Acad Sci U S A.* 2009;106:617–622.
10. Weissman MM, Bland RC, Canino GJ, et al. Cross-national epidemiology of major depression and bipolar disorder. *JAMA.* 1996;276:293–299.
11. Murphy DL, Fox MA, Timpano KR, et al. How the serotonin story is being rewritten by new gene-based discoveries principally related to SLC6A4, the serotonin transporter gene, which functions to influence all cellular serotonin systems. *Neuropharmacology.* 2008;55:932–960.
12. Selvaraj S, Godlewska BR, Norbury R, et al. Decreased regional gray matter volume in S′ allele carriers of the 5-HTTLPR triallelic polymorphism. *Mol Psychiatry.* 2011;16: 471–473.
13. Wendland JR, Moya PR, Kruse MR, et al. A novel, putative gain-of-function haplotype at SLC6A4 associates with obsessive-compulsive disorder. *Hum Mol Genet.* 2008;17: 717–723.

14. Joensuu M, Lehto SM, Tolmunen T, et al. Serotonin-transporter-linked promoter region polymorphism and serotonin transporter binding in drug-naive patients with major depression. *Psychiatry Clin Neurosci.* 2010;64:387–393.

15. Smith GS, Lotrich FE, Malhotra AK, et al. Effects of serotonin transporter promoter polymorphisms on serotonin function. *Neuropsychopharmacology.* 2004;29:2226–2234.

16. Uher R. The implications of gene-environment interactions in depression: will cause inform cure? *Mol Psychiatry.* 2008;13:1070–1078.

17. Kishida I, Aklillu E, Kawanishi C, Bertilsson L, Agren H. Monoamine metabolites level in CSF is related to the 5-HTT gene polymorphism in treatment-resistant depression. *Neuropsychopharmacology.* 2007;32:2143–2151.

18. Gonda X, Fountoulakis KN, Juhasz G, et al. Association of the s allele of the 5-HTTLPR with neuroticism-related traits and temperaments in a psychiatrically healthy population. *Eur Arch Psychiatry Clin Neurosci.* 2009;259:106–113.

19. Munafo MR, Freimer NB, Ng W, et al. 5-HTTLPR genotype and anxiety-related personality traits: a meta-analysis and new data. *Am J Med Genet B Neuropsychiatr Genet.* 2009;150B:271–281.

20. Munafo MR, Clark TG, Roberts KH, Johnstone EC. Neuroticism mediates the association of the serotonin transporter gene with lifetime major depression. *Neuropsychobiology.* 2006;53:1–8.

21. Perez M, Burns AB, Brown JS, Sachs-Ericsson N, Plant A, Joiner TE, Jr. Association of serotonin transporter genotypes to components of the tripartite model of depression and anxiety. *Personal Individ Differ.* 2007;43:107–118.

22. Perez-Edgar K, Bar-Haim Y, McDermott JM, et al. Variations in the serotonin-transporter gene are associated with attention bias patterns to positive and negative emotion faces. *Biol Psychol.* 2010;83:269–271.

23. Pergamin-Hight L, Bakermans-Kranenburg MJ, van Ijzendoorn MH, Bar-Haim Y. Variations in the promoter region of the serotonin transporter gene and biased attention for emotional information: a meta-analysis. *Biol Psychiatry.* 2012;71:373–379.

24. Pluess M, Velders FP, Belsky J, et al. Serotonin transporter polymorphism moderates effects of prenatal maternal anxiety on infant negative emotionality. *Biol Psychiatry.* 2011;69:520–525.

25. Hayden EP, Dougherty LR, Maloney B, et al. Early-emerging cognitive vulnerability to depression and the serotonin transporter promoter region polymorphism. *J Affect Disord.* 2008;107:227–230.

26. Canli T, Lesch KP. Long story short: the serotonin transporter in emotion regulation and social cognition. *Nat Neurosci.* 2007;10:1103–1109.

27. Way BM, Lieberman MD. Is there a genetic contribution to cultural differences? Collectivism, individualism and genetic markers of social sensitivity. *Soc Cogn Affect Neurosci.* 2010;5:203–211.

28. Risch N, Herrell R, Lehner T, et al. Interaction between the serotonin transporter gene (5-HTTLPR), stressful life events, and risk of depression: a meta-analysis. *JAMA.* 2009; 301:2462–2471.

29. Apkarian AV, Bushnell MC, Treede RD, Zubieta JK. Human brain mechanisms of pain perception and regulation in health and disease. *Eur J Pain.* 2005;9:463–484.

30. Pezawas L, Meyer-Lindenberg A, Drabant EM, et al. 5-HTTLPR polymorphism impacts human cingulate-amygdala interactions: a genetic susceptibility mechanism for depression. *Nat Neurosci.* 2005;8:828–834.

31. Hariri AR, Drabant EM, Munoz KE, et al. A susceptibility gene for affective disorders and the response of the human amygdala. *Arch Gen Psychiatry.* 2005;62:146–152.

32. MacLullich AM, Ferguson KJ, Wardlaw JM, Starr JM, Deary IJ, Seckl JR. Smaller left anterior cingulate cortex volumes are associated with impaired hypothalamic-pituitary-adrenal axis regulation in healthy elderly men. *J Clin Endocrinol Metab.* 2006;91: 1591–1594.

33. Baliki MN, Geha PY, Apkarian AV. Spontaneous pain and brain activity in neuropathic pain: functional MRI and pharmacologic functional MRI studies. *Curr Pain Headache Rep.* 2007;11:171–177.

34. Frodl T, Koutsouleris N, Bottlender R, et al. Reduced gray matter brain volumes are associated with variants of the serotonin transporter gene in major depression. *Mol Psychiatry.* 2008;13:1093–1101.

35. Pacheco J, Beevers CG, Benavides C, McGeary J, Stice E, Schnyer DM. Frontal-limbic white matter pathway associations with the serotonin transporter gene promoter region (5-HTTLPR) polymorphism. *J Neurosci.* 2009;29:6229–6233.

36. Beevers CG, Pacheco J, Clasen P, McGeary JE, Schnyer D. Prefrontal morphology, 5-HTTLPR polymorphism and biased attention for emotional stimuli. *Genes Brain Behav.* 2010;9:224–233.

37. O'Hara R, Schroder CM, Mahadevan R, et al. Serotonin transporter polymorphism, memory and hippocampal volume in the elderly: association and interaction with cortisol. *Mol Psychiatry.* 2007;12:544–555.

38. Jedema HP, Gianaros PJ, Greer PJ, et al. Cognitive impact of genetic variation of the serotonin transporter in primates is associated with differences in brain morphology rather than serotonin neurotransmission. *Mol Psychiatry.* 2010;15:512–522, 446.

39. Frodl T, Meisenzahl EM, Zill P, et al. Reduced hippocampal volumes associated with the long variant of the serotonin transporter polymorphism in major depression. *Arch Gen Psychiatry.* 2004;61:177–183.

40. Frodl T, Reinhold E, Koutsouleris N, et al. Childhood stress, serotonin transporter gene and brain structures in major depression. *Neuropsychopharmacology.* 2010;35:1383–1390.

41. Taylor WD, Steffens DC, Payne ME, et al. Influence of serotonin transporter promoter region polymorphisms on hippocampal volumes in late-life depression. *Arch Gen Psychiatry.* 2005;62:537–544.

42. Danese A, Moffitt TE, Harrington H, et al. Adverse childhood experiences and adult risk factors for age-related disease: depression, inflammation, and clustering of metabolic risk markers. *Arch Pediatr Adolesc Med.* 2009;163:1135–1143.

43. Eker MC, Kitis O, Okur H, et al. Smaller hippocampus volume is associated with short variant of 5-HTTLPR polymorphism in medication-free major depressive disorder patients. *Neuropsychobiology.* 2011;63:22–28.

44. Alexopoulos GS, Murphy CF, Gunning-Dixon FM, et al. Serotonin transporter polymorphisms, microstructural white matter abnormalities and remission of geriatric depression. *J Affect Disord.* 2009;119:132–141.

45. Young KA, Holcomb LA, Bonkale WL, Hicks PB, Yazdani U, German DC. 5HTTLPR polymorphism and enlargement of the pulvinar: unlocking the backdoor to the limbic system. *Biol Psychiatry.* 2007;61:813–818.

46. Heinz A, Braus DF, Smolka MN, et al. Amygdala-prefrontal coupling depends on a genetic variation of the serotonin transporter. *Nat Neurosci.* 2005;8:20–21.

47. Fortier E, Noreau A, Lepore F, et al. Early impact of 5-HTTLPR polymorphism on the neural correlates of sadness. *Neurosci Lett.* 2010;485:261–265.

48. Langguth B, Sand P, Marek R, et al. Allelic variation in the serotonin transporter promoter modulates cortical excitability. *Biol Psychiatry.* 2009;66:283–286.

49. Schardt DM, Erk S, Nusser C, et al. Volition diminishes genetically mediated amygdala hyperreactivity. *Neuroimage.* 2010;53:943–951.

50. Lemogne C, Gorwood P, Boni C, Pessiglione M, Lehericy S, Fossati P. Cognitive appraisal and life stress moderate the effects of the 5-HTTLPR polymorphism on amygdala reactivity. *Hum Brain Mapp.* 2011;32:1856–1867.

51. Jonassen R, Endestad T, Neumeister A, Foss Haug KB, Berg JP, Landro NI. Serotonin transporter polymorphism modulates N-back task performance and fMRI BOLD signal intensity in healthy women. *PLoS ONE.* 2012;7:e30564.

52. Matsunaga M, Murakami H, Yamakawa K, et al. Genetic variations in the serotonin transporter gene-linked polymorphic region influence attraction for a favorite person and the associated interactions between the central nervous and immune systems. *Neurosci Lett.* 2010;468:211–215.

53. Gotlib IH, Joormann J, Minor KL, Hallmayer J. HPA axis reactivity: a mechanism underlying the associations among 5-HTTLPR, stress, and depression. *Biol Psychiatry.* 2008; 63:847–851.

54. Ohira H, Matsunaga M, Isowa T, et al. Polymorphism of the serotonin transporter gene modulates brain and physiological responses to acute stress in Japanese men. *Stress.* 2009;12:533–543.

55. Fredericks CA, Drabant EM, Edge MD, et al. Healthy young women with serotonin transporter SS polymorphism show a pro-inflammatory bias under resting and stress conditions. *Brain Behav Immun.* 2010;24:350–357.

56. Lau JY, Goldman D, Buzas B, et al. Amygdala function and 5-HTT gene variants in adolescent anxiety and major depressive disorder. *Biol Psychiatry.* 2009;65:349–355.

57. Dannlowski U, Ohrmann P, Bauer J, et al. 5-HTTLPR biases amygdala activity in response to masked facial expressions in major depression. *Neuropsychopharmacology.* 2008;33:418–424.

58. Wray NR, James MR, Gordon SD, et al. Accurate, large-scale genotyping of 5HTTLPR and flanking single nucleotide polymorphisms in an association study of depression, anxiety, and personality measures. *Biol Psychiatry.* 2009;66:468–476.

59. Brockmann H, Zobel A, Schuhmacher A, et al. Influence of 5-HTTLPR polymorphism on resting state perfusion in patients with major depression. *J Psychiatr Res.* 2011;45: 442–451.

60. Goodyer IM, Bacon A, Ban M, Croudace T, Herbert J. Serotonin transporter genotype, morning cortisol and subsequent depression in adolescents. *Br J Psychiatry.* 2009;195: 39–45.

61. Su S, Zhao J, Bremner JD, et al. Serotonin transporter gene, depressive symptoms, and interleukin-6. *Circul Cardiovasc Genet.* 2009;2:614–620.

62. Haenisch B, Herms S, Mattheisen M, et al. Genome-wide association data provide further support for an association between 5-HTTLPR and major depressive disorder. *J Affect Disord.* 2013;56:155–162.

63. Lasky-Su JA, Faraone SV, Glatt SJ, Tsuang MT. Meta-analysis of the association between two polymorphisms in the serotonin transporter gene and affective disorders. *Am J Med Genet B Neuropsychiatr Genet.* 2005;133B:110–115.

64. Veletza S, Samakouri M, Emmanouil G, Trypsianis G, Kourmouli N, Livaditis M. Psychological vulnerability differences in students—carriers or not of the serotonin transporter promoter allele S: effect of adverse experiences. *Synapse.* 2009;63:193–200.

65. Caspi A, Sugden K, Moffitt TE, et al. Influence of life stress on depression: moderation by a polymorphism in the 5-HTT gene. *Science.* 2003;301:386–389.

66. Wilhelm K, Mitchell PB, Niven H, et al. Life events, first depression onset and the serotonin transporter gene. *Br J Psychiatry.* 2006;188:210–215.

67. Lazary J, Lazary A, Gonda X, et al. New evidence for the association of the serotonin transporter gene (SLC6A4) haplotypes, threatening life events, and depressive phenotype. *Biol Psychiatry.* 2008;64:498–504.

68. Karg K, Burmeister M, Shedden K, Sen S. The serotonin transporter promoter variant (5-HTTLPR), stress, and depression meta-analysis revisited: evidence of genetic moderation. *Arch Gen Psychiatry.* 2011;68:444–454.

69. Zalsman G, Huang YY, Oquendo MA, et al. Association of a triallelic serotonin transporter gene promoter region (5-HTTLPR) polymorphism with stressful life events and severity of depression. *Am J Psychiatry.* 2006;163:1588–1593.

70. Cervilla JA, Molina E, Rivera M, et al. The risk for depression conferred by stressful life events is modified by variation at the serotonin transporter 5HTTLPR genotype: evidence from the Spanish PREDICT-Gene cohort. *Mol Psychiatry.* 2007;12:748–755.

71. Kendler KS, Kuhn KJ, Vittum J, Prescott CA, Riley B. The interaction of stressful life events and a serotonin transporter polymorphism in the prediction of episodes of major depression. *Arch Gen Psychiatry.* 2005;62:529–535.

72. Beaver KM, Wright JP, DeLisi M, Vaughn MG. Dopaminergic polymorphisms and educational achievement: results from a longitudinal sample of Americans. *Dev Psychol.* 2012;48:932–938.

73. Baune BT, Hohoff C, Mortensen LS, Deckert J, Arolt V, Domschke K. Serotonin transporter polymorphism (5-HTTLPR) association with melancholic depression: a female specific effect? *Depress Anxiety.* 2008;25:920–925.

74. Brummett BH, Boyle SH, Siegler IC, et al. Effects of environmental stress and gender on associations among symptoms of depression and the serotonin transporter gene linked polymorphic region (5-HTTLPR). *Behav Genet.* 2008;38:34–43.

75. Munafo MR, Durrant C, Lewis G, Flint J. Gene × environment interactions at the serotonin transporter locus. *Biol Psychiatry.* 2009;65:211–219.

76. Uher R, McGuffin P. The moderation by the serotonin transporter gene of environmental adversity in the aetiology of mental illness: review and methodological analysis. *Mol Psychiatry.* 2008;13:131–146.

77. Uher R, McGuffin P. The moderation by the serotonin transporter gene of environmental adversity in the etiology of depression: 2009 update. *Mol Psychiatry.* 2010;15:18–22.

78. Wankerl M, Wust S, Otte C. Current developments and controversies: does the serotonin transporter gene-linked polymorphic region (5-HTTLPR) modulate the association between stress and depression? *Curr Opin Psychiatry.* 2010;23:582–587.

79. Cutuli JJ, Raby KL, Cicchetti D, Englund MM, Egeland B. Contributions of maltreatment and serotonin transporter genotype to depression in childhood, adolescence, and early adulthood. *J Affect Disord.* 2013;149(1–3):30–37.

80. Roy A, Hu XZ, Janal MN, Goldman D. Interaction between childhood trauma and serotonin transporter gene variation in suicide. *Neuropsychopharmacology.* 2007;32:2046–2052.

81. Fisher HL, Cohen-Woods S, Hosang GM, et al. Interaction between specific forms of childhood maltreatment and the serotonin transporter gene (5-HTT) in recurrent depressive disorder. *J Affect Disord.* 2013;145(1):136–141.

82. Uher R, Caspi A, Houts R, et al. Serotonin transporter gene moderates childhood maltreatment's effects on persistent but not single-episode depression: replications and implications for resolving inconsistent results. *J Affect Disord.* 2011;135:56–65.

83. Brown GW, Ban M, Craig TK, Harris TO, Herbert J, Uher R. Serotonin transporter length polymorphism, childhood maltreatment, and chronic depression: a specific gene-environment interaction. *Depress Anxiety.* 2013;30:5–13.

84. Jenness JL, Hankin BL, Abela JR, Young JF, Smolen A. Chronic family stress interacts with 5-HTTLPR to predict prospective depressive symptoms among youth. *Depress Anxiety.* 2011;28:1074–1080.

85. Brown GW, Harris TO. Depression and the serotonin transporter 5-HTTLPR polymorphism: a review and a hypothesis concerning gene-environment interaction. *J Affect Disord.* 2008;111:1–12.

86. Hamilton JP, Chen G, Thomason ME, Schwartz ME, Gotlib IH. Investigating neural primacy in major depressive disorder: multivariate Granger causality analysis of resting-state fMRI time-series data. *Mol Psychiatry.* 2011;16:763–772.

87. Taylor SE, Way BM, Welch WT, Hilmert CJ, Lehman BJ, Eisenberger NI. Early family environment, current adversity, the serotonin transporter promoter polymorphism, and depressive symptomatology. *Biol Psychiatry.* 2006;60:671–676.

88. Pauli-Pott U, Friedel S, Hinney A, Hebebrand J. Serotonin transporter gene polymorphism (5-HTTLPR), environmental conditions, and developing negative emotionality and fear in early childhood. *J Neural Transm.* 2009;116:503–512.

89. Kaufman J, Yang BZ, Douglas-Palumberi H, et al. Social supports and serotonin transporter gene moderate depression in maltreated children. *Proc Natl Acad Sci U S A.* 2004;101:17316–17321.

90. Kilpatrick DG, Koenen KC, Ruggiero KJ, et al. The serotonin transporter genotype and social support and moderation of posttraumatic stress disorder and depression in hurricane-exposed adults. *Am J Psychiatry.* 2007;164:1693–1699.

91. Olsson CA, Foley DL, Parkinson-Bates M, et al. Prospects for epigenetic research within cohort studies of psychological disorder: a pilot investigation of a peripheral cell marker of epigenetic risk for depression. *Biol Psychol.* 2010;83:159–165.

92. Devlin AM, Brain U, Austin J, Oberlander TF. Prenatal exposure to maternal depressed mood and the MTHFR C677T variant affect SLC6A4 methylation in infants at birth. *PLoS ONE.* 2010;5:e12201.

93. van IMH, Caspers K, Bakermans-Kranenburg MJ, Beach SR, Philibert R. Methylation matters: interaction between methylation density and serotonin transporter genotype predicts unresolved loss or trauma. *Biol Psychiatry.* 2010;68:405–407.

94. Taylor MJ, Sen S, Bhagwagar Z. Antidepressant response and the serotonin transporter gene-linked polymorphic region. *Biol Psychiatry.* 2010;68:536–543.

95. Serretti A, Kato M, De Ronchi D, Kinoshita T. Meta-analysis of serotonin transporter gene promoter polymorphism (5-HTTLPR) association with selective serotonin reuptake inhibitor efficacy in depressed patients. *Mol Psychiatry.* 2007;12:247–257.

96. Arias B, Catalan R, Gasto C, Gutierrez B, Fananas L. 5-HTTLPR polymorphism of the serotonin transporter gene predicts non-remission in major depression patients treated with citalopram in a 12-weeks follow up study. *J Clin Psychopharmacol.* 2003;23:563–567.

97. Serretti A, Mandelli L, Lorenzi C, et al. Serotonin transporter gene influences the time course of improvement of "core" depressive and somatic anxiety symptoms during treatment with SSRIs for recurrent mood disorders. *Psychiatry Res.* 2007;149:185–193.

98. Huezo-Diaz P, Uher R, Smith R, et al. Moderation of antidepressant response by the serotonin transporter gene. *Br J Psychiatry.* 2009;195:30–38.

99. Keers R, Uher R, Huezo-Diaz P, et al. Interaction between serotonin transporter gene

variants and life events predicts response to antidepressants in the GENDEP project. *Pharmacogenomics J.* 2011;11:138–145.

100. Nikisch G, Mathe AA, Czernik A, et al. Stereoselective metabolism of citalopram in plasma and cerebrospinal fluid of depressive patients: relationship with 5-HIAA in CSF and clinical response. *J Clin Psychopharmacol.* 2004;24:283–290.

101. Backman J, Alling C, Alsen M, Regnell G, Traskman-Bendz L. Changes of cerebrospinal fluid monoamine metabolites during long-term antidepressant treatment. *Eur Neuropsychopharmacol.* 2000;10:341–349.

102. Sheline Y, Bardgett ME, Csernansky JG. Correlated reductions in cerebrospinal fluid 5-HIAA and MHPG concentrations after treatment with selective serotonin reuptake inhibitors. *J Clin Psychopharmacol.* 1997;17:11–14.

103. Buckholtz JW, Callicott JH, Kolachana B, et al. Genetic variation in MAOA modulates ventromedial prefrontal circuitry mediating individual differences in human personality. *Mol Psychiatry.* 2008;13:313–324.

104. Kim-Cohen J, Caspi A, Taylor A, et al. MAOA, maltreatment, and gene-environment interaction predicting children's mental health: new evidence and a meta-analysis. *Mol Psychiatry.* 2006;11:903–913.

105. Ducci F, Enoch MA, Hodgkinson C, et al. Interaction between a functional MAOA locus and childhood sexual abuse predicts alcoholism and antisocial personality disorder in adult women. *Mol Psychiatry.* 2008;13:334–347.

106. Dannlowski U, Ohrmann P, Konrad C, et al. Reduced amygdala-prefrontal coupling in major depression: association with MAOA genotype and illness severity. *Int J Neuropsychopharmacol.* 2009;12:11–22.

107. Armbruster D, Mueller A, Strobel A, Lesch KP, Brocke B, Kirschbaum C. Children under stress—COMT genotype and stressful life events predict cortisol increase in an acute social stress paradigm. *Int J Neuropsychopharmacol.* 2012;15:1229–1239.

108. Slifstein M, Kolachana B, Simpson EH, et al. COMT genotype predicts cortical-limbic D1 receptor availability measured with [^{11}C]NNC112 and PET. *Mol Psychiatry.* 2008;13:821–827.

109. Diamond A. Consequences of variations in genes that affect dopamine in prefrontal cortex. *Cereb Cortex.* 2007;17(suppl 1):i161–i170.

110. Harrison PJ, Tunbridge EM. Catechol-*O*-methyltransferase (COMT): a gene contributing to sex differences in brain function, and to sexual dimorphism in the predisposition to psychiatric disorders. *Neuropsychopharmacology.* 2008;33:3037–3045.

111. Cerasa A, Gioia MC, Labate A, Liguori M, Lanza P, Quattrone A. Impact of catechol-*O*-methyltransferase Val(108/158) Met genotype on hippocampal and prefrontal gray matter volume. *Neuroreport.* 2008;19:405–408.

112. Honea R, Verchinski BA, Pezawas L, et al. Impact of interacting functional variants in COMT on regional gray matter volume in human brain. *Neuroimage.* 2009;45:44–51.

113. Mechelli A, Tognin S, McGuire PK, et al. Genetic vulnerability to affective psychopathology in childhood: a combined voxel-based morphometry and functional magnetic resonance imaging study. *Biol Psychiatry.* 2009;66:231–237.

114. Bilder RM, Volavka J, Lachman HM, Grace AA. The catechol-*O*-methyltransferase polymorphism: relations to the tonic-phasic dopamine hypothesis and neuropsychiatric phenotypes. *Neuropsychopharmacology.* 2004;29:1943–1961.

115. Meyer-Lindenberg A, Nichols T, Callicott JH, et al. Impact of complex genetic variation in COMT on human brain function. *Mol Psychiatry.* 2006;11:867–877, 797.

116. Smolka MN, Schumann G, Wrase J, et al. Catechol-*O*-methyltransferase val158met genotype affects processing of emotional stimuli in the amygdala and prefrontal cortex. *J Neurosci.* 2005;25:836–842.

117. Schmack K, Schlagenhauf F, Sterzer P, et al. Catechol-*O*-methyltransferase val158met genotype influences neural processing of reward anticipation. *Neuroimage.* 2008;42: 1631–1638.

118. Domschke K, Baune BT, Havlik L, et al. Catechol-*O*-methyltransferase gene variation: impact on amygdala response to aversive stimuli. *Neuroimage.* 2012;60:2222–2229.

119. Kempton MJ, Haldane M, Jogia J, et al. The effects of gender and COMT Val158Met polymorphism on fearful facial affect recognition: a fMRI study. *Int J Neuropsychopharmacol.* 2009;12:371–381.

120. Chen C, Chen C, Moyzis R, et al. Sex modulates the associations between the COMT gene and personality traits. *Neuropsychopharmacology.* 2011;36:1593–1598.

121. Felten A, Montag C, Markett S, Walter NT, Reuter M. Genetically determined dopamine availability predicts disposition for depression. *Brain Behav.* 2011;1:109–118.

122. Hettema JM, An SS, Neale MC, van den Oord EJ, Kendler KS, Chen X. Lack of association between the amiloride-sensitive cation channel 2 (ACCN2) gene and anxiety spectrum disorders. *Psychiatr Genet.* 2008;18:73–79.

123. Massat I, Kocabas NA, Crisafulli C, et al. COMT and age at onset in mood disorders: a replication and extension study. *Neurosci Lett.* 2011;498:218–221.

124. Nyman ES, Sulkava S, Soronen P, et al. Interaction of early environment, gender and genes of monoamine neurotransmission in the aetiology of depression in a large population-based Finnish birth cohort. *BMJ Open.* 2011;1:e000087.

125. Aberg E, Fandino-Losada A, Sjoholm LK, Forsell Y, Lavebratt C. The functional Val-158Met polymorphism in catechol-*O*-methyltransferase (COMT) is associated with depression and motivation in men from a Swedish population-based study. *J Affect Disord.* 2011;129:158–166.

126. Jabbi M, Kema IP, van der Pompe G, te Meerman GJ, Ormel J, den Boer JA. Catechol-*O*-methyltransferase polymorphism and susceptibility to major depressive disorder modulates psychological stress response. *Psychiatr Genet.* 2007;17:183–193.

127. Evans J, Xu K, Heron J, et al. Emotional symptoms in children: the effect of maternal depression, life events, and COMT genotype. *Am J Med Genet B Neuropsychiatr Genet.* 2009;150B:209–218.

128. Baune BT, Hohoff C, Berger K, et al. Association of the COMT val158met variant with antidepressant treatment response in major depression. *Neuropsychopharmacology.* 2008;33:924–932.

129. Tsai SJ, Gau YT, Hong CJ, Liou YJ, Yu YW, Chen TJ. Sexually dimorphic effect of catechol-*O*-methyltransferase val158met polymorphism on clinical response to fluoxetine in major depressive patients. *J Affect Disord.* 2009;113:183–187.

130. Frokjaer VG, Mortensen EL, Nielsen FA, et al. Frontolimbic serotonin 2A receptor binding in healthy subjects is associated with personality risk factors for affective disorder. *Biol Psychiatry.* 2008;63:569–576.

131. Jokela M, Keltikangas-Jarvinen L, Kivimaki M, et al. Serotonin receptor 2A gene and the influence of childhood maternal nurturance on adulthood depressive symptoms. *Arch Gen Psychiatry.* 2007;64:356–360.

132. Jokela M, Lehtimaki T, Keltikangas-Jarvinen L. The influence of urban/rural residency on depressive symptoms is moderated by the serotonin receptor 2A gene. *Am J Med Genet B Neuropsychiatr Genet.* 2007;144B:918–922.

133. Paddock S. Genetic variation in GRIK4 and the implications for antidepressant treatment. *Pharmacogenomics.* 2008;9:133–135.

134. Xu Z, Zhang Z, Shi Y, et al. Influence and interaction of genetic polymorphisms in catecholamine neurotransmitter systems and early life stress on antidepressant drug response. *J Affect Disord.* 2011;133:165–173.

135. Kato M, Zanardi R, Rossini D, et al. 5-HT2A gene variants influence specific and different aspects of antidepressant response in Japanese and Italian mood disorder patients. *Psychiatry Res.* 2009;167:97–105.

136. McMahon FJ, Buervenich S, Charney D, et al. Variation in the gene encoding the serotonin 2A receptor is associated with outcome of antidepressant treatment. *Am J Hum Genet.* 2006;78:804–814.

137. Kato M, Fukuda T, Wakeno M, et al. Effect of 5-HT1A gene polymorphisms on antidepressant response in major depressive disorder. *Am J Med Genet B Neuropsychiatr Genet.* 2009;150B:115–123.

138. Frodl T, Moller HJ, Meisenzahl E. Neuroimaging genetics: new perspectives in research on major depression? *Acta Psychiatr Scand.* 2008;118:363–372.

139. Carlson P, Bain, R., Tinsley A, et al. Serotonin-1A receptor binding in depression: Correlates with interleukin-6 and the hypothalamic-pituitary-adrenal axis. *Neuroimage.* 2006;31:T44-T186.

140. Anttila S, Huuhka K, Huuhka M, et al. Interaction between 5-HT1A and BDNF genotypes increases the risk of treatment-resistant depression. *J Neural Transm.* 2007;114: 1065–1068.

141. Illi A, Setala-Soikkeli E, Viikki M, et al. 5-HTR1A, 5-HTR2A, 5-HTR6, TPH1 and TPH2 polymorphisms and major depression. *Neuroreport.* 2009;20:1125–1128.

142. Zhang K, Xu Q, Xu Y, et al. The combined effects of the 5-HTTLPR and 5-HTR1A genes modulates the relationship between negative life events and major depressive disorder in a Chinese population. *J Affect Disord.* 2009;114:224–231.

143. Haghighi F, Bach-Mizrachi H, Huang YY, et al. Genetic architecture of the human tryptophan hydroxylase 2 Gene: existence of neural isoforms and relevance for major depression. *Mol Psychiatry.* 2008;13:813–820.

144. Ansorge MS, Hen R, Gingrich JA. Neurodevelopmental origins of depressive disorders. *Curr Opin Pharmacol.* 2007;7:8–17.

145. Munoz KE, Hyde LW, Hariri AR. Imaging genetics. *J Am Acad Child Adolesc Psychiatry.* 2009;48:356–361.

146. Haavik J, Blau N, Thony B. Mutations in human monoamine-related neurotransmitter pathway genes. *Hum Mutat.* 2008;29:891–902.

147. Levinson DF. The genetics of depression: a review. *Biol Psychiatry.* 2006;60:84–92.

148. Flint J, Shifman S, Munafo M, Mott R. Genetic variants in major depression. *Novartis Found Symp.* 2008;289:23–42, 87–93.

149. Xu Z, Zhang Z, Shi Y, et al. Influence and interaction of genetic polymorphisms in the serotonin system and life stress on antidepressant drug response. *J Psychopharmacol.* 2012;26:349–359.

150. Serretti A, Cusin C, Rossini D, Artioli P, Dotoli D, Zanardi R. Further evidence of a combined effect of SERTPR and TPH on SSRIs response in mood disorders. *Am J Med Genet B Neuropsychiatr Genet.* 2004;129B:36–40.

151. Xu Y, Li F, Huang X, et al. The norepinephrine transporter gene modulates the relationship between urban/rural residency and major depressive disorder in a Chinese population. *Psychiatry Res.* 2009;168:213–217.

152. Jonsson EG, Nothen MM, Gustavsson JP, et al. Polymorphisms in the dopamine, serotonin, and norepinephrine transporter genes and their relationships to monoamine metabolite concentrations in CSF of healthy volunteers. *Psychiatry Res.* 1998;79:1–9.

153. Kim H, Lim SW, Kim S, et al. Monoamine transporter gene polymorphisms and antidepressant response in Koreans with late-life depression. *JAMA.* 2006;296:1609–1618.

154. Houston JP, Lau K, Aris V, et al. Association of common variations in the norepinephrine transporter gene with response to olanzapine-fluoxetine combination versus continued-fluoxetine treatment in patients with treatment-resistant depression: a candidate gene analysis. *J Clin Psychiatry.* 2012;73:878–885.

155. Kirchheiner J, Grundemann D, Schomig E. Contribution of allelic variations in transporters to the phenotype of drug response. *J Psychopharmacol.* 2006;20:27–32.

156. Lavretsky H, Siddarth P, Kumar A, Reynolds CF 3rd. The effects of the dopamine and serotonin transporter polymorphisms on clinical features and treatment response in geriatric depression: a pilot study. *Int J Geriatr Psychiatry.* 2008;23:55–59.

157. Nagappan G, Zaitsev E, Senatorov VV Jr, Yang J, Hempstead BL, Lu B. Control of extracellular cleavage of proBDNF by high frequency neuronal activity. *Proc Natl Acad Sci U S A.* 2009;106:1267–1272.

158. Duman RS, Monteggia LM. A neurotrophic model for stress-related mood disorders. *Biol Psychiatry.* 2006;59:1116–1127.

159. Linker R, Gold R, Luhder F. Function of neurotrophic factors beyond the nervous system: inflammation and autoimmune demyelination. *Crit Rev Immunol.* 2009;29:43–68.

160. Chen ZY, Bath K, McEwen B, Hempstead B, Lee F. Impact of genetic variant BDNF (Val66Met) on brain structure and function. *Novartis Found Symp.* 2008;289:180–188; discussion 188–195.

161. Manji HK, Duman RS. Impairments of neuroplasticity and cellular resilience in severe mood disorders: implications for the development of novel therapeutics. *Psychopharmacol Bull.* 2001;35:5–49.

162. Charney DS, Manji HK. Life stress, genes, and depression: multiple pathways lead to increased risk and new opportunities for intervention. *Sci STKE.* 2004;2004:re5.

163. Sublette ME, Baca-Garcia E, Parsey RV, et al. Effect of BDNF val66met polymorphism on age-related amygdala volume changes in healthy subjects. *Prog Neuropsychopharmacol Biol Psychiatry.* 2008;32:1652–1655.

164. Bueller JA, Aftab M, Sen S, Gomez-Hassan D, Burmeister M, Zubieta JK. BDNF Val-66Met allele is associated with reduced hippocampal volume in healthy subjects. *Biol Psychiatry.* 2006;59:812–815.

165. Pezawas L, Verchinski BA, Mattay VS, et al. The brain-derived neurotrophic factor val66met polymorphism and variation in human cortical morphology. *J Neurosci.* 2004;24:10099–10102.

166. Frodl T, Schule C, Schmitt G, et al. Association of the brain-derived neurotrophic factor Val66Met polymorphism with reduced hippocampal volumes in major depression. *Arch Gen Psychiatry.* 2007;64:410–416.

167. Harris SE, Fox H, Wright AF, et al. The brain-derived neurotrophic factor Val66Met polymorphism is associated with age-related change in reasoning skills. *Mol Psychiatry.* 2006;11:505–513.

168. Hariri AR, Goldberg TE, Mattay VS, et al. Brain-derived neurotrophic factor val66met polymorphism affects human memory-related hippocampal activity and predicts memory performance. *J Neurosci.* 2003;23:6690–6694.

169. Egan MF, Kojima M, Callicott JH, et al. The BDNF val66met polymorphism affects

activity-dependent secretion of BDNF and human memory and hippocampal function. *Cell.* 2003;112:257–269.

170. Szeszko PR, Lipsky R, Mentschel C, et al. Brain-derived neurotrophic factor val66met polymorphism and volume of the hippocampal formation. *Mol Psychiatry.* 2005;10:631–636.

171. Cardoner N, Soria V, Gratacos M, et al. Val66met BDNF genotypes in melancholic depression: effects on brain structure and treatment outcome. *Depress Anxiety.* 2013;30(3):225–233.

172. Maletic V, Robinson M, Oakes T, Iyengar S, Ball SG, Russell J. Neurobiology of depression: an integrated view of key findings. *Int J Clin Pract.* 2007;61:2030–2040.

173. Maletic V, Raison CL. Neurobiology of depression, fibromyalgia and neuropathic pain. *Front Biosci.* 2009;14:5291–5338.

174. Schule C, Zill P, Baghai TC, et al. Brain-derived neurotrophic factor Val66Met polymorphism and dexamethasone/CRH test results in depressed patients. *Psychoneuroendocrinology.* 2006;31:1019–1025.

175. Menon V. Large-scale brain networks and psychopathology: a unifying triple network model. *Trends Cogn Sci.* 2011;15:483–506.

176. Sheline YI, Price JL, Yan Z, Mintun MA. Resting-state functional MRI in depression unmasks increased connectivity between networks via the dorsal nexus. *Proc Natl Acad Sci U S A.* 2010;107:11020–11025.

177. Thomason ME, Yoo DJ, Glover GH, Gotlib IH. BDNF genotype modulates resting functional connectivity in children. *Front Hum Neurosci.* 2009;3:55.

178. Hamilton JP, Furman DJ, Chang C, Thomason ME, Dennis E, Gotlib IH. Default-mode and task-positive network activity in major depressive disorder: implications for adaptive and maladaptive rumination. *Biol Psychiatry.* 2011;70:327–333.

179. Clasen PC, Wells TT, Knopik VS, McGeary JE, Beevers CG. 5-HTTLPR and BDNF Val-66Met polymorphisms moderate effects of stress on rumination. *Genes Brain Behav.* 2011;10:740–746.

180. Licinio J, Dong C, Wong ML. Novel sequence variations in the brain-derived neurotrophic factor gene and association with major depression and antidepressant treatment response. *Arch Gen Psychiatry.* 2009;66:488–497.

181. Ribeiro L, Busnello JV, Cantor RM, et al. The brain-derived neurotrophic factor rs6265 (Val66Met) polymorphism and depression in Mexican-Americans. *Neuroreport.* 2007;18:1291–1293.

182. Jonsson EG, Saetre P, Edman-Ahlbom B, et al. Brain-derived neurotrophic factor gene variation influences cerebrospinal fluid 3-methoxy-4-hydroxyphenylglycol concentrations in healthy volunteers. *J Neural Transm.* 2008;115:1695–1699.

183. Dwivedi Y, Rizavi HS, Conley RR, Roberts RC, Tamminga CA, Pandey GN. Altered gene expression of brain-derived neurotrophic factor and receptor tyrosine kinase B in postmortem brain of suicide subjects. *Arch Gen Psychiatry.* 2003;60:804–815.

184. Perroud N, Uher R, Ng MY, et al. Genome-wide association study of increasing suicidal ideation during antidepressant treatment in the GENDEP project. *Pharmacogenomics J.* 2012;12:68–77.

185. McGregor S, Strauss J, Bulgin N, et al. p75(NTR) gene and suicide attempts in young adults with a history of childhood-onset mood disorder. *Am J Med Genet B Neuropsychiatr Genet.* 2007;144B:696–700.

186. Kunugi H, Hashimoto R, Yoshida M, Tatsumi M, Kamijima K. A missense polymorphism (S205L) of the low-affinity neurotrophin receptor p75NTR gene is associated

with depressive disorder and attempted suicide. *Am J Med Genet B Neuropsychiatr Genet.* 2004;129B:44–46.

187. Binder EB, Nemeroff CB. The CRF system, stress, depression and anxiety-insights from human genetic studies. *Mol Psychiatry.* 2010;15:574–588.

188. Klengel T, Mehta D, Anacker C, et al. Allele-specific FKBP5 DNA demethylation mediates gene-childhood trauma interactions. *Nat Neurosci.* 2013;16:33–41.

189. Wasserman D, Wasserman J, Sokolowski M. Genetics of HPA-axis, depression and suicidality. *Eur Psychiatry.* 2010;25:278–280.

190. Wang SS, Kamphuis W, Huitinga I, Zhou JN, Swaab DF. Gene expression analysis in the human hypothalamus in depression by laser microdissection and real-time PCR: the presence of multiple receptor imbalances. *Mol Psychiatry.* 2008;13:786–799, 741.

191. Oberlander TF, Weinberg J, Papsdorf M, Grunau R, Misri S, Devlin AM. Prenatal exposure to maternal depression, neonatal methylation of human glucocorticoid receptor gene (NR3C1) and infant cortisol stress responses. *Epigenetics.* 2008;3:97–106.

192. Tyrka AR, Price LH, Marsit C, Walters OC, Carpenter LL. Childhood adversity and epigenetic modulation of the leukocyte glucocorticoid receptor: preliminary findings in healthy adults. *PLoS ONE.* 2012;7:e30148.

193. McGowan PO, Sasaki A, D'Alessio AC, et al. Epigenetic regulation of the glucocorticoid receptor in human brain associates with childhood abuse. *Nat Neurosci.* 2009;12: 342–348.

194. Simic I, Maric NP, Mitic M, et al. Phosphorylation of leukocyte glucocorticoid receptor in patients with current episode of major depressive disorder. *Prog Neuropsychopharmacol Biol Psychiatry.* 2013;40:281–285.

195. Zimmermann P, Bruckl T, Nocon A, et al. Interaction of FKBP5 gene variants and adverse life events in predicting depression onset: results from a 10-year prospective community study. *Am J Psychiatry.* 2011;168:1107–1116.

196. Binder EB, Salyakina D, Lichtner P, et al. Polymorphisms in FKBP5 are associated with increased recurrence of depressive episodes and rapid response to antidepressant treatment. *Nature Genet.* 2004;36:1319–1325.

197. Hsu DT, Mickey BJ, Langenecker SA, et al. Variation in the corticotropin-releasing hormone receptor 1 (CRHR1) gene influences fMRI signal responses during emotional stimulus processing. *J Neurosci.* 2012;32:3253–3260.

198. Liu Z, Zhu F, Wang G, et al. Association of corticotropin-releasing hormone receptor1 gene SNP and haplotype with major depression. *Neurosci Lett.* 2006;404:358–362.

199. Helm C, Bradley B, Mletzko TC, Deveau TC, Musselman DL, Nemeroff CB, Ressler KJ, Binder EB. Effect of childhood trauma on adult depression and neuroendocrine function: sex-specific moderation by CRH receptor 1 gene. *Front Behav Neurosci.* 2009;3: Article 41.

200. Polanczyk G, Caspi A, Williams B, et al. Protective effect of CRHR1 gene variants on the development of adult depression following childhood maltreatment: replication and extension. *Arch Gen Psychiatry.* 2009;66:978–985.

201. Ressler KJ, Bradley B, Mercer KB, et al. Polymorphisms in CRHR1 and the serotonin transporter loci: gene × gene × environment interactions on depressive symptoms. *Am J Med Genet B Neuropsychiatr Genet.* 2010;153B:812–824.

202. Liu Z, Zhu F, Wang G, et al. Association study of corticotropin-releasing hormone receptor1 gene polymorphisms and antidepressant response in major depressive disorders. *Neurosci Lett.* 2007;414:155–158.

203. Binder EB, Owens MJ, Liu W, et al. Association of polymorphisms in genes regulating

the corticotropin-releasing factor system with antidepressant treatment response. *Arch Gen Psychiatry.* 2010;67:369–379.

204. Gillespie CF, Phifer J, Bradley B, Ressler KJ. Risk and resilience: genetic and environmental influences on development of the stress response. *Depress Anxiety.* 2009;26: 984–992.

205. Raison CL, Capuron L, Miller AH. Cytokines sing the blues: inflammation and the pathogenesis of depression. *Trends Immunol.* 2006;27:24–31.

206. Shelton RC, Claiborne J, Sidoryk-Wegrzynowicz M, et al. Altered expression of genes involved in inflammation and apoptosis in frontal cortex in major depression. *Mol Psychiatry.* 2011;16:751–762.

207. Alesci S, Martinez PE, Kelkar S, et al. Major depression is associated with significant diurnal elevations in plasma interleukin-6 levels, a shift of its circadian rhythm, and loss of physiological complexity in its secretion: clinical implications. *J Clin Endocrinol Metab.* 2005;90:2522–2530.

208. Raison CL, Rutherford RE, Woolwine BJ, et al. A randomized controlled trial of the tumor necrosis factor antagonist infliximab for treatment-resistant depression: the role of baseline inflammatory biomarkers. *JAMA Psychiatry.* 2013;70:31–41.

209. Wong ML, Dong C, Maestre-Mesa J, Licinio J. Polymorphisms in inflammation-related genes are associated with susceptibility to major depression and antidepressant response. *Mol Psychiatry.* 2008;13:800–812.

210. Traks T, Koido K, Eller T, et al. Polymorphisms in the interleukin-10 gene cluster are possibly involved in the increased risk for major depressive disorder. *BMC Med Genet.* 2008;9:111.

211. Mamdani F, Berlim MT, Beaulieu MM, Labbe A, Merette C, Turecki G. Gene expression biomarkers of response to citalopram treatment in major depressive disorder. *Translat Psychiatry.* 2011;1:e13.

212. Jun TY, Pae CU, Hoon H, et al. Possible association between -G308A tumour necrosis factor-alpha gene polymorphism and major depressive disorder in the Korean population. *Psychiatr Genet.* 2003;13:179–181.

213. Beste C, Heil M, Domschke K, Baune BT, Konrad C. Associations between the tumor necrosis factor alpha gene (-308G→A) and event-related potential indices of attention and mental rotation. *Neuroscience.* 2010;170:742–748.

214. Bedrosian TA, Weil ZM, Nelson RJ. Chronic dim light at night provokes reversible depression-like phenotype: possible role for TNF. *Mol Psychiatry.* 2013;18(8):930–936.

215. Oxenkrug GF. Genetic and hormonal regulation of tryptophan kynurenine metabolism: implications for vascular cognitive impairment, major depressive disorder, and aging. *Ann N Y Acad Sci.* 2007;1122:35–49.

216. Kim JM, Stewart R, Kim SW, et al. Physical health and incident late-life depression: modification by cytokine genes. *Neurobiol Aging.* 2013;34:356 e351–359.

217. Bosker FJ, Hartman CA, Nolte IM, et al. Poor replication of candidate genes for major depressive disorder using genome-wide association data. *Mol Psychiatry.* 2011;16:516–532.

218. Lio D, Scola L, Crivello A, et al. Inflammation, genetics, and longevity: further studies on the protective effects in men of IL-10 -1082 promoter SNP and its interaction with TNF-alpha -308 promoter SNP. *J Med Genet.* 2003;40:296–299.

219. Clerici M, Arosio B, Mundo E, et al. Cytokine polymorphisms in the pathophysiology of mood disorders. *CNS Spectr.* 2009;14:419–425.

220. Sanacora G, Treccani G, Popoli M. Towards a glutamate hypothesis of depression: an

emerging frontier of neuropsychopharmacology for mood disorders. *Neuropharmacology.* 2012;62:63–77.

221. Zhao J, Bao AM, Qi XR, et al. Gene expression of GABA and glutamate pathway markers in the prefrontal cortex of non-suicidal elderly depressed patients. *J Affect Disord.* 2012;138:494–502.

222. Lee M, McGeer EG, McGeer PL. Mechanisms of GABA release from human astrocytes. *Glia.* 2011;59:1600–1611.

223. Lee M, Schwab C, McGeer PL. Astrocytes are GABAergic cells that modulate microglial activity. *Glia.* 2011;59:152–165.

224. Miller AH, Maletic V, Raison CL. Inflammation and its discontents: the role of cytokines in the pathophysiology of major depression. *Biol Psychiatry.* 2009;65:732–741.

225. Shah A, Silverstein PS, Singh DP, Kumar A. Involvement of metabotropic glutamate receptor 5, AKT/PI3K signaling and NF-kappaB pathway in methamphetamine-mediated increase in IL-6 and IL-8 expression in astrocytes. *J Neuroinflamm.* 2012;9:52.

226. Steiner J, Walter M, Gos T, et al. Severe depression is associated with increased microglial quinolinic acid in subregions of the anterior cingulate gyrus: evidence for an immune-modulated glutamatergic neurotransmission? *J Neuroinflamm.* 2011;8:94.

227. O'Riordan KJ, Huang IC, Pizzi M, et al. Regulation of nuclear factor kappaB in the hippocampus by group I metabotropic glutamate receptors. *J Neurosci.* 2006;26:4870–4879.

228. Ghosh M, Yang Y, Rothstein JD, Robinson MB. Nuclear factor-kappaB contributes to neuron-dependent induction of glutamate transporter-1 expression in astrocytes. *J Neurosci.* 2011;31:9159–9169.

229. Pace TW, Miller AH. Cytokines and glucocorticoid receptor signaling. Relevance to major depression. *Ann N Y Acad Sci.* 2009;1179:86–105.

230. Barger SW, Moerman AM, Mao X. Molecular mechanisms of cytokine-induced neuroprotection: NFkappaB and neuroplasticity. *Curr Pharm Des.* 2005;11:985–998.

231. Koo JW, Russo SJ, Ferguson D, Nestler EJ, Duman RS. Nuclear factor-kappaB is a critical mediator of stress-impaired neurogenesis and depressive behavior. *Proc Natl Acad Sci U S A.* 2010;107:2669–2674.

232. Sequeira A, Mamdani F, Ernst C, et al. Global brain gene expression analysis links glutamatergic and GABAergic alterations to suicide and major depression. *PLoS ONE.* 2009;4:e6585.

233. Fiori LM, Turecki G. Broadening our horizons: gene expression profiling to help better understand the neurobiology of suicide and depression. *Neurobiol Dis.* 2012;45:14–22.

234. Bernard R, Kerman IA, Thompson RC, et al. Altered expression of glutamate signaling, growth factor, and glia genes in the locus coeruleus of patients with major depression. *Mol Psychiatry.* 2011;16:634–646.

235. Lee PH, Perlis RH, Jung JY, et al. Multi-locus genome-wide association analysis supports the role of glutamatergic synaptic transmission in the etiology of major depressive disorder. *Translat Psychiatry.* 2012;2:e184.

236. Chiesa A, Crisafulli C, Porcelli S, et al. Influence of GRIA1, GRIA2 and GRIA4 polymorphisms on diagnosis and response to treatment in patients with major depressive disorder. *Eur Arch Psychiatry Clin Neurosci.* 2012;262:305–311.

237. Utge S, Kronholm E, Partonen T, et al. Shared genetic background for regulation of mood and sleep: association of GRIA3 with sleep duration in healthy Finnish women. *Sleep.* 2011;34:1309–1316.

238. Whalley HC, Pickard BS, McIntosh AM, et al. Modulation of hippocampal activation by genetic variation in the GRIK4 gene. *Mol Psychiatry*. 2009;14:465.

239. Frodl TS, Koutsouleris N, Bottlender R, et al. Depression-related variation in brain morphology over 3 years: effects of stress? *Arch Gen Psychiatry*. 2008;65:1156–1165.

240. Klempan TA, Sequeira A, Canetti L, et al. Altered expression of genes involved in ATP biosynthesis and GABAergic neurotransmission in the ventral prefrontal cortex of suicides with and without major depression. *Mol Psychiatry*. 2009;14:175–189.

241. Yamada K, Watanabe A, Iwayama-Shigeno Y, Yoshikawa T. Evidence of association between gamma-aminobutyric acid type A receptor genes located on 5q34 and female patients with mood disorders. *Neurosci Lett*. 2003;349:9–12.

242. Henkel V, Baghai TC, Eser D, et al. The gamma amino butyric acid (GABA) receptor alpha-3 subunit gene polymorphism in unipolar depressive disorder: a genetic association study. *Am J Med Genet B Neuropsychiatr Genet*. 2004;126B:82–87.

243. Hettema JM, An SS, Neale MC, et al. Association between glutamic acid decarboxylase genes and anxiety disorders, major depression, and neuroticism. *Mol Psychiatry*. 2006; 11:752–762.

244. Agrawal A, Nelson EC, Littlefield AK, et al. Cannabinoid receptor genotype moderation of the effects of childhood physical abuse on anhedonia and depression. *Arch Gen Psychiatry*. 2012;69:732–740.

245. Juhasz G, Chase D, Pegg E, et al. CNR1 gene is associated with high neuroticism and low agreeableness and interacts with recent negative life events to predict current depressive symptoms. *Neuropsychopharmacology*. 2009;34:2019–2027.

246. Mickey BJ, Zhou Z, Heitzeg MM, et al. Emotion processing, major depression, and functional genetic variation of neuropeptide Y. *Arch Gen Psychiatry*. 2011;68:158–166.

247. Wong ML, Whelan F, Deloukas P, et al. Phosphodiesterase genes are associated with susceptibility to major depression and antidepressant treatment response. *Proc Natl Acad Sci U S A*. 2006;103:15124–15129.

248. Zubenko GS, Maher B, Hughes HB, et al. Genome-wide linkage survey for genetic loci that influence the development of depressive disorders in families with recurrent, early-onset, major depression. *Am J Med Genet B Neuropsychiatr Genet*. 2003;123B: 1–18.

249. Zubenko GS, Hughes HB, 3rd, et al. Sequence variations in CREB1 cosegregate with depressive disorders in women. *Mol Psychiatry*. 2003;8:611–618.

250. Perlis RH, Purcell S, Fagerness J, et al. Clinical and genetic dissection of anger expression and CREB1 polymorphisms in major depressive disorder. *Biol Psychiatry*. 2007; 62:536–540.

251. Miller AL. The methylation, neurotransmitter, and antioxidant connections between folate and depression. *Alt Med Rev*. 2008;13:216–226.

252. Haroon E, Raison CL, Miller AH. Psychoneuroimmunology meets neuropsychopharmacology: translational implications of the impact of inflammation on behavior. *Neuropsychopharmacology*. 2012;37:137–162.

253. Cunnington C, Channon KM. Tetrahydrobiopterin: pleiotropic roles in cardiovascular pathophysiology. *Heart*. 2010;96:1872–1877.

254. Felger JC, Li L, Marvar PJ, et al. Tyrosine metabolism during interferon-alpha administration: association with fatigue and CSF dopamine concentrations. *Brain Behav Immun*. 2013;31:153–160.

255. McHugh PC. Tetrahydrobiopterin pathway may provide novel molecular targets for

acute and long term efficacy of mood-regulating drugs. *Curr Pharmacogenom Pers Med.* 2010;8:1–8.

256. McGuffin P, Knight J, Breen G, et al. Whole genome linkage scan of recurrent depressive disorder from the depression network study. *Hum Mol Genet.* 2005;14:3337–3345.

257. Lopez-Leon S, Janssens AC, Gonzalez-Zuloeta Ladd AM, et al. Meta-analyses of genetic studies on major depressive disorder. *Mol Psychiatry.* 2008;13:772–785.

258. Peerbooms OL, van Os J, Drukker M, et al. Meta-analysis of MTHFR gene variants in schizophrenia, bipolar disorder and unipolar depressive disorder: evidence for a common genetic vulnerability? *Brain Behav Immun.* 2011;25:1530–1543.

259. Gaysina D, Cohen S, Craddock N, et al. No association with the 5,10-methylenetetrahydrofolate reductase gene and major depressive disorder: results of the depression case control (DeCC) study and a meta-analysis. *Am J Med Genet B Neuropsychiatr Genet.* 2008;147B:699–706.

260. Lan WH, Yang AC, Hwang JP, et al. Association of MTHFR C677T polymorphism with loneliness but not depression in cognitively normal elderly males. *Neurosci Lett.* 2012;521:88–91.

261. Hong ED, Taylor WD, McQuoid DR, et al. Influence of the MTHFR C677T polymorphism on magnetic resonance imaging hyperintensity volume and cognition in geriatric depression. *Am J Geriatr Psychiatry.* 2009;17:847–855.

262. Kim JM, Stewart R, Kim SW, Yang SJ, Shin IS, Yoon JS. Modification by two genes of associations between general somatic health and incident depressive syndrome in older people. *Psychosom Med.* 2009;71:286–291.

263. Mischoulon D, Lamon-Fava S, Selhub J, et al. Prevalence of MTHFR C677T and MS A2756G polymorphisms in major depressive disorder, and their impact on response to fluoxetine treatment. *CNS Spectr.* 2012;17:76–86.

264. Sun X, Zhang Z, Shi Y, Xu Z, Pu M, Geng L. [Influence of methylenetetrahydrofolate reductase gene polymorphisms on antidepressant response]. *Zhonghua Yi Xue Yi Chuan Xue Za Zhi [Chin J Med Genet]*. 2013;30:26–30.

265. Cross-Disorder Group of the Psychiatric Genomics Consortium. Identification of risk loci with shared effects on five major psychiatric disorders: a genome-wide analysis. *Lancet.* 2013;381(9875):1371–1379.

266. Keers R, Farmer AE, Aitchison KJ. Extracting a needle from a haystack: reanalysis of whole genome data reveals a readily translatable finding. *Psychol Med.* 2009;39:1231–1235.

267. Dao DT, Mahon PB, Cai X, et al. Mood disorder susceptibility gene CACNA1C modifies mood-related behaviors in mice and interacts with sex to influence behavior in mice and diagnosis in humans. *Biol Psychiatry.* 2010;68:801–810.

268. Bhat S, Dao DT, Terrillion CE, et al. CACNA1C (Ca(v)1.2) in the pathophysiology of psychiatric disease. *Prog Neurobiol.* 2012;99:1–14.

269. Bigos KL, Mattay VS, Callicott JH, et al. Genetic variation in CACNA1C affects brain circuitries related to mental illness. *Arch Gen Psychiatry.* 2010;67:939–945.

270. Raison CL, Miller AH. The evolutionary significance of depression in Pathogen Host Defense (PATHOS-D). *Mol Psychiatry.* 2013;18:15–37.

271. Kaufman J, Yang BZ, Douglas-Palumberi H, et al. Brain-derived neurotrophic factor-5-HTTLPR gene interactions and environmental modifiers of depression in children. *Biol Psychiatry.* 2006;59:673–680.

272. Wichers M, Kenis G, Jacobs N, et al. The BDNF Val(66)Met × 5-HTTLPR × child adver-

sity interaction and depressive symptoms: an attempt at replication. *Am J Med Genet B Neuropsychiatr Genet.* 2008;147B:120–123.

273. Aguilera M, Arias B, Wichers M, et al. Early adversity and 5-HTT/BDNF genes: new evidence of gene-environment interactions on depressive symptoms in a general population. *Psychol Med.* 2009;39:1425–1432.

274. Pezawas L, Meyer-Lindenberg A, Goldman AL, et al. Evidence of biologic epistasis between BDNF and SLC6A4 and implications for depression. *Mol Psychiatry.* 2008; 13:709–716.

275. Chen CH, Ridler K, Suckling J, et al. Brain imaging correlates of depressive symptom severity and predictors of symptom improvement after antidepressant treatment. *Biol Psychiatry.* 2007;62:407–414.

276. Dannlowski U, Ohrmann P, Bauer J, et al. Amygdala reactivity predicts automatic negative evaluations for facial emotions. *Psychiatry Res.* 2007;154:13–20.

277. Jabbi M, Korf J, Kema IP, et al. Convergent genetic modulation of the endocrine stress response involves polymorphic variations of 5-HTT, COMT and MAOA. *Mol Psychiatry.* 2007;12:483–490.

278. Conway CC, Hammen C, Brennan PA, Lind PA, Najman JM. Interaction of chronic stress with serotonin transporter and catechol-*O*-methyltransferase polymorphisms in predicting youth depression. *Depress Anxiety.* 2010;27:737–745.

279. Benedetti F, Dallaspezia S, Lorenzi C, et al. Gene-gene interaction of glycogen synthase kinase 3-beta and serotonin transporter on human antidepressant response to sleep deprivation. *J Affect Disord.* 2012;136:514–519.

280. Zhang K, Yang C, Xu Y, et al. Genetic association of the interaction between the BDNF and GSK3B genes and major depressive disorder in a Chinese population. *J Neural Transm.* 2010;117:393–401.

281. Juhasz G, Dunham JS, McKie S, et al. The CREB1-BDNF-NTRK2 pathway in depression: multiple gene-cognition-environment interactions. *Biol Psychiatry.* 2011;69:762–771.

282. GENDEP Investigators, MARS Investigators, STAR*D Investigators. Common genetic variation and antidepressant efficacy in major depressive disorder: a meta-analysis of three genome-wide pharmacogenetic studies. *Am J Psychiatry.* 2013;170:207–217.

283. Manji HK, Drevets WC, Charney DS. The cellular neurobiology of depression. *Nat Med.* 2001;7:541–547.

284. Carlson PJ, Singh JB, Zarate CA Jr, Drevets WC, Manji HK. Neural circuitry and neuroplasticity in mood disorders: insights for novel therapeutic targets. *NeuroRx.* 2006; 3:22–41.

285. Wichers MC, Barge-Schaapveld DQ, Nicolson NA, et al. Reduced stress-sensitivity or increased reward experience: the psychological mechanism of response to antidepressant medication. *Neuropsychopharmacology.* 2009;34(4):923–931.

CHAPTER 5

Depression and the Brain-Body Dance
Roles of Neuroendocrine, Autonomic, and Immune Pathways

What we feel and think and are is to a great extent determined by the state of our ductless glands and viscera.

Aldous Huxley

Good for the body is the work of the body, and good for the soul is the work of the soul, and good for either is the work of the other.

Henry David Thoreau

At the time of this writing, the National Institute of Mental Health has gone on record as saying that mental disorders are brain disorders. At first blush this might seem so obvious to those of us who work in mental health that it hardly needs saying. But it would have surprised many philosophers and doctors in the ancient and medieval world, who tended to give primacy to the heart as the seat of thought and feeling. And we think it might have surprised many early scientists studying the biology of Major Depression, because paradoxically almost all the early discoveries regarding the pathophysiology of depression that have passed the test of time involved abnormalities not in the brain but in the body.

At the risk of oversimplifying, we suggest that, when it comes to mood disorders, biological psychiatry was born with three observations: (a) that medications with effects on neurotransmitters worked as antidepressants, (b) that depressed individuals showed reduced time latency to enter rapid-eye-movement sleep, and (c) that depressed individuals had complex abnormalities in the functioning of the hypothalamic-pituitary-adrenal (HPA) axis. Of these three observations, the only one that has bred true—despite accruing complications and some contradictions over the years—is the one involving the HPA axis. The first observation, that medications with neurotransmitter effects work as antidepressants, has spawned a multibillion dollar industry and helped many people with depression, but all the early conceptions of how these antidepressants worked (e.g., by simply increasing serotonin or norepinephrine) have been largely discredited. Similarly, with the passage of time, although shortened rapid-eye-movement latency has held up fairly well as a marker for depression and related conditions, other sleep abnormalities, such as reduced slow-wave sleep or impaired sleep continuity, have come to be recognized as equally common and perhaps more detrimental.

On the other hand, the discovery that many patients with severe depression have circulating levels of the glucocorticoid stress hormone cortisol that were as high as those typically seen in Cushing's disease opened a line of research that has, if anything, become increasingly relevant with the passing years. Of even greater importance than the finding of hypercortisolemia was the discovery that many patients with major depressive disorder (MDD)—especially those with elevated levels of circulating cortisol—were also resistant to the effects of cortisol at the level of the pituitary as measured by the dexamethasone (DEX) suppression test (DST) and at the level of immune cells as measured by various in vitro techniques.[1,2]

Before delving more deeply into the HPA axis and other pathways by which mind, brain, and body are interconnected, it is important to emphasize a key fact about reduced cortisol sensitivity that is so common in depression. (Following convention, we will refer to cortisol sensitivity or resistance with the term *glucocorticoid*, which describes the larger class of hormones of which cortisol is a member.) DEX, the synthetic glucocorticoid used to probe for this reduced sensitivity in the DST, does not cross the blood–brain barrier and so exerts its effects primarily at the level of the pituitary gland. This means that one of the most reproducible findings in biological psychiatry, based on a test that was briefly held to be the future of psychiatric diagnosis, comes from the body and not the brain, leaving us to ponder the fact that the biological study of mood disorders in modern times began to a large degree based on an often unacknowledged truth: that depression exists in the body as much as in the brain.

Perhaps this shouldn't surprise us, given our discussion in Chapter 3 regarding the ability of inflammatory molecules (e.g., interferon-alpha [IFN-α]) introduced into the periphery of the body to reliably produce depressive symptoms.[3] Of course, in the case of peripheral inflammation or glucocorticoid resistance, it may be that these physiological changes have no causal capacity to produce depression in and of themselves but, rather, merely induce brain changes that are the real cause of depression. We will not argue the likelihood of this but point out that causality becomes a slippery slope when too rigid a line is drawn between the central nervous system (CNS) and periphery of the body. Consider a study done by our group in which we gave medically stable/healthy individuals with treatment-resistant MDD three infusions of either a saltwater placebo or infliximab, a very powerful antagonist of the proinflammatory cytokine tumor necrosis factor.[4] While infliximab did not perform any better than placebo overall, in subjects with high levels of peripheral inflammation at baseline it worked as well compared with placebo as do standard antidepressants. Importantly, infliximab is too large to cross the blood–brain barrier, meaning that it treated depression in these people by reducing inflammation in the body and not by any direct effects on the brain. Said differently, the brains of subjects entering the study with increased levels of peripheral inflammation were constantly receiving signals from their bodies that they were in danger of dying from infection and should feel sick (i.e., given the role of inflammation in signaling these dangers to the brain). Turn off that peripheral signal and that reason for the brain to be depressed goes away, and the depression improves. So from one point of view, we might truly say that the cause of depression in these people was in their bodies, and their brains were just responding reasonably to the signals they were receiving.

We encourage keeping this perspective in mind as we move now into a more detailed discussion of the types of bidirectional interactions between brain and the rest of the body that have been repeatedly implicated in the pathogenesis of depression.

Brain-Body Interactions Implicated in Depression I: Meeting the Players

In Chapter 3 we attempted to demonstrate that the environmental risk factors for depression are not random but, rather, cluster around events and situations that reduce reproductive fitness in the environments in which humans and our mammalian forbearers evolved. What all these situations/events shared in common was that they signaled danger to survival, reproduction, or both. As an outgrowth of the fact that humans are supremely social animals who long ago overcame most of the risk of death by predation (except from one another), it is not surprising that many of the most depressogenic dangers are social in nature. Similarly, because infection has been a primary driver of human mortality far back into our evolutionary past, it is not surprising that, as we discussed in Chapter 3, inflammatory signals from the immune system that signal likely infection should also be profoundly depressogenic, as indeed they are.

From these observations one would predict that brain areas most essential for social interactions and for recognizing danger, both from within and from without, should be those areas most likely to be implicated in the pathogenesis of depression. And, as we discuss in Chapter 8, this is the case. By the same logic, brain-body communication pathways especially relevant to the detecting and surviving danger should be the ones most implicated in pathogenesis of depression. Again, overwhelming evidence suggests this is the case and that, to the degree that depression "lives in the body," it does so first and foremost in the body's three primary danger pathways: the HPA axis, the autonomic nervous system (ANS), and the immune system. Moreover, although individual cases vary widely, in general depression is characterized by a clear pattern in this extended "danger circuit," consisting of insufficient signaling by cortisol (the glucocorticoid hormone end product of the HPA axis), increased sympathetic tone, diminished parasympathetic tone, and increased inflammation.[5] This constellation of changes is also characteristic of chronic stress states and is seen in both animals and humans. In this way, depression can yet again be seen as a state in which the brain-body complex perceives itself to be in a state of chronic danger, loss, or both. The degree to which this perception corresponds with what others would perceive as reality varies among depressed individuals, but the biological changes that characterize bodily systems in depression seem as likely to occur from depressogenic misperceptions of reality as from truth.

THE HPA AXIS

People have debated exact definitions of the concept of "stress" for decades, but if we accept it at face value the way most of us conceive of it, then we can say that stress begins when the brain perceives a change in the internal or external environment that offers either danger or opportunity, with the intensity of the stressor generally linked to its relevance to the survival and reproduction of the organism (or, more exactly, to the relevance of the stressor to proximal goals that serve these evolutionary ends, as we discuss in Chapter 3).

Upon perceiving stress, the brain's first move is to activate the ANS (discussed further below). But concurrent with this, via multiple pathways the brain stimulates the production of two closely related neuropeptides in the pariventricular nucleus (PVN) of the hypothalamus: corticotropin-releasing hormone (CRH) and arginine vasopressin. Although both of these chemicals (often called secretagogues because they stimulate the secretion of other hormones) produce subtly different biological effects, in general their actions are redundant and serve to turn on the HPA axis. Here we focus on CRH because it has been the most intensively studied and to date appears to be the more relevant of the two for the pathophysiology of MDD.[6]

Like many substances that operate as hormones in the body, CRH works more like a neurotransmitter in the CNS. So in addition to activating the HPA axis, CRH induces brain effects via receptors located in the brain, especially in limbic areas such as the amygdala and the bed nucleus of the stria terminalis. Although the exact behavioral effects of CRH depend on the mix of CRH receptor subtypes in any given brain region, in general CRH's effects are anxiogenic and depressogenic, and agents that block CRH in the CNS show antianxiety and antidepressant effects in animals,[7] although for reasons that are not entirely clear they have failed to reliably demonstrate the same effects in humans.[8]

Perhaps the easiest way to envision the primary activities of CRH is to picture it sitting at the bottom of the brain awaiting the arrival of a stressor. When a stressor arrives, CRH has upward action into the brain itself, where it produces a range of effects that promote fear, anxiety, vigilance, and other states reasonable in the context of danger. CRH has what might be thought of a "lateral" action in that it has a direct connection with the locus ceruleus in the brainstem, which is the primary activator of the sympathetic nervous system (SNS). The SNS does not require CRH to activate, but CRH stimulation powerfully reinforces other SNS activators.

Finally, and most famously, CRH is the primary activator of the HPA axis, which is the quintessential hormonal stress system in the body (Figure 5.1). Stressors of all sorts, both psychological and physical, promote the production and release of CRH from the PVN. From there CRH is transported by a specialized portal circulatory system to the anterior portion of the pituitary gland, where it stimulates the release of adrenocorticotropic hormone (ACTH). ACTH, in turn, enters the bloodstream and stimulates the outer portion of the adrenal glands (i.e., the zona fasciculate of the adrenal cortex) to release glucocorticoids (cortisol in humans and the closely related corticosterone in rodents). Glucocorticoids have the capacity to impact the functioning of every cell.

Although glucocorticoids have been shown to have rapid effects mediated by cell surface receptors, their primary effects—and those most relevant to depression—result from the actions of glucocorticoids on receptors that, when quiescent, reside in the cytosolic compartment of cells. When unstimulated, these receptors exist within a topologically complex assembly of heat-shock proteins that stabilize the unbound receptor and have been shown to play important roles in relationship to depression, as we discuss below. Glucocorticoids passively diffuse through the membranes of cells and bind to these receptors, which frees up the receptor from its heat-shock protein moorings, allowing it to translocate to the cellular nucleus. Within the nucleus these ligand-activated receptors induce effects primarily by interacting with other transcription factors or by binding to specific DNA response elements, which results in either the up- or downregulation of a host of other genes.

Upon diffusing through the cell membrane, glucocorticoids interact with two distinct types of intracellular receptors. Mineralocorticoid receptors (MRs) have a high affinity for cortisol and corticosterone (i.e., naturally occurring glucocorticoids), as well as the salt-regulating hormone aldosterone. In contrast, glucocorticoid receptors (GRs) bind avidly to synthetic glucocorticoids such as DEX but have a much lower affinity for cortisol or corticosterone, which means they are activated only when cortisol levels are high, such as occurs during stress. In contrast, MRs play a primary role in mediating glucocorticoid effects under basal conditions when hormone levels are low. As glucocorticoid levels rise, either in response to stressor or as a function of the HPA circadian cycle, MRs saturate and GRs become the primary transducers of glucocorticoid signaling to tissues in the body and brain. For this reason, far more research has been done on the role of

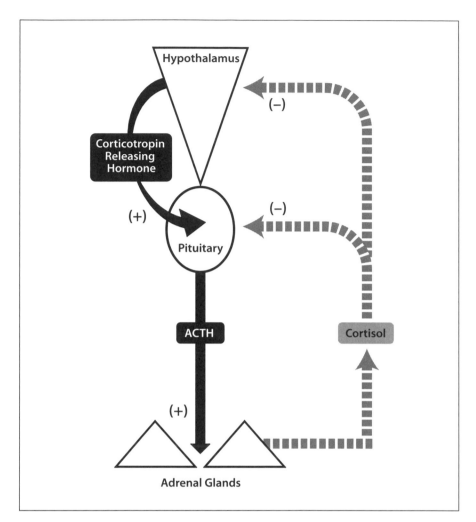

FIGURE 5.1. This schematic of the hypothalamic-pituitary-adrenal (HPA) axis shows that a variety of stressors, both psychological and physical, activate the hypothalamus to produce corticotrophin releasing hormone (CRH). CRH then passes via a specialized vascular pathway to the anterior portion of the pituitary gland, where it stimulates the release of adrenocortico-tropin (ACTH). ACTH is released into the general circulation through which it travels to the adrenal glands where it stimulates the release of cortisol, the body's primary stress hormone. However, although cortisol has many stress-producing effect it also plays a key role in damp-ening stress responses because it feeds back on all levels of the HPA axis to turn off its own production.

GRs than MRs in the pathogenesis of depression. Accordingly, our discussion here focuses primarily on the role of GRs in mediating HPA axis effects relevant to MDD.

Cortisol in humans and corticosterone in rodents are the quintessential stress hormones that have multiple effects that enhance the fight-or-flight response.

They stimulate the breakdown of amino acids in muscles, which are then converted to glucose for rapid energy utilization by the body, while at the same time promoting insulin resistance. They increase blood pressure and enhance the ability of stress-released catecholamines to increase cardiac output, which also increases energy available to the organism for coping with stress. The effects of glucocorticoids on the brain are complex, but in response to acute stress they narrow and focus attention and enhance memory formation for the circumstances that promoted their release. Finally, as we discuss at some length below, glucocorticoids have powerful and diverse immune effects. They are powerfully antiinflammatory, which is why synthetic glucocorticoids have been the mainstay of treatment for so many inflammatory conditions, but they also play important roles in redirecting immune cells to areas of the body, such as the skin, where they would be of most likely benefit in the case of wounding.

We know of few things in biology as remarkable as the fact that glucocorticoids are both the body's primary stress hormone and its primary antistress hormone. Can you imagine a car built with a single pedal that is both the gas pedal and the brake? And yet in a very real sense this is how the HPA axis is constructed. CRH from the hypothalamus stimulates the release of ACTH from the pituitary, which stimulates release of glucocorticoids from the adrenal glands, which then feed back at the hypothalamus to shut off CRH, at the pituitary to shut off ACTH, and at the adrenal glands to shut off those glands. Unlike machines designed by humans in which opposing functions are housed in separate systems, most bodily processes contain within themselves built-in restraining mechanisms, but even amidst this biological complexity it is rare for a single chemical to perform such diametrically opposed tasks as do glucocorticoids.

We believe this complexity has played much havoc in psychiatry's understanding of the role of the HPA axis in depression over the years, a topic that we address at some length below. But for now consider this: if depressed patients have elevated levels of cortisol in their blood, does this represent a detrimentally overactive stress response, or does it reflect the fact that they do not have sufficient cortisol signaling to turn off the production of cortisol? Said more simply, do they have too much cortisol signal, as one would predict from their hypercortisolism, or do they have too little cortisol signal, given that without this signal they also would not be able to turn off the production of cortisol and so would demonstrate the same type of hypercortisolemia?

THE AUTONOMIC NERVOUS SYSTEM

Just as key elements of the HPA axis significantly impact brain functioning in addition to their endocrine effects, the primary neurotransmitters of the ANS (norepinephrine [NE] for the SNS and acetylcholine for the parasympathetic nervous system [PNS]) are also important neurotransmitters in the CNS, from where they have multiple effects relevant to every aspect of cognition, emotion, and behavior.

Moreover, many psychiatric medicines over the years have putatively worked by altering the functioning of these neurotransmitter systems in the CNS. Whereas we tend to think of cortisol as being a bodily chemical, in psychiatry at least it is hard for us not to hear the word *norepinephrine* and immediately think of the brain. Our task here is to overcome this bias and consider catecholaminergic and cholinergic signaling within the body and to consider how these autonomic effects might promote emotional disease or well-being.

The word *autonomic* suggests the word *automatic*, which gets at a key characteristic of the ANS. Unlike the somatic motor system, by which bodily movements of all types, both voluntary and reflexive, are generated, the ANS generally functions below the level of consciousness to maintain all the visceral functions of the body that are essential for life but that largely occur without our conscious awareness or control (exceptions include the central role of the ANS in sexual activity, urination, and defecation). Classically, the ANS is considered to have two primary subsystems, the SNS and PNS, which work collaboratively for some biological functions, such as sexual arousal and orgasm, but often have opposing effects on the visceral functions they impact. Ignoring multiple complexities, it is generally true that the SNS subserves fight-or-flight responses and thus can be considered a paradigmatic "danger pathway" by which the brain marshals bodily resources to best survive threat and/or maximize the chances of reward from antagonistic encounters. In contrast, the PNS is essential for many of the body's restorative and maintenance activities, and for situations of cooperation as opposed to challenge or threat. Thus, if the SNS is "fight or flight," the PNS might be characterized as "rest and digest" or "feed and breed."

Consistent with this characterization, activation of the SNS rapidly produces many physiological effects that evolved to help cope with threat, including increased blood flow to skeletal muscles, the heart, and the lungs, dilation of lung bronchioles, increased heart rate and contraction strength, and dilation of the pupils to allow more light to enter the eye and enhance far vision. At the same time, SNS activation diverts blood flow away from the gastrointestinal tract and skin by stimulating vasoconstriction and inhibits gastrointestinal peristalsis. Conversely, activation of the PNS increases blood flow to the gastrointestinal tract and stimulates salivary gland secretion and peristalsis to enhance food digestion. The PNS also reduces heart rate and contractility, constricts lung bronchioles, constricts the pupils to aid in close vision, and stimulates sexual arousal.

To accomplish these effects, the SNS and PNS use different primary effector transmitters. Although both systems utilize acetylcholine stimulation of nicotinic receptors for preganglionic signaling, for postganglionic (i.e., end-organ) signaling the SNS uses NE whereas the PNS uses acetylcholine stimulation of muscarinic receptors. Exceptions exist, however. For example, the SNS utilizes nicotinic receptors in the adrenal medulla to drive epinephrine release. NE and epinephrine signal through two broad classes of receptors, termed alpha and beta, which often have opposing effects (especially in terms of constriction or dilation of blood vessels). Most sympathetic modulation of the heart occurs via beta type 1 and type 2 receptors, whereas alpha receptors modulate blood pressure.

Both the SNS and PNS have rich connections with various brain areas, but the CNS neurons specific for these pathways lie within discrete areas of the brainstem and spinal cord, with cell bodies for the PNS located in the brainstem and sacral spinal cord, and cell bodies for the SNS sandwiched between these PNS areas within the lateral horn of the spinal cord from the first thoracic vertebrae in the neck to the second and third lumbar vertebrae in the lower back. Unlike somatic neurons, which project directly to their peripheral targets, CNS neurons of the ANS are preganglionic, meaning that they synapse with one additional and final postganglionic neuron that then projects to any given visceral target. In the SNS, the cell bodies for these postganglionic nuclei form two chains on either side of the spinal cord. In the PNS, these cell bodies tend to be located adjacent to the organ/viscera to be innervated. Several exceptions to these organizational patterns exist. For example, CNS sympathetic neurons project monosynaptically to the adrenal medulla to stimulate the release of the hormone epinephrine, which greatly augments the stress response in general and NE effects in particular. You have experienced this augmentation if you have ever had a near miss with some dangerous occurrence and then 30–60 seconds after the event suddenly felt your heart pound for no apparent reason. That is epinephrine being released and stimulating cardiac function.

We tend to think of the ANS as primarily an output system from the brain, but it also has afferent fibers that provide a feedback loop by providing information on the state of bodily organs, thereby also allowing the body to serve as a "sounding board" for CNS perceptions of the risks and benefits of any given situation. Anyone who has ever taken a beta-blocker to quiet the sympathetic activation of the heart in response to performance anxiety knows how subtly powerful the impact of body is on the brain. Without the signal that one's heart is racing, it is difficult to be convinced that one is nervous, even if the mind recognizes that it should feel that way.

Thus far we have presented the ANS as it appears in most textbooks, is taught in medical school, and is generally understood in psychiatry and related mental health disciplines. As we have suggested, in this conceptualization PNS activity predominates for activities requiring some degree of safety, such as digesting food, excreting wastes, and engaging in rest and sexual activity, whereas in the face of threat the PNS activity recedes and the SNS is activated to provide energy and focus to help the organism either flee from danger or fight. But intriguingly, this schema leaves out a third response to environmental conditions that is readily apparent in humans and animals and is captured in the colloquial phrase "like a deer in the headlights." In the face of extreme danger, mammals often evince a freezing response that is neither vegetative nor fight-flight in nature but, rather, represents a shutdown of the organism. In many prey animals this response is so profound that it can be characterized as feigning death, and indeed sometimes the act is so physiologically effective that the animal actually dies. In humans this type of behavioral paralysis in response to severe trauma or danger often portends the development of later maladaptive psychological responses, such as posttraumatic stress disorder (PTSD).

In response to data indicating that this third state often appeared at odds with other vagal effects, as measured by a heart rate variability (HRV) metric known as respiratory sinus arrhythmia, Stephen Porges in the early 1990s articulated the much debated but highly influential polyvagal theory, which postulates that vagal activity may not be a unified phenomenon but may in fact arise from two anatomically and functionally distinct branches of the efferent vagal system.[9–11] This conceptualization splits the ANS into three subsystems instead of two, with these subsystems being phylogenetically ordered, meaning that they evolved in sequence as vertebrate behavioral repertoires became more complex.

The oldest system is exemplified by an unmyelinated branch of the vagus nerve that originates from the dorsal motor nucleus of the vagus and primarily innervates organs below the diaphragm. This system is found in most vertebrates and when activated produces physical and emotional immobilization. Second, to survive all vertebrates need a system to mobilize in the face of danger, and this is the task of the SNS from a polyvagal perspective. Finally, present only in mammals is a myelinated branch of the vagus nerve that originates in the nucleus ambiguous and is conceptualized as being part of a far more extensive, integrated social communication system that through its evolution allowed mammals to tolerate levels of intimacy in their associations with others that are strikingly lacking in reptiles and fish. Signaling through the myelinated vagus is integrated by the brain with somatosensory nerves that control muscles important for eye gaze and facial expression and that allow the muscles of the inner ear to be optimally tuned for the frequency of species-specific communications, the human voice in our case.

The polyvagal perspective suggests that perceptions of safety (whether from the external world by the senses or from the internal milieu via hormonal and afferent autonomic signals) enhance signaling in the myelinated vagus, which can be "read out" as increased HRV, captured in the frequency domain measure of respiratory sinus arrhythmia. Increased signaling through the myelinated vagus allows the bodily state to be regulated in an efficient manner that promotes growth and restoration. This is accomplished by slowing heart rate below the intrinsic level of the cardiac pacemaker, inhibiting the SNS and the HPA axis, and reducing inflammation (as we discuss below). As a result of this vagal influence, our heart rate at rest is controlled by increases and decreases in vagal signaling to the heart, allowing rapid adjustments in heart rate in response to environmental conditions without incurring the metabolic costs of activating the SNS. It is only when stress/danger levels exceed this moment-by-moment modulatory influence that the phylogentically older SNS kicks in and a full-blown stress response is under way. Research has provided support for several aspects of the polyvagal theory, and if this continues it may well be that our standard view of the ANS as composed of two subsystems will be replaced with this more elegant tripartite view of its organization and functioning.

THE IMMUNE SYSTEM

Whereas the HPA axis and ANS have been linked to depressive pathophysiology since the beginning of biological psychiatry and to emotional states longer than that, the immune system is the new kid on the block. In the 1980s when we went to medical school the words *immune* and *brain* never came up in the same sentence unless it was to emphasis that the brain was an "immune-protected organ" because of the blood–brain barrier and was therefore beyond the reach of immune cells and chemicals (which we now know isn't true),[12] all of which did their work in the periphery of the body. We knew that the adaptive immune system had the capacity to remember pathogens to which it had been exposed in the past and so could be said, like the brain, to learn from experience, but that is as far as it went.

Looking back, it is remarkable how rapidly all this has changed. We now know that the immune system and CNS are better thought of as one extended network, with each element requiring the other to function properly. Brain activity profoundly impacts immune functioning and vice versa. More recently, it has become apparent that immune cells (e.g., microglia) and molecules (e.g., cytokines) play essential roles in guiding the formation of the brain during development.[13] And many chemicals important for brain functioning (i.e., brain-derived neurotrophic factor [BDNF]) display immune properties when present in the body. These insights have given rise to the field of psychoneuroimmunology, dedicated to studying the multidirectional connections that exist among the brain, neuroendocrine and autonomic pathways, and the immune system.

Chapter 3 covered the innate immune inflammatory response and its relation to stress. Missing from that discussion was any consideration of the other major arm of the mammalian immune system, referred to alternately as specific or acquired immunity. This is the immune system as most of us think of it, the target of vaccines, the culprit behind human immunodeficiency virus, the B cells that produce antibodies, and the T cells that work as antigen-driven killing machines or that coordinate the body's overall immune response. When researchers first began examining brain–immune connections in the late 1970s and early 1980s, it was to the adaptive immune system that they turned, in part because it was so much better understood than innate immunity in those years and in part because its impact on life and death in the context of infection was so apparent.[14]

But with the discovery that chemicals secreted by cells of both the innate and acquired immune systems had the capacity to profoundly change brain chemistry and behavior, the emphasis switched in the 1990s away from studying the effect of stress on the composition of immune cells to examining how cytokines and chemokines impacted the brain and were in turn impacted by CNS responses to stress. But now the tide of scientific fashion is turning once again, and there is a renewed interest in the role that peripheral immune cell functioning may play both in developmental disorders such as autism and in predisposing toward the development of depression and anxiety in the context of stress.

An Overview of the Immune System in Action: The Body Meets a Bug

Recognizing that what follows is by necessity a simplification, let's examine what happens when a pathogen invades the body, typically through the respiratory system, the gastrointestinal tract, the reproductive system, or a tear in the skin—all those places of vulnerability where the body meets and communicates with the outside world. All these areas are enriched with immune patrol cells, the most important of which are macrophages and dendritic cells that continually monitor their local environment for the presence of foreign objects that might pose a danger. These patrol cells have surface receptors that bind to a variety of molecules that are commonly found on the surface of pathogens but that are missing from mammalian cells. Unlike the activities of T cells and B cells (which we discuss below), the receptors on innate immune patrol cells like macrophages and dendritic cells are much more nonspecific. They recognize general patterns of foreignness, equivalent to a person who can recognize that a stranger is speaking a romance language but can't tell whether it is Spanish, French, or Italian. These molecular clusters are known as pathogen-associated molecular patterns (PAMPs). The best-characterized PAMP receptors are known as Toll-like (which sit on the surface of patrol cells) and NOD-like (which exist within cells). Interestingly, these receptors can be activated and launch an innate immune response not just after exposure to PAMPs but also after detecting molecules from within the host that suggest tissue damage (not surprisingly these molecules are known as DAMPs, or danger-associated molecular patterns).[15]

Once activated, these receptors in turn activate the patrol cells to perform an array of functions essential for host defense. We have already discussed in Chapter 3 their role in innate immunity. In this capacity these cells secrete cytokines and chemokines that have profound effects at the site of pathogen invasion or tissue damage and more widely in the body and brain. Macrophages, especially, are efficient also at directly attacking invading organisms. By engulfing pathogens, this phagocytic activity helps rid the body of infection. Innate immune cells also secrete chemicals essential for wound repair once the damage has been done and the infectious risk has passed.

In lower vertebrates these activities, in concert with other innate immune mechanisms, are all that are available to provide host defense. However, in mammals a second, much more efficient and specific, or acquired, immune response has evolved. Unlike innate immunity, which responds to pathogens in only a generalized way, acquired immunity has a remarkable ability to recognize and destroy specific pathogens and to remember prior exposure to these pathogens so that when they are encountered again a far more rapid and effective immune response can be mounted. However, as with all evolved systems, these innovations did not arise by discarding processes already in place but, rather, by building upon them. Thus, the innate and acquired immune systems interdigitate at multiple points, and both cooperate and compete.

A key point of cooperation occurs at the start of an acquired immune response, which can be launched only when phagocytic cells of the innate immune system (especially dendritic cells) engulf an invading pathogen, and then digest, process and present molecules from the invader on their cell surfaces. These molecules are invariably associated with one of two types of host cell surface molecules known as type I or type II major histocompatibility molecules (MHC). MHC molecules serve as a type of security system to prevent T cells from mistakenly orchestrating immune attacks against the self, because T cells will respond to these pathogen products only when they are "presented" by an MHC molecule. When thus presented, the pathogen particles (which are usually proteins) are known as antigens because they elicit robust responses from T cells that have receptors specific for that particular pathogen molecule.

How T cells are able to have receptors specific for the nearly infinite pathogen-derived chemical arrangements placed on the surface of antigen presenting cells such as macrophages and dendritic cells was one of the great mysteries of immunology when we were in medical school. It seemed miraculous. The answer, as it turns out, is a perfect example of the process of natural selection in a microcosm because it involves the generation of a huge array of random variations that then either die or live and reproduce or not depending on whether they are selected by the environment. Early in life a huge array of T cells are generated in the thymus, each with a slightly different, randomly arranged antigen receptor confirmation. Early in this process T cells with receptors that just happen to recognize (i.e., run the risk of binding to) molecules found in the body are destroyed so that autoimmunity does not occur, or is at least minimized. For the rest, T cells circulate through the body and/or reside in immune organs such as lymph nodes or the spleen in an unstimulated, "naïve" state.

These T cells remain in this state until they happen to meet up with an antigen being presented on the surface of a dendritic cell or macrophage that happens to have a pattern that corresponds with T cell receptor. When this happens the T cell is activated, leading to the production of a huge number of copies of itself, all with the ability to bind to, and thereby destroy, cells with that same antigen. From an evolutionary perspective this can be seen as a type of "survival of the fittest," with fitness being defined as having—by sheer accident—a receptor that becomes immunologically valuable because it matches the shape of an antigen on a pathogen. Although most of these T cell progeny will perish once the pathogen danger has been eliminated, a subset of these cells will develop into memory T cells, which will live on for extended periods, ready to recognize the same pathogen should it enter the body again and respond rapidly by again producing a huge number of copies of itself, each with the capacity to fight the invading organism. This process of natural selection in miniature explains why vaccines work. Vaccines introduce a pathogen-related antigen that produces a small army of memory T cells ready to spring to life and rapidly clear that antigen from the body should it ever appear again (this time attached to a dangerous pathogen).

T cells come in two primary types, based on the pattern of molecules on their surfaces (which are known as clusters of differentiation, or CD) and their attendant functional capacities. CD4 T cells are known as T helper cells, whereas CD8 T cells are known as effector T cells. Although CD8 T cells, when activated, do much of the actual work of killing pathogens, CD4 T cells play an even more primary role in shaping overall immune responses. That they are absolutely essential to the proper functioning of the immune system has been made apparent by the lethality of the human immunodeficiency virus, which causes AIDS by selectively killing off CD4 T cells.

It is increasingly clear that the shape of any given acquired immune response results to a large degree from a complex interaction between antigen-presenting cells (especially dendritic cells) and CD4 T helper cells. This interaction guides CD4 cells to differentiate along one of a number of lines of functional activity characterized largely by the types of cytokines produced. We have known for several decades that when confronted with viruses and bacteria that exist within cells, CD4 cells differentiate into what is known as a type 1, or Th1, response, whereas when confronted with bacteria that exist outside cells or worms and other extracellular parasites, CD4 cells differentiate along Th2 lines. More recently, other lines of CD4 differentiation have been identified, the most important of which is the highly proinflammatory Th17 profile. Classic Th1 cytokines include interferon-gamma (IFN-γ) and interleukin-2 (IL-2); classic Th2 cytokines include IL-4 and IL-5; and classic Th17 cytokines include IL-17 and IL-23.

Although most interest in the role of acquired immunity in psychological functioning has focused on T cells, they represent only half of the acquired immune armamentarium. The other half of acquired immune antipathogen activity is conducted by B cells (so named because they were first identified in the bursa organ of birds). When activated by T cells and by exposure to antigens, these cells differentiate to produce antibodies that bind to the surface of infected cells and to extracellular pathogens and greatly facilitate their killing by CD8 effector T cells. In many ways antibodies can be thought of as similar to the receptors on T cells; these are simply shed into the external environment by B cells. Like T cells, B cells that respond to any given pathogen do so because the antibodies they produce are shaped to respond to specific antigens. In another example of innate-acquired immune collaboration, the work of antibodies is greatly enhanced by the production of complement proteins by the innate immune system. These proteins, in addition to having intrinsic antipathogen effects, coat extracellular bacteria and by doing so make it far easier for antibodies to "grab" of them and promote their destruction. Finally, although all acquired immune responses include a B cell component, Th2 responses especially favor antibody production, consistent with their focus on killing extracellular organisms.

As we noted in regard to the HPA axis, bodily processes almost always contain built-in mechanisms that constrain or oppose the primary activity of the process in question. Said differently, they almost always have a built-in brake to keep them from overshooting. Acquired immune responses are no different. When we were in medical school several decades ago we learned about supposed T suppressor cells that developed to turn off acquired immune responses. Subsequent studies suggested these cells were more mythic than real, and thus they fell out of scientific favor. However, in one of the most remarkable turnarounds in the history of immunology, the idea of suppressor cells has come roaring back in the form of regulatory T (Treg) cells, which are currently one of the hottest areas of investigation in the field. Treg cells are in the CD4, T helper cell lineage. They form a subset of cells that also express the cell surface activation marker CD25 but are best distinguished by the intracellular expression of Foxp3 (Forkhead box 3), an important T cell immunoregulatory transcription factor.[16] Treg cells are an important source of IL-10, once considered a Th2 cytokine but now recognized as being more generally immunoregulatory and anti-inflammatory. Treg cells also produce transforming growth factor-beta, a cytokine with complex and somewhat contradictory actions but with a profile that is generally anti-inflammatory.[17]

Given the general rule that physiological systems in the body have built-in restraining mechanisms, it should perhaps not be surprising that the discovery of Tregs has prompted the search for regulatory cells in other immune lineages. And indeed, although they are not as well characterized as Tregs, it is now clear that such cells exist and are important for proper immune functioning. Such cells include regulatory dendritic and B cells and M2-type macrophages. It is increasingly recognized that inflammatory and autoimmune conditions are promoted when these regulatory cells function suboptimally. On the other hand, increasing data suggest that these cells can also pose a risk of inducing patterns of immune suppression that are not always health promoting. For example, regulatory cells have been implicated in vulnerability to cancer development and spread. Of more direct relevance to our interests, increasing evidence suggests that suboptimal immunoregulatory functioning may be a common feature of Major Depression and may in fact contribute to the proinflammatory state often observed in MDD.[15]

Brain-Body Interactions Implicated in Depression II: The Centrality of Danger Pathways to Depressive Pathogenesis

THE HPA AXIS IN DEPRESSION

Studies conducted over many years suggest that, as a group, people with MDD demonstrate various indices of HPA axis hyperactivity. Almost all work in this area has focused on CRH, the primary secretagogue of the HPA axis , and cortisol, its primary end-product hormone. The role of ACTH, the hormone that links CRH to cortisol via stimulation of the adrenal glands, in depression is far less understood. Below we discuss the complexities of cortisol signaling in depression at some length. Prior to this, we briefly comment on CRH.

Abnormal activity in CRH pathways has been repeatedly observed in medically healthy patients with Major Depression.[18–21] Many,[22–27] but not all,[28–30] studies report that patients with Major Depression demonstrate increased cerebrospinal (CSF) concentrations of CRH, consistent with increased release of CRH from extrahypothalamic (i.e., limbic/cortical) areas of the brain.[31] Several studies indicate that CSF concentrations of CRH normalize when patients recover from a depressive episode.[32–34] Moreover, patients who normalize CSF CRH concentrations in concert with recovering from depression are more likely to relapse if CRH concentrations begin to increase in the subsequent six months.[35] Also consistent with increased CRH activity in Major Depression are postmortem studies reporting increased CRH mRNA expression in the PVN of patients with depression and decreased CRH binding sites in the frontal cortex of suicide victims (presumably secondary to hypersecretion of CRH), as well as blunted ACTH responses following CRH administration, consistent with CRH receptor downregulation in the pituitary in the face of hypersecretion of hypothalamic CRH.[36,37] Finally, medications that block the CRH type 1 receptor have been repeatedly shown to have antidepressant effects in animal model systems, although their promise in humans, while suggestive, has never fully materialized.[7]

GLUCOCORTICOID INSUFFICIENCY IN THE PATHOGENESIS OF DEPRESSION

For those of us familiar with the huge data set of physiological abnormalities that have been repeatedly associated with MDD, it is hard to imagine the excitement generated in the 1970s by the discovery that cortisol levels were elevated in depression. The discovery that monoamines were involved in depression generated more national news, but the evidence of their involvement was more indirect, based almost entirely on the effectiveness of the first generation of antidepressants, all of which to one degree or other block the reuptake of serotonin or NE. Moreover, with the technology available at the time, evidence that monoamine neurotransmitters were actually abnormal in MDD was hard to come by, generating a literature with subtle findings and conflicting results.

On the other hand, in those early years the differences in cortisol levels between depressed and nondepressed individuals were stunning. The problem was not separating depressed from nondepressed but, rather, trying to determine how to reliably differentiate MDD from Cushing's syndrome. And as we noted at the start of this chapter, hypercortisolemia in the context of MDD, as in Cushing's, is often associated with an inability of cortisol to efficiently turn off the HPA axis and hence its own production. This failure has been often referred to as glucocorticoid resistance, although we prefer the term *insufficient glucocorticoid signaling* to highlight the fact that the reduced glucocorticoid sensitivity observed in MDD is not absolute but, rather, relative to the optimal biological and mental needs of the person at the time.[38]

The circularity of HPA functioning allows for several possible explanations of these two findings (i.e., hypercortisolemia and insufficient glucocorticoid signaling). As in Cushing's syndrome, depressed people may have HPA overdrive, either at the level of the hypothalamus, with too much CRH production, or at the level of the pituitary, with too much ACTH production. This state of overdrive would then overcome the ability of cortisol to turn the system off, which would manifest as glucocorticoid resistance of the HPA axis and chronic overproduction of cortisol. On the other hand, the primary problem may lie at the level of glucocorticoid signaling itself. In this scenario, insufficient glucocorticoid signaling, due to poor functioning of GRs, leads to hypercortisolemia as a side effect of the fact that, despite the high levels of cortisol, the glucocorticoid signal is too weak to turn itself off. Because cortisol exerts negative feedback at all levels of the HPA axis, including the hippocampus (more on this shortly), this insufficient signaling would be predicted to increase concentrations of CRH and ACTH because these hormones would be released from cortisol-mediated inhibitory control. Finally, a third possibility incorporates both these ideas by suggesting that increased central HPA axis drive leads to increased CRH, increased ACTH, and increased cortisol, with subsequent downregulation of GR sensitivity as a physiological response to the chronically heightened levels of cortisol. Paradoxically, this downregulation only makes things worse because it diminishes the ability of cortisol to turn off CRH, ACTH, and itself.

Early on, the related fields of biological psychiatry and neuroendocrinology opted for the first and third options above, which implicate hypercortisolemia in the pathophysiology of MDD, based on both their apparent obviousness and the fact that animal studies had demonstrated that very high levels of glucocorticoids can damage the brain. Enshrined in a concept known as the cascade hypothesis,[39] these ideas exerted a profound and, we believe, mostly unfortunate effect on research into the biology of mood disorders because they encouraged a huge amount of research based on the assumption that depression was driven by too much cortisol. Much evidence accumulated over the last 15 years or so suggests that these ideas are exactly backward and that in fact MDD is far more typically a condition associated with insufficient, rather than excessive, glucocorticoid signaling.[5]

It should have been obvious from the very beginning that something was wrong with the theory that depression is associated too much cortisol in the body, or in the theory's more definitive forms, that hypercortisolemia was causing, or contributing to the development of, depression. If depression is associated with hypercortisolemia, and if depressed people have cortisol levels in the range of patients with Cushing's syndrome, why don't people with depression look like they have Cushing's syndrome? With the exception of an unrestrained source of HPA axis overdrive (usually the pituitary gland), the bodily tissues of people with Cushing's are sensitive to cortisol, so they take the full brunt of excess cortisol. And it shows: Cushing's is one of the most distinctive looking of medical disorders. People with the condition gain tremendous weight, all in the trunk, leaving them with enormous bellies and thin legs and arms. They develop a characteristic hump on their upper bank (known as a buffalo hump) and a round face (known as moon facies). Their skin thins, and they get long purplish streaks on their abdomen, known as striae. They are at great risk of developing hypertension and diabetes, all known effects of overly intense cortisol signaling to the various bodily organs involved in these conditions.

The majority of people with depression could hardly be more different in many key ways. This is even truer, on average, for depressed people with hypercortisolemia, who tend to show melancholic and/or psychotic features. Whereas the depression associated with Cushing's syndrome tends to be characterized by eating and sleeping too much, melancholic and/or psychotic depression is uniformly characterized by loss of appetite, weight loss, and reduced sleep. Moreover, depressed people do not develop buffalo humps and round faces, and they don't suffer skin thinning. Although depression is associated with mild increases in blood pressure and insulin resistance, these changes are nothing like the far more profound changes in these variables routinely observed in Cushing's syndrome. And although Cushing's syndrome, with its chronic hypercortisolemia, is associated with increased rates of depression, the most common reaction to the administration of cortisol analogs, such as prednisone, for medical reasons is not depression but, rather, various shades of mania.

How do we understand these contradictions within a framework that views MDD as a disorder of "too much cortisol"? In fact, we don't think you can. The most obvious explanation for why hypercortisolemic MDD does not look like Cushing's syndrome is that, unlike Cushing's, in which most of the body remains sensitive to the effects of cortisol, MDD is associated with widespread glucocorticoid resistance in the tissues of the body. In this scenario, although cortisol levels are high, the message is not getting through. Moreover, the very increased cortisol is a signal not only that is the message not getting through but that it is not getting through at anywhere near the level needed for the individual's physiological circumstances, precisely because not enough cortisol signaling is occurring for cortisol to turn itself off via its inhibitory effects on the HPA axis.

Although this explanation is a straightforward way of reconciling the hypercortisolemia of MDD with the fact that MDD doesn't look like Cushing's syndrome, it failed to get any traction in the twentieth century for several reasons. First, because exposure to very high (i.e., nonphysiological) doses of glucocorticoids had been shown to cause brain changes in animals that resemble those that were beginning to be identified in MDD, it seemed obvious that cortisol was the link between stress and depression. Second, because cortisol was widely understood to have immunosuppressive effects (and indeed, glucocorticoids are among the most powerfully anti-inflammatory molecules in nature—hence their widespread use for inflammatory and autoimmune conditions), the fact that early studies showed depression was associated with immune suppression also bolstered the case for cortisol as the agent provocateur in the relationship between changes in the HPA axis and the development of MDD. Finally, in those early years it was totally unclear what could be causing the damage that cortisol was believed to be capable of causing if it wasn't cortisol.

But developments in immunology in the 1990s set the groundwork for reversing these ways of thinking and for providing an alternative "bad guy" that might account for at least some of the changes in the brain and body seen in depression. Prior to discussing these developments it is important to understand the state of the field at the start of the twenty-first century. Guided by the understanding of glucocorticoids as immunosuppressive, and bolstered by findings that activation of the SNS also attenuated certain immune responses, researchers expected that stress should suppress immune functioning, and they found multiple lines of evidence to suggest that this was the case. Moreover, because stress is a primary risk factor for MDD, and because MDD is associated with apparent hyperactivity of stress pathways (e.g., hypercortisolemia), it made sense to assume that the immune changes seen in depression should parallel those seen with stress in general and chronic stress in particular. Again, multiple lines of evidence demonstrated that this was the case. Both chronic stress and MDD were shown in many studies to be associated with reductions in measures of immune functioning in vitro, including decreased nonspecific mitogen-stimulated lymphocyte proliferation, attenuated natural killer cell cytotoxic activity, and reductions in circulating lymphocytes and numbers of various lymphocyte subsets, including B cells and T cells.[40–42] Studies suggested that depression was also associated with impairments in more naturalistic measures of immune functioning, such as delayed-type hypersensitivity (DTH), which measures the capacity of CD4 T helper cells to react to immunogenic antigens in the skin.[40]

As with the idea that depression is associated with too much glucocorticoid signaling, the idea that stress routinely induces reduced immune functioning was based on data that are subject to multiple interpretations. For example, because all human studies examined immune cells from the blood, reductions of lymphocytes in this bodily compartment might not reflect absolute reductions but, rather, might reflect movement out of the blood into other areas of the body, where they might be more effective in providing host defense. In fact, this is exactly what Firdaus Dhabhar and colleagues demonstrated in a highly influential series of animal studies in which they showed that acute stressors led to the movement of lymphocytes from immune tissues into the blood and then to areas where an invading organism would be most likely to be first encountered, in particular the skin.[43–46] In an image that conjures associations with nineteenth-century Paris, Dhabhar has written that acute stressors drive lymphocytes from the barracks to the boulevards and then on to battle stations.[47] Dhabhar and colleagues demonstrated this process most conclusively for the DTH reaction. Unlike chronic stress, acute stressors in animals increase the DTH response via the cortisol-mediated trafficking of CD4+ T helper cells from the blood to the skin. Blocking cortisol abrogates this effect, clearly demonstrating that, although glucocorticoids have powerful anti-inflammatory properties, in the context of acute stress they may serve immune-enhancing roles as a result of their effects on where leukocytes go in the body.[48] On the other hand, Dhabhar and colleagues have shown that chronic stress, like depression, suppresses DTH in a process at least partly dependent on glucocorticoid signaling, suggesting that glucocorticoids promote different physiological responses to stress based on the temporal nature of the danger.[49]

While Dhabhar was publishing his initially counterintuitive studies, an even more paradoxical set of findings was beginning to emerge. In those years, when everyone in mental health research "knew" that stress and depression suppressed immune functioning, reports began to appear suggesting that MDD was associated with increases in a variety of measures associated with inflammation.[50] Although a surprise from the perspective of psychiatry, these results were entirely consistent with animal data that had emerged over the preceding decade demonstrating that many of the newly discovered inflammatory cytokines (as well as factors that activate cytokine production, e.g., bacterial cell wall lipopolysaccharide [LPS]) produced a behavioral state that has come to be known as "sickness syndrome."[51] This syndrome is behaviorally and biologically similar to states induced by psychological stressors and in many of its features resembles MDD in humans.

Glucocorticoids had long been known to play an important role in stress-induced immune trafficking, so Dhabhar's finding that cortisol contributed to enhanced adaptive immunity in the skin did not pose a direct challenge to the idea that conditions associated with increased cortisol (i.e., stress and MDD) were also pathologies of glucocorticoid excess. However, the repeated observation of increased inflammation in MDD posed a direct challenge to orthodox understandings of the role of the HPA axis in the disorder. Philip Hench and his colleagues were awarded the Nobel Prize in Physiology or Medicine in 1950 for the discovery of the stunning anti-inflammatory effects of cortisol, and since that time related (mostly synthetic) glucocorticoids have been the mainstay of treatment for a whole galaxy of conditions dominated by inflammation, from skin rashes to the most serious of autoimmune conditions.

Glucocorticoids reduce inflammatory activity via a number of mechanisms. For example, following the binding of glucocorticoids to the GR, this "glucocorticoid-GR" complex translocates from the cytoplasm to the cellular nucleus, where it interferes with the DNA binding activity of the major inflammatory transcription factor nuclear factor kappa-beta (NFκB).[52] And just to make the matter more acute, Michael Maes had observed that it was exactly the depressed patients with increased cortisol who also were most likely to demonstrate increased peripheral inflammatory biomarkers.[53] So how could it be possible for MDD to be a condition characterized by both hypercortisolemia and inflammation? To the best of our knowledge, the answer to this conundrum was first articulated explicitly by Andrew H. Miller and Gregory E. Miller (no relation), and their colleagues, who independently recognized that glucocorticoid resistance provided an easy solution to the enigma.[54] If glucocorticoid resistance in MDD results from reduced GR signaling, this would explain both the increased plasma cortisol levels (because of inefficient negative feedback on the HPA axis) and inflammation (because of reduced cortisol-mediated anti-inflammatory signal) that characterize the condition.

Before examining why glucocorticoid resistance (or, more exactly, insufficiency) might develop and prior to reviewing the multiple lines of evidence that support this idea, it is worth pausing to recognize what a revolutionary concept this was when first proposed. With one theoretical shift depression, had gone from being a disease driven by too much HPA axis activity to an illness characterized by insufficient glucocorticoid signaling—too little HPA axis activity in the ways that matter most. Rather than potentially causing the disorder, the hypercortisolemia of MDD was now an epiphenomenon, resulting from the inability of the cortisol message to "get through" to the relevant bodily tissues, a classic example of the Ancient Mariner's "water, water everywhere, nor any drop to drink." Indeed, more than this, hypercortisolemia could be seen as a failed homeostatic effort to increase hormone levels to induce increased GR signaling, which would then feed back at multiple levels of the HPA axis to turn further cortisol release.

According to the standard notions of the 1970s and 1980s, encapsulated in the cascade hypothesis made famous by Robert Sapolsky,[39] stress activates the HPA axis, which leads to the production of cortisol, which while beneficial acutely becomes toxic when chronically elevated. Such chronic elevation was understood to occur either as a result of ongoing stress or as a result of individual physiological vulnerabilities that promote HPA axis hyperactivity. Chronic excess cortisol over time was believed to damage the structure and thus impair functioning of the hippocampus, the brain area (along with the PVN) most important in rodent models for restraining HPA axis activity. Lacking the inhibitory control provided by a fully functional hippocampus, the HPA axis was thought to be released from proper feedback and thus subject to chronic hyperactivity, leading to more cortisol release, with resultant ongoing damage to the tissues of the brain and body. This damage manifests behaviorally as depression.

Contrast this with the glucocorticoid insufficiency model, in which the primary pathogenic mechanism is reduced functionality of the GR in the brain and various bodily tissues, which results in secondary hyperactivity of the HPA axis, which manifests as increased production/release of CRH in the CNS and overproduction of cortisol by the adrenal glands as a result of inadequate inhibitory feedback from GR-mediated signaling. In this scenario, the damage to brain and body ascribed to cortisol in the cascade hypothesis results from downstream effects of insufficient cortisol signaling, especially the activation of innate immune pathways in the brain and body that have been shown in numerous studies to induce many of the same pathogenic changes observed in animals exposed to very high doses of glucocorticoids (e.g., metabolic abnormalities, alterations of brain structure, loss of bone mineral density, cardiac damage).[5]

Putting Glucocorticoid Insufficiency to the Test

The circular nature of HPA axis functioning makes it impossible to determine from hormonal output of the axis alone which of these diametrically opposed views (cascade vs. glucocorticoid insufficiency) is more relevant to the majority of people suffering with MDD, but fortunately these theories make a number of testable hypotheses that provide more support for one view or the other. Here we examine a few of the most important of predictions that would support the primacy of glucocorticoid insufficiency:

- The two major risk factors for MDD around the world, psychosocial stress and sickness, should promote glucocorticoid insufficiency, even when not promoting increased cortisol production.
- MDD should be associated with reduced GR signaling in the brain and periphery of the body.
- Genetic and epigenetic factors that reduce glucocorticoid sensitivity should increase the risk for depression.
- Antidepressant modalities should increase, not decrease, GR signaling, and increased GR signaling should, in the main, be associated with antidepressant effects.

Stress and Sickness Promote Glucocorticoid Insufficiency

Although we have thus far discussed glucocorticoid insufficiency only in terms of reduced receptor functioning, it might develop in other ways, including, most obviously, reduced production/release of cortisol. In this regard, it is intriguing that in humans chronic stress appears to be as likely to reduce as to increase concentrations of cortisol. Indeed, as early as the 1960s researchers noted that medically healthy people living in conditions of chronic stress frequently exhibited lower urinary and plasma cortisol concentrations than matched controls, with cortisol concentrations decreasing further during periods of heightened stress.[55] Although the data are not entirely consistent, decreased plasma, salivary, and urinary cortisol concentrations have also been reported in subjects suffering from PTSD, whether the syndrome developed as a result of combat exposure, severe environmental trauma such as an earthquake, or sexual and/or physical abuse in childhood.[56] Reduced levels of cortisol have also been observed in adults with a history of early-life adversity (ELA), both "at rest" and in response to laboratory psychosocial stressors.[57–59] Importantly, like MDD, both PTSD and ELA are associated with increased measures of peripheral inflammation, strongly suggesting that the lowered cortisol levels in these conditions reflect not just reduced hormone levels but reduced glucocorticoid signaling capacity, or glucocorticoid insufficiency.[5]

In addition to evidence that chronic stress can both raise and lower cortisol concentrations depending on a variety of circumstances, significant animal and human data demonstrate that chronic stress promotes the development of glucocorticoid resistance, even when other changes in HPA axis activity are not observed.[60] Interestingly, in animal studies this phenomenon is more robustly induced by the types of naturalistic social stressors that mirror depressogenic conditions in humans than by more artificial stressors. For example, as we discuss again toward the end of this section, chronic social disruption paradigms, in which stable rodent hierarchies are repeatedly disrupted, induce glucocorticoid resistance in immune tissues, an effect not seen with restraint stress.[61]

One of the best demonstrations of the ability of chronic stress to induce glucocorticoid resistance in humans comes from a longitudinal study of individuals caring for family members with cancer. Over the course of the patients' treatment, caregivers demonstrated reduced sensitivity of their inflammatory systems to the inhibitory effects of glucocorticoids compared with control subjects, as assessed in vitro by the ability of DEX to inhibit LPS-stimulated production of IL-6, as well as by the sensitivity of circulating monocytes to glucocorticoid signaling, based on a reduction in GR gene expression. During this same time period no changes were observed in either the amount or rhythm of circulating cortisol, suggesting that while glucocorticoid resistance and hypercortisolism may co-occur in 60 percent of depressed individuals with one or the other of these changes, the two mechanisms represent separate physiological responses. Importantly, while no changes in circulating cortisol were seen, individuals undergoing chronic caregiver stress demonstrated increased levels plasma concentrations of C-reactive protein and IL-1 receptor antagonist, as well as decreased expression of anti-inflammatory genes, including I-kappa B, and the ratio of the active to the inactive isoform of the GR (alpha/beta isoforms).[62,63] More recently, monocytes in cancer caregivers have been found to demonstrate increased expression of genes with response elements for NFκB and reduced expression of genes with response elements for the GR, while showing no changes in diurnal cortisol profiles.[64] These studies all point to a pattern of reduced glucocorticoid signaling with increased inflammation that is exactly what one would predict if the loss of GR signaling was releasing peripheral inflammatory processes from HPA axis inhibitory control, consistent with the known role of glucocorticoid resistance in increasing inflammatory reactions to psychosocial stress in animal studies.

If stress is one route into depression, sickness is the other. Data from the World Health Organization suggest that medical illness is probably the most powerful driver of MDD worldwide, irrespective of culture, age, sex, or financial status.[65] As such, one would predict that sickness should also be associated with reduced sensitivity to glucocorticoids, if indeed insufficient glucocorticoid signaling contributes to the pathogenesis of MDD. In fact, overwhelming data demonstrate that a wide range of medical diseases are associated with glucocorticoid resistance and that the development of such resistance portends poor clinical outcomes.

At the back of almost all disease states, whether they result from chronic tissue damage (e.g., cardiovascular disease), neoplasm, autoimmunity, metabolic derangements (e.g., diabetes), or infection, is the inflammatory system. Inflammation is the sine qua non of sickness. One might expect, therefore, that many of the associations observed between sickness and HPA axis functioning might be mediated by inflammation. And in fact, many studies suggest this is the case. Just as stress activates inflammation, inflammation, especially when acute, robustly activates the stress system and does so in a manner that resembles the effects of psychological stress on these same pathways (i.e., CRH-induced stimulation of the HPA axis and activation of the SNS). For example, administration of inflammatory cytokines to laboratory animals profoundly stimulates not only ACTH and cortisol but also the expression and release of CRH from the hypothalamus.[66–68] Similar effects pertain in humans, based on studies showing that a first injection of the cytokine IFN-α robustly activates ACTH and cortisol production/release (presumably due to activation of CRH pathways).[69] Highlighting the depressogenic relevance of these effects is the fact that increased ACTH/cortisol release in response to an initial IFN-α dose (but not to subsequent doses) strongly predicted the subsequent development of depressive symptoms while on IFN-α therapy.[69] In contrast to acute administration, chronic IFN-α administration results in a flattening of the diurnal cortisol rhythm and increased evening corti-sol concentrations, both of which correlate with the development of depression and fatigue.[70] Flattening of the diurnal cortisol rhythm has been reported in a number of medical disorders associated with inflammation, including cardiovas-cular disease and cancer, where it has been associated with a worse out come in these conditions.[70,71]

Flattening of the diurnal cortisol rhythm, or slope, and increased evening plasma cortisol concentrations are also hallmarks of MDD that have been associ-ated repeatedly with insufficient glucocorticoid signaling. Given that inflamma-tory cytokines flatten the cortisol slope and increase evening cortisol levels, one might predict that they would also promote glucocorticoid resistance. This prediction has been borne out by numerous studies, which suggest that gluco-corticoid and inflammatory signaling exist in the type of complex relationship of cooperation and conflict/competition that characterizes most evolved systems. Thus, although the immune system relies on glucocorticoids to shape and termi-nate its efforts for the benefit of the organism, it also competes with glucocorti-coids and via multiple pathways seeks to attenuate glucocorticoid signaling to its own benefit (with benefit here defined as an increase in its own inflammatory processes).

Many studies demonstrate that inflammatory cytokines disrupt GR function while decreasing GR expression.[72] For example, IFN-α has been shown to inhibit GR function by activating STAT5 (signal transducer and activator of transcription 5), which in turn binds to the activated GR in the nucleus, thus disrupting GR-DNA binding.[73] A similar protein-protein interaction between the GR and the primary intracellular inflammatory mediator NFκB in the nucleus has also been described.[74] Clinically, in patients with hepatitis C virus infection, treatment with IFN-α has been shown to reduce glucocorticoid negative feedback sensitiv-ity (i.e., to induce glucocorticoid resistance) as measured by increased cortisol concentrations following the DST, with this increased cortisol correlating with both flattening of the diurnal slope and with the development of depressive symp-toms.[75]

In addition to interfering with GR signaling in the nucleus, inflammatory cytokines are also capable of impeding the ability of the activated GR to enter the nucleus in the first place. For example, IL-1α and IL-1β have been shown both in vitro and in vivo to inhibit GR translocation from the cytoplasm to the nucleus through activation of p38 mitogen-activated protein kinase.[76] Consistent with our increasing understanding of how inflammatory pathways mediate many of the effects of psychosocial stress, stress-induced alterations in GR translocation lead-ing to glucocorticoid resistance in laboratory mice have been found to be medi-ated by IL-1 through the use of IL-1 knockout mice that fail to exhibit impaired GR translocation following social disruption stress.[77] Finally, in addition to reducing overall glucocorticoid gene expression, exposure to inflammatory cytokines increases expression of the beta-isoform of the GR, which has a distinct hormone binding domain (and is unable to bind known glucocorticoids), a unique pattern of gene regulation and the physiological effect of attenuating glucocorticoid signaling.[72]

A mistake often made in psychiatry, as well as in other relevant mind-body disciplines, is to see bodily systems as complete in themselves rather than as open-ended communication pathways evolved to help the organism cope with the threats and opportunities of its larger interdependent environment. As we discuss at length in Chapter 9, no risks are more serious or, we believe, more relevant to Major Depression than infection.[78] And despite the fact that the immune system evolved to help organisms cope with the microbial and parasitic world within and without them, many microbes and parasites have nonetheless devised very clever ways of manipulating and thereby benefiting from immune mechanisms initially evolved to combat them. One might predict that the same type of effects would be apparent within the HPA axis, given its centrality in constraining and molding inflammatory and other immune responses. And indeed, studies show that infectious agents such as viruses are capable of inducing glucocorticoid resistance upon infection. For example, in an in vitro study of human bronchial epithelial cells, rhinovirus RV-16 infection impaired the ability of the synthetic glucocorticoid DEX to (a) inhibit IL-1β–induced release of the inflammatory chemokine IL-8, (b) induce gene expression of the proinflammatory intracellular signaling element of mitogen-activated protein kinase phosphatase 1, and (c) promote the binding of the GR to its DNA response elements (thereby interfering with its ability to impact gene expression). Infection also impaired the ability of the active alpha-isoform of the GR to translocate from the cytoplasm to the nucleus. These effects appeared to be dependent upon viral actions on I-kappa B kinase and c-Jun N-terminal kinase, two pathways important for the regulation of inflammation, because inhibitors of these pathways completed restored glucocorticoid sensitivity in rhinovirus-infected cells.[79] Thus, although we think of inflammation as a protective response in the face of infection, this is an example of a microorganism appropriating the ability of inflammation to induce glucocorticoid resistance to serve its own ends.

Insufficient Glucocorticoid Signaling in MDD

Glucocorticoids have the capacity to impact the functioning of almost all bodily tissues. So when we discuss glucocorticoid resistance or, more correctly, insufficient glucocorticoid signaling, a first question to ask is not just what we mean but where we mean it. This is especially relevant for MDD because the issue has been examined with any rigor only within the immune system and the HPA axis itself. Whether other bodily tissues become resistant to the effects of cortisol in the context of MDD is an open question, although one study intriguingly shows that the skin of depressed individuals may also be resistant to the physiological effects of glucocorticoids.[80]

Two tests are routinely used to assess glucocorticoid sensitivity within the HPA axis in humans, and both rely on the fact that the strength of the cortisol signal can be measured, paradoxically enough, by its ability to silence its own signal. The first test developed around this idea was the DST.[81] Most psychiatrists take a dim view toward the DST without fully understanding how much it has taught us about depression, because it is best known for its failure to deliver on its early promise as a diagnostic test for MDD. This failure occurred for two reasons that now confirm key points in our understanding of depression. First, only a subset of depressed individuals differed from nondepressed people, consistent with our current understanding of depression as a biologically and behaviorally heterogeneous condition. Second, other conditions were found to be associated with an increased risk of abnormal DST results. What was not fully appreciated at the time was that all these conditions (i.e., illness, psychological stress, sleep loss, family loading for mood disorders) are robust risk factors for depression, highlighting the fact that MDD is not really a discrete disease state but, rather, a process that blends in with both its environmental and genetic antecedents and its behavioral sequolac.

The DST has several versions, but all rely on the fact that DEX is a highly potent GR-specific hormone that operates at the level of the pituitary and adrenals to inhibit cortisol release via glucocorticoid-receptor-mediated inhibitory feedback. Typically a dose of DEX is taken by mouth in the evening. and plasma or saliva concentrations of cortisol are measured at various time points the next day. A normal DST result is one in which cortisol levels are profoundly reduced the day after the DEX pill. People with abnormal DST results are usually referred to as "nonsuppressors" because the prior administration of DEX failed to suppress subsequent cortisol release in the body.

The second test for assessing glucocorticoid sensitivity within the HPA axis in humans is known as the DEX-CRH stimulation test.[82] Although more elaborate than the DST, it is built around the same physiological principle that glucocorticoids should suppress their subsequent production. As with the DST, in the DEX-CRH stimulation test the subject ingests a dose of DEX in the evening and then has cortisol levels measured repeatedly the following day. The difference is that during the afternoon of the following day (typically at 3 p.m. by convention) the subject is administered a dose of intravenous CRH. As the primary secretagogue of the HPA axis, CRH powerfully stimulates the production of ACTH and then cortisol. But in normal individuals pretreatment with DEX powerfully inhibits the ACTH/cortisol response to CRH. As with the DST, in people with reduced sensitivity to glucocorticoids, the cortisol response "escapes" DEX inhibition, so a large cortisol spike is seen in response to the administration of CRH, even with the DEX pretreatment.

Rates of impaired glucocorticoid responsiveness during MDD (as assessed by nonsuppression of cortisol on the DST or DEX-CRH stimulation test) vary from approximately 25 to 80 percent,[19] depending on depressive symptomatology. Highest rates are found in patients with melancholic or psychotic symptoms and in older individuals.[83] In addition, rates of insufficient signaling are higher when the DEX-CRH stimulation test is used rather than the DST. In addition to being cross-sectionally associated with depression, DST and DEX-CRH test results have also shown to powerfully predict clinical response,[84,85] and in the case of the DEX-CRH test, there is evidence that impaired glucocorticoid responsiveness represents a genetically based risk factor for the development of depression, given that family members of severely depressed individuals are themselves more likely than the general population to show reduced glucocorticoid sensitivity, even when they have not suffered from MDD themselves.[86]

One criticism of both the DST and DEX-CRH stimulation test is that DEX does not easily enter the CNS, and therefore these tests do not reflect much about the known importance of the brain in restraining HPA axis activity. In rodents the hippocampus appears to play a central role in this process; in primates frontal regions of the brain appear to be of increased relative importance in this regard. In either case, the bulk of the evidence suggests that the DST and DEX-CRH tests tell us nothing about whether depression is more associated with increased or decreased glucocorticoid signaling within the CNS. Fortunately, however, several lines of indirect evidence suggest that, as with the periphery, reductions, not increases, in glucocorticoid signaling are likely the norm in depression and contribute to disease pathophysiology.

For example, researchers have created a mouse line characterized by time-limited disruption of GR functioning confined to frontal areas of the brain. Under conditions of forebrain GR dysfunction these mice develop HPA axis hyperactivity paired with insufficient glucocorticoid signaling based on DST nonsuppression.[87] In concert with the development of these mood disorder-relevant HPA changes, the mice demonstrate depressive-like behavior that can be reversed with chronic antidepressant treatment. A second line of evidence comes from convergent animal and human data showing that ELA promotes epigenetic changes in the GR gene within neurons in the hippocampus that are known to reduce GR functionality.[88,89]

Although GRs are the most important final transduction elements for stress-relevant levels of cortisol in the brain and body, glucocorticoid signaling is best understood not as synonymous with GR activity only but, rather, with the summed output of the HPA axis as this translates into strength of the glucocorticoid signal in any tissue of interest. Moreover, it appears that changes at other levels of the HPA axis can impact sensitivity to glucocorticoids. For example, two single-nucleotide polymorphisms (SNPs) in the gene that codes for the type 1 CRH receptor that have been associated with an increased risk for developing depression as an adult in response to ELA also promote glucocorticoid resistance, as measured by the DEX-CRH stimulation test, in individuals with the risk alleles, but not in individuals with protective alleles.[90,91] Because CRH confers its behavior-relevant effects within the CNS, these data are additional circumstantial evidence that brain changes that promote depression also induce insufficient glucocorticoid signaling.

After the HPA axis, the second most exhaustively studied physiological pathway that shows evidence of impaired glucocorticoid signaling in MDD is the immune system. And as with the HPA axis, the bulk of the evidence for glucocorticoid resistance comes from a small number of tests that share basic procedures and assumptions. However, unlike the HPA axis, tests of the glucocorticoid/immune relations in depression have been done almost entirely in vitro using immune cells, as opposed to the in vivo tests that dominate or HPA axis knowledge base.[20]

Given the centrality of GRs in cortisol signaling, an obvious first question to ask is whether their signaling capacity is changed in MDD. Such changes could be supported by any number of mechanisms, but the two most obvious possibilities are a reduction in the number of available GRs or reduced functional capacity of the receptors themselves. Strongly suggesting that reduced numbers of GRs in the brain might contribute to insufficient signaling and to depression are studies using mice that have been genetically altered to produce fewer GRs either in specific brain areas (e.g., the forebrain-specific GR-knockout mouse) or throughout the CNS (GR+/GR− mice that produce only 50 percent as many GRs in the brain as do normal mice).[92] These altered mice demonstrate depressive behavior either at baseline or following stress exposure that can be reversed by antidepressants.[87] Moreover, as in depressed humans, these mice fail to suppress glucocorticoid production using the DEX-CRH stimulation test, demonstrating that reduced CNS glucocorticoid signaling is capable of also inducing reduced glucocorticoid sensitivity in the peripheral elements of the HPA axis, where it is typically measured in depressed humans. GR+/GR− mice also demonstrate reduced BDNF and reduced neurogenesis within the hippocampus, both of which are believed to be of central relevance to depressogenesis in humans.[93]

Given these findings one might expect to see that reduced numbers of GRs in the brain and body would be commonly reported abnormalities in humans with MDD. While older data on GR numbers/density on immune cells in MDD are contradictory,[20] more recent data examining both protein and mRNA expression of GRs in the postmortem human brain are fairly consistent in reporting reduced overall GRs or reductions in the active alpha-isoform of the GR in multiple brain regions repeatedly implicated in MDD, including the hippocampus, amygdala, and cingulate cortex,[94-96] although not all studies have found this,[97] and these findings do not appear to be specific to MDD but are associated with mental illness more generally.[98] And although most studies have focused on the GR, a study found that mRNA expression levels of the active isoform of the MR was reduced in the hippocampus and inferior frontal cingulate cortices,[96] which would be expected to promote reduced glucocorticoid sensitivity when hormone levels are low.

Of course, as we have noted, GR functioning appears to be impacted by many factors other than receptor number. Indeed, alterations in multiple other bodily systems appear to impact GR activity and hence glucocorticoid sensitivity. Given this, the deeper question in relation to the immune system is whether evidence exists for reduced glucocorticoid signaling in depression. Unlike the situation with numbers or density of GRs in immune or brain cells, the story with glucocorticoid signaling on immune cells in depression is one of the most consistent we know of in all psychiatry. As a group, depressed individuals show reductions in immune system sensitivity to the inhibitory effects of glucocorticoids.[20]

These reductions have been shown in several ways. Studies investigating changes in GR binding following in vivo or in vitro treatment with GR agonists have found a remarkable lack of response in depressed patients, especially in those who are nonsuppressors to the DST (i.e., who demonstrate in vivo reductions in glucocorticoid sensitivity within the HPA axis). For example, one study found that control subjects exhibited decreased GR numbers after oral DEX administration, whereas depressed patients did not—with the reductions signifying translocation of the bound GRs from the cytoplasm to the nucleus of the immune cells.[99] Similarly, several research groups reported that only depressed DST suppressors (i.e., those without HPA axis resistance to glucocorticoids) showed a decrease in GR binding after DEX administration, whereas nonsuppressors showed no effect of DEX administration.[100,101] Also of note are two studies in which cortisol secretion was inhibited by metyrapone, a glucocorticoid synthesis inhibitor. In these studies, healthy control subjects exhibited an increase in the number of lymphocyte GRs after metyrapone treatment, whereas depressed patients showed no difference. Since the authors analyzed whole-cell GR binding, these findings suggest that GRs from depressed patients may have a reduced ability to respond to acute changes in circulating cortisol concentrations.[102,103]

If changes in binding are one way of measuring the strength of the GR signal in immune cells, another is to examine whether these cells show normal reductions in functional activity when exposed to GR agonists (primarily DEX) in vitro. Most studies that have tackled this issue have been built around the well-documented capacity of glucocorticoids to inhibit the ability of peripheral blood mononuclear cells to produce proinflammatory cytokines in response to an inflammatory stimulus such as LPS or to proliferate in response to polyclonal mitogens, such as concanavalin A, phytohemaglutinin, and pokeweed mitogen.

Results from these studies have consistently shown reduced responses to DEX in Major Depression. In several studies these reductions correlated with increased levels of plasma cortisol.[20] After clinical recovery, hypercortisolemia resolved and the sensitivity of lymphocytes to DEX returned to control levels, suggesting that, indeed, hypercortisolemia in depression likely represents a compensatory mechanism for reducing signaling rather than a primary abnormality driving disease pathogenesis or pathology.[104,105] However, as in all things psychiatric, results do not always follow along straightforward diagnostic lines. For example, several studies conducted in the 1980s found that patients who were glucocorticoid resistant (i.e., nonsuppressors on the DST) showed no decrease in the lymphoproliferative response to phytohemaglutinin and concanavalin A after overnight oral DEX administration, whereas depressed subjects with normal HPA axis responses (i.e., DST suppressors) exhibited significantly decreased lymphocyte proliferation.[101,106] Moreover, lymphocytes from DST-nonsuppressor subjects were more resistant to the inhibitory effect of DEX administered in vitro. Glucocorticoid resistance in lymphocytes was not present when the depressed group was compared with the control group and emerged only when nonsuppressors from the two groups were pooled together and compared with suppressors.[101]

These older data have been supplemented in more recent years by other, novel methods of assessing insufficient glucocorticoid signaling that do not rely upon functional in vitro immune assays. An early attempt at these types of analyses found that, despite having higher plasma cortisol concentrations relative to control subjects, melancholic depressed patients exhibited no increase in plasma sialyltransferase levels.[107] Sialytransferases are enzymes that participate in oligosaccharide chain metabolism and are known to be stimulated by glucocorticoids via the GR. Similar results have been observed more recently using genome-wide mRNA expression analyses after exposing peripheral blood mononuclear cell to DEX in vitro. Using this technique, Elisabeth Binder and colleagues found that depressed individuals showed significantly less activation of GR-responsive genes in response to DEX stimulation than did normal controls. In fact, using this procedure they were able to sort depressed from nondepressed individuals with a high degree of accuracy, especially among depressed patients with evidence of glucocorticoid resistance in the HPA axis, as assessed by the DST.[108] Importantly, several of the genes that were significantly more activated by DEX in normal individuals than in depressed patients, such as FKBP5, which codes for a GR chaperone protein, have been associated with glucocorticoid resistance using other methodologies.

Several studies, using very different methodologies, provide corroborating evidence of reduced glucocorticoid signaling not just in the immune system but also in the brain of depressed individuals. For example, mRNA levels of a GR-inducible target gene (glucocorticoid-induced leucine zipper) were found to be significantly decreased in the prefrontal cortex and amygdala, but not hippocampus, of depressed teenagers who had committed suicide.[94] On a functional level, several studies suggest that the brains of individuals with MDD are less responsive to the behavioral effects of glucocorticoids than are those of nondepressed comparison subjects. Consider response inhibition, an executive function that relies on the integrity of the prefrontal cortex. Whereas normal individuals show improvements in response inhibition in response to acute cortisol administration, this effect is not seen in depressed patients taken as a group.[109] Similar results have been documented for memory function. When administered acutely to normal individuals, hydrocortisone impairs declarative memory, an effect not observed in patients with MDD even though they show larger rises in salivary cortisol levels after hydrocortisone administration (again suggesting that despite higher levels the cortisol signal is not "getting through").[109]

Genetic and Epigenetic Factors That Reduce Glucocorticoid Sensitivity Increase the Risk for Depression

Several years ago one of us gave a lecture on the genetics of depression, making the argument linking depressogenic genes with immune functioning that forms the centerpiece of Chapter 9 in this book. At the end of the lecture one of the world's foremost researchers on the genetics of depression came up to us and said, "Ingenious lecture! The only problem with your ideas is that there are no genes for depression." In a way this was an overstatement—we know that depression gets passed down in families. But in another very important way the researcher was right. Using the most rigorous methodologies currently at our disposal, no one has been able to identify any gene or SNP within a gene that unequivocally promotes the development of depression, even in huge populations of patients and controls.[110] And when associations are found using the most rigorous methodologies, they tend not to replicate from one ethnic group to another.[111] This situation mandates that, in discussing the impact of HPA axis genes reported to be associated with depression that also impact glucocorticoid sensitivity, all conclusions must be held tentatively.

Having said this, many studies that employ less rigorous methodologies—especially the candidate gene approach—suggest that polymorphisms within HPA axis genes are relevant to the pathophysiology of MDD. An obvious first place to look for such polymorphisms is within the gene for the GR itself (NR3C1). And indeed, a number of studies suggest that functionally relevant SNPs and haplotypes (a collection of SNPs usually inherited together, i.e., in linkage disequilibrium) within the GR gene are overrepresented in individuals with MDD. Moreover, many of these SNPs and haplotypes have been shown to impact glucocorticoid sensitivity in ways relevant to depression.[112]

GR polymorphisms. Two haplotypes within the GR gene are especially interesting in illustrating the complexities of relationships between glucocorticoid sensitivity and health. Haplotype 4 (which includes the genes TthIII1 and 9-beta) and haplotype 5 (TthIII1, 9-beta, and ER22/23EK) have been shown to be associated with reduced glucocorticoid sensitivity in several studies, using various in vitro and in vivo measures.[112,113] Given this, one would expect these variants to be associated with many of the immune and metabolic stigmata of chronic inflammation, but in fact carriers of these haplotypes have been shown to have reduced inflammation and more optimal metabolic measures.[114] These findings likely reflect the fact that carriers are thinner and have less abdominal fat (presumably because they are not experiencing the full effects of glucocorticoids on these measures).[115] Consistent with the importance of glucocorticoid signaling for restraining inflammatory processes, individuals with either of these semiresistant haplotypes (or with the individual SNPs that comprise the haplotype, i.e., 9-beta) are at increased risk for rheumatoid arthritis and reduced cardiac function and demonstrate a more aggressive disease course when afflicted with multiple sclerosis.[113,116–118] People with these haplotypes, or the SNPs comprising them, have also been repeatedly found to be at increased risk for depression, whether they be healthy or suffering with cardiovascular disease.[119,120] As is being increasingly observed for SNPs across the genome, polymorphisms in the GR (9-beta, ER22/23EK) have also been associated with an increased risk of depression in individuals who report ELA.[121]

Because the SNPs/haplotypes discussed thus far have reduce glucocorticoid sensitivity, their association with depression fits nicely glucocorticoid insufficiency models of the condition. But several studies have also linked a BclI polymorphism with an increased risk of depression.[122] This SNP has been shown to enhance glucocorticoid sensitivity as measured by standard in vitro and in vivo (i.e., DST) tests.[112] Based on our discussion thus far, one would have predicted that this SNP should have been protective against depression. It is possible, as some have suggested, that both too much and too little glucocorticoid signaling is depressogenic, and this might certainly be possible. However, a closer inspection of the physiological effects of BclI points to another possibility that highlights the complexity underlying simple notions like glucocorticoid resistance. Specifically, whereas the depressogenic GG variant at BclI increases glucocorticoid sensitivity in the context of standard tests, all of which utilize pharmacological doses of glucocorticoid far higher than those that occur naturally within the body, one study suggests that this variant actually reduces glucocorticoid effects on immune functioning—and hence reduces glucocorticoid signaling—in response to levels of glucocorticoid exposure that more closely parallel those found under naturalistic stress conditions.[123]

CRH receptor polymorphisms. Significant data implicate CRH signaling through its type 1 receptor in the pathogenesis of MDD. While allelic differences within the CRH gene itself have not been consistently associated with depression, SNPs within the type 1 CRH receptor appear to be more promising candidates. In particular, a haplotype consisting of several SNPs has been repeatedly associated with either an increased risk for—or protection against, depending on the variant—MDD in individuals exposed to ELA.[90,124] As one would predict from a glucocorticoid insufficiency model, individuals with two copies of the risk allele at these SNPs (GG carriers at rs110402 and rs24924) and a history of ELA show increased cortisol production in response to the DEX/CRH stimulation test, consistent with glucocorticoid resistance. These findings suggest that genetic variants of the type 1 CRH receptor that predispose to the development of depression in response to ELA may do so, at least in part, by downregulating GR signaling, consistent with overwhelming data from animal models demonstrating that ELA reduces glucocorticoid sensitivity.[125]

FKBP5 polymorphisms.   FKBP5 is an immunophillin and heat-shock protein 90 co-chaperone that interacts with the GR to reduce glucocorticoid sensitivity. When FKBP5 is bound to the GR receptor complex in the cellular cytosol, cortisol is less able to promote GR activation and subsequent translocation of the ligand-GR complex to the cellular nucleus where it exerts most of its effects. In addition to these effects, GR activation leads to increased production of FKBP5, which happens rapidly and serves as an ultrafast mechanism for negative feedback on cortisol signaling. Genetic variants within the FKBP5 gene have been shown to reduce FKBP5 mRNA expression following GR activation and in that way to impair the inhibitory effects of cortisol on its own functioning (which is a hallmark of glucocorticoid resistance). Multiple studies have reported that these variants are associated with an increased risk for depression. More recently, Elisabeth Binder and colleagues reported that only depressed individuals with FKBP5 risk variants (and not depressed individuals without these variants) show glucocorticoid resistance of the FKBP5-mediated ultrafast inhibitory feedback mechanism in vivo.[126]

Epigenetic changes impacting glucocorticoid sensitivity.   Nothing has caused researchers to begin taking the role of the environment in shaping adult behavior and biology more strongly than a series of studies that commenced in the 1990s showing that postnatal rearing conditions induce lifelong changes in rodent behavior and biology that look eerily like the abnormalities that characterize MDD. The first wave of these studies focused on the effect of stress, typically prolonged separation of the rat pup from its mother. But in doing these studies researchers noticed something strange: separating a rat pup from its mother for 3 hours a day produced the expected depressive-like phenotype, but separating rat pups from their mothers for 15 minutes produced exactly opposite effects—that is, these brief separations induced an antidepressant-like phenotype. At first researchers suspected that the 15-minute separations were mild stressors that "toughened" the system, but more observant eyes noticed that rat pups separated for 15 minutes received a dollop of "super love" from their mothers when reunited, whereas 3 hours of separation seemed to confuse the mothers, often leading them to ignore the returned infants. Realizing this, Paul Plotsky, Michael Meaney, and other scientists began examining the degree to which maternal behavior accounted for the neurological and neuroendocrine phenotypes that had been observed in the adult offspring exposed to various degrees of maternal separation.

The results were definitive and transformative. It turned out that the variable effects of maternal separation stress could be replicated in their entirety by observing how much maternal care a given rat pup received, with maternal care in rats consisting of amount of licking and grooming. Whether occurring naturally or as a result of researcher-driven manipulation, pups that receive high amounts of licking and grooming grow up to show behavioral and physiological responses that in humans are associated with stress resilience and protection from mood disorders. As adults, high licking and grooming pups show an antidepressant-like phenotype on a variety of tests that are often used to identify novel compounds as potential antidepressants. When grown these pups show increased hippocampal GR mRNA and protein expression, enhanced glucocorticoid negative feedback sensitivity, and reduced hypothalamic mRNA levels of CRH (presumably as a result of enhanced ability of glucocorticoids to feed back and shut off CRH activity both in the brain and HPA axis). Blocking GR signaling abolishes all these effects of maternal licking and grooming on adult offspring, strongly suggesting that increased GR signaling (and hence increased glucocorticoid sensitivity) plays a pivotal role of converting an early nurturing environment into a lifelong behaviorally and physiologically resilient phenotype.[127]

Although GR signaling may be a necessary final pathway for the effects of maternal behavior in this model, the impact of licking and grooming on rat pup behavior and on the GR is in turn mediated by the effect of these behaviors on serotonin activity in the hippocampus, and specifically on the ability of licking and grooming to increase serotonin signaling through the 5HT-7 serotonin receptor, with subsequent activation of cyclic adenosine monophosphate and a resultant increase in the expression of a transcription factor called nerve-growth factor-inducible factor-A (NGFI-A). NGFI-A binds to a neuron-specific variant of the 5′ noncoding variable exon 1 region of the GR gene and promotes GR gene expression.[127]

It is increasingly clear that environmental influences are able to exert enduring biological effects via epigenetic modifications that alter the degree to which various genes are expressed in any given tissue. So it should not come as a surprise that maternal licking and grooming are associated with epigenetic changes in the gene that codes for the GR, or that these changes appear to account for differences between pups that received high versus low licking and grooming in their adult functioning of their brains and stress systems. Specifically, increased maternal licking and grooming lead to lifelong reductions in methylation of the 5′ CpG dinucleotide of the NGFI-A consensus sequence in the promoter region of the GR gene in the rat pups lucky enough to receive this extra attention from their mothers, whereas lower levels of maternal licking and grooming lead to lifelong increases in methylation at this site.[128] Because methylation silences gene expression, this means that high licking and grooming pups, with lower levels of methylation, have increased expression of the GR, which leads to increased GR signaling and hence to increased glucocorticoid sensitivity. Histone deacetylase inhibitors, which release genes from methylation-based inhibition, reverse maternal effects on offspring hippocampal GR gene expression in adult offspring.[128] More remarkable, chronic CNS infusion of a histone deacetylase inhibitor to adult offspring that received low levels of licking and grooming as pups has been reported to mimic all relevant effects of high licking and grooming early in life, including increased GR gene expression and reduced HPA axis responses to stress.[128]

As we have emphasized repeatedly throughout this book, what we call depression is clearly not one homogeneous biological or behavioral condition but, rather, is very likely nothing but a gloss for many different environmental, genetic, epigenetic, and biological conditions that manifest in a final common behavioral pathway. Multiple lines of evidence suggest that individuals who come to their depression via ELA are more likely than depressed individuals without a history of ELA to have many of the same physiological abnormalities that are observed in animal models of ELA.[129]

This has been demonstrated pointedly by Michael Meaney's group in their work with postmortem brain tissue from suicide completers and control subjects who died via sudden involuntary means. Suicide completers with well-validated histories of ELA had reduced hippocampal GR gene expression that corrected with increased DNA methylation in the exon 1F sequence of the GR gene, which is the human analog of the region that is hypermethylated in rats exposed to minimal maternal care, as assessed by licking and grooming.[89] NGFI-A binding was also reduced in this region of GR in the hippocampus of humans with ELA.

Corroboration for these CNS findings comes from several studies that have examined associations between ELA and GR gene exon 1F methylation in peripheral immune cells. One study found that prenatal exposure to maternal depressed or anxious mood was associated with increased methylation at the predicted NGFI-A binding site on the exon 1F area of the GR gene. In turn, increased methylation at this site, as assessed using mononuclear cells from cord blood at birth, predicted increased salivary cortisol stress responses at three months of age.[130] In a study that compared patients with borderline personality disorder, patients with MDD, and normal controls, increased methylation at exon 1F in immune cells correlated with the presence and severity of childhood sexual abuse. This study did not evaluate whether this increase in methylation might predict reduced immune cell sensitivity to the inhibitory effects of glucocorticoids, but this would be a strong prediction.[131]

Importantly, increased methylation of the 1F exon of the GR gene in adults in these studies was accounted for by ELA and not by the presence or absence of depression at the time of death or clinical assessment, raising the intriguing possibility that different subpopulations of patients with MDD may come to their glucocorticoid resistance via different pathways. Consistent with this possibility, a postmortem brain study of individuals with MDD not selected for a history of ELA showed many of the functional changes in GR activity associated with increased methylation of the 1F exon of the GR but did not find increased 1F methylation.[95] Thus, increased methylation of the GR gene may be one pathway especially driven by early-life circumstances rather than genetic predisposition.

This notion is supported by animal work demonstrating that the impact of licking and grooming on glucocorticoid sensitivity is entirely environmental, and by the fact that the effects of postnatal licking and grooming on GR methylation are not associated with any known polymorphisms in the GR gene.[127]

These findings are quite different from those observed in another gene with epigenetic changes that have been linked to glucocorticoid sensitivity, the glucocorticoid receptor chaperone protein FKBP5. As noted above, risk alleles for this gene (specifically the AG/AA alleles at rs1360780, an SNP near a glucocorticoid response element in intron 7) have been shown repeatedly to increase the risk for mood and anxiety symptoms in individuals exposed to ELA, but not in individuals without ELA.[132] FKBP5 decreases cortisol binding to the GR and plays a pivotal role in an ultrafast feedback loop that terminates GR signaling. Given these activities, one would predict—correctly—that decreased methylation of the FKBP5 gene would inhibit GR signaling, because it would increase the anti-GR activities of FKBP5, and by reducing GR signaling would be associated with increased risk for psychopathology. This possibility has been confirmed in a study that finds that ELA leads to decreased intron 7 methylation, but only in carriers of the rs1360780 risk allele. To quote the investigators directly: "This suggests that, as expected, less methylation of intron 7 CpGs is associated with higher induction of FKBP5 by glucocorticoid receptor activation, especially in risk allele carriers, representing an enhancement of the ultrashort feedback loop leading to increased glucocorticoid receptor resistance"—and also, by extension, to increased stress-related depression and PTSD in risk allele carriers subjected to ELA.

The gene–environment interaction that leads to methylation (epigenetic) changes in the FKBP5 gene is worth pondering for a moment, as it provides a salient example of the complexities inherent in even so seemingly straightforward a concept as glucocorticoid resistance. Both directly and via the promotion of reduced methylation, the FKBP5 risk allele promotes overall glucocorticoid resistance precisely because it makes the FKBP5 gene itself more sensitive to GR signaling. That is, an allele that makes its gene more sensitive to glucocorticoids has the paradoxical long-term effect of making the organism as a whole more resistant to glucocorticoids.

Antidepressant Modalities Increase Glucocorticoid Signaling, Associated With Antidepressant Effects

Two powerful, highly replicated findings appear to contradict our argument that glucocorticoid signaling is best seen as an antidepressant pathway. First, animal and human studies demonstrate that exposure of the brain to high levels of glucocorticoids results in many changes either that are seen in MDD or that are counter to the effects of antidepressants. For example, chronic exposure to high doses of glucocorticoids in animal models or humans with Cushing's syndrome results in significant hippocampal atrophy, and in both rodents and primates high doses of glucocorticoids impair hippocampal neurogenesis. MDD has been repeatedly associated with reductions in hippocampal volume, and antidepressants reliably increase hippocampal neurogenesis in animal models. Second, when administered chronically antidepressants reduce cortisol concentrations in the blood and CSF of patients with MDD.[81]

Because antidepressants also reduce CSF concentrations and the amount of gene expression of CRH, the "head-gate" hormone of the HPA axis, one simple explanation of how antidepressants work is that they turn down CRH, which then leads to a reduction in cortisol and a concomitant improvement in symptoms. ("Head-gate" is a term borrowed from irrigation. It means the start of a system.) Because hormones and their receptors exist in a yin-yang relationship (i.e., when one goes up the other goes down), one might predict that antidepressants would secondarily increase the number or activity of GRs and MRs to compensate for the reduction in cortisol. And indeed, antidepressants have been shown in multiple animal studies to increase the binding capacity and/or gene expression of both MRs and GRs in hippocampal, limbic, and cortical brain areas.[20]

But here is the wrinkle: if antidepressants exert their effect by turning down CRH activity, with a subsequent reduction in cortisol production one would predict that changes in CRH and circulation cortisol should precede changes in GR/MR activity. However, the exact opposite appears to be the case: antidepressants increase MR signaling prior to reducing CRH activity and prior to lowering circulating levels of cortisol.[133–135] Although we have focused on GRs in this chapter, several lines of evidence suggest that antidepressants first upregulate MR activity and only secondarily sensitize GR. In one particularly telling study, depressed patients were treated with the tricyclic antidepressant amitriptyline plus the MR-specific antagonist spironolactone or placebo.[136] Subjects receiving spironolactone showed a markedly reduced response to amitriptyline, demonstrating that enhancement of MR activity early in antidepressant therapy contributes to symptomatic improvement.

These findings are consistent with many other studies suggesting that antidepressants turn down HPA axis activity by paradoxically initially increasing HPA axis signaling via sensitization of MRs and GRs. This increased receptor activity then subsequently, as a result of negative feedback, turns the axis off. Said in lay terms, the best way to lower cortisol levels and protect against any negative effects that might be conferred by long-term exposure to the hormone is not to directly reduce hormone levels but, rather, to actually increase hormonal signaling, which appears to "reset the dial," making the HPA axis more sensitive to glucocorticoids, which in turn prompts a reduction in further CRH and cortisol production and release.

Many animal and cell-culture studies suggest that antidepressants enhance glucocorticoid signaling by increasing activity of the MR and GR, with the majority of studies focusing on the GR.[20] Antidepressants of all classes appear capable of enhancing the transit (or translocation) of cortisol-GR complexes from the cytoplasm to the cellular nucleus, which is where the cortisol-GR complex exerts its effects on gene expression and, by that mechanism, on cellular function. Interesting, some studies suggest that certain antidepressants (e.g., desipramine) are able to directly induce translocation of the GR into the nucleus even in the absence of a glucocorticoid ligand.[137] Many antidepressants are also substrates for a protein known as the multidrug resistance transporter, or P-glycoprotein.[138] By blocking this transporter at the blood–brain barrier, antidepressants increase the concentration of cortisol within cells in the CNS, which secondarily leads to increased glucocorticoid signaling and an enhanced ability to thereby attenuate further HPA axis activity.

Again a paradox: by increasing MR and GR signaling, antidepressants eventually downregulate MR and GR mRNA production. While this could be interpreted as reducing glucocorticoid signaling, we suggest that it more likely reflects optimization of HPA activity such that less hormone and fewer receptors are needed to "get the job done." We base this on the fact that short- and longer-term treatment with antidepressants enhances glucocorticoid-mediated inhibitory feedback on the HPA axis and on the in vitro stimulated inflammatory responses of immune cells.[5,139] Moreover, patients with MDD who achieve symptomatic improvement following antidepressant treatment but who do not normalize glucocorticoid-mediated inhibitory control of the HPA axis (as assessed by the DEX-CRH stimulation test) are at an increased risk of depressive relapse compared with patients who achieve both symptomatic improvement and enhanced in vivo glucocorticoid sensitivity.[85] All these findings indicate that, when examined in functional terms, the overall effect of antidepressants is to increase the potency of the glucocorticoid message, at least in its role of suppressing HPA function and inflammatory activation. Nonetheless, this very increase in signaling may also blunt other aspects of cortisol activity. For example, Carmine Pariante and his colleagues have reported that four days of treatment with the selective serotonin reuptake inhibitor citalopram attenuated the impact of a dose of cortisol on EEG alpha power and working memory, two factors known to be powerfully impacted by glucocorticoid signaling.[140]

Let us turn now from the question of whether antidepressants increase or decrease glucocorticoid functionality and ask the more direct question of whether glucocorticoids have primarily pro- or antidepressant effects when given to humans. To our way of thinking, this is the ultimate test for establishing the relative veracity of our glucocorticoid insufficiency model, which sees cortisol as primarily a "good guy," versus the more widely embraced (in psychiatry at least) glucocorticoid cascade model, which envisions cortisol as a primary contributor to depression and its associated pathological changes in brain function and structure.

If the hypercortisolemia seen in depression is in some ultimate sense a primary cause of the disorder, one would certainly not expect glucocorticoids to demonstrate antidepressant effects, but in fact they do. Although never confirmed in large-scale clinical trials, many smaller studies suggest that both acute and short-term (i.e., two weeks) treatment with glucocorticoids produces a respectable antidepressant response. For example, Alan Schatzberg's group at Stanford randomized depressed patients not on other medications to a single infusion of cortisol, CRH, or placebo and followed changes in depressive symptoms for three days. While placebo and CRH had no effect, cortisol produced an average 37 percent decrease in depressive symptoms.[141] Similarly, four days of treatment with oral DEX produced a 37 percent response rate (defined as a ≥50 percent reduction in baseline depression score) 10 days later, as opposed to a mere 6 percent response to placebo.[142]

As we have highlighted repeatedly thus far in this book, stress is a major environmental driver of depression. Because cortisol is the quintessential stress hormone, it is easy to see how early investigators began their studies with the presumption that cortisol, therefore, must be depressogenic. One can immediately make two predictions if this assumption is true: (a) people who respond to a stress or trauma with increased cortisol should be at increased risk of developing stress-related mood and anxiety disorders down the road; and (b) treating recently traumatized individuals with cortisol should worsen their clinical course. However, both predictions are dead wrong.

Many studies now confirm that people who demonstrate low, not high, levels of cortisol immediately after a trauma are more likely than others to subsequently develop symptoms of PTSD, which is highly comorbid with MDD.[143,144] Moreover, patients who develop PTSD have been reported in many studies to maintain lower levels of cortisol in a variety of bodily tissues (i.e., hair, blood, saliva) than individuals without PTSD.[145–147] Although we have focused thus far on glucocorticoid insufficiency arising from reduced receptor activity (because this is the most germane cause for depression), there are other possible routes to glucocorticoid insufficiency, and certainly reduced cortisol is one of these routes.[5] Thus, it may be that individuals who respond to environmental adversities with insufficient cortisol production/release (or who are resistant at the level of receptors) are at increased risk for the development of mood and anxiety disturbances, and this, in turn, may account for at least some of the connection between insufficient glucocorticoid signaling and MDD.

If insufficient cortisol production contributes to psychopathology in the context of stress, it should be the case that, rather than making things worse, cortisol administration would make people more stress resilient and less likely to develop psychiatric sequelae. Think of how completely illogical this possibility is from the perspective of the glucocorticoid cascade. From this perspective, stress activates cortisol, which then over time damages the brain and body in ways that make a person anxious and depressed. People who respond to stressors with higher levels of cortisol should be most at risk, and strategies that block cortisol signaling should be protective.

In fact, many studies report that the administration of cortisol (or hydrocortisone) enhances emotional stress resilience. Several studies using standardized laboratory psychosocial stress tests (typically a combination of public speaking and mental arithmetic in front of an emotionally nonresponsive panel) have shown that the administration of hydrocortisone prior to the stressor significantly reduces emotional upset following the ordeal.[148,149] Similarly, glucocorticoid administration during or in the immediate aftermath of a traumatic experience reduces the risk of subsequent mood and anxiety difficulties. This has been observed naturalistically in hospital settings, where it has been repeatedly observed that patients who receive stress doses of hydrocortisone (or other glucocorticoids, e.g., prednisone) as part of their medical treatment have lower rates of subsequent PTSD development than do similarly ill patients not receiving glucocorticoids.[150,151] More recently, two prospective, randomized trials have shown that the administration of either a single bolus or chronic lower doses of cortisol immediately following trauma (typically an automobile accident) significantly reduces the development of both PTSD and depressive symptoms.[152,153] Consistent with these findings, cortisol administration has been shown to reduce symptoms in patients with already existent PTSD,[154–156] suggesting that enhanced glucocorticoid signaling may treat, as well as prevent, stress-induced psychopathology.

These findings strongly support a glucocorticoid insufficiency model of depression, but we would be remiss if we did not mention that other findings provide at least potential support for viewing cortisol as a pathogenic agent in MDD. Specifically, if cortisol promotes depression, then blocking its signaling or reducing its production should improve depressive symptomatology. Based on this idea, several cortisol synthesis inhibitors (e.g., metyrapone and ketoconazole) and the GR antagonist mifepristone (RU486) have been evaluated as antidepressants. Most of these studies are small, open-label" efforts. However, a randomized, double-blind, placebo-controlled study found that metyrapone outperformed placebo as an augmenting strategy to standard antidepressants.[157] However, in this study the addition of metyrapone had no impact on circulating cortisol levels, making it less likely that this clinical effect resulted directly from reduced glucocorticoid signaling.

By far the most intensively studied antiglucocorticoid strategy involves use of mifepristone. In fact, a company was formed (Corcept) to test and develop this product as an antidepressant, with an special focus on treating psychotic depression. This effort was abandoned several years ago when it became clear that, in fact, mifepristone showed no evidence of antidepressant efficacy.[158] Combined with evidence that blocking MRs actually attenuates response to standard antidepressants, the negative findings with mifepristone make a strong case that MDD is not in any simple way a disorder of "too much cortisol" but do support the possibility that glucocorticoid insufficiency contributes significantly to at least some cases of depression.

As we have noted, a traditional bulwark of the glucocorticoid cascade hypothesis has been the many animal studies showing that high doses of glucocorticoids negatively impact the functioning and architecture of the brain. Assuming that glucocorticoids do indeed have the potential to cause CNS mayhem when they are chronically present at high levels (which has never been fully established in humans), what evidence is there that glucocorticoids might have positive effects on brain functioning to account for their apparent antidepressant properties? We can begin this search with a study that exposed mice to the scent of a cat, which is a powerful, ecologically valid stressor for small rodents.[152] An hour after this "trauma" exposure, the mice were injected with either hydrocortisone or a saline placebo. When the researchers examined the morphology of the dendrite gyrus in these animals eight days later, they found that the hydrocortisone injection had markedly attenuated the reduction in dendritic length and synaptic spine density and complexity induced by the stressor. Animals that received hydrocortisone shortly after the stressor also had higher levels of hippocampal BDNF and demonstrated less anxiety-like behavior than the stressed mice that received placebo.

These findings are in line with other data showing that, when delivered to the brains of in living animals or to cultures of hippocampal and cortical neurons, glucocorticoids are capable of activating tyrosine receptor kinase B (TrkB) receptors via signaling through GR.[159] TrkB receptors are best known for conferring the neuroprotective effects of trophic factors, such as BDNF, that have been repeatedly shown to be reduced in depression and increased by antidepressant treatment. Thus at least in some circumstances, rather than damaging neuronal structure and functional integrity, glucocorticoids can actually function as neuroprotective agents. Interestingly, the ability of glucocorticoids to activate TrkB receptors was independent of any need for additional neurotrophic factors and protected neurons from death in the absence of other neurotrophic factors.

At a higher level of brain function, glucocorticoids have also shown effects relevant to depression. For example, Israel Liberzon and colleagues showed happy, sad, and neutral faces to healthy control subjects undergoing functional MRI. Prior to the imaging session subjects received either a single 100 mg dose of hydrocortisone, 25 mg/day hydrocortisone for four days, or placebo. Subjects receiving either dosing schedule of hydrocortisone showed significantly less activation of the subgenual anterior cingulate cortex (sgACC) in response to viewing sad faces.[160] These results are intriguing, given that sgACC hyperactivity is a classic functional MRI finding associated with MDD.[161] Moreover, inflammatory stimuli (i.e., a typhoid vaccine), which are suppressed by glucocorticoids, have been shown to activate the sgACC, with the amount of activation being associated with the increased depressive symptoms induced by the stimuli.[162]

Summary of the Role of the HPA Axis in MDD

We often like to think of the HPA axis as being like a Möbius strip—one of those twisted pieces of paper that turn out to have only one side. A simple twist of the paper and two sides become one without a place of start or ending. In a similar way, the HPA axis abnormalities that characterize MDD are easy to enumerate but hard to understand, because in a very real way the axis is an infinite loop with no clear beginning or end and with directionality effects that are almost incomprehensibly complex. How can we understand the simple fact that cortisol is both the body's primary stress and antistress hormone, a chemical whose primary functions include turning itself off? Because of this, if you don't have enough cortisol signaling via MRs and GRs, you will wind up with too much cortisol. Paradoxically, if you increase glucocorticoid signaling even further, as happens with antidepressants, the cortisol message gets through and cortisol levels drop. Should this be seen as increasing or decreasing HPA axis functioning?

We feel that findings regarding glucocorticoids and depression make most sense if characterized as reflecting insufficient glucocorticoid signaling, but we recognize that increased signaling has the effect of turning down the signaling, or at least optimizing it so that lower levels of glucocorticoids are necessary to get the message through. It is clear that, when this message is not optimized, glucocorticoids can induce many symptoms seen in Major Depression. We know this from naturalistic observations of people who develop Cushing's syndrome, either as result of taking glucocorticoid medications or from a biological abnormality such as a pituitary or adrenal tumor. Although initial pathological responses to high doses of glucocorticoids tend to be manic more often than depressive (in keeping with the acute antidepressant effects of hydrocortisone and DEX), over time chronic exposure to high doses of glucocorticoids increasingly promotes depression,[163] but it also induces a compensatory downregulation of receptor functioning, leading to glucocorticoid resistance. In fact, the classic test of glucocorticoid resistance, the DST, was invented not for depression but to help diagnose the likely cause for any given case of Cushing's syndrome. This again raises the perpetual conundrum: is the depressive pathology associated with Cushing's a reflection of too much or too little cortisol signaling in the areas of the brain and body that matter most in this regard?

We don't know the answer, but an intriguing study in patients with multiple sclerosis suggests that the high doses of glucocorticoids that cause Cushing's aren't able to get enough of the cortisol message through to shut the system down (and so in that way can be seen as insufficient).[164] In this study, patients with a multiple sclerosis exacerbation were treated with high doses of the glucocorticoid fluocortolone and either placebo or the reversible monoamine oxidase inhibitor antidepressant moclobemide. At several points across two and a half months of fluocortolone therapy the patients underwent DEX-CRH stimulation testing to evaluate sensitivity of the HPA axis to glucocorticoid negative feedback. Interestingly, the high-dose glucocorticoid alone produced glucocorticoid resistance (compared with a group of normal control subjects), whereas the addition of moclobemide normalized the DEX-CRH stimulation test response, suggesting that antidepressants enhanced the inhibitory feedback effects of the glucocorticoid. We suggest it is this inability of chronically high glucocorticoids to optimize inhibitory feedback that explains why prolonged exposure to high levels of glucocorticoids promotes depression, not because cortisol is a depressogenic substance in and of itself.

The Autonomic Nervous System

In many fields of medicine that study stress-related conditions, such as coronary artery disease, the ANS easily trumps the HPA axis as an object of general attention and study. In contrast, our lack of understanding of the role of the ANS in the pathogenesis of MDD is quite striking, especially given that researchers have investigated this question off and on for more than 40 years. Prior to writing this book we hadn't given much thought to this striking disparity, but now that we have, let us start this section by offering a few possible reasons for our relative ignorance regarding the ANS in MDD.

We begin with the simple observation that cortisol, the hormonal end product of HPA activation, is produced in only one place, the adrenal cortex, from whence it disperses throughout the body and the brain. Fully recognizing the many CNS actions of CRH, the primary secretagogue of the HPA axis, it is nonetheless fair to say that many of the primary actions of the HPA axis on the brain and body are directly driven by the amount of free cortisol circulating in blood and other bodily fluids such as saliva. Thus, when one measures cortisol, one is measuring "the thing itself." Moreover, although cortisol's activities vary somewhat within different brain and bodily organs, on the surface it is quite accurate to say that cortisol orchestrates the stress response.

Compare this with the situation that pertains in the ANS. In response to a stressor several things happen sequentially. First parasympathetic tone is withdrawn. If this is inadequate to the perceived danger, the SNS is then activated. It begins with an increase in SNS nerve fiber signaling, with a resultant release of the neurotransmitter NE. One SNS channel connects brain with the adrenal medulla, from whence epinephrine is released. The release of epinephrine is much faster than the release of cortisol, but slower than the release of NE. If you've ever had your heart start racing 30 seconds or so after narrowly escaping some danger (when all is safe) that is epinephrine coming online—in this case "a day late and a dollar short."

Note that, with the exception of epinephrine, the amount of the primary molecular agents of the ANS (i.e., NE and acetylcholine) in the blood is only a pale reflection of what might be actually happening at the all-important ANS synapse. So, unlike for cortisol, the concentrations of NE or acetylcholine in the blood (or any other fluid) can give us only a hint at the operation of the ANS in MDD and tell us nothing about whether the condition is associated with different ANS reactions in different bodily compartments. Hypercortisolemia means too much cortisol everywhere that blood goes (to a first approximation—other factors influence how much gets into the brain). On the other hand, increased NE in the blood could mean increased SNS signaling to the heart, to the skin, to the gut, to the immune system, or to all these areas/organs.

HRV provides a more direct measure of ANS signaling, but only to the heart, leaving unanswered the question of whether abnormalities in this metric in MDD reflect a more widespread, whole-body disturbance in ANS function or a localized cardiac dysfunction. Moreover, despite years of debate, not everyone agrees on what various HRV measures mean in terms of reflecting SNS versus PNS activity. There is fairly strong consensus that among the spectral metrics—which are the most commonly used ones in research—high-frequency HRV (also known as respiratory sinus arrhythmia) reflects parasympathetic tone to the heart. But how best to interpret other commonly employed spectral measures, such as low-frequency HRV and very low-frequency HRV, remains more contentious. While some evidence suggests that these metrics reflect primarily SNS activity, other data indicate that they are at least partly a reflection of vagal, parasympathetic signaling. For example, low-frequency HRV can be abolished by administration of the cholinergic muscarinic antagonist atropine.[11]

As we've discussed at some length, the HPA axis is awash in complexities because of its circular nature and the fact that CRH, ACTH, and cortisol have different effects on the brain/body complex, not all of which, in the case of CRH, are part of HPA axis functionality (i.e., CRH operates as a neurotransmitter in the brain). Nonetheless, despite these complexities, the molecular players in the HPA axis mostly function as a team to expedite the mammalian stress response.

On the other hand, catecholamines (i.e., NE and epinephrine) and acetylcholine play very different roles as neurotransmitters in the brain than they do as purveyors of ANS signaling. Consider acetylcholine: as the end-product neurotransmitter of the PNS it promotes behaviors and physiological responses essential to social interactions, bodily repair, food digestion, and key aspects of the sexual response, all of which are suppressed by SNS activation. One might almost think of it as the relaxation system, and indeed it was made famous by Herbert Benson as the "relaxation response." Given the ubiquity of anxiety in MDD, as well as disruptions in exactly the vegetative functions subserved by the PNS, it is no surprise that the bulk of available evidence points to reduced activity of this system in depressed individuals. Given this, one might predict that increasing acetylcholine levels would improve depressive symptoms. But here is where the logic fails. In fact, although never really embraced by psychiatry, evidence has existed for more than a generation that depression is associated with increased cholinergic signaling. Studies confirm this by showing that the muscarinic cholinergic receptor antagonist produces robust, and very rapid, antidepressant effects. The solution to this discrepancy lies in the fact that, unlike cortisol, acetylcholine has very different effects in the brain than it does in the PNS.

Early evidence for increased SNS activity in MDD came from studies reporting increased plasma concentrations of NE, which presumably reflects spillover into the blood from increased SNS synaptic activity.[165–168] However, other early studies provided conflicting findings, such as reduced concentrations of urinary NE.[169,170] A more recent study that measured whole-body SNS activity may help explain these contradictory findings. Whereas in this study normal controls demonstrated a unimodal distribution of SNS activity, people with depression tended to segregate along a bimodal distribution, such that one contingent of the depressed cohort had very low SNS activity and the other had very high activity.[171] Unfortunately, this finding has yet to be replicated, so we do not know how generalizable it is, nor do we know what other biological changes might manifest the high- or low-SNS group. Given evidence that SNS activation can promote peripheral inflammation,[172] we might expect that the high-SNS group would comprise people with elevated levels of inflammation, but this is only a conjecture at this point.

In recent years measures of plasma concentrations of NE and epinephrine have given way to more complex functional assessments. As with most things related to depression, findings are not entirely consistent but in general support the notion that MDD is a condition characterized by increased SNS and reduced PNS activity. A major caveat, however, is that many of the studies in this area have examined depressed patients on antidepressants, which represents a significant confound given that these agents (and especially those with noradrenergic effects, e.g., the tricyclics and serotonin and NE reuptake inhibitors) can themselves induce or worsen the same types of ANS alterations associated with MDD.

With these caveats in mind, many studies support that general notion that SNS activity is increased and PNS signaling is diminished in MDD. For example, in a cohort of depressed individuals (two-thirds of whom were on antidepressants), the sympathetic skin response to a noxious electrical stimulus was characterized by reduced latency and increased amplitude compared with the response in normal controls.[173] This study is intriguing, because in contradistinction to HRV studies, the skin response is purely sympathetic and thus supports the notion that changes in the sympathetic/parasympathetic balance in MDD may occur as a result of changes in both arms of the ANS.

In decreasing order of certainty are the following facts: (a) MDD is associated with alterations in HRV; (b) time-based HRV is reduced in MDD; (c) among spectral measures of HRV, respiratory sinus arrhythmia (or high frequency) is reduced in MDD; (d) low-frequency HRV, as well as the ratio of low-frequency to high-frequency HRV, is increased in MDD; (e) various more complex, nonlinear measures of HRV may be abnormal in MDD; and (f) the association of MDD with altered HRV results from the disease state itself and not its treatment with antidepressants. Although not found in every study, many reports link depression with reduced HRV, whether measured via time domain or frequency methods. A number of studies also report increases in the low-frequency/high-frequency ratio, which many take to be a marker of sympathetic to parasympathetic balance. For example, a study that is important because it examined depressed individuals not taking antidepressants found reductions in a variety of indicators of vagal function when 75 nonmedicated depressed patients were compared with 75 psychiatrically and medically healthy age- and sex-matched controls.[174] In addition, depressed subjects showed an increase in the QT variability index, which has been shown to reflect sympathetic input to the heart. Although most studies have examined HRV, at rest at least one study has examined the impact of depression on HRV responses to emotion-relevant stimuli. In this study, depressed women were shown to have less of an increase in respiratory sinus arrhythmia while engaged in relationship-focused imagery compared with nondepressed control subjects.[175]

The great question regarding HRV in depression is the extent to which findings reflect the disease state itself or its treatment with antidepressants, given ample evidence that several classes of antidepressants induce many of the same changes in HRV that have been ascribed to MDD.[176] On one side of the ledger is a meta-analysis of 18 studies (673 patients with depression, 407 controls) showing that MDD is associated with reduced time-domain HRV, low-frequency HRV, and valsalva ratio, all consistent with reduced vagal, parasympathetic signaling to the heart.[177] Moreover, in this meta-analysis the more severe the depression, the greater the reduction in HRV measures of vagal tone. However, these results need to be balanced against the largest study of HRV in depression that we know of, conducted in the Netherlands. In this study, the reductions in time and frequency-domain measures of HRV linked to vagal function were almost entirely accounted for by the use of antidepressant medications, with the impact of antidepressants on HRV increasing with increasing medication doses.[176] Although a very small association between reduced respiratory sinus arrhythmia (i.e., high-frequency HRV) remained after adjusting for antidepressant use, this hardly supports a significant role for vagal changes in the pathophysiology of MDD.

So where does this leave us? Unlike the situation with the HPA axis, where changes in MDD are consistent enough we feel to be considered established fact, when it comes to the ANS we must hold our conclusions loosely and not be overly surprised if the future provides no great insights. Nonetheless, we suspect that in general MDD is indeed a condition characterized by various degrees of SNS activation and parasympathetic withdrawal because so many convergent lines of evidence point in this direction.

References

1. Carroll BJ. The dexamethasone suppression test for melancholia. *Br J Psychiatry.* 1982; 140:292–304.

2. Pariante CM, Nemeroff CB, Miller AH. Glucocorticoid receptors in depression. *Isr J Med Sci.* 1995;31(12):705–712.

3. Raison CL, Demetrashvili M, Capuron L, Miller AH. Neuropsychiatric adverse effects of interferon-alpha: recognition and management. *CNS Drugs.* 2005;19(2):105–123.

4. Raison CL, Rutherford RE, Woolwine BJ, et al. A randomized controlled trial of the tumor necrosis factor antagonist infliximab for treatment-resistant depression: the role of baseline inflammatory biomarkers. *Arch Gen Psychiatry.* 2012:1–11.

5. Raison CL, Miller AH. When not enough is too much: the role of insufficient glucocorticoid signaling in the pathophysiology of stress-related disorders. *Am J Psychiatry.* 2003;160(9):1554–1565.

6. Owens MJ, Nemeroff CB. The role of corticotropin-releasing factor in the pathophysiology of affective and anxiety disorders: laboratory and clinical studies. *Ciba Found Symp.* 1993;172:296–316.

7. Zobel AW, Nickel T, Kunzel HE, et al. Effects of the high-affinity corticotropin-releasing hormone receptor 1 antagonist R121919 in major depression: the first 20 patients treated. *J Psychiatr Res.* 2000;34(3):171–181.

8. Schule C, Baghai TC, Eser D, Rupprecht R. Hypothalamic-pituitary-adrenocortical system dysregulation and new treatment strategies in depression. *Expert Rev Neurother.* 2009;9(7):1005–1019.

9. Porges SW. Making the world safe for our children: down-regulating defence and up-regulating social engagement to optimise the human experience. *Children Australia.* 2015;40:114–123.

10. Porges SW. The polyvagal theory: phylogenetic substrates of a social nervous system. *Int J Psychophysiol.* 2001;42(2):123–146.

11. Porges SW. The polyvagal perspective. *Biol Psychol.* 2007;74(2):116–143.

12. Louveau A, Harris TH, Kipnis J. Revisiting the mechanisms of CNS immune privilege. *Trends Immunol.* 2015;36(10):569–577.

13. Tay TL, Savage J, Hui CW, Bisht K, Tremblay ME. Microglia across the lifespan: from origin to function in brain development, plasticity and cognition. *J Physiol.* 2016 (epub ahead of print, 1–17).

14. Ader R, Felten DL, Cohen N, eds. *Psychoneuroimmunology.* 3rd ed. San Diego: Academic Press; 2001.

15. Miller AH, Raison CL. The role of inflammation in depression: from evolutionary imperative to modern treatment target. *Nat Rev Immunol.* 2015;16(1):22–34.

16. Freier E, Weber CS, Nowottne U, et al. Decrease of CD4(+)FOXP3(+) T regulatory cells in the peripheral blood of human subjects undergoing a mental stressor. *Psychoneuroendocrinology.* 2010;35(5):663–673.

17. Travis MA, Sheppard D. TGF-beta activation and function in immunity. *Annu Rev Immunol.* 2014;32:51–82.

18. Plotsky P, Owens MJ, Nemeroff CB. Neuropeptide alterations in affective disorders. In:

Bloom FE, Kupfer DJ, eds. *Psychopharmacology: The Fourth Generation of Progress.* New York: Raven Press; 1995:971–981.

19. Holsboer F. The corticosteroid hypothesis of depression. *Neuropsychopharmacology.* 2000;23:477–501.

20. Pariante CM, Miller AH. Glucocorticoid receptors in major depression: relevance to pathophysiology and treatment. *Biol Psychiatry.* 2001;49(5):391–404.

21. Arborelius L, Owens MJ, Plotsky PM, Nemeroff CB. The role of corticotropin-releasing factor in depression and anxiety disorders. *J Endocrinol.* 1999;160(1):1–12.

22. Nemeroff CB, Widerlov E, Bissette G, et al. Elevated concentrations of CSF corticotropin-releasing factor-like immunoreactivity in depressed patients. *Science.* 1984;226(4680):1342–1344.

23. France RD, Urban B, Krishnan KR, et al. CSF corticotropin-releasing factor-like immunoactivity in chronic pain patients with and without major depression. *Biol Psychiatry.* 1988;23(1):86–88.

24. Benca RM. Sleep in psychiatric disorders. *Neurol Clin.* 1996;14(4):739–764.

25. Widerlov E, Bissette G, Nemeroff CB. Monoamine metabolites, corticotropin releasing factor and somatostatin as CSF markers in depressed patients. *J Affect Disord.* 1988;14(2):99–107.

26. Arato M, Banki CM, Bissette G, Nemeroff CB. Elevated CSF CRF in suicide victims. *Biol Psychiatry.* 1989;25(3):355–359.

27. Banki CM, Bissette G, Arato M, O'Connor L, Nemeroff CB. CSF corticotropin-releasing factor-like immunoreactivity in depression and schizophrenia. *Am J Psychiatry.* 1987;144(7):873–877.

28. Kling MA, Roy A, Doran AR, et al. Cerebrospinal fluid immunoreactive corticotropin-releasing hormone and adrenocorticotropin secretion in Cushing's disease and major depression: potential clinical implications. *J Clin Endocrinol Metab.* 1991;72(2):260–271.

29. Molchan SE, Hill JL, Martinez RA, et al. CSF somatostatin in Alzheimer's disease and major depression: relationship to hypothalamic-pituitary-adrenal axis and clinical measures. *Psychoneuroendocrinology.* 1993;18(7):509–519.

30. Pitts AF, Samuelson SD, Meller WH, Bissette G, Nemeroff CB, Kathol RG. Cerebrospinal fluid corticotropin-releasing hormone, vasopressin, and oxytocin concentrations in treated patients with major depression and controls. *Biol Psychiatry.* 1995;38(5):330–335.

31. Kalin NH. Behavioral and endocrine studies of corticotropin-releasing hormone in primates. In: De Souza EB, Nemeroff CB, eds. *Corticotropin-Releasing Factor: Basic and Clinical Studies of a Neuropeptide.* Boca Raton, FL: CRC Press; 1990:275–289.

32. Nemeroff CB, Bissette G, Akil H, Fink M. Neuropeptide concentrations in the cerebrospinal fluid of depressed patients treated with electroconvulsive therapy: corticotrophin-releasing factor, beta-endorphin and somatostatin. *Br J Psychiatry.* 1991;158:59–63.

33. Kling MA, Geracioti TD, Licinio J, Michelson D, Oldfield EH, Gold PW. Effects of electroconvulsive therapy on the CRH-ACTH-cortisol system in melancholic depression: preliminary findings. *Psychopharmacol Bull.* 1994;30(3):489–494.

34. De Bellis MD, Gold PW, Geracioti TD Jr, Listwak SJ, Kling MA. Association of fluoxetine treatment with reductions in CSF concentrations of corticotropin-releasing hormone and arginine vasopressin in patients with major depression. *Am J Psychiatry.* 1993;150(4):656–657.

35. Banki CM, Karmacsi L, Bissette G, Nemeroff CB. CSF corticotropin-releasing hormone

and somatostatin in major depression: response to antidepressant treatment and relapse. *Eur Neuropsychopharmacol.* 1992;2(2):107–113.

36. Raadsheer FC, Hoogendijk WJ, Stam FC, Tilders FJ, Swaab DF. Increased numbers of corticotropin-releasing hormone expressing neurons in the hypothalamic paraventricular nucleus of depressed patients. *Neuroendocrinology.* 1994;60(4):436–444.

37. Nemeroff CB, Owens MJ, Bissette G, Andorn AC, Stanley M. Reduced corticotropin releasing factor binding sites in the frontal cortex of suicide victims. *Arch Gen Psychiatry.* 1988;45(6):577–579.

38. Raison CL, Miller AH. When not enough is too much: the role of insufficient glucocorticoid signaling in the pathophysiology of stress-related disorders. *Am J Psychiatry.* 2003;160:1554–1565.

39. Sapolsky RM, Krey LC, McEwen BS. The neuroendocrinology of stress and aging: the glucocorticoid cascade hypothesis. *Endocr Rev.* 1986;7(3):284–301.

40. Raison CL, Gumnick JF, Miller AH. Neuroendocrine-immune interactions: implications for health and behavior. In: Pfaff D, Arnold A, Etgen A, Fahrbach S, Rubin RT, eds. *Hormones, Brain and Behavior.* Vol 5. San Diego: Academic Press; 2002:209–261.

41. Herbert TB, Cohen S. Depression and immunity: a meta-analytic review. *Psychol Bull.* 1993;113(3):472–486.

42. Herbert TB, Cohen S. Stress and immunity in humans: a meta-analytic review. *Psychosom Med.* 1993;55(4):364–379.

43. Dhabhar FS, McEwen BS. Stress-induced enhancement of antigen-specific cell-mediated immunity. *J Immunol.* 1996;156(7):2608–2615.

44. Dhabhar FS, McEwen BS. Enhancing versus suppressive effects of stress hormones on skin immune function. *Proc Natl Acad Sci U S A.* 1999;96(3):1059–1064.

45. Viswanathan K, Daugherty C, Dhabhar FS. Stress as an endogenous adjuvant: augmentation of the immunization phase of cell-mediated immunity. *Int Immunol.* 2005;17(8):1059–1069.

46. Dhabhar FS. Enhancing versus suppressive effects of stress on immune function: implications for immunoprotection and immunopathology. *Neuroimmunomodulation.* 2009;16(5):300–317.

47. Miller AH, Spencer RL, Pearce BD, et al. 1996 Curt P. Richter Award: effects of viral infection on corticosterone secretion and glucocorticoid receptor binding in immune tissues. *Psychoneuroendocrinology.* 1997;22(6):455–474.

48. Dhabhar FS, Miller AH, McEwen BS, Spencer RL. Stress-induced changes in blood leukocyte distribution: role of adrenal steroid hormones. *J Immunol.* 1996;157(4):1638–1644.

49. Dhabhar FS. Stress, leukocyte trafficking, and the augmentation of skin immune function. *Ann N Y Acad Sci.* 2003;992:205–217.

50. Maes M. Cytokines in major depression. *Biol Psychiatry.* 1994;36(7):498–499.

51. Kent S, Bluthe RM, Kelley KW, Dantzer R. Sickness behavior as a new target for drug development. *Trends Psychosom Med Pharmacol Sci.* 1992;13(1):24–28.

52. McKay LI, Cidlowski JA. Molecular control of immune/inflammatory responses: interactions between nuclear factor-kappa B and steroid receptor-signaling pathways. *Endocr Rev.* 1999;20(4):435–459.

53. Maes M, Scharpe S, Meltzer HY, et al. Relationships between interleukin-6 activity, acute phase proteins, and function of the hypothalamic-pituitary-adrenal axis in severe depression. *Psychiatry Res.* 1993;49(1):11–27.

54. Miller GE, Cohen S, Ritchey AK. Chronic psychological stress and the regulation of pro-

inflammatory cytokines: a glucocorticoid-resistance model. *Health Psychol.* 2002;21(6): 531–541.

55. Friedman SB, Mason JW, Hanburg DA. Urinary 17-hydroxycorticosteroid levels in parents of children with neoplastic disease: a study of chronic psychological stress. *Psychosom Med.* 1963;25:364–376.

56. Yehuda R. Biology of posttraumatic stress disorder. *J Clin Psychiatry.* 2001;62(suppl 17):41–46.

57. Heim C, Newport DJ, Heit S, et al. Pituitary-adrenal and autonomic responses to stress in women after sexual and physical abuse in childhood. *JAMA.* 2000;284(5):592–597.

58. Heim C, Newport DJ, Bonsall R, Miller AH, Nemeroff CB. Altered pituitary-adrenal axis responses to provocative challenge tests in adult survivors of childhood abuse. *Am J Psychiatry.* 2001;158(4):575–581.

59. Loevinger BL, Shirtcliff EA, Muller D, Alonso C, Coe CL. Delineating psychological and biomedical profiles in a heterogeneous fibromyalgia population using cluster analysis. *Clin Rheumatol.* 2012;31(4):677–685.

60. Rohleder N. Acute and chronic stress induced changes in sensitivity of peripheral inflammatory pathways to the signals of multiple stress systems—2011 Curt Richter Award Winner. *Psychoneuroendocrinology.* 2012;37(3):307–316.

61. Avitsur R, Padgett DA, Sheridan JF. Social interactions, stress, and immunity. *Neurol Clin.* 2006;24(3):483–491.

62. Rohleder N, Marin TJ, Ma R, Miller GE. Biologic cost of caring for a cancer patient: dysregulation of pro- and anti-inflammatory signaling pathways. *J Clin Oncol.* 2009;27(18): 2909–2915.

63. Miller GE, Chen E, Sze J, et al. A functional genomic fingerprint of chronic stress in humans: blunted glucocorticoid and increased NF-kappaB signaling. *Biol Psychiatry.* 2008;64(4):266–272.

64. Miller GE, Murphy ML, Cashman R, et al. Greater inflammatory activity and blunted glucocorticoid signaling in monocytes of chronically stressed caregivers. *Brain Behav Immun.* 2014;41:191–199.

65. Moussavi S, Chatterji S, Verdes E, Tandon A, Patel V, Ustun B. Depression, chronic diseases, and decrements in health: results from the World Health Surveys. *Lancet.* 2007; 370(9590):851–858.

66. Berkenbosch F, van Oers J, del Rey A, Tilders F, Besedovsky H. Corticotropin-releasing factor-producing neurons in the rat activated by interleukin-1. *Science.* 1987;238(4826): 524–526.

67. Besedovsky H, del Rey A, Sorkin E, Dinarello CA. Immunoregulatory feedback between interleukin-1 and glucocorticoid hormones. *Science.* 1986;233(4764):652–654.

68. Sapolsky R, Rivier C, Yamamoto G, Plotsky P, Vale W. Interleukin-1 stimulates the secretion of hypothalamic corticotropin-releasing factor. *Science.* 1987;238(4826):522–524.

69. Capuron L, Raison CL, Musselman DL, Lawson DH, Nemeroff CB, Miller AH. Association of exaggerated HPA axis response to the initial injection of interferon-alpha with development of depression during interferon-alpha therapy. *Am J Psychiatry.* 2003;160(7): 1342–1345.

70. Raison CL, Borisov AS, Woolwine BJ, Massung B, Vogt G, Miller AH. Interferon-alpha effects on diurnal hypothalamic-pituitary-adrenal axis activity: relationship with proinflammatory cytokines and behavior. *Mol Psychiatry.* 2010;15(5):535–547.

71. Sephton SE, Sapolsky RM, Kraemer HC, Spiegel D. Diurnal cortisol rhythm as a predictor of breast cancer survival. *J Natl Cancer Inst.* 2000;92(12):994–1000.

72. Pace TW, Hu F, Miller AH. Cytokine-effects on glucocorticoid receptor function: relevance to glucocorticoid resistance and the pathophysiology and treatment of major depression. *Brain Behav Immun.* 2007;21(1):9–19.

73. Hu F, Pace TW, Miller AH. Interferon-alpha inhibits glucocorticoid receptor-mediated gene transcription via STAT5 activation in mouse HT22 cells. *Brain Behav Immun.* 2009;23(4):455–463.

74. Smoak KA, Cidlowski JA. Mechanisms of glucocorticoid receptor signaling during inflammation. *Mech Ageing Dev.* 2004;125(10–11):697–706.

75. Felger JC, Haroon E, Woolwine BJ, Raison CL, Miller AH. Interferon-alpha-induced inflammation is associated with reduced glucocorticoid negative feedback sensitivity and depression in patients with hepatitis C virus. *Physiol Behav.* 2016;166:14–21.

76. Wang X, Wu H, Miller AH. Interleukin 1alpha (IL-1alpha) induced activation of p38 mitogen-activated protein kinase inhibits glucocorticoid receptor function. *Mol Psychiatry.* 2004;9(1):65–75.

77. Engler H, Bailey MT, Engler A, Stiner-Jones LM, Quan N, Sheridan JF. Interleukin-1 receptor type 1-deficient mice fail to develop social stress-associated glucocorticoid resistance in the spleen. *Psychoneuroendocrinology.* 2008;33(1):108–117.

78. Raison CL, Miller AH. The evolutionary significance of depression in Pathogen Host Defense (PATHOS-D). *Mol Psychiatry.* 2013;18(1):15–37.

79. Papi A, Contoli M, Adcock IM, et al. Rhinovirus infection causes steroid resistance in airway epithelium through nuclear factor kappaB and c-Jun N-terminal kinase activation. *J Allergy Clin Immunol.* 2013;132(5):1075–1085 e1076.

80. Cotter PA, Mulligan OF, Landau S, Papadopoulos A, Lightman SL, Checkley SA. Vasoconstrictor response to topical beclomethasone in major depression. *Psychoneuroendocrinology.* 2002;27(4):475–487.

81. Carroll BJ. Use of the dexamethasone suppression test in depression. *J Clin Psychiatry.* 1982;43(11 pt 2):44–50.

82. Ising M, Kunzel HE, Binder EB, Nickel T, Modell S, Holsboer F. The combined dexamethasone/CRH test as a potential surrogate marker in depression. *Prog Neuropsychopharmacol Biol Psychiatry.* 2005;29(6):1085–1093.

83. Maes M, Maes L, Suy E. Symptom profiles of biological markers in depression: a multivariate study. *Psychoneuroendocrinology.* 1990;15(1):29–37.

84. Greden JF, Gardner R, King D, Grunhaus L, Carroll BJ, Kronfol Z. Dexamethasone suppression tests in antidepressant treatment of melancholia: the process of normalization and test-retest reproducibility. *Arch Gen Psychiatry.* 1983;40(5):493–500.

85. Zobel AW, Nickel T, Sonntag A, Uhr M, Holsboer F, Ising M. Cortisol response in the combined dexamethasone/CRH test as predictor of relapse in patients with remitted depression. a prospective study. *J Psychiatr Res.* 2001;35(2):83–94.

86. Modell S, Lauer CJ, Schreiber W, Huber J, Krieg JC, Holsboer F. Hormonal response pattern in the combined DEX-CRH test is stable over time in subjects at high familial risk for affective disorders. *Neuropsychopharmacology.* 1998;18(4):253–262.

87. Boyle MP, Brewer JA, Funatsu M, et al. Acquired deficit of forebrain glucocorticoid receptor produces depression-like changes in adrenal axis regulation and behavior. *Proc Natl Acad Sci U S A.* 2005;102(2):473–478.

88. Meaney MJ, Diorio J, Francis D, et al. Early environmental regulation of forebrain glucocorticoid receptor gene expression: implications for adrenocortical responses to stress. *Dev Neurosci.* 1996;18(1–2):49–72.

89. McGowan PO, Sasaki A, D'Alessio AC, et al. Epigenetic regulation of the glucocorticoid

receptor in human brain associates with childhood abuse. *Nat Neurosci.* 2009;12(3): 342–348.

90. Bradley RG, Binder EB, Epstein MP, et al. Influence of child abuse on adult depression: moderation by the corticotropin-releasing hormone receptor gene. *Arch Gen Psychiatry.* 2008;65(2):190–200.

91. Heim C, Bradley B, Mletzko TC, et al. Effect of childhood trauma on adult depression and neuroendocrine function: sex-specific moderation by CRH receptor 1 gene. *Front Behav Neurosci.* 2009;3:41.

92. Chourbaji S, Vogt MA, Gass P. Mice that under- or overexpress glucocorticoid receptors as models for depression or posttraumatic stress disorder. *Prog Brain Res.* 2008;167: 65–77.

93. Kronenberg G, Kirste I, Inta D, et al. Reduced hippocampal neurogenesis in the GR(+/-) genetic mouse model of depression. *Eur Arch Psychiatry Clin Neurosci.* 2009;259(8): 499–504.

94. Pandey GN, Rizavi HS, Ren X, Dwivedi Y, Palkovits M. Region-specific alterations in glucocorticoid receptor expression in the postmortem brain of teenage suicide victims. *Psychoneuroendocrinology.* 2013;38(11):2628–2639.

95. Alt SR, Turner JD, Klok MD, et al. Differential expression of glucocorticoid receptor transcripts in major depressive disorder is not epigenetically programmed. *Psychoneuroendocrinology.* 2010;35(4):544–556.

96. Klok MD, Alt SR, Irurzun Lafitte AJ, et al. Decreased expression of mineralocorticoid receptor mRNA and its splice variants in postmortem brain regions of patients with major depressive disorder. *J Psychiatr Res.* 2011;45(7):871–878.

97. Lopez JF, Chalmers DT, Little KY, Watson SJ. A.E. Bennett Research Award. Regulation of serotonin1A, glucocorticoid, and mineralocorticoid receptor in rat and human hippocampus: implications for the neurobiology of depression. *Biol Psychiatry.* 1998;43(8): 547–573.

98. Webster MJ, Knable MB, O'Grady J, Orthmann J, Weickert CS. Regional specificity of brain glucocorticoid receptor mRNA alterations in subjects with schizophrenia and mood disorders. *Mol Psychiatry.* 2002;7(9):985–994, 924.

99. Wassef A, Smith EM, Rose RM, Gardner R, Nguyen H, Meyer WJ. Mononuclear leukocyte glucocorticoid receptor binding characteristics and down-regulation in major depression. *Psychoneuroendocrinology.* 1990;15(1):59–68.

100. Gormley GJ, Lowy MT, Reder AT, Hospelhorn VD, Antel JP, Meltzer HY. Glucocorticoid receptors in depression: relationship to the dexamethasone suppression test. *Am J Psychiatry.* 1985;142(11):1278–1284.

101. Lowy MT, Reder AT, Gormley GJ, Meltzer HY. Comparison of in vivo and in vitro glucocorticoid sensitivity in depression: relationship to the dexamethasone suppression test. *Biol Psychiatry.* 1988;24(6):619–630.

102. Rupprecht M, Rupprecht R, Kornhuber J, et al. Elevated glucocorticoid receptor concentrations before and after glucocorticoid therapy in peripheral mononuclear leukocytes of patients with atopic dermatitis. *Dermatologica.* 1991;183(2):100–105.

103. Rupprecht R, Kornhuber J, Wodarz N, et al. Disturbed glucocorticoid receptor autoregulation and corticotropin response to dexamethasone in depressives pretreated with metyrapone. *Biol Psychiatry.* 1991;29(11):1099–1109.

104. Wodarz N, Rupprecht R, Kornhuber J, et al. Normal lymphocyte responsiveness to lectins but impaired sensitivity to in vitro glucocorticoids in major depression. *J Affect Disord.* 1991;22(4):241–248.

105. Wodarz N, Rupprecht R, Kornhuber J, Schmitz B, Wild K, Riederer P. Cell-mediated immunity and its glucocorticoid-sensitivity after clinical recovery from severe major depressive disorder. *J Affect Disord.* 1992;25(1):31–38.

106. Lowy MT, Reder AT, Antel JP, Meltzer HY. Glucocorticoid resistance in depression: the dexamethasone suppression test and lymphocyte sensitivity to dexamethasone. *Am J Psychiatry.* 1984;141(11):1365–1370.

107. Maguire TM, Thakore J, Dinan TG, Hopwood S, Breen KC. Plasma sialyltransferase levels in psychiatric disorders as a possible indicator of HPA axis function. *Biol Psychiatry.* 1997;41(11):1131–1136.

108. Menke A, Arloth J, Putz B, et al. Dexamethasone stimulated gene expression in peripheral blood is a sensitive marker for glucocorticoid receptor resistance in depressed patients. *Neuropsychopharmacology.* 2012;37(6):1455–1464.

109. Schlosser N, Wolf OT, Fernando SC, et al. Effects of acute cortisol administration on response inhibition in patients with major depression and healthy controls. *Psychiatry Res.* 2013;209(3):439–446.

110. Cross-Disorder Group of the Psychiatric Genomics Consortium, Lee SH, Ripke S, et al. Genetic relationship between five psychiatric disorders estimated from genome-wide SNPs. *Nat Genet.* 2013;45(9):984–994.

111. CONVERGE Consortium. Sparse whole-genome sequencing identifies two loci for major depressive disorder. *Nature.* 2015;523(7562):588–591.

112. van Rossum EF, van den Akker EL. Glucocorticoid resistance. *Endocr Dev.* 2011;20:127–136.

113. Derijk RH, Schaaf MJ, Turner G, et al. A human glucocorticoid receptor gene variant that increases the stability of the glucocorticoid receptor beta-isoform mRNA is associated with rheumatoid arthritis. *J Rheumatol.* 2001;28(11):2383–2388.

114. van Rossum EF, Koper JW, Huizenga NA, et al. A polymorphism in the glucocorticoid receptor gene, which decreases sensitivity to glucocorticoids in vivo, is associated with low insulin and cholesterol levels. *Diabetes.* 2002;51(10):3128–3134.

115. van Rossum EF, Lamberts SW. Polymorphisms in the glucocorticoid receptor gene and their associations with metabolic parameters and body composition. *Rec Prog Horm Res.* 2004;59:333–357.

116. van Oosten MJ, Dolhain RJ, Koper JW, et al. Polymorphisms in the glucocorticoid receptor gene that modulate glucocorticoid sensitivity are associated with rheumatoid arthritis. *Arthritis Res Ther.* 2010;12(4):R159.

117. van Winsen LM, Manenschijn L, van Rossum EF, et al. A glucocorticoid receptor gene haplotype (TthIII1/ER22/23EK/9beta) is associated with a more aggressive disease course in multiple sclerosis. *J Clin Endocrinol Metab.* 2009;94(6):2110–2114.

118. van den Akker EL, Koper JW, van Rossum EF, et al. Glucocorticoid receptor gene and risk of cardiovascular disease. *Arch Intern Med.* 2008;168(1):33–39.

119. Otte C, Wust S, Zhao S, Pawlikowska L, Kwok PY, Whooley MA. Glucocorticoid receptor gene and depression in patients with coronary heart disease: the Heart and Soul Study-2009 Curt Richter Award Winner. *Psychoneuroendocrinology.* 2009;34(10):1574–1581.

120. Spijker AT, van Rossum EF. Glucocorticoid sensitivity in mood disorders. *Neuroendocrinology.* 2012;95(3):179–186.

121. Bet PM, Penninx BW, Bochdanovits Z, et al. Glucocorticoid receptor gene polymorphisms and childhood adversity are associated with depression: new evidence for a gene-environment interaction. *Am J Med Genet B Neuropsychiatr Genet.* 2009;150B(5):660–669.

122. van Rossum EF, Binder EB, Majer M, et al. Polymorphisms of the glucocorticoid receptor gene and major depression. *Biol Psychiatry.* 2006;59(8):681–688.

123. Xiang L, Marshall GD Jr. Glucocorticoid receptor BclI polymorphism associates with immunomodulatory response to stress hormone in human peripheral blood mononuclear cells. *Int J Immunogenet.* 2013;40(3):222–229.

124. Polanczyk G, Caspi A, Williams B, et al. Protective effect of CRHR1 gene variants on the development of adult depression following childhood maltreatment: replication and extension. *Arch Gen Psychiatry.* 2009;66(9):978–985.

125. Ladd CO, Huot RL, Thrivikraman KV, Nemeroff CB, Meaney MJ, Plotsky PM. Long-term behavioral and neuroendocrine adaptations to adverse early experience. *Prog Brain Res.* 2000;122:81–103.

126. Menke A, Klengel T, Rubel J, et al. Genetic variation in FKBP5 associated with the extent of stress hormone dysregulation in major depression. *Genes Brain Behav.* 2013; 12(3):289–296.

127. Zhang TY, Labonte B, Wen XL, Turecki G, Meaney MJ. Epigenetic mechanisms for the early environmental regulation of hippocampal glucocorticoid receptor gene expression in rodents and humans. *Neuropsychopharmacology.* 2013;38(1):111–123.

128. Weaver IC, Cervoni N, Champagne FA, et al. Epigenetic programming by maternal behavior. *Nat Neurosci.* 2004;7(8):847–854.

129. Danese A, Moffitt TE, Pariante CM, Ambler A, Poulton R, Caspi A. Elevated inflammation levels in depressed adults with a history of childhood maltreatment. *Arch Gen Psychiatry.* 2008;65(4):409–415.

130. Oberlander TF, Weinberg J, Papsdorf M, Grunau R, Misri S, Devlin AM. Prenatal exposure to maternal depression, neonatal methylation of human glucocorticoid receptor gene (NR3C1) and infant cortisol stress responses. *Epigenetics.* 2008;3(2):97–106.

131. Perroud N, Paoloni-Giacobino A, Prada P, et al. Increased methylation of glucocorticoid receptor gene (NR3C1) in adults with a history of childhood maltreatment: a link with the severity and type of trauma. *Translat Psychiatry.* 2011;1:e59.

132. Klengel T, Mehta D, Anacker C, et al. Allele-specific FKBP5 DNA demethylation mediates gene-childhood trauma interactions. *Nat Neurosci.* 2013;16(1):33–41.

133. Brady LS, Whitfield HJ Jr, Fox RJ, Gold PW, Herkenham M. Long-term antidepressant administration alters corticotropin-releasing hormone, tyrosine hydroxylase, and mineralocorticoid receptor gene expression in rat brain: therapeutic implications. *J Clin Invest.* 1991;87(3):831–837.

134. Reul JM, Stec I, Soder M, Holsboer F. Chronic treatment of rats with the antidepressant amitriptyline attenuates the activity of the hypothalamic-pituitary-adrenocortical system. *Endocrinology.* 1993;133(1):312–320.

135. Reul JM, Labeur MS, Grigoriadis DE, De Souza EB, Holsboer F. Hypothalamic-pituitary-adrenocortical axis changes in the rat after long-term treatment with the reversible monoamine oxidase-A inhibitor moclobemide. *Neuroendocrinology.* 1994;60(5):509–519.

136. Holsboer F. The rationale for corticotropin-releasing hormone receptor (CRH-R) antagonists to treat depression and anxiety. *J Psychiatr Res.* 1999;33(3):181–214.

137. Pariante CM, Pearce BD, Pisell TL, Owens MJ, Miller AH. Steroid-independent translocation of the glucocorticoid receptor by the antidepressant desipramine. *Mol Pharmacol.* 1997;52(4):571–581.

138. Pariante CM. The role of multi-drug resistance p-glycoprotein in glucocorticoid function: studies in animals and relevance in humans. *Eur J Pharmacol.* 2008;583(2–3): 263–271.

139. Pariante CM, Papadopoulos AS, Poon L, et al. Four days of citalopram increase suppression of cortisol secretion by prednisolone in healthy volunteers. *Psychopharmacology (Berl).* 2004;177(1–2):200–206.

140. Pariante CM, Alhaj HA, Arulnathan VE, et al. Central glucocorticoid receptor-mediated effects of the antidepressant, citalopram, in humans: a study using EEG and cognitive testing. *Psychoneuroendocrinology.* 2012;37(5):618–628.

141. DeBattista C, Posener JA, Kalehzan BM, Schatzberg AF. Acute antidepressant effects of intravenous hydrocortisone and CRH in depressed patients: a double-blind, placebo-controlled study. *Am J Psychiatry.* 2000;157(8):1334–1337.

142. Arana GW, Santos AB, Laraia MT, et al. Dexamethasone for the treatment of depression: a randomized, placebo-controlled, double-blind trial. *Am J Psychiatry.* 1995;152(2):265–267.

143. Delahanty DL, Raimonde AJ, Spoonster E. Initial posttraumatic urinary cortisol levels predict subsequent PTSD symptoms in motor vehicle accident victims. *Biol Psychiatry.* 2000;48(9):940–947.

144. McFarlane AC, Atchison M, Yehuda R. The acute stress response following motor vehicle accidents and its relation to PTSD. *Ann N Y Acad Sci.* 1997;821:437–441.

145. Steudte S, Kirschbaum C, Gao W, et al. Hair cortisol as a biomarker of traumatization in healthy individuals and posttraumatic stress disorder patients. *Biol Psychiatry.* 2013;74(9):639–646.

146. Bicanic IA, Postma RM, Sinnema G, et al. Salivary cortisol and dehydroepiandrosterone sulfate in adolescent rape victims with post traumatic stress disorder. *Psychoneuroendocrinology.* 2013;38(3):408–415.

147. Rohleder N, Joksimovic L, Wolf JM, Kirschbaum C. Hypocortisolism and increased glucocorticoid sensitivity of pro-Inflammatory cytokine production in Bosnian war refugees with posttraumatic stress disorder. *Biol Psychiatry.* 2004;55(7):745–751.

148. Het S, Wolf OT. Mood changes in response to psychosocial stress in healthy young women: effects of pretreatment with cortisol. *Behav Neurosci.* 2007;121(1):11–20.

149. Het S, Schoofs D, Rohleder N, Wolf OT. Stress-induced cortisol level elevations are associated with reduced negative affect after stress: indications for a mood-buffering cortisol effect. *Psychosom Med.* 2012;74(1):23–32.

150. Schelling G, Stoll C, Kapfhammer HP, et al. The effect of stress doses of hydrocortisone during septic shock on posttraumatic stress disorder and health-related quality of life in survivors. *Crit Care Med.* 1999;27(12):2678–2683.

151. Schelling G, Kilger E, Roozendaal B, et al. Stress doses of hydrocortisone, traumatic memories, and symptoms of posttraumatic stress disorder in patients after cardiac surgery: a randomized study. *Biol Psychiatry.* 2004;55(6):627–633.

152. Zohar J, Yahalom H, Kozlovsky N, et al. High dose hydrocortisone immediately after trauma may alter the trajectory of PTSD: interplay between clinical and animal studies. *Eur Neuropsychopharmacol.* 2011;21(11):796–809.

153. Delahanty DL, Gabert-Quillen C, Ostrowski SA, et al. The efficacy of initial hydrocortisone administration at preventing posttraumatic distress in adult trauma patients: a randomized trial. *CNS Spectr.* 2013;18(2):103–111.

154. Aerni A, Traber R, Hock C, et al. Low-dose cortisol for symptoms of posttraumatic stress disorder. *Am J Psychiatry.* 2004;161(8):1488–1490.

155. Miller MW, McKinney AE, Kanter FS, Korte KJ, Lovallo WR. Hydrocortisone suppression of the fear-potentiated startle response and posttraumatic stress disorder. *Psychoneuroendocrinology.* 2011;36(7):970–980.

156. Suris A, North C, Adinoff B, Powell CM, Greene R. Effects of exogenous glucocorticoid on combat-related PTSD symptoms. *Ann Clin Psychiatry.* 2010;22(4):274–279.

157. Jahn H, Schick M, Kiefer F, Kellner M, Yassouridis A, Wiedemann K. Metyrapone as additive treatment in major depression: a double-blind and placebo-controlled trial. *Arch Gen Psychiatry.* 2004;61(12):1235–1244.

158. Blasey CM, Block TS, Belanoff JK, Roe RL. Efficacy and safety of mifepristone for the treatment of psychotic depression. *J Clin Psychopharmacol.* 2011;31(4):436–440.

159. Jeanneteau F, Garabedian MJ, Chao MV. Activation of Trk neurotrophin receptors by glucocorticoids provides a neuroprotective effect. *Proc Natl Acad Sci U S A.* 2008; 105(12):4862–4867.

160. Sudheimer KD, Abelson JL, Taylor SF, et al. Exogenous glucocorticoids decrease sub-genual cingulate activity evoked by sadness. *Neuropsychopharmacology.* 2013;38(5): 826–845.

161. Drevets WC, Price JL, Simpson JR Jr, et al. Subgenual prefrontal cortex abnormalities in mood disorders. *Nature.* 1997;386(6627):824–827.

162. Harrison NA, Brydon L, Walker C, Gray MA, Steptoe A, Critchley HD. Inflammation causes mood changes through alterations in subgenual cingulate activity and meso-limbic connectivity. *Biol Psychiatry.* 2009;66(5):407–414.

163. Dorn LD, Burgess ES, Dubbert B, et al. Psychopathology in patients with endogenous Cushing's syndrome: "atypical" or melancholic features. *Clin Endocrinol (Oxf).* 1995; 43(4):433–442.

164. Then Bergh F, Kumpfel T, Grasser A, Rupprecht R, Holsboer F, Trenkwalder C. Combined treatment with corticosteroids and moclobemide favors normalization of hypothalamo-pituitary-adrenal axis dysregulation in relapsing-remitting multiple sclerosis: a randomized, double blind trial. *J Clin Endocrinol Metab.* 2001;86(4): 1610–1615.

165. Lechin F, van der Dijs B, Orozco B, et al. Plasma neurotransmitters, blood pressure, and heart rate during supine-resting, orthostasis, and moderate exercise conditions in major depressed patients. *Biol Psychiatry.* 1995;38(3):166–173.

166. Roy A, Pickar D, Linnoila M, Potter WZ. Plasma norepinephrine level in affective disorders. Relationship to melancholia. *Arch Gen Psychiatry.* 1985;42(12):1181–1185.

167. Esler M, Turbott J, Schwarz R, et al. The peripheral kinetics of norepinephrine in depressive illness. *Arch Gen Psychiatry.* 1982;39(3):295–300.

168. Veith RC, Lewis N, Linares OA, et al. Sympathetic nervous system activity in major depression: basal and desipramine-induced alterations in plasma norepinephrine kinetics. *Arch Gen Psychiatry.* 1994;51(5):411–422.

169. Schildkraut JJ. The catecholamine hypothesis of affective disorders: a review of supporting evidence. *Am J Psychiatry.* 1965;122(5):509–522.

170. Linnoila M, Karoum F, Calil HM, Kopin IJ, Potter WZ. Alteration of norepinephrine metabolism with desipramine and zimelidine in depressed patients. *Arch Gen Psychiatry.* 1982;39(9):1025–1028.

171. Barton DA, Dawood T, Lambert EA, et al. Sympathetic activity in major depressive disorder: identifying those at increased cardiac risk? *J Hypertens.* 2007;25(10): 2117–2124.

172. Powell ND, Sloan EK, Bailey MT, et al. Social stress up-regulates inflammatory gene expression in the leukocyte transcriptome via beta-adrenergic induction of myelopoi-esis. *Proc Natl Acad Sci U S A.* 2013;110(41):16574–16579.

173. Boettger MK, Greiner W, Rachow T, Bruhl C, Bar KJ. Sympathetic skin response fol-

lowing painful electrical stimulation is increased in major depression. *Pain.* 2010; 149(1):130–134.

174. Koschke M, Boettger MK, Schulz S, et al. Autonomy of autonomic dysfunction in major depression. *Psychosom Med.* 2009;71(8):852–860.

175. Cyranowski JM, Hofkens TL, Swartz HA, Salomon K, Gianaros PJ. Cardiac vagal control in nonmedicated depressed women and nondepressed controls: impact of depression status, lifetime trauma history, and respiratory factors. *Psychosom Med.* 2011; 73(4):336–343.

176. Licht CM, de Geus EJ, Zitman FG, Hoogendijk WJ, van Dyck R, Penninx BW. Association between major depressive disorder and heart rate variability in the Netherlands Study of Depression and Anxiety (NESDA). *Arch Gen Psychiatry.* 2008;65(12):1358–1367.

177. Kemp AH, Quintana DS, Gray MA, Felmingham KL, Brown K, Gatt JM. Impact of depression and antidepressant treatment on heart rate variability: a review and meta-analysis. *Biol Psychiatry.* 2010;67(11):1067–1074.

CHAPTER 6

The Immune System
Relationships with the Stress System and Major Depression

We often lecture to psychiatrists and other mental health professionals about the role of the immune system in psychiatric disease. Just to warm the audience up we often ask for a show of hands for how many people received in-depth training in the immune system as part of their training to be a mental health professional. The typical response rate—even in rooms with several hundred audience members—is zero. Although we do this exercise for fun, it belies a remarkable truth, which is that even a decade ago most clinicians and scientists did not use the words "immune" and "brain" very often in the same sentence, and so no one in mental health got any training in the complexities of immune function. How times have changed. It is increasingly clear that the immune system and the brain really form one larger super-organ with so many bi-directional interconnections that it makes less and less sense to think of them as operating in separate domains. This chapter provides an overview of this new way of seeing immune system and brain functioning in relation to depression. But first, we turn briefly to a lingering question from the last chapter, showing how the immune system provides an intriguing answer.

Why Does Depression Have the HPA and Autonomic Changes It Does?

Consider a prototypical depressed person, based on our discussion thus far. Compared with average values for her age, our depressed patient shows increased cortisol production, and release, a flattening of the diurnal cortisol rhythm and a reduction in glucocorticoid sensitivity. She also has various findings suggesting an autonomic balance skewed toward sympathetic overdrive and parasympathetic nervous system (PNS) withdrawal. Why do so many depressed individuals share this constellation of physiological findings? Most of us involved in clinical work would probably answer with a tautology: depressed people have these findings because depression is an illness characterized by these findings. Or, if we were bolder, we might suggest that these changes produce depression, case closed.

This type of answer works very well for diseases that result from age-related failures of bodily organs or processes or for very rare genetic conditions, but as we discuss at length in Chapter 9, this type of circular reasoning fails spectacularly for conditions that have strong genetic and/or environmental antecedents and that are very common, as is the case with major depressive disorder (MDD). The reason for this is straightforward: evolutionary logic dictates that alleles that promote a nonadaptive condition in response to common environmental circumstances (e.g., stress or sickness) should be (and are) culled over time from the genome by natural selection. Conversely, if an apparently nonadaptive condition like depression is at least partly genetic and also very common, the genes that promote the condition, and/or the condition itself, must confer survival/reproductive benefits that offset the costs of the disorder. Given this, might it be that hypothalamic-pituitary-adrenal (HPA) axis and autonomic changes common in MDD have conferred survival benefits over mammalian evolution? And if so, where might these advantages lie? We ask these questions as an introduction to our discussion of immune system changes that have been reported in MDD, because, as it turns out, HPA and autonomic changes common in depression share a proclivity to increase activity in the body's inflammatory response.

INFLAMMATORY EFFECTS OF STRESS SYSTEM CHANGES SEEN IN MDD

Through their inhibitory effects on the proinflammatory transcription factor nuclear factor kappa-beta (NFκB) and other signaling pathways, glucocorticoids potently antagonize inflammatory activity. Given this, one would predict that the reduced sensitivity to cortisol observed in both the HPA axis and the immune system associated with depression would also promote increased inflammation in the disorder. And indeed, some data indicate that glucocorticoid insufficiency—as assessed by either in vivo tests such as the dexamethasone suppression test or in vitro tests such as dexamethasone suppression of inflammatory cytokine stimulation—predicts increased inflammation in depressed individuals or in those with posttraumatic stress symptoms (which have large overlap with depressive symptoms) in adults with histories of early-life adversity.[1,2]

Whereas the impact of glucocorticoid insufficiency on inflammation appears to be longer lasting and tonic in nature, many lines of evidence indicate that autonomic nervous system (ANS) changes play a more primary role in the increases in inflammation that can be seen in humans and animals in response to acute stress. However, one challenge in better understanding these findings results from the fact that the easiest ANS indices to measure (heart rate, blood pressure, heart rate variability [HRV]) do not easily allow one to disentangle sympathetic nervous system (SNS) activation from PNS withdrawal. For example, reduced high-frequency and low-frequency HRV has been repeatedly associated with increased concentrations of circulating inflammatory biomarkers, usually inter-leukin-6 (IL-6) or C-reactive protein (CRP).[3,4] For example, although we never published these findings, we have observed a strong association between amount of decline in low- and high-frequency HRV at the beginning of a laboratory stress test involving public speaking and mental arithmetic and subsequent stress-induced increases in blood levels of IL-6. While most scientists agree that high-frequency HRV reflects vagal input to the heart, low-frequency HRV, which showed a stronger association with inflammation in our study and many others, is more contested, with some lines of evidence suggesting it reflects mostly SNS activity and others indicating that it also reflects vagal (or PNS) activity.

Although many studies are saddled with these types of physiological measures that do not easily demonstrate how much of the association between ANS activity and inflammation is due to which arm of the system, significant work suggests that, in general, SNS activation increases inflammatory activity in the brain and body, whereas PNS activation dampens it. For example, catecholamines (i.e., norepinephrine and epinephrine) acting through alpha- and beta-adrenergic receptors have been shown to increase cytokine expression in both the brain and the periphery of rats,[5] and alpha-adrenergic antagonists were noted to block the increased peripheral blood concentrations of IL-6 induced by altitude stress in humans.[6] In addition, alpha- and beta-adrenergic agonists have been shown to directly activate NFκB in vitro,[7] which then leads to activation of the entire inflammatory response.

On the other hand, PNS activation dampens inflammation. This was first shown by Kevin Tracey's group with the striking demonstration that stimulation of efferent PNS fibers, including the motor vagus, reduced mortality secondary to endotoxin administration in laboratory rats while also reducing the endotoxin-induced activation of NFκB, as well as the proinflammatory cytokine tumor necrosis factor-alpha (TNF).[8] These inhibitory effects on the inflammatory response are mediated by the vagal release of acetylcholine, which in turn activates the alpha-7 subunit of the nicotinic acetylcholine receptor, which can regulate both cytokine transcription and translation (often referred to as the cholinergic anti-inflammatory pathway).[8] In addition, there appears to be a cellular component to this inhibitory cholinergic reflex. Indeed, adoptive transfer of T effector cells from vagotomized mice was shown to aggravate colitis in association with increased inflammatory scores and reduced anti-inflammatory regulatory T cells.[9]

WHY STRESSED MICE LOOK LIKE DEPRESSED HUMANS

Because many initial studies examined immune indices that seemed to be reduced in response to acute and chronic stress, it came as something of a surprise in the 1990s when these same stressors were shown to reliably activate other aspects of immunity, both innate and acquired. What could be the adaptive value of adversities routinely and universally turning down immune defenses in response to exactly the kinds of risks that would be likely to lead to wounding and hence a markedly increased risk of infection and, by this route, to reduced reproductive success? We now know from literally hundreds of studies that both acute and chronic stressors increase inflammatory activity, and that multiple classes of acute stressors in animals actually enhance host defense against pathogens. On the other hand, it is also clear that stress, especially when chronic, impairs other types of immunity, especially adaptive immunity mediated by T cells. In fact, inflammation itself, while essential for the initial phases of host defense, can itself reduce T cell function in ways that increase an organism's risk for failing to adequately cope with certain types of infection. In Chapter 9 we offer a novel theory to account for why depression should be associated with the types of immune changes commonly observed, and why these changes are similar to those seen when animals are exposed to psychosocial stress. In this chapter, we delve more deeply into the evidence that immune processes in general, and inflammatory activity in particular, are important for the development, maintenance and treatment of MDD.

Evidence Linking Inflammation with Depression

PEOPLE WITH DEPRESSION HAVE INCREASES IN INFLAMMATORY BIOMARKERS

The fact that depression is associated with increased inflammation was initially met with surprise and more than a little skepticism,[10] because this discovery occurred in the context of a preexisting literature on the immune system in depression that was dominated by reports of decreased cellular (lymphocyte) responses and reduced natural killer cell activity.[11] Although we now know that these types of T cell changes can be induced by inflammation, and especially the via cytokine effects on T cell receptors,[12,13] this was not known when the first reports of immune activation in MDD appeared.

However, since these first reports, published in the 1990s, a vast literature has reproduced these findings, and meta-analyses confirm that peripheral blood elevations in the cytokines IL-6, TNF, and acute-phase reactant CRP are reliably associated with depression, whether depression is measured by the diagnostic criteria of MDD or as severity of depressive symptoms.[14–16] Increases in peripheral blood chemokines and cellular adhesion molecules, as well as increased stress-induced NFκB, an important signaling molecule in the inflammatory response, have also been reported in patients with MDD.[17] Further strengthening the association of depression and increased inflammation is the fact that many studies have also found significant associations between blood concentrations of inflammatory factors and the severity of depressive symptoms.[18–21]

Although some studies find that individuals with a history of MDD show elevations in inflammatory biomarkers even when clinically improved, most of the data suggest that levels of inflammation are significantly higher when patients are symptomatic. Thus, inflammation seems to be primarily a state-dependent phenomenon in MDD, especially given evidence that inflammatory markers in depressed patients return to control levels following successful antidepressant treatment.[22] These findings suggest that failure to respond to antidepressant treatment should be associated with ongoing elevations in inflammatory biomarkers, and indeed several studies support this.[23,24] Moreover, a corollary prediction would be that elevations in inflammation prior to treatment might predict poor response. And indeed, patients with increased inflammatory markers at baseline have been repeatedly reported to be less likely to show a response to a variety of treatments, both pharmacological and behavioral, suggesting a relationship between inflammation and treatment resistance.[23–26] Finally, although the association of depression and inflammation seems to be primarily a state-dependent as opposed to a trait-dependent phenomenon, most known risk factors for MDD (see Table 3.1), including chronic personality styles, are also associated with increased inflammation, suggesting that in addition to being a correlate of depression, inflammation may cause the disorder.

INFLAMMATORY STIMULI CAUSE DEPRESSION

If inflammation plays a causative role in depression, as opposed to being merely a side effect of other biological changes that more directly cause the condition, one would expect that exposure to inflammatory cytokines should induce the disorder. In fact, as discussed in Chapter 3, data incontrovertibly demonstrate that this is the case. Acute exposure to inflammatory stimuli, such as endotoxin and typhoid vaccination, in humans produces a host of behavioral changes associated with MDD, including sadness, fatigue, cognitive dysfunction, and feelings of social isolation.[27–30] The depressogenic proclivity of inflammation is even more striking when the source of immune stimulation is chronic. For example, long-term treatment with the inflammatory cytokine interferon-alpha (IFNα) induces clinically relevant depressive symptoms in most individuals undergoing therapy, with as many as 30–50 percent of treated individuals meeting symptom criteria for MDD.[31] Moreover, a comparison of symptoms in patients with IFNα-induced depression versus medically healthy depressed patients revealed a large degree of overlap in both symptom expression and severity.[32] Further supporting the similarity between the depression associated with IFNα and depression in other populations is the fact that IFNα-induced depression can be prevented and/or treated by conventional antidepressants.[33–36]

Mechanisms by Which Inflammation Causes Depression

The color plate section is schematic for many of the mechanisms by which cytokines are known to impact central nervous system (CNS) and neuroendocrine function in ways relevant to the pathophysiology of MDD. Of the mechanisms by which cytokines promote depression, probably best studied are their effects on neurotransmitter metabolism. Numerous human and laboratory animal studies have shown that multiple neurotransmitter systems are affected by acute and chronic administration of cytokines including dopamine, serotonin, and glutamate.[22]

CYTOKINE EFFECTS ON DOPAMINE AND SEROTONIN

Cytokines significantly impact dopamine signaling in the brain and, in fact, appear to have a tropism for the basal ganglia, one of the primary sites of dopaminergic activity in the CNS. Studies in humans have repeatedly observed altered blood flow and metabolic activity in basal ganglia nuclei during exposure to inflammatory stimuli.[28,37,38] In rhesus macaques, reduced cerebrospinal fluid (CSF) concentrations of the dopamine metabolite homovanillic acid have been associated with depressive-like huddling behavior secondary to chronic IFNα administration.[39] That such huddling behavior reflects, at least in part, an effect of cytokines on CNS monoamine signaling is supported by the fact that similar huddling behavior is observed following chronic administration of the monoamine-depleting drug reserpine.[40] Inflammatory cytokines target the basal ganglia and dopamine pathways in rodents, suggesting that this effect is phylogenetically ancient.[41] Moreover, in rodents chronic administration of high-dose endotoxin into the brain was associated with a 70 percent reduction of nigral dopaminergic neurons within 10 weeks.[42]

The repeatedly observed fact that serotonin reuptake inhibitors prevent and/or treat depressive symptoms during chronic exposure to IFNα provides strong evidence that serotonin pathways are involved in cytokine effects on behavior.[33,34] Genetic studies have complemented this work by suggesting that polymorphisms in the promoter region of the serotonin transporter gene 5-HTTLPR that increase the risk of developing depression in response to stress may be associated with IFNα-induced depressive symptoms.[43,44] Additional evidence supporting a role for serotonin metabolism in cytokine-induced depression comes from one of our studies showing that IFNα-associated increases in CSF concentrations of IL-6 are inversely correlated with the serotonin metabolite 5-hydroxyindoleacetic acid, which in turn negatively correlate with IFNα-induced depression severity.[45]

MECHANISMS BY WHICH CYTOKINES AFFECT MONOAMINE METABOLISM

The enzyme indoleamine 2,3-dioxygenase (IDO) is activated by a various cytokines alone or in combination.[46,47] IDO catabolizes tryptophan, the primary amino acid precursor of serotonin, into kynurenine. Depletion of tryptophan provides protection against a variety of pathogens (because they also need tryptophan) but also inhibits effector T cell responses and thereby contributes to immune tolerance.[48] Evidence of a role of IDO in cytokine-induced depression comes from a number of studies that have demonstrated associations between IFNα-induced depression and decreases in tryptophan and increases in kynurenine and/or the kynurenine:tryptophan ratio.[49,50] Although much of the attention regarding IDO was initially focused on the depletion of tryptophan, and in turn serotonin, multiple lines of evidence have increasingly pointed to the relevance of increased production of kynurenine and its metabolites for immune-induced depression.[51–53] For example, we showed that chronic treatment with IFNα profoundly increased levels of kynurenine and its metabolites quinolinic and kynurenic acid in CSF while having no impact on CSF levels of tryptophan. Moreover, levels of all three kynurenine pathway products correlated with severity of IFNα-induced depressive symptoms, while levels of tryptophan were not associated with depression.[53]

Cytokines can also influence monoamine metabolism via activation of the p38 mitogen-activated protein kinase (MAPK). Both in vitro and in vivo data demonstrate that stimulation of the p38 MAPK pathway increases the expression and function of the serotonin transporter, which in animal studies has been shown to increase depressive-like behavior in response to inflammatory stimuli.[54] In humans, increased phosphorylation of p38 MAPK following the first injection of IFNα was associated with the subsequent development of IFNα-induced depression and fatigue.[55] In addition to effects on serotonin metabolism, MAPK pathways have also been found to influence the dopamine transporter.[56]

Finally, proinflammatory cytokines promote the generation of reactive oxygen and nitrogen species that degrade tetrahydrobiopterin (BH4), a key enzyme cofactor required for the synthesis of all monoamine neurotransmitters, which is highly sensitive to oxidation.[57] While only limited data support a reduction of BH4 in MDD,[58] our group found evidence that decreased BH4 availability may be especially relevant for the link between depression and inflammation. We have shown in patients undergoing IFNα treatment that CSF concentrations of IL-6 are associated with reduced CSF concentrations of BH4.[59] Moreover, the ratio of plasma phenylalanine to tyrosine (an indirect measure of BH4 activity) was shown to correlate with CSF concentrations of dopamine, as well as symptoms of depression, in IFNα-treated patients.[59]

CYTOKINE EFFECTS ON GLUTAMATE METABOLISM

In addition to affecting monoamine neurotransmitters, inflammatory cytokines are known to profoundly impact glutamatergic functioning in the CNS. For example, cytokines have been shown to decrease the expression of glutamate transporters on glial cells and to increase the release of glutamate from astrocytes.[60–64] This astrocyte-derived glutamate preferentially binds to extrasynaptic N-methyl-D-aspartate (NMDA) receptors, which can mediate excitotoxicity and lead to decreased production of trophic factors, including brain-derived neurotrophic factor (BDNF).[65,66] Moreover, inflammation-induced quinolinic acid can augment glutamatergic excitotoxicity through direct activation of the NMDA receptor while also contributing to oxidative stress that can further damage oligodendrocytes, which are responsible for white matter production and are especially vulnerable to oxidative damage and overactivation of calcium-permeable glutamate receptors.[64,67] Interestingly, loss of glial elements such as oligodendrocytes in multiple mood relevant brain regions, including the subgenual anterior cingulate cortex and amygdala, has emerged as a fundamental morphological abnormality in Major Depression.[68]

CYTOKINE EFFECTS ON NEUROGENESIS AND NEUROTROPHIC FACTORS

Many lines of evidence testify to the importance of impaired neurogenesis in the development of depression and the activity of antidepressant medications.[69] When released in the CNS, cytokines suppress neurogenesis. The relevance of this for stress-related conditions such as MDD is highlighted by findings that stress-induced decreases in neurogenesis (as well as the expression of relevant nerve growth factors, including BDNF, that support neurogenesis) can be reversed by administration of the IL-1 receptor antagonist, transplantation of neural precursor cells that secrete IL-1 receptor antagonist into the hippocampus, or the use of IL-1 receptor knockout mice.[70–72] In vitro studies indicate that the inhibitory effect of IL-1 on neurogenesis is mediated by activation of NFκB.[72] In humans, treatment with IFNα has been associated with reduced levels of peripheral BDNF, which are known to correlate well with BDNF availability in the CNS.[73] In turn, reduced BDNF during IFNα treatment has been associated with increased depression.[73]

CYTOKINE EFFECTS ON NEUROENDOCRINE FUNCTION

As we've highlighted at some length, alterations in the HPA axis are among the most reproducible findings in patients with Major Depression. As a group, patients with Major Depression exhibit increased concentrations of the HPA axis hormones adrenocorticotropic hormone (ACTH) and cortisol, as well as increases in CSF measures of the HPA axis regulatory neuropeptide corticotropin-releasing hormone (CRH).[74,75] Depression is also associated with glucocorticoid resistance and with flattening of the diurnal cortisol rhythm. One of the strong arguments for a role for inflammation in the pathogenesis of depression is the fact that inflammatory processes are capable of producing all these HPA axis changes.

Administration of inflammatory cytokines to laboratory animals and to humans has been shown to profoundly stimulate not only ACTH and cortisol but also the expression and release of CRH.[76] For example, in humans the acute ACTH and cortisol response to the first injection of IFNα (presumably due to activation of CRH pathways) is large and correlates with the subsequent development of depressive symptoms two months later during IFNα therapy.[77] In contrast to acute IFNα, chronic IFNα administration is associated with flattening of the diurnal cortisol curve and with increased evening cortisol concentrations, both of which correlate with the development of depression and fatigue during treatment.[78] Flattening of the diurnal cortisol rhythm is common in a number of medical conditions associated with inflammation, including cardiovascular disease and cancer, and when present is associated with a worse outcome.[78] For example, patients with metastatic breast cancer with a flattened cortisol slope were noted to have decreased natural killer cell number and activity and to die sooner than similar patients with a steeper cortisol slopes.[79]

Studies in depressed patients have shown that flattening of the cortisol rhythm is associated with nonsuppression of cortisol by dexamethasone in the dexamethasone suppression test.[80] Inflammatory cytokines appear capable of producing the same pattern of findings. In patients receiving IFNα, we found that reductions in HPA axis sensitivity to cortisol-driven inhibitory feedback correlated strongly with flattening of the diurnal slope during treatment, again highlighting the capability of cytokines to induce linked changes in HPA axis activity that are common in MDD.[81] A final piece of evidence demonstrating a link between inflammation and insufficient glucocorticoid signaling comes from a human study that reported increased TNF associated with glucocorticoid resistance in the skin as measured by reduced cutaneous blanching in response to topically applied glucocorticoids.[24]

As we've discussed, it is generally believed that glucocorticoid resistance results primarily from decreased expression and/or function of the receptor for glucocorticoids. Of relevance in this regard, many studies demonstrate that inflammatory cytokines can disrupt glucocorticoid receptor (GR) function while decreasing GR expression.[82] For example, by activating the intracellular STAT5 (signal transducer and activator of transcription 5) pathway, which in turns binds to the activated GR in the nucleus, disrupting GR-DNA binding, IFNα inhibits GR functioning.[83] A similar protein–protein interaction between the GR and NFκB in the nucleus has also been described and represents another pathway by which inflammation impairs GR function.[84] IL-1α and IL-1β have been shown both in vitro and in vivo to inhibit GR translocation from the cytoplasm to the nucleus through activation of the p38 MAPK pathway.[85–87] Finally, chronic exposure to inflammatory cytokines has been shown to increase the expression the beta-isoform of the GR, which has a distinct hormone-binding domain (which is unable to bind known glucocorticoids) and a unique pattern of gene regulation.[82,88] Of note, expression of the beta-isoform is increased in patients with inflammatory disorders, bronchial asthma and rheumatoid arthritis (RA).[88] Given the potent anti-inflammatory effects of glucocorticoids, it is not surprising that glucocorticoid resistance secondary to stress in mice is associated with increased lethality in response to endotoxin administration.[89] Thus, the effects of cytokines on GR function may lead to a feed-forward cascade whereby increased inflamma-tion through its effects of the GR undercuts the well-known ability of glucocor-ticoids to restrain inflammatory responses,[90] leading to further increases in inflammation and reduced GR function.

IMPACT OF CYTOKINES ON NEURAL CIRCUITRY

In concert with other lines of evidence implicating inflammatory processes in the pathogenesis of MDD, an increasing number of neuroimaging studies are provid-ing a remarkably consistent body of data showing that both acute and chronic exposure to inflammatory stimuli impact both the structure and function of brain areas of direct relevance to depression, including the anterior cingulate cortex and basal ganglia.

Anterior Cingulate Cortex

Various regions of the cingulate cortex are especially sensitive to cytokine expo-sure. In particular, several studies identify the dorsal anterior cingulate cortex (dACC), which plays an important role in error detection and conflict monitor-ing,[91] as a primary CNS target for peripheral cytokine signaling. For example, chronic exposure to IFNα in patients with hepatitis C specifically activates the dACC (Brodmann area 24), based on a study that used functional MRI and a task of visuospatial attention.[92] A strong correlation was found in this study between activation of the dACC in IFNα-treated patients and the number of errors made during the task. The error rate was quite low for the task, and no such correlation was found in control subjects. This pattern of dACC activation in response to triv-ial errors is also seen in individuals with high state anxiety.[93] In addition, increased activation of the dACC has been observed in subjects with neuroticism and obses-sive compulsive disorder, both of which are associated with increases in anxiety as well as arousal.[94,95] Findings similar to these with IFNα (i.e., increased dACC activation) have also been observed in response to a high-demand color–word Stroop task in patients administered typhoid vaccination.[29]

Moreover, increased activation of the dACC in response to a social rejection task was correlated with increased activation of peripheral blood IL-6 in response to a psychosocial stress test, suggesting a role for stress-induced inflammation in an individual's sensitivity to social stress.[96] Indeed, functional MRI studies uti-lizing this social rejection task suggest that the cingulate cortex in general, and the dACC in particular, plays a role not only in error detection and conflict mon-itoring but also in the processing of social pain.[97] Given the connection of the dACC with downstream autonomic nervous system arousal pathways, it is fur-ther hypothesized that the dACC may serve as a "neural alarm system" that can both detect and respond (with arousal and distress) to threatening environmental stimuli in the social domain.[97] Thus, cytokines may sensitize the responsivity of the dACC, thereby contributing to the anxiety, arousal, and alarm that often accompany chronic exposure to inflammatory stimuli such as IFNα. Finally, different areas of the cingulate cortex may be differentially impacted by inflammation, depending on the nature of the task employed. Just as inflammation increases dACC activity in response to error detection tasks that are more cognitive in nature, an inflammatory stimulus (typhoid vaccination) has been associated with activation of the subgenual ACC, an area central to emotional processing that is also the target of deep brain stimulation strategies in patients with treatment resistant depression.[98]

Basal Ganglia

Using positron emission tomography, early studies in patients undergoing IFNα therapy for cancer or hepatitis C revealed marked increases in glucose metabolic activity in the basal ganglia, which correlated with symptoms of fatigue.[37,38] These increases are consistent with metabolic changes in the basal ganglia seen in patients with Parkinson's disease and are believed to reflect increased oscillatory burst activity in relevant basal ganglia nuclei as a result of dopamine depletion. Consistent with this notion, increased metabolic activity in the basal ganglia of Parkinson's disease patients can be reversed by the administration of levodopa.[99] Using functional MRI, typhoid vaccination was also found to alter activation in the basal ganglia. In particular, vaccinated volunteers (compared with a control condition) exhibited increased evoked activity in the substantia nigra that was associated with both prolonged reaction times and increased peripheral blood concentrations of IL-6.[28] Finally, administration of endotoxin to healthy volunteers led to reduced activation in the ventral striatum during a monetary reward task.[100]

A study strongly suggests that these associations between inflammation and striatal function are not limited to individuals undergoing exogenous cytokine stimulation. In medically healthy individuals with MDD, increased CRP was associated with decreased connectivity between ventral striatum and ventromedial prefrontal cortex, which in turn correlated with increased anhedonia.[101] Increased CRP also predicted decreased connectivity of the dorsal striatal to the ventromedial prefrontal cortex and presupplementary motor area, which correlated with decreased motor speed and increased psychomotor slowing. Finally, decreased connectivity between striatum and ventromedial prefrontal cortex was associated with increased plasma IL-6, IL-1β, and IL-1 receptor antagonist.

As we discuss at some length in Chapter 9, cytokine-induced changes in brain function may serve evolved adaptive purposes. Thus, cytokine-driven increases in dACC activity (and the resultant heightened sensitivity to social threat) may subserve the survival priority of vigilance against attack in an animal that is otherwise vulnerable due to infection and/or wounding.[102] Taken together with the effects of inflammation on the basal ganglia, the effects of inflammation on neural circuitry in the brain appear to subserve two competing evolutionary survival priorities: to "lay low" to conserve energy resources for fighting infection and wound healing and to be vigilant for protection against future attack.[102]

Is Depression an Inflammatory Condition?

As a thought experiment, suppose you are a rheumatologist seeing a middle-aged patient who complains of a painful right knee. To help diagnose the condition, you aspirate synovial fluid from the offending knee and submit it for analysis. Suspecting RA, you are surprised when the results come back completely normal in terms of inflammatory markers in the synovial fluid. Had inflammatory measures been high, that would not have confirmed RA because other autoimmune and infectious causes for arthritis are also characterized by increased synovial inflammation. However, knowing that concentrations of an inflammatory cytokine such as IL-6 are typically 1,000 times higher in the synovial fluid of an affected RA joint than in the blood of a healthy adult, what would be your conclusion regarding the likelihood of RA in this patient? Most likely it would be no joint inflammation, no RA. That is more or less what we mean when we say that RA is an inflammatory disorder.

Now compare this with an analogous clinical situation, but this time you are a psychiatrist seeing a middle-aged patient complaining of severe depression. Hearing that MDD is an inflammatory condition, you measure plasma concentrations of inflammatory cytokines and the acute-phase reactant CRP. Believing MDD to be a brain disease, you also go beyond the call of duty and perform a lumbar puncture in your office to measure CSF concentrations of the same inflammatory markers. A few days later the patient returns, and you hold the laboratory results in your hands. There is no evidence of increased inflammation in the CNS or periphery. The patient is weeping and says he can think of nothing but killing himself. Would you decide that, because the patient's inflammatory measures are normal, that he cannot be depressed?

Based on these scenarios, we think the answer to the question of whether depression is an inflammatory disorder is a resounding no. Even with a nod of recognition toward the fact that all disease processes have an inherent "sloppiness" that precludes absolute one-to-one correspondences between putative causes and observed symptomatic outcomes, it is clear that inflammation is neither necessary nor sufficient to cause MDD. Desperately depressed people often have low levels of systemic inflammation, and individuals with ragingly high inflammatory activity are often, but less commonly, able to retain a good mood and hopeful stance toward their lives.

WHO HAS THE INFLAMMATORY SUBTYPE?

There are a couple of ways of answering this question. One is to address how much inflammation one needs to qualify for an inflammatory subtype. The other way is to consider which depressed subjects came to their condition from conditions that first produced chronic inflammatory activation. Regarding the first question, as good an answer as any comes from research done by our group looking at whether agents that block peripheral inflammatory activity might show promise as novel antidepressants. Working with Andrew H. Miller, at Emory University, we conducted a randomized, placebo-controlled trial of the TNF antagonist infliximab in medically healthy/stable individuals with treatment-resistant depression.[103] After an assessment of symptoms and of peripheral inflammation (indexed by plasma concentrations of CRP and TNF), subjects were randomized to receive three infusions of either infliximab or saltwater delivered at baseline, study week 2, and study week 6. Mood and inflammatory markers were followed for 12 weeks (i.e., during the 6-week infusion period and for 6 subsequent weeks).

This study yielded several revealing surprises. First, in contrast to our expectations, infliximab did not outperform the saltwater placebo: both groups showed an approximate 50 percent response rate. If replicated in future studies, this suggests that blocking peripheral inflammatory cytokine activity does not hold significant promise as a general antidepressant strategy. A second surprise came when we tested our hypothesis that people with increased levels of plasma CRP or TNF at baseline would have stronger antidepressant responses to infliximab but not to placebo. As we expected, people with elevated pretreatment inflammation did indeed have a significantly larger response than did those with lower levels. But what we did not expect was that depressed people with low levels of peripheral inflammation actually did much worse on infliximab than they did on placebo. Much of the effect of antidepressants is known to be carried by the placebo effect of taking the pill. Infliximab seemed to antagonize the placebo effect in depressed individuals with low levels of inflammation. Said differently, lowering levels of inflammation in depressed individuals without increased inflammation made them worse, which explains why infliximab did not perform better than placebo: it worked better in the subgroup of depressed people with increased inflammation but worked worse in those with low levels. Although the relationship between response (and nonresponse) to infliximab and pretreatment levels of inflammation was strikingly linear, the cut-point for inflammation at which infliximab began outperforming placebo was at 5 mg/L CRP; that is, patients with ≥5 mg/L CRP did better in infliximab, and those with <5 mg/L CRP did worse.

Thus, seems to us that ≥5 mg/L CRP is as good as any to identify a subgroup of depressed people for whom inflammatory processes are likely to be especially relevant to MDD pathogenesis. On the other hand, although we don't fully understand it, our data suggest that depressed people with low levels of inflammation may actually need the levels of inflammation they have to avoid doing worse. How else might we explain that infliximab did worse than placebo in this group? Moreover, animal data support the notion that, at lower levels, inflammatory cytokines, especially TNF, may function as neurotrophic agents important for long-term potentiation and synaptic scaling, both of which are essential for learning.[104,105] A CRP of 5 mg/L is high, but not that high. During an acute infection, for

Data suggest that ELA may also sensitize people to the depressogenic effects of inflammation. Greg Miller and Steve Cole analyzed data from a longitudinal study of 147 adolescent girls with family histories or cognitive styles that put them at high risk for developing depression.[113] Plasma concentrations of IL-6 and depressive symptoms were assessed every six months over a thirty-month period to evaluate whether inflammation at any given assessment predicted depression six months later, and vice versa. In fact, increased IL-6 at any given time point did predict increased depressive symptoms, but only in the girls with a history of ELA. In girls lacking an ELA history, increased inflammation at any given time point actually predicted reduced levels of depression six months later.

As with ELA, obesity has been repeatedly associated with increased levels of a variety of peripheral inflammatory biomarkers and is a risk factor for the development of depression, especially in females.[114,115] The strength of the connection between obesity and inflammation is such that adjusting for it often reduces associations between depression and inflammation to nonsignificance.[116] And just as with ELA, some evidence suggests that obesity may sensitize individuals to the depressogenic effects of inflammation. In one of the larger studies to examine associations between inflammation and Major Depression, levels of both IL-6 and CRP were higher in depressed subjects who were obese but not in normal-weight depressed subjects.[19]

It is likely that ELA and obesity individually contribute in a disproportionate manner to the inflammatory subtype of depression. But it would be a mistake to view these factors as unrelated, given that ELA promotes adulthood obesity (and related metabolic derangements that also promote inflammation). Therefore, to some significant degree we can collapse these factors into a single pathway characterized by a maladaptive feed-forward loop involving ELA, inflammation, obesity, more inflammation, and, at some point in this cycle, depression, which may in turn promote patterns of stress sensitivity that further aggravate inflammatory responses to the daily travails of life.

References

1. Maes M, Scharpe S, Meltzer HY, et al. Relationships between interleukin-6 activity, acute phase proteins, and function of the hypothalamic-pituitary-adrenal axis in severe depression. *Psychiatry Res.* 1993;49(1):11–27.
2. Pace TW, Wingenfeld K, Schmidt I, Meinlschmidt G, Hellhammer DH, Heim CM. Increased peripheral NF-kappaB pathway activity in women with childhood abuse-related posttraumatic stress disorder. *Brain Behav Immun.* 2012;26(1):13–17.
3. Frasure-Smith N, Lesperance F, Irwin MR, Talajic M, Pollock BG. The relationships among heart rate variability, inflammatory markers and depression in coronary heart disease patients. *Brain Behav Immun.* 2009;23(8):1140–1147.
4. Thayer JF, Fischer JE. Heart rate variability, overnight urinary norepinephrine and C-reactive protein: evidence for the cholinergic anti-inflammatory pathway in healthy human adults. *J Intern Med.* 2009;265(4):439–447.

5. Johnson JD, Campisi J, Sharkey CM, et al. Catecholamines mediate stress-induced increases in peripheral and central inflammatory cytokines. *Neuroscience.* 2005;135(4): 1295–1307.

6. Mazzeo RS, Donovan D, Fleshner M, et al. Interleukin-6 response to exercise and high-altitude exposure: influence of alpha-adrenergic blockade. *J Appl Physiol.* 2001;91(5): 2143–2149.

7. Bierhaus A, Wolf J, Andrassy M, et al. A mechanism converting psychosocial stress into mononuclear cell activation. *Proc Natl Acad Sci U S A.* 2003;100(4):1920–1925.

8. Tracey KJ. Reflex control of immunity. *Nat Rev Immunol.* 2009;9(6):418–428.

9. O'Mahony C, van der Kleij H, Bienenstock J, Shanahan F, O'Mahony L. Loss of vagal anti-inflammatory effect: in vivo visualization and adoptive transfer. *Am J Physiol Regul Integr Comp Physiol.* 2009;297(4):R1118–R1126.

10. Maes M. Major depression and activation of the inflammatory response system. *Adv Exp Med Biol.* 1999;461:25–46.

11. Irwin MR, Miller AH. Depressive disorders and immunity: 20 years of progress and discovery. *Brain Behav Immun.* 2007;21(4):374–383.

12. Clark J, Vagenas P, Panesar M, Cope AP. What does tumour necrosis factor excess do to the immune system long term? *Ann Rheum Dis.* 2005;64(suppl 4):iv70–iv76.

13. Blume J, Douglas SD, Evans DL. Immune suppression and immune activation in depression. *Brain Behav Immun.* 2011;25(2):221–229.

14. Zorilla E, Luborsky L, McKay J, Roesnthal R, et al. The relationship of depression and stressors to immunological assays: a meta-analytic review. *Brain Behav Immun.* 2001; 15:199–226.

15. Dowlati Y, Herrmann N, Swardfager W, et al. A meta-analysis of cytokines in major depression. *Biol Psychiatry.* 2010;67(5):466–457.

16. Howren MB, Lamkin DM, Suls J. Associations of depression with C-reactive protein, IL-1, and IL-6: a meta-analysis. *Psychosom Med.* 2009;71(2):171–186.

17. Haroon E, Raison CL, Miller AH. Psychoneuroimmunology meets neuropsychopharmacology: translational implications of the impact of inflammation on behavior. *Neuropsychopharmacology.* 2012;37(1):137–162.

18. Bower JE, Ganz PA, Aziz N, Fahey JL. Fatigue and proinflammatory cytokine activity in breast cancer survivors. *Psychosom Med.* 2002;64(4):604–611.

19. Miller GE, Stetler CA, Carney RM, Freedland KE, Banks WA. Clinical depression and inflammatory risk markers for coronary heart disease. *Am J Cardiol.* 2002;90(12): 1279–1283.

20. Alesci S, Martinez PE, Kelkar S, et al. Major depression is associated with significant diurnal elevations in plasma interleukin-6 levels, a shift of its circadian rhythm, and loss of physiological complexity in its secretion: clinical implications. *J Clin Endocrinol Metab.* 2005;90(5):2522–2530.

21. Motivala SJ, Sarfatti A, Olmos L, Irwin MR. Inflammatory markers and sleep disturbance in major depression. *Psychosom Med.* 2005;67:187–194.

22. Miller AH, Maletic V, Raison CL. Inflammation and its discontents: the role of cytokines in the pathophysiology of major depression. *Biol Psychiatry.* 2009;65(9):732–741.

23. Lanquillon S, Krieg JC, Bening-Abu-Shach U, Vedder H. Cytokine production and treatment response in major depressive disorder. *Neuropsychopharmacology.* 2000;22(4): 370–379.

24. Fitzgerald P, O'Brien SM, Scully P, Rijkers K, Scott LV, Dinan TG. Cutaneous glucocorticoid receptor sensitivity and pro-inflammatory cytokine levels in antidepressant-resistant depression. *Psychol Med.* 2006;36(1):37–43.

25. Benedetti F, Lucca A, Brambilla F, Colombo C, Smeraldi E. Interleukine-6 serum levels correlate with response to antidepressant sleep deprivation and sleep phase advance. *Prog Neuropsychopharmacol Biol Psychiatry.* 2002;26(6):1167–1170.

26. Harley J, Luty S, Carter J, Mulder R, Joyce P. Elevated C-reactive protein in depression: a predictor of good long-term outcome with antidepressants and poor outcome with psychotherapy. *J Psychopharmacol.* 2010;24(4):625–626.

27. Reichenberg A, Yirmiya R, Schuld A, et al. Cytokine-associated emotional and cognitive disturbances in humans. *Arch Gen Psychiatry.* 2001;58(5):445–452.

28. Brydon L, Harrison NA, Walker C, Steptoe A, Critchley HD. Peripheral inflammation is associated with altered substantia nigra activity and psychomotor slowing in humans. *Biol Psychiatry.* 2008;63(11):1022–1029.

29. Harrison NA, Brydon L, Walker C, Gray MA, Steptoe A, Critchley HD. Inflammation causes mood changes through alterations in subgenual cingulate activity and mesolimbic connectivity. *Biol Psychiatry.* 2009;66(5):407–414.

30. Eisenberger NI, Inagaki TK, Mashal NM, Irwin MR. Inflammation and social experience: an inflammatory challenge induces feelings of social disconnection in addition to depressed mood. *Brain Behav Immun.* 2010;24(4):558–563.

31. Raison CL, Demetrashvili M, Capuron L, Miller AH. Neuropsychiatric side effects of interferon-alpha: recognition and management. *CNS Drugs.* 2005;19(2):1–19.

32. Capuron L, Fornwalt FB, Knight BT, Harvey PD, Ninan PT, Miller AH. Does cytokine-induced depression differ from idiopathic major depression in medically healthy individuals? *J Affect Disord.* 2009;119(1–3):181–185.

33. Musselman DL, Lawson DH, Gumnick JF, et al. Paroxetine for the prevention of depression induced by high-dose interferon alfa. *N Engl J Med.* 2001;344(13):961–966.

34. Raison CL, Woolwine BJ, Demetrashvili MF, et al. Paroxetine for prevention of depressive symptoms induced by interferon-alpha and ribavirin for hepatitis C. *Aliment Pharmacol Ther.* 2007;25(10):1163–1174.

35. Kraus MR, Schafer A, Schottker K, et al. Therapy of interferon-induced depression in chronic hepatitis C with citalopram: a randomised, double-blind, placebo-controlled study. *Gut.* 2008;57(4):531–536.

36. Hauser P, Khosla J, Aurora H, et al. A prospective study of the incidence and open-label treatment of interferon-induced major depressive disorder in patients with hepatitis C. *Mol Psychiatry.* 2002;7(9):942–947.

37. Juengling FD, Ebert D, Gut O, et al. Prefrontal cortical hypometabolism during low-dose interferon alpha treatment. *Psychopharmacology.* 2000;152(4):383–389.

38. Capuron L, Pagnoni G, Demetrashvili MF, et al. Basal ganglia hypermetabolism and symptoms of fatigue during interferon-alpha therapy. *Neuropsychopharmacology.* 2007;32(11):2384–2392.

39. Felger JC, Alagbe O, Hu F, et al. Effects of interferon-alpha on rhesus monkeys: a nonhuman primate model of cytokine-induced depression. *Biol Psychiatry.* 2007;62(11):1324–1333.

40. McKinney WT Jr, Eising RG, Moran EC, Suomi SJ, Harlow HF. Effects of reserpine on the social behavior of rhesus monkeys. *Dis Nerv Syst.* 1971;32(11):735–741.

41. Qin L, Wu X, Block ML, et al. Systemic LPS causes chronic neuroinflammation and progressive neurodegeneration. *Glia.* 2007;55(5):453–462.

42. Gao HM, Jiang J, Wilson B, Zhang W, Hong JS, Liu B. Microglial activation-mediated delayed and progressive degeneration of rat nigral dopaminergic neurons: relevance to Parkinson's disease. *J Neurochem.* 2002;81(6):1285–1297.

43. Bull SJ, Huezo-Diaz P, Binder EB, et al. Functional polymorphisms in the interleukin-6

and serotonin transporter genes, and depression and fatigue induced by interferon-alpha and ribavirin treatment. *Mol Psychiatry.* 2009;14(12):1095–1104.

44. Lotrich FE, Ferrell RE, Rabinovitz M, Pollock BG. Risk for depression during interferon-alpha treatment is affected by the serotonin transporter polymorphism. *Biol Psychiatry.* 2009;65(4):344–348.

45. Raison CL, Borisov AS, Majer M, et al. Activation of central nervous system inflammatory pathways by interferon-alpha: relationship to monoamines and depression. *Biol Psychiatry.* 2009;65(4):296–303.

46. Pemberton LA, Kerr SJ, Smythe G, Brew BJ. Quinolinic acid production by macrophages stimulated with IFN-gamma, TNF-alpha, and IFN-alpha. *J Interferon Cytokine Res.* 1997;17(10):589–595.

47. Fujigaki H, Saito K, Fujigaki S, et al. The signal transducer and activator of transcription 1alpha and interferon regulatory factor 1 are not essential for the induction of indoleamine 2,3-dioxygenase by lipopolysaccharide: involvement of p38 mitogen-activated protein kinase and nuclear factor-kappaB pathways, and synergistic effect of several proinflammatory cytokines. *J Biochem.* 2006;139(4):655–662.

48. Huang L, Baban B, Johnson BA 3rd, Mellor AL. Dendritic cells, indoleamine 2,3 dioxygenase and acquired immune privilege. *Int Rev Immunol.* 2010;29(2):133–155.

49. Bonaccorso S, Marino V, Puzella A, et al. Increased depressive ratings in patients with hepatitis C receiving interferon-alpha-based immunotherapy are related to interferon-alpha-induced changes in the serotonergic system. *J Clin Psychopharmacol.* 2002;22(1):86–90.

50. Capuron L, Neurauter G, Musselman DL, et al. Interferon-alpha-induced changes in tryptophan metabolism: relationship to depression and paroxetine treatment. *Biol Psychiat.* 2003;54(9):906–914.

51. O'Connor JC, Lawson MA, Andre C, et al. Lipopolysaccharide-induced depressive-like behavior is mediated by indoleamine 2,3-dioxygenase activation in mice. *Mol Psychiatry.* 2009;14(5):511–522.

52. Schwarcz R, Pellicciari R. Manipulation of brain kynurenines: glial targets, neuronal effects, and clinical opportunities. *J Pharmacol Exp Ther.* 2002;303(1):1–10.

53. Raison CL, Dantzer R, Kelley KW, et al. CSF concentrations of brain tryptophan and kynurenines during immune stimulation with IFN-alpha: relationship to CNS immune responses and depression. *Mol Psychiatry.* 2010;15(4):393–403.

54. Zhu CB, Blakely RD, Hewlett WA. The proinflammatory cytokines interleukin-1beta and tumor necrosis factor-alpha activate serotonin transporters. *Neuropsychopharmacology.* 2006;31(10):2121–2131.

55. Felger JC, Alagbe O, Pace TW, et al. Early activation of p38 mitogen activated protein kinase is associated with interferon-alpha-induced depression and fatigue. *Brain Behav Immun.* 2011;25(6):1094–1058.

56. Moron JA, Zakharova I, Ferrer JV, et al. Mitogen-activated protein kinase regulates dopamine transporter surface expression and dopamine transport capacity. *J Neurosci.* 2003;23(24):8480–8488.

57. Neurauter G, Schrocksnadel K, Scholl-Burgi S, et al. Chronic immune stimulation correlates with reduced phenylalanine turnover. *Curr Drug Metab.* 2008;9(7):622–627.

58. Knapp S, Irwin M. Plasma levels of tetrahydrobiopterin and folate in major depression. *Biol Psychiatry.* 1989;26(2):156–162.

59. Felger JC, Li L, Marvar PJ, et al. Tyrosine metabolism during interferon-alpha administration: association with fatigue and CSF dopamine concentrations. *Brain Behav Immun.* 2013;31:153–160.

60. Bezzi P, Domercq M, Brambilla L, et al. CXCR4-activated astrocyte glutamate release via TNFalpha: amplification by microglia triggers neurotoxicity. *Nat Neurosci.* 2001;4(7): 702–710.

61. Pitt D, Nagelmeier IE, Wilson HC, Raine CS. Glutamate uptake by oligodendrocytes: implications for excitotoxicity in multiple sclerosis. *Neurology.* 2003;61(8):1113–1120.

62. Volterra A, Meldolesi J. Astrocytes, from brain glue to communication elements: the revolution continues. *Nat Rev Neurosci.* 2005;6(8):626–640.

63. Tilleux S, Hermans E. Neuroinflammation and regulation of glial glutamate uptake in neurological disorders. *J Neurosci Res.* 2007;85(10):2059–2070.

64. Ida T, Hara M, Nakamura Y, Kozaki S, Tsunoda S, Ihara H. Cytokine-induced enhancement of calcium-dependent glutamate release from astrocytes mediated by nitric oxide. *Neurosci Lett.* 2008;432(3):232–236.

65. Hardingham GE, Fukunaga Y, Bading H. Extrasynaptic NMDARs oppose synaptic NMDARs by triggering CREB shut-off and cell death pathways. *Nat Neurosci.* 2002; 5(5):405–414.

66. Haydon PG, Carmignoto G. Astrocyte control of synaptic transmission and neurovascular coupling. *Physiol Rev.* 2006;86(3):1009–1031.

67. Matute C, Domercq M, Sanchez-Gomez MV. Glutamate-mediated glial injury: mechanisms and clinical importance. *Glia.* 2006;53(2):212–224.

68. Rajkowska G, Miguel-Hidalgo JJ. Gliogenesis and glial pathology in depression. *CNS Neurol Disord Drug Targets.* 2007;6(3):219–233.

69. Duman RS, Monteggia LM. A neurotrophic model for stress-related mood disorders. *Biol Psychiatry.* 2006;59(12):1116–1127.

70. Barrientos RM, Sprunger DB, Campeau S, et al. Brain-derived neurotrophic factor mRNA downregulation produced by social isolation is blocked by intrahippocampal interleukin-1 receptor antagonist. *Neuroscience.* 2003;121(4):847–853.

71. Ben Menachem-Zidon O, Goshen I, Kreisel T, et al. Intrahippocampal transplantation of transgenic neural precursor cells overexpressing interleukin-1 receptor antagonist blocks chronic isolation-induced impairment in memory and neurogenesis. *Neuropsychopharmacology.* 2008;33(9):2251–2262.

72. Koo JW, Duman RS. IL-1beta is an essential mediator of the antineurogenic and anhedonic effects of stress. *Proc Natl Acad Sci U S A.* 2008;105(2):751–756.

73. Kenis G, Prickaerts J, van Os J, et al. Depressive symptoms following interferon-alpha therapy: mediated by immune-induced reductions in brain-derived neurotrophic factor? *Int J Neuropsychopharmacol.* 2011;14(2):247–253.

74. Pariante CM, Makoff A, Lovestone S, et al. Antidepressants enhance glucocorticoid receptor function in vitro by modulating the membrane steroid transporters. *Br J Pharmacol.* 2001;134(6):1335–1343.

75. Pariante CM. The role of multi-drug resistance p-glycoprotein in glucocorticoid function: studies in animals and relevance in humans. *Eur J Pharmacol.* 2008;583(2–3):263–271.

76. Besedovsky HO, del Rey A. Immune-neuro-endocrine interactions: facts and hypotheses. *Endocr Rev.* 1996;17(1):64–102.

77. Capuron L, Raison CL, Musselman DL, Lawson DH, Nemeroff CB, Miller AH. Association of exaggerated HPA axis response to the initial injection of interferon-alpha with development of depression during interferon-alpha therapy. *Am J Psychiatry.* 2003;160(7): 1342–1345.

78. Raison CL, Borisov AS, Woolwine BJ, Massung B, Vogt G, Miller AH. Interferon-alpha effects on diurnal hypothalamic-pituitary-adrenal axis activity: relationship with proinflammatory cytokines and behavior. *Mol Psychiatry.* 2010;15(5):535–547.

79. Sephton SE, Sapolsky RM, Kraemer HC, Spiegel D. Diurnal cortisol rhythm as a predictor of breast cancer survival. *J Natl Cancer Inst.* 2000;92(12):994–1000.

80. Spiegel D, Giese-Davis J, Taylor CB, Kraemer H. Stress sensitivity in metastatic breast cancer: analysis of hypothalamic-pituitary-adrenal axis function. *Psychoneuroendocrinology.* 2006;31(10):1231–1244.

81. Felger JC, Haroon E, Woolwine BJ, Raison CL, Miller AH. Interferon-alpha-induced inflammation is associated with reduced glucocorticoid negative feedback sensitivity and depression in patients with hepatitis C virus. *Physiol Behav.* 2016;166:14–21.

82. Pace TW, Hu F, Miller AH. Cytokine-effects on glucocorticoid receptor function: relevance to glucocorticoid resistance and the pathophysiology and treatment of major depression. *Brain Behav Immun.* 2007;21(1):9–19.

83. Hu F, Pace TW, Miller AH. Interferon-alpha inhibits glucocorticoid receptor-mediated gene transcription via STAT5 activation in mouse HT22 cells. *Brain Behav Immun.* 2009;23(4):455–463.

84. Smoak KA, Cidlowski JA. Mechanisms of glucocorticoid receptor signaling during inflammation. *Mech Ageing Dev.* 2004;125(10–11):697–706.

85. Wang X, Wu H, Miller AH. Interleukin 1alpha (IL-1alpha) induced activation of p38 mitogen-activated protein kinase inhibits glucocorticoid receptor function. *Mol Psychiatry.* 2004;9(1):65–75.

86. Engler H, Bailey MT, Engler A, Stiner-Jones LM, Quan N, Sheridan JF. Interleukin-1 receptor type 1-deficient mice fail to develop social stress-associated glucocorticoid resistance in the spleen. *Psychoneuroendocrinology.* 2008;33(1):108–117.

87. Pariante CM, Pearce BD, Pisell TL, et al. The proinflammatory cytokine, interleukin-1alpha, reduces glucocorticoid receptor translocation and function. *Endocrinology.* 1999;140(9):4359–4366.

88. Kino T, Manoli I, Kelkar S, Wang Y, Su YA, Chrousos GP. Glucocorticoid receptor (GR) beta has intrinsic, GRalpha-independent transcriptional activity. *Biochem Biophys Res Commun.* 2009;381(4):671–675.

89. Quan N, Avitsur R, Stark JL, et al. Social stress increases the susceptibility to endotoxic shock. *J Neuroimmunol.* 2001;115(1–2):36–45.

90. Rhen T, Cidlowski JA. Antiinflammatory action of glucocorticoids—new mechanisms for old drugs. *N Engl J Med.* 2005;353(16):1711–1723.

91. Carter CS, Braver TS, Barch DM, Botvinick MM, Noll D, Cohen JD. Anterior cingulate cortex, error detection, and the online monitoring of performance. *Science.* 1998;280(5364):747–749.

92. Capuron L, Pagnoni G, Demetrashvili M, et al. Anterior cingulate activation and error processing during interferon-alpha treatment. *Biol Psychiatry.* 2005;58(3):190–196.

93. Paulus MP, Feinstein JS, Simmons A, Stein MB. Anterior cingulate activation in high trait anxious subjects is related to altered error processing during decision making. *Biol Psychiatry.* 2004;55(12):1179–1187.

94. Eisenberger NI, Lieberman MD, Satpute AB. Personality from a controlled processing perspective: an fMRI study of neuroticism, extraversion, and self-consciousness. *Cogn Affect Behav Neurosci.* 2005;5(2):169–181.

95. Ursu S, Stenger VA, Shear MK, Jones MR, Carter CS. Overactive action monitoring in obsessive-compulsive disorder: evidence from functional magnetic resonance imaging. *Psychol Sci.* 2003;14(4):347–353.

96. Slavich GM, Way BM, Eisenberger NI, Taylor SE. Neural sensitivity to social rejection is

associated with inflammatory responses to social stress. *Proc Natl Acad Sci U S A.* 2010;107(33):14817–14822.

97. Eisenberger NI, Lieberman MD. Why rejection hurts: a common neural alarm system for physical and social pain. *Trends Cogn Sci.* 2004;8(7):294–300.

98. Lozano AM, Mayberg HS, Giacobbe P, Hamani C, Craddock RC, Kennedy SH. Subcallosal cingulate gyrus deep brain stimulation for treatment-resistant depression. *Biol Psychiatry.* 2008;64(6):461–467.

99. Feigin A, Ghilardi MF, Fukuda M, et al. Effects of levodopa infusion on motor activation responses in Parkinson's disease. *Neurology.* 2002;59(2):220–226.

100. Eisenberger NI, Berkman ET, Inagaki TK, Rameson LT, Mashal NM, Irwin MR. Inflammation-induced anhedonia: endotoxin reduces ventral striatum responses to reward. *Biol Psychiatry.* 2010;68(8):748–754.

101. Felger JC, Li Z, Haroon E, et al. Inflammation is associated with decreased functional connectivity within corticostriatal reward circuitry in depression. *Mol Psychiatry.* 2016;21(10)1358–1365.

102. Miller AH. Mechanisms of cytokine-induced behavioral changes: psychoneuroimmunology at the translational interface. *Brain Behav Immun.* 2009;23(2):149–158.

103. Raison CL, Rutherford RE, Woolwine BJ, et al. A randomized controlled trial of the tumor necrosis factor antagonist infliximab for treatment-resistant depression: the role of baseline inflammatory biomarkers. *JAMA Psych.* 2013;70(1):31–41.

104. Kreisel T, Frank MG, Licht T, et al. Dynamic microglial alterations underlie stress-induced depressive-like behavior and suppressed neurogenesis. *Mol Psychiatry.* 2014; 19(6):699–709.

105. Yirmiya R, Goshen I. Immune modulation of learning, memory, neural plasticity and neurogenesis. *Brain Behav Immun.* 2011;25(2):181–213.

106. Raison CL, Lowry CA, Rook GA. Inflammation, sanitation, and consternation: loss of contact with coevolved, tolerogenic microorganisms and the pathophysiology and treatment of major depression. *Arch Gen Psychiatry.* 2010;67(12):1211–1224.

107. Danese A, Caspi A, Williams B, et al. Biological embedding of stress through inflammation processes in childhood. *Mol Psychiatry.* 2011;16(3):244–246.

108. Danese A, Moffitt TE, Harrington H, et al. Adverse childhood experiences and adult risk factors for age-related disease: depression, inflammation, and clustering of metabolic risk markers. *Arch Pediatr Adolesc Med.* 2009;163(12):1135–1143.

109. Danese A, Moffitt TE, Pariante CM, Ambler A, Poulton R, Caspi A. Elevated inflammation levels in depressed adults with a history of childhood maltreatment. *Arch Gen Psychiatry.* 2008;65(4):409–415.

110. Danese A, Pariante CM, Caspi A, Taylor A, Poulton R. Childhood maltreatment predicts adult inflammation in a life-course study. *Proc Natl Acad Sci U S A.* 2007;104(4): 1319–1324.

111. Pace TW, Mletzko TC, Alagbe O, et al. Increased stress-induced inflammatory responses in male patients with major depression and increased early life stress. *Am J Psychiatry.* 2006;163(9):1630–1633.

112. Carpenter LL, Gawuga CE, Tyrka AR, Lee JK, Anderson GM, Price LH. Association between plasma IL-6 response to acute stress and early-life adversity in healthy adults. *Neuropsychopharmacology.* 2010;35(13):2617–2623.

113. Miller GE, Cole SW. Clustering of depression and inflammation in adolescents previously exposed to childhood adversity. *Biol Psychiatry.* 2012;72(1):34–40.

114. Pan A, Sun Q, Czernichow S, et al. Bidirectional association between depression and obesity in middle-aged and older women. *Int J Obes (Lond).* 2012;36(4):595–602.

115. Beydoun MA, Wang Y. Pathways linking socioeconomic status to obesity through depression and lifestyle factors among young US adults. *J Affect Disord.* 2010;123(1–3): 52–63.

116. O'Connor MF, Bower JE, Cho HJ, et al. To assess, to control, to exclude: effects of biobehavioral factors on circulating inflammatory markers. *Brain Behav Immun.* 2009;23(7): 887–897.

CHAPTER 7

Neuroplastic, Inflammatory, and Cellular Changes in Depression

When Werner Heisenborg formulated his uncertainty principle in 1927, he pointed out a fundamental challenge inherent in observation of any phenomena with dual properties, in this instance the matter–wave nature of quantum objects: it is nearly impossible to simultaneously ascertain position and movement of a given wave/ particle with an equal precision. We face a similarly daunting challenge in our attempt to provide a cogent summary of cellular and subcellular perturbations in the context of major depressive disorder (MDD).

The function and structure of neural elements are inextricably interwoven. Increased activation of pyramidal neurons precipitates elevation of second messengers and, subsequently, transcription factors regulating neurotrophic factor synthesis. Neurotrophins influence the synthesis of skeletal proteins via mediating molecules (e.g., mTOR, the mammalian mechanistic target of rapamyacin) and thus future synaptic function. This brief description of neural signaling illustrates a smooth dynamic transition from function to structure and back to function.

A more accurate representation of neural signaling would include interactions among multiple cell types, such as neurons, astroglia, microglia, oligodendroglia, and even T lymphocytes. Myriad neurotransmitters, modulators, chemokines, cytokines, and neurotrophic molecules converge on cellular membranes and generate synergistic and antagonistic intracellular cascades, all funneling toward regulation of transcription factors. Decoding the cellular and subcellular signature of depression involves not only grasping the alterations in the numbers and function of cellular elements but also identifying aberrations in the dynamic between the cells and their signaling molecules. In other words, understanding depression relies on our ability to capture quantitative, qualitative, and dynamic changes simultaneously.

The best didactic strategy might dictate that we sequentially introduce the relevant cellular elements and signaling molecules and then point out their deviations in the context of depression. Unfortunately, if one follows this recipe, it is at the expense of describing alternations in the more dynamic aspects of the process, such as changes in the complex interactions between the signaling molecules and cellular elements. This second strategy also has its shortcomings, focusing on the intricate dynamic without providing a previous knowledge of the function of various elements. We attempt to address this duality through a compromise. After a functional description of the relevant components, we highlight their dynamic interactions in the context of MDD. As we have previously explored changes in neurotransmission in MDD, we now endeavor to shed light on cellular, neuroplastic, and inflammatory processes relevant to understanding the pathophysiology of MDD.

An Overview of Glial Architecture and Function

Accumulating evidence suggests that pathology in glial cell density and function may be the primary cytological substrate in MDD. The human nervous system is composed of approximately 100 billion neurons and 1 trillion glia cells.[1] Thus, glia cells outnumber neurons at a ratio of approximately 10:1. Traditionally, glia cells have been cast in a supportive role, as a passive supportive matrix for neurons.[1] However, in a dramatic shift from prior assumptions, contemporary research has established astroglia and oligodendroglia as full-fledged neuronal partners in the dynamic signaling processes.[2]

Indeed, the brain architecture is primarily defined by astrocytes. Astrocytes are not only the most numerous cell type in the brain but also quite diverse. While protoplasmatic astrocytes reside in the gray matter, fibrous astrocytes inhabit the white matter.[3] A protoplasmic astrocyte is a "master" of its own territory, enveloping portions of all the neural elements within its domain.[4] Astrocytes create glial networks communicating with each other via gap junctions utilizing adenosine triphosphate (ATP)-induced calcium signaling.[5] Each human astrocyte contacts and encases approximately 2 million synapses.[4] In addition to managing the content of the synaptic cleft by actively taking up the "excess" neurotransmitter, astroglia may have a role in synchronizing the activity of all neurons within their domains.[5] Furthermore, astrocytes provide conditions for unfettered synaptic activity. Rapid synaptic signaling, accompanied by propagation of active potentials and membrane depolarization, generates an accumulation of K^+ ions in the extracellular compartment. Astrocytes are capable of rapid K^+ uptake, thus reestablishing K^+ gradients conducive to continued synaptic activity.[6]

Intense synaptic signaling also mandates a sustained energy supply and adequate cerebral perfusion. Astroglia form a live metabolic bridge coupling the synapse with the cerebral vasculature. On one end, astroglial extensions encapsulate the synapse and "sense" its activity; on the other end, their distal processes, or perivascular "end feet," modulate vascular tone and capillary permeability.[7,8] Half of the glucose that reaches the brain is taken up by neurons; the other half, by astrocytes. During peak synaptic activity, astroglia mobilize their glycogen supply to provide "accessory" energy by releasing lactate in the neuronal vicinity. Magnetic resonance spectroscopy has provided evidence that the "lactate shuttle" can also work in the opposite direction: excessive lactate generated during intense neural activity can be taken up by astrocytes.[9] Additionally, glycogen metabolism provides the energy for astrocytic K^+ pumps to keep pace with heightened synaptic activity.[10–12] Aquaporin-4 is a protein, forming water channels in astrocytic end feet, which helps maintain water and ion homeostasis. Appropriate astrocytic contribution is also essential for the proper functioning of the blood–brain barrier (BBB). Astrocyte-mediated neurovascular coupling allows fine microcirculatory adjustments to accommodate increased metabolic and oxygen demand in the face of robust neural activity.[3,13,14]

ASTROGLIAL RECEPTORS AND TRANSPORTERS

The multitude of receptors and uptake sites reflect the importance of astrocytes as the neuronal partners in transmission. Astroglial cell membranes express almost all classes of receptors for serotonin (5HT), norepinephrine (NE), dopamine (DA), cholines, histamines, substance P (SP), opioids, purines, gamma-aminobutyric acid (GABA), glutamate, glycine, vasopressin, neurotrophins, and cytokines.[2,5,15–18] Additionally, astroglial membranes express transporters of monoamines (5HT, NE, DA, histamine), GABA, and glutamate.[15,16] Unlike the conventional neuronal monoamine transporters, which are located predominantly in the synaptic cleft and depend on the Na^+/Cl^- gradient, glia cells mostly utilize low-affinity, high-capacity plasma membrane transporters.[19] Transport of monoamines, including histamine, across the astrocyte plasma membrane is conducted by the low-affinity Organic Cation Transporter-3 (OCT-3) and Plasma Membrane Monoamine Transporter (PMAT) transporters.[19,20]

Monoamine Receptors on Astrocytes

The ramifications of astrocyte receptor activation remain to be fully elucidated. Preclinical studies have found that activation of the 5HT receptor 5HT1A induces release of S100B, a glial trophic factor, which promotes neuronal cytoskeletal and synaptic development.[21] Several preclinical studies have focused on the consequences of astrocyte signaling with the 5HT receptor 5HT2B. Researchers have noted consequent 5HT2B-mediated elevation in extracellular regulated kinase 1/2 and subsequent increase in synthesis of calcium-dependant phospholipase A2. Additionally activation of the same receptor has been associated with transactivation of epidermal growth factor. The cumulative downstream effects of these endo-cellular messengers may be upregulation of specific genes, glycogenolysis, increased cell proliferation, and eventual modulation of brain plasticity and memory.[18,22,23]

In addition to 5HT2A, adrenergic alpha-2 receptors have also been implicated in the transactivation of epidermal growth factor, with all the ensuing neuroplas-tic effects. Moreover, alpha-2 astrocytic signaling has also been linked with a cyclical adenosine monophosphate (cAMP) response element binding protein (CREB)-dependent increase in glial-cell-line–derived neurotrophic factor (GDNF) release.[24] (Neuroplastic and neurotrophic aspects of GDNF are discussed in more detail later in this chapter.) In addition to alpha-1, preclinical studies suggest that astrocyte alpha-2 adrenergic receptors also have a role in neuroplastic processes by aiding short-term and intermediate memory consolidation in the hippocam-pus.[25] (See table 7.1 for a list of abbreviations used throughout this chapter.)

In further support of astrocyte noradrenergic receptor involvement in neuro-plasticity and learning are animal research findings pointing to joint alpha-1, beta-1, and beta-2 mediation of brain-derived neurotrophic factor (BDNF) synthe-sis in astrocytes.[25] Moreover, beta-2 adrenergic agonists in combination with phosphodiesterase 4 antagonists appear capable of elevating intercellular cAMP, causing subsequent downregulation of inflammatory mediators monocyte che-motactic protein-1 (MCP-1) and interleukin-6 (IL-6).[26] Beyond its role in modulat-ing neurotrophic and inflammatory signaling, NE also regulates the release of glia transmitters, such as ATP. One of the principal downstream consequences of astroglial ATP release and subsequent binding of the receptor P2X7 is insertion of alpha-amino-3-hydroxy-5-methyl-4-isoxazolepropionic acid (AMPA) glutamate receptors into neural membranes.[27]

In vitro manipulation of astrocytic dopaminergic D1 receptors has consis-tently produced increased synthesis and release of GDNF and nerve growth fac-tor (NGF); D2 agonism either had no effect or suppressed BDNF synthesis, while its impact on GDNF synthesis release has not been consistent across studies. Pos-sibly due to methodological differences, some D2 agonists have caused suppres-sion of GDNF synthesis in astrocytes, while others have had the opposite effect.[28–31] DA may have an effect on astrocyte function that is independent of its receptor activation. Metabolism of DA by monoamine oxidase with resulting reactive oxy-gen species (ROS) production has been shown to stimulate phospholipase C and subsequently mobilize endoplasmic calcium ions (Ca^{2+}).[32] This finding is of par-ticular relevance, since Ca^{2+} release from astrocyte endoplasmic stores may pre-cipitate exocytosis of glial transmitters.

Glutamate and GABA Receptors on Astrocytes

Astroglial cells also express both ionotropic glutamate receptors of the AMPA and N-methyl-D-aspartate (NMDA) variety, as well as metabotropic glutamate recep-tors mGluR3 and mGluR5. These receptors are localized mostly in astroglial pro-cesses, where they are believed to modulate multiple metabolic functions via

TABLE 7.1. Abbreviations Used in this Chapter

AMP	adenosine monophosphate
AMPA	alpha-amino-3-hydroxy-5-methyl-4 isoxazolepropionic acid glutamatergic receptor
ATP	adenosine triphosphate
BDNF	Brain-derived neurotrophic factor
CaMK II	Ca^{2+}-calmodulin-dependent protein kinase II
cAMP	cyclical adenosinemonophosphate
CB-1 and CB-2	cannabinoid receptors 1 and 2
COX-2	cyclo-oxygenase-2
CREB	cAMP response element binding protein
CSF	cerebro-spinal fluid
EAAT	excitatory amino acid transporter
ECT	electroconvulsive treatment
ERK	extracellular signal-regulated kinase
GABA	gamma aminobutyric acid
GAT-3	GABA transporter-3
GDNF	glial cell-derived neurotrophic factor
GSK-3	glycogen synthase kinase-3
HAMD also HDRS	Hamilton depression rating scale
IGF-1	insulin-like growth factor-1
IL-6	interleukin-6
MAPK	mitogen-activated protein kinase
MCP-1	monocyte chemotractant protein-1
mGlu, also mGluR	metabotropic glutamate receptor
nAchR	nicotinic acetylcholine receptor
NFkB	nuclear factor kappa-beta
NGF	nerve growth factor
NMDA	*N*-methyl-D-aspartate glutamatergic receptor
NO	nitric oxyde
NOS	nitricnoxyde synthase
NRI	norepinephrine (NE) reuptake inhibitor
NT-3	neurotrophin-3
p75 NTR	p75 neurotrophin receptor
PG	prostaglandin
PKA	protein kinase-A
PKC	protein kinase-C
PLC	phospholipase-C
RNS	reactive nitrogen species
ROS	reactive oxygen species
SNRI	serotonin/norepinephrine reuptake inhibitor
SP	substance-P
SSRI	selective serotonin reuptake inhibitor
TGF-beta	transforming growth factor-beta
TLR	toll-like receptors
TNF-alpha	tumor necrosis factor-alpha
Trk-B	tropomyosin receptor kinase-B
TSP	thrombospondin
VEGF	vascular endothelial growth factor

activation of cAMP and regulation of Ca^{2+} trafficking. Astroglial GABA-B receptors may play an important role in complex regulatory hippocampal loops. Increased GABA release from hippocampal interneurons leads to activation of astroglial GABA-B receptors and subsequent increase in Ca^{2+} in glial cells. The elevation in Ca^{2+} induces astrocytes to release glutamate. Glutamate of astrocytic origin interacts with kainate receptors on the interneurons, causing them to discharge more GABA, thereby inhibiting pyramidal neuron. This interneuron–astrocyte–interneuron–pyramidal neuron loop acts as an amplifier of GABA inhibitory signaling in hippocampus.[33]

Purinergic, Neurotrophin, and Cytokine Receptors on Astrocytes

Purinergic (pertaining to ATP) signaling, especially via P2X7 receptors, is very important for regulation of ion channel function, gene expression, and ongoing transmitter "dialogue" with neurons, microglia, and oligodendroglia.[16] Astrocytes are additionally endowed with multiple other receptor types, including receptors for inflammatory cytokines and neurotrophic factors. Activation of the astrocytic, truncated version of BDNF receptors, tyrosine receptor kinase B (TrkB), has a different consequence than binding with a more elaborate neuronal TrkB receptor. The main outcome of BDNF signaling to astrocytes is a rapid release of Ca^{2+} from the intercellular stores, with consequent downstream regulation of other types of glia cells and neuronal activity.[34] Both epidermal growth factor and transforming growth factor-beta (TGFβ), interacting with their respective astrocytic receptors, have been identified as determinants of astrocyte differentiation.[35]

In summary, activation of astrocytic receptors is a significant modulator of neuronal excitability and synaptic signaling and may have an even more enduring impact by sculpting synaptic structure and function via neurotrophin release and modification of gene function.[36] One may even conclude that brain connectivity is effectively shaped by astrocytes through regulation of adaptive synaptic plasticity. All these processes are likely to be highly relevant in primary brain functions, such as learning and memory.

Astrocyte Transmitters

It has been unequivocally established that astrocytes are not just passive, silent partners in neural transmission but very active participants. Astrocytes are capable of releasing glutamate, GABA, ATP, D-serine, and taurine.[16] Both neurons and astrocytes rely on exocytosis as the primary mechanism of transmitter release from the secretory vesicles, although the mechanics of this process differ between them. While neurons mostly rely on immediate entry of Ca^{2+} from extracellular space to cytosol to trigger transmitter exocytosis, astrocytes can additionally mobilize Ca^{2+} from its internal store in the endoplasmic reticulum.[16]

In addition to the more conventional vesicular release, glia transmitters can be released in several other ways. Negatively charged transmitters such as glutamate, GABA, and ATP can be released through membrane channels and transporters, which specialize in exchanging transmitters with other molecules across cell membranes. Intensive stimulation of purinergic P2X7 receptor can cause the receptor structure to morph into a pore, spanning the membrane and allowing glutamate to "escape" into the extracellular space. Finally, in special circumstances membrane transporters such as astroglial GABA transporter-3 can be induced into changing the direction of their activity and start pumping GABA out of the cell. A similar process is theoretically possible with astroglial glutamate transporters (excitatory amino acid transporters EAAT-1 and -2) but is much less likely to occur in physiological circumstances.[16]

Once released from the astroglia, glutamate seems to be an influential modulator of synaptic strength and a regulator of neuronal excitability.[37] It is believed that release of glutamate from astrocytes is one of the key events in establishing long-term potentiation (LTP), widely considered to be the neural basis for memory and learning. Exocytosis of D-serine leads to enhancement of NMDA-based glutamate signaling.[16] Juxtaposed to their ability to positively modulate excitatory transmission, astroglia can also turn down neuronal activity via release of ATP and GABA. When a 2011 paper reported that as many as a half of the GABA cells in the brain may be astrocytes, it created quite a stir in the neuroscience circles.[38,39] Astrocytes possess a complete set of metabolic enzymes necessary for GABA synthesis, as well as GABA transporters and receptors.[40] Since astrocytes have a capacity to generate glutamine from glutamate and then supply it to either GABA or glutamatergic neurons as the building block for their respective neurotransmitters, and also scale and strengthen either glutamate or GABA synapses, they can be construed, figuratively speaking, as the guardians of the yin–yang balance in the brain.[37,39,41]

Astrocytes have an alternative path to providing an inhibitory influence on neighboring neurons. Generally speaking, ATP of astrocytic origin has an inhibitory impact on the release of excitatory neurotransmitters, as well as a stabilizing influence on microglia and endothelial cells. As ATP becomes metabolized into adenosine in the extracellular space, it emerges as one of the main circadian and sleep/wakefulness regulators.[16,37] Interestingly, preliminary preclinical evidence suggests that astrocytes also possess a capability to synthesize melatonin.[42] The physiological relevance of this discovery remains yet to be established. There is another intriguing parallel between the roles of astrocytic GABA and ATP: they both exert an anti-inflammatory influence on microglia cells.[16,39] Finally, astrocytes may regulate GABA-A receptor activity by releasing neurosteroids, including estradiol and progesterone.[36]

ASTROCYTES AS REGULATORS OF NEUROPLASTICITY

Brain connectivity is effectively shaped by astroglia through regulation of synaptogenesis, synaptic strength, plasticity, and elimination.[4,43] Astrocytes sculpt the neurocircuitry in the developing brain by promoting the formation of new synapses but also by pruning away the less functional ones.[44] Both neurons and astrocytes originate from common precursor cells. Astrocytes can use soluble, diffusible signals and contact-mediated cues to assist in synaptic development. Interestingly, astrocytic assignment to synaptogenesis and neuronal repair in the sectors of brain tissue seems to be specific and to coincide with their common embryonic site of origin. In other words, astrocytes assist neurons that originate from the same periventricular zone "neighborhood" as they do.[45]

Thrombospondins (TSPs) and hevin have been identified as key astroglia-secreted chemicals involved in excitatory synaptogenesis. Binding of TSPs to the alpha2-delta subunit of voltage-gated Ca^{2+} channels initiates the synthesis of scaffolding and adhesion molecules, supporting synaptic formation.[43,44] Hevin appears to increase the synaptic size and is more involved with maturation and maintenance of synapses.[43] Although astroglia have a documented role in formation of inhibitory GABA synapses, it appears that a different, thus far not fully identified set of modulatory molecules is utilized.[43] While astrocytic-origin TSPs, ATP, and tumor necrosis factor-alpha (TNF) have a significant role in AMPA receptor insertion and ensuing strengthening of glutamate signaling, it appears that BDNF may have a more significant role in modulation of GABA signaling.[33,44,46]

The Role of Astrocytes in Synapse Formation and Maintenance

Astrocytes have been reported to influence both excitatory and inhibitory synapse formation by direct contact with neurons via activation of integrin receptors. Researchers have also described an intriguing "dance" between fine astrocytic processes (filopodia) and dendritic spines.[43,44] The dynamics of these interactions can be quite rapid: glutamate can precipitate cytoskeletal changes within astrocytes, causing the emergence of filopodia within minutes.[47] Dendritic spines are extremely dynamic and sensitive to changes in neuronal signaling and the microenvironment. They can quickly appear, grow in size, or disappear depending on the signaling dynamic.

Astrocytes have a principal role in stabilizing the spines and changing their size, thus amplifying or reducing the strength of synaptic signaling. Spines that have more sustained contact with astrocytic processes become larger and more stable.[43,44] Communication between the highly motile astrocytic processes and dendritic spines is mediated by ephrine and involves subsequent activation of the corresponding neuronal receptors EphA4.[33,43,44] This type of signaling involving the close contact of cell membranes, also referred to as ephrine/Eph or juxtacrine signaling, has been reported to have a significant role in neurogenesis. Ephrine B of astrocytic origin was reported to support neural stem cell differentiation in the adult hippocampus.[48]

Neuronal–glial juxtaposition and synaptic sealing, involving multiple soluble and juxtacrine factors, is a powerful modulator of synaptic remodeling and regulation of synaptic strength. Neuron–glia interactions induce a rapid response. Within a matter of hours, the number and density of inhibitory (GABA) and excitatory (glutamate) synapses, as well as GABA-A and -B, glutamate, NMDA, and mGlu receptors, are significantly altered.[49,50]

Astrocyte Release of D-Serine Modulates Glutamatergic Transmission and Neuroplasticity

Astrocytes indirectly influence glutamatergic transmission and neuroplasticity by regulating D-serine, a cotransmitter in NMDA-mediated signaling. Astrocytes contain serine racemase, an enzyme responsible for the conversion of L-serine to D-serine.[6] Compromised astrocytic function in MDD may therefore lead to altered D-serine release. D-serine is an endogenous ligand of the glycine receptor and therefore a comodulator of NMDA function and synaptic plasticity.[6] Astroglial coverage of the synapse determines the extent of D-serine available to synaptic NMDA receptors. If astrocytic processes retract from the synapse, the amount of D-serine is reduced, resulting in long-term depression of synaptic function.[8] Conversely, excessive astrocytic release of D-serine and consequent NMDA overstimulation may be toxic to neurons.[7] In support of this view, a study reported that elevation of plasma L-serine and glutamate in depressed patients was directly associated with symptom severity, possibly hinting at astrocytic insufficiency of converting L-serine to D-serine.[51]

Astrocytes Play a Role in Synaptic Elimination

Elimination of unnecessary synapses to improve the efficiency of neural circuitry may also be within the scope of astrocyte activity. Astrocytes may direct the phagocytic cells by tagging the synapses targeted for elimination with C1q, a component of the classical complement cascade. Tagged synapses are subsequently eliminated by phagocytic cells, including microglia, and possibly even astrocytes themselves.[43,44,52]

Astrocytes as the Source of Neurotrophic Signaling

Evidence suggests that neurotrophic factors, such as BDNF and GDNF, as well as cytokines (e.g., TNF), are synthesized within glia cells.[2,15] GDNF released by astroglia has been reported to have neuroprotective properties,[53] especially in the context of NMDA-mediated excitotoxicity. In that context, GDNF supports neuronal survival, at least in part, by stabilizing microglia.[54] Separate research has revealed that astrocytes intervene at the time of elevated inflammatory signaling by releasing GABA, which has a "settling" effect on microglia. Reports indicate that, in addition to a neuroprotective impact of GDNF release, astrocytes also enhance their own survival through autocrine GDNF signaling, that is, influencing the cell that has released the GDNF.[55]

Astrocytes Regulate Microglial Cytokine Signaling

Most likely astrocytic GABA diminishes microglial TNF and IL-6 discharge by exacting an inhibitory influence on their transcription at the nuclear factor kappa-beta (NFκB) level.[39] Several cell types, including lymphocytes, mononuclear cells, neurons, and astrocytes, are capable of secreting TGFβ. TGFβ is related to cytokines and has multiple roles, from supporting neurogenesis and astrocyte proliferation and maturation to regulation of axonal growth and stabilization of microglia in the face of inflammatory signaling.[35,56]

OLIGODENDROGLIA

Research suggests that, beyond their well-established role in axon myelination, oligodendroglia have an independent and instrumental role in the long-term maintenance of axonal functional integrity.[57] Oligodendrocytes, in addition to their small round bodies, possess about half a dozen processes capable of jointly myelinating up to sixty neural axons. Myelin is mostly composed of lipids (70 percent) and, to a lesser extent, proteins (30 percent), including myelin basic protein. The myelin sheath is wrapped around bare axons in concentric layers, called lamellae, much like the rings in the cross section of a tree trunk. Up to one hundred lamellae wrap around an axon, eventually become fused, allowing for more rapid conduction of nerve impulses.[58] Furthermore, oligodendrocytes have a principal role in the development of the nodes of Ranvier—uncovered sections of the axon containing ion channels—which have a key role in saltatory (leaping) propagation of the action potential down the axon.[58]

Oligodendroglia Interact With Neurotransmitters

Membranes of the oligodendrocytes are endowed with multiple ion channels and transmitter receptors, including glutamatergic AMPA, kainate, and NMDA receptors, GABA-A receptors, DA receptors, and purinergic P2X receptors.[58,59] Unlike the opposing influence of these transmitters on neural and astrocytic function, it appears that glutamate, GABA, and ATP all promote depolarization of oligodendroglia, thus hastening the propagation of nerve impulses. Reports indicate that increased K^+ concentration due to neuronal excitation also contributes to oligodendroglia depolarization. Due to the small volume of the myelinating processes, ion influx precipitates osmotic swelling of the myelin sheath, causing significant changes in axonal conduction velocity.[59] Thus, oligodendroglia, by synchronizing the activity of several axons and regulating the pace of impulse propagation, play a major role in regulating neural plasticity, which underpins learning and other adaptive processes in the brain.[58,59]

Oligodendroglia, Glutamate, and Inflammation

Oligodendroglia appear to have a primary role in glutamate clearance from white matter in humans. Oligodendroglia express higher levels of mRNA and protein forms of EAAT-1 and EAAT-2 (the main glial glutamate uptake sites) than even white matter astrocytes. Oligodendrocyte ability to modulate glutamate transmission can be substantially altered by inflammatory cytokines. Incubation of oligodendrocytes with TNF substantially reduced expression of the glutamate transporters, with ensuing accumulation of the excitatory neurotransmitter. Therefore, excessive exposure of oligodendroglia to inflammatory cytokines may underpin glutamate excitotoxicity and axonal damage in the white matter tracts.[60,61]

Inflammatory mediators have an additional way of harming oligodendrocytes. Excessive elevation of TNF, often released by mononuclear cells, microglia, and astrocytes, may reduce the activity of survival pathways within oligodendroglia, while at the same time inducing pro-apoptotic caspase-1 signaling. Such imbalance in activity between pro-apoptotic and survival pathways has been observed to cause oligodendroglial death in vitro and may be a precipitant of demyelination in vivo in the context of pathological states.[62,63]

Oligodendroglia Participate in Neuroplastic Processes

Neurotrophic factors, including BDNF, that are generated and released by oligodendroglia have a significant role in axonal resilience and recovery.[64] Furthermore, neurotrophins such as NGF, BDNF, and neurotrophin-3 (NT-3), via tyrosine receptor kinase (Trk) and p75 neurotrophin receptor (p75NTR) receptors, activate intracellular signaling cascades leading to myelination and cell proliferation.[65–67] Loss of oligodendroglial support appears to promote axonal degeneration and local inflammation, a known pathophysiological substrate for a number of central nervous system (CNS) disorders.[57]

MICROGLIA

Microglia represent 10–12 percent of all the brain cells, making them one of the most numerous cellular populations in the brain, arguably outnumbering the neurons themselves.[68,69] Unlike astrocytes and oligodendrocytes, which share an ectodermal lineage and have a common glial precursor, microglia are the only cell population in the brain of mesodermal origin.[70] As the matter of fact, microglial ancestors have migrated from the yolk sack and joined the development of the neural tube, predating the arrival of the astrocyte/oligodendrocyte predecessors.[69] While microglia have branched away from their peripheral mononuclear bone-marrow-borne cousins early in embryogenesis, it is most likely that subsequent local microenvironments had a decisive role in determining the developmental trajectory of astrocytes and oligodendroglia.[69,71] The early partnership between neurons and microglia bespeaks of its cardinal role in brain development. Sometimes unfairly accused of being the neuronal executioner or cleaner-upper of "apoptotic mess," microglia have a much more complex role in early brain development and its adult function.

Microglia have two distinct phenotypical and functional manifestations. "Resting" microglia may be more appropriately called "surveying" microglia since they act as resident macrophages, constantly screening the CNS environment for any remarkable changes in the molecular environment or neurotransmission.[72] Aside from the two functional phenotypes, microglia are also characterized by significant regional morphological diversity. While surveying microglia have a reticulated morphology, with multiple fine processes detecting the changes in the milieu and synaptic function, activated microglia take on an amoeboid shape of a phagocytic cell.[68,72–74]

Microglia as Synaptic Architects

We mentioned above that microglia are present during early neural development. They have a key role in detecting and removing injured neurons and dysfunctional synapses, thus setting the stage for unencumbered development of neural circuits. Microglial processes are highly motile, making them the fastest-moving cellular structures in the brain. These processes are in continuous contact with presynaptic boutons and perpetually developing dendritic spines. One can conceive of microglia as the hand of Darwinian selection at the cellular level. Synaptic elements of active circuits are allowed to persist; in contrast, low activity or aberrant development will cause microglia-precipitated demise of the affected structures. Elements of the complement system like C1q are expressed by neurons and cause microglial activation; additionally dysfunctional synapses can also be tagged by astroglia—either way, microglia will sense these doomed synaptic structures and engulf and subsequently eliminate them.[69,72–74]

Extended contact between microglia and synapses can either be a good sign or a bad omen for synaptic structures. Researchers have noted that prolonged contact between microglia and dendritic spines can lead to either their growth or their disappearance. Microglial participation in synaptic remodeling has also been dubbed "synaptic stripping." MCP-1 appears to be the principal chemical signal initiating the microglial synaptic stripping. Electron microscopy has identified undigested synaptic structural elements inside microglia, providing direct evidence of their involvement in synaptic destruction.[69,72,73] In addition to synaptic pruning, microglia also partner with T lymphocytes to facilitate neurogenesis in response to an enriched environment.[73]

Microglia Are a Source of Neurotrophic Factors

Microglia are a known source of such neurotrophic factors as BDNF, NT-3, TGFβ1, GDNF, fibroblast growth factor, and NGF, all of which assist in synaptic differentiation, development of neurocircuitry, and neuroplasticity.[69,72–75] Preclinical research has identified microglial-origin BDNF as a key contributor to phosphorylation of neuronal TrkB (a BDNF receptor) and ensuing changes in synaptic plasticity. Thus, microglial BDNF release appears to have a central role in learning and memory-related synaptic plasticity[76] (see figure 7.1). A more balanced view of microglia would suggest that, depending on the circumstances, microglia perform

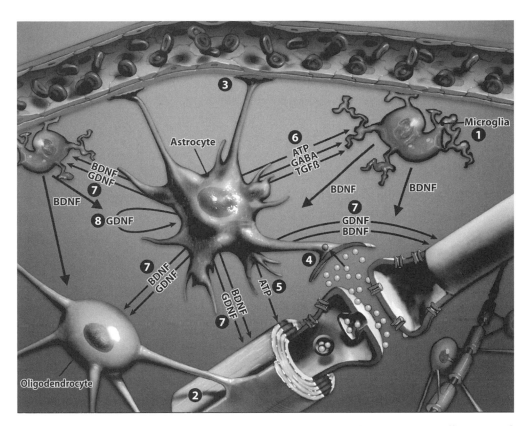

FIGURE 7.1. Glial–neuronal interactions in physiological conditions. Figure illustrates the relationship between glial cells and a glutamate neuron. Numbers in legend refer to corresponding numbers on image. Glial cell functioning is critical to sustaining and optimizing neuronal functioning in the CNS. There are three types of glial cells in the brain: microglia, oligodendrocytes, and astroglia. Microglia are the principal immune cells in the brain. (1) They are involved in monitoring and responding to peripheral inflammatory signals. Oligodendrocytes optimize neuronal signaling by myelination of neuronal axons. (2). Astrocytes serve a number of functions including: maintenance of the blood–brain barrier and facilitation of neurovascular coupling (3); protection of the neuronal synapse (4) by removing excess ions and glutamate before it can diffuse out of the synapse and bind to extrasynaptic NMDA glutamate receptors (which are implicated in neurotoxicity); (5) release of ATP as a modulator of neuronal glutamate release; (6) preventing microglial transformation and stabilizing microglia via release of ATP, GABA, and TGF-β; providing trophic support via BDNF and GDNF to neurons, microglia, and oligodendrocytes (7). GDNF released by the astrocyte also supports the functioning of astrocytes themselves via an autocrine signaling pathway (8). Abbreviations: NMDA, *N*-methyl-d-aspartate; GABA, gamma aminobutyric acid; TGFβ, transforming growth factor beta; BDNF, brain-derived neurotrophic factor; GDNF, glial cell-derived neurotrophic factor; ATP, adenosine triphosphate.

a variety of roles, including the apparently opposing functions of neuroprotection and neural elimination, as well as support of oligodendrogliogenesis and astroglial function.[72,74,77,78]

Microglia Are Recipients and Propagators of Inflammatory Signaling

Microglia are thought to serve as detectors of peripheral stress signals in the CNS. Under usual circumstances, microglia have a protective role; however, in pathological conditions these cells amplify and perpetuate stress signals, contributing to oligodendroglia and neuronal damage.[79–81] Neurotoxicity and apoptosis, as well as oligodendrocyte damage, seem to be instantiated by excessive microglial release of inflammatory cytokines such as IL-1β, IL-6, TNF, ROS, and reactive nitrogen species (nitric oxide synthase [NOS]), combined with diminished neurotrophic support[68,75,77,79,82,83] (figure 7.1). Thus complex neuron–astrocyte–oligodendroglia–microglia interactions have an organizing role in the development of neural circuitry, as well as in processes that underlie learning and memory.[78,82]

Microglial Receptors

Like astrocytes and oligodendroglia, microglia are endowed with a wide variety of receptors, including those for chemokines, cytokines, GABA, glutamate, acetylcholine (ACh), NE, DA, 5HT, SP, and opioids. Adrenergic receptors, including alpha-1 and -2 and beta-1 and -2, have a bivalent role in regulating microglia activation; for the most part they have a stabilizing effect, attenuating an inflammatory response, much like alpha-7 nicotinic ACh receptors (nAChRs).[84,85] Norepinephrine receptor activation stimulates cAMP synthesis, which in turn attenuates NFκB, a well-known transcription factor regulating cytokine synthesis, subsequently downgrading IL-1 and TNF signaling, in addition to decreasing NO and MCP-1 release.[86] 5HT1, 5HT2, 5HT5, and 5HT7 receptors have also been identified in vitro on microglial cells (see figure 7.2). The role of microglial 5HT receptors has not been very well characterized, but they are believed to have a role in modulation of chemotaxis and phagocytic activity.[86] DA-like receptors have also been identified on the surface of microglial membranes, where they may have a role in regulating NO release.[85,86] Activation of microglial cannabinoid receptors (CB1 and CB2), as well as kappa opioid receptors, suppresses neurotoxic effect of microglia and the release of inflammatory mediators. Glutamate and GABA receptors on the microglial membranes have a more nuanced and intricate role.

GABA released from either astrocytes or neurons interacts with microglial GABA-A and GABA-B receptors, diminishing the risk of their transformation into the proinflammatory phenotype. It appears that GABA receptor activation initiates an intracellular cascade that downregulates NFκB, a key transcription factor involved in cytokine synthesis.[38,39,85] Providing almost a yin–yang kind of symmetry, glutamate signaling via mGlu2 receptors induces release of TNF and microglial transformation into neurotoxic phenotype. The relevance of microg-

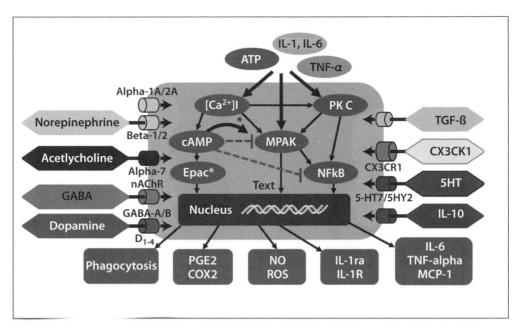

FIGURE 7.2. Microglia may be activated by a number of chemical signals, including proinflammatory cytokines (e.g., IL-1 and TNF-alpha), endogenous and exogenous antigens), or ATP. Once activated microglia produce proinflammatory cytokines, chemokines and ROS and RNS (nitric oxide). Synthesis of inflammatory compounds is mediated by mobilization of signaling pathways such as MAPK and NFk B via PKC or intracellular calcium signaling. Norepinephrine may inhibit microglial inflammatory transformation via mobilization of cAMP and suppression of downstream MAPK and/or NFk B. Alternatively, NE (possibly via alpha-1B receptors) may also activate MAPK and/or NFk B, and aid production of pro-inflammatory compounds. Stimulated microglia produce various substances such as inflammatory cytokines, prostaglandins, chemokines (MCP-1 and CX3CK-1) and participate in phagocytosis. Acetylcholine via alpha-7 nAChRs, GABA via GABA-A and -B receptors, dopamine via D1-4 receptors, CX3CK1 (also known as fractalkine), TGF-beta and IL-10, via their corresponding receptors all stabilize microglia, while 5HT via 5HT2 and -7 receptors may facilitate its proinflammatory transformation. For a list of abbreviations see Table 7.1.

lial ionotropic glutamatergic AMPA and NMDA receptors remains to be established.[85] Not only can dysregulated and excessive glutamate signaling precipitate TNF release, but the reverse is also true. TNF activation of its microglial receptors may induce glutamate release from these cells.[85,87]

Furthermore, immune activation of microglia mediated by toll-like receptor-4 precipitates the release of ATP from microglia. Microglial ATP, via astrocytic purinergic P2Y1R receptors, in a feed-forward fashion, induces astrocytes to discharge additional ATP, which feeds back to purinergic receptors, causing astrocytes to release glutamate. Astrocytic glutamate interacts with the presynaptic neuronal mGlu-5 receptors leading to augmentation of excitatory glutamatergic transmission.[73,88]

There is another example where microglia and astrocytes cooperate to amplify glutamate signaling. The stroma-cell-derived factor CXC is a chemokine that signals to CXCR-4 receptors located both on microglia and astrocytes. Microglia again act as a signal amplifier by releasing copious amounts of TNF, eliciting a robust release of glutamate from astrocytes, possibly inducing neurotoxicity.[89] Although in vitro studies have identified ionotropic glutamatergic and GABAergic receptors on microglia, in vivo evidence suggests that constitutional GABA and glutamate signals indirectly influence microglia function by the way of ATP mediation.[90]

Microglial On and Off Signals

ATP and its derivatives, including adenosine diphosphate and adenosine, are important components of the microglial signaling repertoire used for communication with other neural elements including astroglia and oligodendroglia. ATP, acting in an autocrine as well as paracrine manner, participates in on and off signaling regulating microglial activation. In addition to purinergic metabotropic P2Y and ionotropic P2X receptors, microglia are also equipped with adenosine A2 and A3 receptors.[85,91] ATP signaling, conveyed by subclasses of P2Y receptors, modulates the motility of microglial processes and, by its beacon-like chemotactic action, microglial response to neuronal injury, which includes phagocytosis. "On" signaling via P2X receptors, in addition "off" chemotactic influence, initiates the microglial metamorphosis, as well as release of inflammatory mediators such as TNF and superoxide, and growth factors, which contribute to establishment of neuropathic pain.[85,91] Adenosine, by engaging its receptors, further contributes to the on signal by inducing cyclooxygenase-2 with ensuing prostaglandin (PG) synthesis.[85] SP offers its contribution to the on signal by activating its neurokinin-1 receptors, resulting in chemotaxis, NO, and prostaglandin E2 (PGE2) release.[85] We have already discussed the role of glutamate AMPA- and mGlu2/3-mediated microglial activation and TNF release. Furthermore, preclinical studies have provided evidence that 5HT7 signaling may provoke microglial activation and IL-6 release[92] (see figure 7.2).

Other important on signals remind us that microglia are, after all, career immune cells. Toll-like receptors, which respond to a wide range of microbial antigens and substances of endogenous origin, are probably one of the principal microglial activators in the physiological circumstances. Pattern recognition receptors, most likely originally designed to sense pathogen-related molecular patterns, have achieved notoriety due to one of its members' involvement in the pathophysiology of Alzheimer's disease, diabetes, and assorted malignancies.[68] Microglia also respond to an array of environmental toxins, pesticides and heavy metals.[68]

Some of the on signaling is conducted through direct contact between neural and microglial membranes. Developing synapses express complement proteins, such as C3a, C5a, and C1q, which interact with their matching receptors on microglial membranes, precipitating phagocytosis of the "marked" synapses.[72,78] This is an essential component of developmental pruning, resulting in greater efficiency of brain circuitry.

Microglia can also be activated due to inadequate presence of the off signals. One of the key neuronal "stay at rest" signals, fractalkine or CX3CL1, is constitutively expressed by healthy neurons and received by CX3CR1 microglial receptors.[72,73,78] Additionally, neurons express CD200, a membrane glycoprotein that interacts with corresponding microglial CD200 receptor, thus providing a calming influence and preventing neurotoxicity.[78,93] Other prominent off signals are delivered to microglia by NE acting through beta and alpha-2 receptors; by ACh via alpha-7 nAChRs; by endogenous cannabinoids through CB1 and CB2 receptors; by anti-inflammatory cytokines such as TGFβ and IL-10; by growth factors, including BDNF, NGF, and NT-3 interacting with their respective receptors; by endogenous opioids via kappa receptors; by GABA activation of GABA-A and GABA-B receptors; and by steroids, including estrogen and glucocorticoids.[68,84,85,94]

Microglia Are a Source of Multiple Chemical Signals

Microglial cells have a capacity to synthesize and release PGs, proinflammatory cytokines, ROS and RNS, ATP, growth factors, glutamate, and quinolinic acid (QUIN).[73,85] (A more detailed discussion regarding aberrant astroglial and microglial tryptophan (TRP) metabolism in the context of MDD is given below.) BDNF is released from microglial cells in response to ATP signaling via P2X4 receptors. Once released, BDNF may partake in autocrine signaling by interacting with a truncated version of the neurotrophin TrkB receptor, suppressing microglia activation and NO release.[86] Additionally, BDNF of microglial origin may compromise neuronal K^+/Cl^- exchange transporters, reducing the effect of inhibitory GABA signaling.[73]

SUMMARY

This brief review of the cellular function in the brain may leave us with a different understanding of cerebral organization. It is becoming increasing clear that the concept of the synapse as the main functional signaling unit in the brain needs an update. Even the slightly newer concept of the tripartite synapse, incorporating astrocytes, may have been transcended. An alternative view is to consider a neural–glial junction, comprising pre- and postsynaptic neurons, synapse, astroglia, microglia, and oligodendroglia, as the key processing/homeostatic unit in the brain. All these cellular elements have their specialties but also share a common language. Microglia are immune cells that are also proficient in the language of neural signaling. They can process a great array of molecules informing them of environmental change. Microglia's varied output in the form of cytokines, ATP, glutamate, ROS, RNS, and growth factors is accepted and deciphered primarily by astrocytes but also by neurons and oligodendroglia. In physiological circumstances their conversation, including inflammatory cytokine signaling, subserves homeostatic adjustments and neuroplasticity—in other words, it is the basis for adaptation, learning, and memory. This is nature's processing chip, composed of the neuron–glial junction, which can make fine adjustments in GABA/glutamate balance, influencing not only the key inhibitory/excitatory transmitter balance but also the relationship between inflammatory and anti-inflammatory signaling in the brain. (GABA has an anti-inflammatory, and glutamate, an inflammatory potential.)

This is also as good a time as any to disabuse ourselves of the outdated distinctions between "inflammatory molecules" and neurotrophic factors. In physiological circumstances, typical "inflammatory" cytokines, such as IL-6 and TNF, participate in neural scaling and regulation of neuroplasticity, principal elements of learning and memory.[95] The relationship between glia and neurons is ancient in evolutionary terms. Even the roundworm *Caenorhabditis elegans*, along with its modest 302 neurons, possesses glia cells. Glia allow it to harmoniously integrate information from the external environment and make subtle adjustments in its humble nervous system.[96] In the human brain, intricate communication at the neuron–glia junction influences not only neural plasticity but, through adjustments of oligodendroglia function, myelination of white matter tracts. Therefore, aberrant glia–neuronal relationships are likely to contribute to malformation and dysfunction of neural circuitry, causing cognitive problems.[78,79,82]

Glia–neuronal interaction may be a key element of mind-body communication, including the stress response. Preclinical studies have established that stress may increase microglial concentration and prime the CNS for an inflammatory response, either by glucocorticoid-induced escalation in NMDA–glutamate transmission or by suppression of the CD200 regulatory off signaling between neurons and microglia.[80,83,97]

Contributions of Glial Pathology to MDD

The role of glia cells in etiopathogenesis of MDD has been unduly neglected for a long time. The last three decades of research have generated a body of evidence suggesting that glia cells may be the cornerstone of MDD-related pathohistology.[2,5,6,15,87,98–100] Earlier studies did not emphasize the cytological differences in the glia cells involved in the MDD neuropathology.

Alterations in glial cell density and morphology have been reported in the subgenual anterior cingulate cortex (sgACC), dorsolateral prefrontal cortex (dlPFC), orbitofrontal cortex (OFC), and amygdala of unmedicated MDD patients,[2,100–103] and it appears that both astroglia and oligodendroglia may be affected. One study noted a significant reduction of glia density in the dlPFC and OFC of MDD subjects.[98] Further supporting glial involvement in mood disorders,[104] another study observed a significant alteration in glial density and neuronal morphology in the dentate gyrus of the hippocampus in MDD subjects.[105]

While some studies noted changes in neuronal density in conjunction with morphological and numerical changes in glia population in the orbital PFC,[98] others have had discrepant findings. Some researchers noted only morphological neuronal changes in the ACC of depressed patients,[106] others reported both changes in glia density and numbers as well as a decrease in ACC neuronal size and density,[107] while yet others described reduction in glia density in sgACC in familial MDD patients with no concomitant changes in neuronal morphology or numbers.[104]

Preclinical findings in rodents provide further support to the hypothesis of glial dysfunction as the primary cytopathology in MDD. Studies utilized a neurotoxin and glial toxin to selectively deplete their respective cell populations in the rodent PFC. Glial damage, unlike neuronal loss, was associated with impaired performance in several animal models of depression, including ones reflecting learned helplessness (forced swim test), harm avoidance, and anhedonia (sucrose preference test.) Researchers concluded that glial loss in the PFC may be sufficient to induce depressive behaviors in rodents.[108]

ALTERATIONS IN OLIGODENDROGLIA STRUCTURE AND FUNCTION IN MDD

In addition to morphological changes, one study describes a prominent 19 percent reduction in oligodendroglia, due to apoptosis and necrosis, in the dlPFC (Brodmann area [BA] 9) of MDD patients.[100] Further extending these findings, the same group reported a substantial reduction (19–25 percent) in oligodendrocyte densities in the pregenual ACC and dlPFC of depressed patients relative to control subjects.[100,109] Keeping in mind the pivotal role that the dlPFC and pregenual ACC play in executive function and "top-down" limbic regulation, the implications of this finding are striking, because it may provide a neurobiological explanation for emotional dysregulation and cognitive dysfunction, both commonly observed in MDD. Another study found a reduction in oligodendrocyte density in the amygdala of depressed patients, without concomitant changes in astrocyte and microglia density, relative to control group. This is an intriguing finding, possibly pointing to the primacy of oligodendroglial changes in MDD cellular pathology.[110] Alteration in oligodendrocyte function in the dlPFC of MDD patients was further confirmed in a study that found less intense myelin staining in the deep white matter of depressed subjects compared with controls.[111] All of these formations have an important role in the stress response, emotional regulation, and executive function.

We mentioned in Chapter 8 that several diffusion tensor imaging studies, aimed at evaluating the integrity of white matter tracts, found aberrant connectivity in corticolimbic pathways in MDD patients. A five-year prospective study reported impaired functional integrity of white matter in adolescents who have experienced childhood maltreatment and subsequently developed depression. Superior longitudinal fasciculi, connecting frontal, parietal, temporal, and occipital lobes, believed to play an important role in executive function and emotional regulation, had greater disruption of integrity, as measured by fractional anisotropy, in maltreated depressed adolescents compared with their healthy counterparts.[112] There was a parallel finding in the cingulo-hippocampal white matter tract involved in emotional regulation, especially in stressful circumstances.[112]

Several genetic studies have provided accumulating evidence of dysfunction in oligodendroglia-related genes in the temporal cortex and subcortical regions of deceased MDD patients relative to unaffected individuals.[113-115] A transcriptional profiling study identified aberrant expression of 17 oligodendroglia-related genes in MDD subjects compared with healthy controls.[113] Furthermore, another study noted an antidepressant dose-related increase in genetic expression of Olig-1, an oligodendoglial transcription factor, in depressed subjects; elevated gene expression was presumed to be of compensatory nature.[116]

ALTERATIONS IN S100B, AN ASTROGLIA AND OLIGODENDROGLIA MARKER, IN MDD

Age-dependent decrements in astroglial markers were reported in a group of MDD subjects.[105,117,118] Several studies have assessed serum levels of S100B, a protein expressed by oligodendrocytes and astrocytes. S100B is a glia-expressed calcium-binding protein, which can have a bivalent effect in the CNS, depending on its concentration. In nanomolar concentrations S100B confers multiple neurotrophic and neuroprotective benefits; in contrast, in micromolar concentrations it can be a harbinger of neural degenerative processes.[119]

In vitro studies have demonstrated a reciprocal relationship between proinflammatory cytokines and S100B. Higher concentrations of S100B induced the release of IL-1 and IL-6 from neurons and microglial cells;[120,121] conversely IL-1β, IL-6, IL-8, and TNF all stimulate glial S100B secretion mediated by the mitogen-activated protein kinase (MAPK) pathway.[122,123] Postmortem studies have reported decreased S100B-immunoreactive astrocytes in both MDD and bipolar disorder, while lower density of immunoreactive oligodendroglia was a characteristic only of bipolar illness, possibly reflecting subtle differences in cytopathology between these two conditions.[124]

Depressed patients tend to manifest an elevation of serum and plasma S100B relative to healthy controls. Higher peripheral concentrations of S100B correlated with female gender, a greater number of previous depressive episodes, family history of depression, severity of depressive symptoms on admission, and cognitive disturbance scores.[125-127] Serum levels of S100B subsided with effective antidepressant treatment and resolution of depressive symptomatology.[125,128] One has to be reserved in interpreting these peripheral oligodendroglia/astroglia markers, since they are significantly influenced by body mass index, as well as markers of adipose tissue dysfunction, such as leptin and adipocyte-type fatty acid binding protein.[129] Boundaries may be a bit blurry in attempting to dissect the influence of stress and adiposity versus MDD on peripheral levels of S100B, as they appeared to have a shared pathophysiological signature.[130–132]

As is the case with several other biomarkers, the "Goldilocks principle" applies to levels of S100B in cerebrospinal fluid (CSF) and the risk of depression. Either too much or too little S100B may be problematic. A study examined S100B levels in a group of neurological patients with noninflammatory disorders. Lower CSF S100B levels were associated with higher Beck Depression Inventory–II scores, reflecting a greater symptom severity.[133] Some authors have gone as far as to suggest that MDD may be a consequence of astroglial bioenergetics dysfunction.[134]

ALTERATIONS IN ASTROGLIA DENSITY AND FUNCTION IN MDD

We have previously described the glia–synaptic junction, composed of pre- and postsynaptic neurons, astroglia, oligodendroglia, and microglia, as the main information- processing "chip" in the brain. Arguably, astroglia have a key role in regulating the glia–synaptic microenvironment in terms of neurotransmitter, ion, energy, neurotrophin, and cytokine trafficking. Additionally, astroglia are the main regulator of neurovascular coupling, ensuring adequate vascularization of the busy brain tissue. Postmortem studies have detected significant differences in astroglial markers such as glial fibrillary acidic protein (GFAP), gap junction proteins (connexin 40 and 43), and water channel aquaporin-4 in depressed patients relative to the control group. These differences were noted in the ACC, OFC, medial PFC (mPFC), dlPFC, amygdala, hippocampus, thalamic structures, basal ganglia, and the NE-producing locus coeruleus.[3,117,135] One study investigated the influence of age and MDD on the packing density of GFAP-positive astrocytes in the dlPFC. Individuals afflicted with MDD had a much steeper correlation between reduction of GFAP levels and age relative to healthy controls, suggesting a synergy between the aging process and disease state in reducing glia density in the dlPFC.[118,136] These brain areas are the same ones implicated by imaging studies as having altered structure and function in MDD. These "usual suspects" are also the key components of the executive cognitive, salience, and default-mode functional networks. Moreover, expression of mRNA and proteins of the glial glutamate transporters EAAT-1 and -2, as well as glutamine synthase, is also altered in the PFC, ACC, hippocampus, and amygdala of depressed patients compared with control group.[3]

Magnetic resonance spectroscopic studies have also found indirect evidence of astroglia-related glutamatergic dysfunction in depressed patients, which improved after successful antidepressant treatment.[137] Widespread astrocyte-associated disturbances in glutamate signaling are one of the key pathophysiological underpinnings of MDD. Furthermore, astrocytic contribution to aberrant neurovascular coupling has been suggested by imunofluorescent staining of aquaporin-4, an astroglial marker in the ventromedial PFC of depressed patients. Compared with control group, depressed individuals had a 50 percent reduction in astrocyte end-foot coverage of cerebral blood vessels, most likely impacting water homeostasis, blood flow, and glucose metabolism.[138]

MICROGLIAL CHANGES IN MDD

A study using immunohistochemistry assessed microglia density in the dlPFC, ACC, mediodorsal thalamus, and hippocampus of depressed patients. The authors suggested that significant microgliosis (i.e., increased number of microglia) in depressed patients who committed suicide relative to healthy controls may be a marker of presuicidal stress. They hypothesized that proinflammatory mediators released from microglia may have altered 5HT and NE transmission and contributed to suicidality.[139] A more recent study from the same group found elevated immunoreactivity related to QUIN in sgACC and anterior mid-cingulate microglia of acutely depressed, suicidal subjects compared with healthy controls.[119] Given that QUIN is a known antagonist of glutamatergic NMDA and alpha-7 nAChRs, this study may provide additional insight into microglia-related glutamate and ACh dysfunction underlying the cognitive and emotional symptoms of MDD. Deficient alpha-7 nicotinic ACh and NE signaling in MDD may also promote microglial activation and ensuing CNS inflammation.[84] A genetic study associating a vulnerability allele of a gene coding for purinergic P2RX7 receptor with MDD provides further evidence of compromised ATP signaling, which has a stabilizing influence on microglia.[78]

NEURONAL CHANGES IN MDD

In contrast to relatively consistent findings of widespread glial abnormalities, neuronal changes appear to be subtler and more discrete in MDD. Several authors have noted decreased pyramidal somal size in hippocampus,[105] ACC,[106] dlPFC (BA 9),[102] and OFC (BA 47) in postmortem studies of MDD patients compared with unaffected controls.[103] Reduction in neuronal size is much more pronounced in elderly depressed patients than in younger cohorts.

One study found 20–60 percent decreases in density of pyramidal glutamatergic neurons in the OFC in a group of depressed patients older than 60 compared with matched controls. This is a particularly intriguing finding, given that layers III and V of the OFC give rise to multiple corticolimbic projections and also act as principal recipients of thalamocortical pathways.[140] Furthermore, decreased neuronal density was reported in the dlPFC, ventral PFC, and ACC.[98,135,141,142] A 50 percent reduction in the density and 18 percent decrease in size of a subset of GABAergic interneurons immunoreactive for calcium binding proteins were reported in the dlPFC, accompanied by less pronounced changes in the OFC of depressed individuals relative to unaffected controls.[143] However, most of the postmortem pathohistological studies of depression did not find a decrease in neuronal numbers or density.[3]

Several reports indicate reductions in dendritic branching in the ACC of depressed suicide victims,[144] dendritic length in the dlPFC of depressed subjects, and synaptic density in the PFC of MDD patients, compared with control groups.[141,145] The distribution of glial and neuronal pathology in MDD remarkably overlaps with the findings from structural and functional imaging studies.

NEUROTROPHIC FACTORS

Multiple lines of convergent evidence including preclinical, imaging, biochemical, and pathological studies all point to abnormalities in neuroplasticity and neurotrophic signaling in MDD. Before we begin our discussion of neurotrophic changes in the disease state, we briefly review physiological function and regulation of the neuroplasticity mediators.

BDNF is by far the most researched neuroplasticity modulator in the context of MDD. In addition to its role in neuroplastic processes, BDNF also acts as a resilience factor, assists the maturation and differentiation of the nerve cell progenitors,[146] and even acts as an immunomodulator in the periphery.[147] BDNF is released from neurons in two forms, as pro-BDNF and its chemically abbreviated version, mature BDNF. These two molecules exercise opposing functions. Pro-BDNF binds to p75 receptor, initiating apoptosis, manifested initially by retraction and shriveling of neuronal processes, followed by programmed death of the neurons. By contrast, mature BDNF has primary affinity for TrkB receptors, which mediate maturation of neuronal progenitor cells, neuroplasticity, and resilience.[148] The tissue-type plasminogen activator–plasminogen–plasmin cascade is crucial for the cleavage of pro-BDNF into mature BDNF. Preclinical research has provided evidence that application of electroconvulsive therapy (ECT) to produce an electroconvulsive seizure will increase synthesis of pro-BDNF and tissue-type plasminogen activator and subsequently elevate conversion into mature BDNF in the rodent hippocampus.[149]

INTERACTIONS BETWEEN BDNF AND IMMUNE SIGNALING

The immune system and neuroplasticity are involved in a very intricate dance of mutual regulation. Proinflammatory cytokines induce NOS, a pivotal enzyme mediating nitrogen oxide (NO) synthesis. NOS induction following exposure to inflammatory cytokines has been observed in microglial, astrocytic, and neuronal preparations.[150–152] Moreover, postmortem research has revealed elevated NOS in hippocampal neurons of deceased depressed patients.[152] Additionally, preclinical studies have reported a suppressant effect of NO on BDNF synthesis.[153] In contrast, constitutively released TNF and IL-6 may enhance BDNF secretion from human monocytes.[154] There is even evidence of "cooperation" among TNF, NGF, and BDNF in stimulating NFκB, a principal transcription factor mediating cytokine synthesis.[155]

Evidence points to participation of several inflammatory mediators in regulation of neuroplasticity and learning. Neural injury caused by proinflammatory cytokines may be in part attributed to induction of cyclooxygenase and ensuing PG synthesis and release.[156] Reports have implicated PGs in memory processes. Direct injection of PG into the rodent dorsal hippocampus was sufficient to impair memory and reduce postconditioning BDNF levels.[156] Furthermore, cyclooxygenase-2 activation includes induction of NOS with ensuing accumulation of NO, and potentially inhibitory effects on BDNF synthesis.[153,157]

HORMONES AND NEUROTRANSMITTERS INFLUENCE BDNF SIGNALING

Multiple signaling pathways have a convergent influence on neurotrophic factor synthesis. Preclinical data also demonstrate that a loss of diurnal rhythm of corticosterone secretion impairs BDNF function.[158] Altered astroglia function in MDD may have significant ramifications on neurotrophic signaling. Researchers have demonstrated a significant increase of BDNF in astroglial cultures treated with NE, DA and 5HT, establishing an important relationship between monoaminergic neuronal activity and astroglial neurotrophic support.[159] In physiological circumstances astroglia regulate synaptic glutamate content by taking up the excessive neurotransmitter. Glutamate released from astroglia has a bivalent influence on BDNF synthesis. However, astroglia stimulated by inflammatory cytokines or oxidative stress release glutamate almost exclusively into the extrasynaptic space, where it binds to extrasynaptic NMDA receptors.[8] Unlike activation of synaptic NMDA receptors, which promotes BDNF release, activation of extrasynaptic NMDA receptors powerfully suppresses BDNF synthesis through a CREB-dependent mechanism.[160] Thus, local balance of glutamate, GABA, and monoamines and its influence on the glia–synaptic junction is very influential in determining BDNF tone and neuroplasticity.

THE ROLE OF BDNF IN MDD AND ITS TREATMENT

Indirect evidence pointing to the relevance of BDNF in the etiology of MDD comes from treatment studies. Multiple treatment interventions with proven efficacy in MDD, also influence BDNF signaling. Different antidepressant classes, including tricyclic and heterocyclic antidepressants, monoamine oxidase inhibitors, selective 5HT reuptake inhibitors (SSRIs), 5HT-NE reuptake inhibitors (SNRIs), and NE reuptake inhibitors (NRIs), and ketamine (an NMDA receptor antagonist), as well as ECT, repetitive transcranial magnetic stimulation, exercise, and even psychotherapy have been implicated in modulation of BDNF, neuroplasticity, and neurogenesis.[161–166] Both peripheral and central administration of BDNF, in preclinical models, produces behavioral anxiolytic- and antidepressant-like effects accompanied by modulation of glutamate, 5HT, and NE transmission, as well as increased synaptic signaling survival of newborn neural progenitors.[161,163,167]

Antidepressant effects on BDNF signaling are, at least in part, mediated by their ability to elevate monoamine transmission thus activating different classes of NE and 5HT receptors. Activation of the beta-adrenergic receptors may be necessary for elevation in BDNF mRNA induced by monoamine oxidase inhibitors and exercise, while 5HT2A/2C binding provides minor contribution in exercise-mediated BDNF increase.[167] Some of the 5HT-receptor-related enhancement in BDNF signaling might be due to its ability to modulate GABA and glutamate transmission and thus influence BDNF synthesis.[168] Additionally, autocrine BDNF signaling via its TrkB receptor may be required for antidepressant action.[169]

Several intracellular pathways, including monoamine receptor–G-protein-coupled cAMP–protein kinase A–CREB; Wnt–GSK; Ras–MAPK–extracellular regulated kinase–CREB; and phosphoinositide 3-kinase (PI3K)–Akt, seem to be involved in transducing the signal from the surface of the cell to transcription factors regulating the BDNF synthesis.[161,162] Binding of BDNF to its TrkB receptor initiates several intracellular signaling cascades, including CaMK-II, MAPK, PLC-gamma, and PI3K/Akt-mediated signaling. The PI3K–Akt intracellular signaling cascade is particularly important for the antiapoptotic BDNF benefits, as its downstream action includes increased activation of Bcl-2 (a resilience-boosting, antiapoptotic molecule) and inhibition of caspase-9 and GSK-3 (which brings on cellular demise).[161] Thus, autocrine BDNF signaling, where BDNF engages the TrkB receptors on the same cell that has released it, may play an important role in the feed-forward loop that propagates antiapoptotic effect and neural resilience.

A substantial body of preclinical research provides indirect support to the neurotrophic theory of depression. Ability of antidepressants to promote BDNF signaling appears to vary by pharmacological class of the agent, dose, and timing. Due to substantial differences in methodology, studies have generated divergent data, which are often difficult to interpret. Several investigators have reported a biphasic effect of antidepressants, whereby administration of the agent in the short term (hours) negatively impacts BDNF synthesis, unlike long-term influence (weeks), which facilitates it.[168,170,171] Different antidepressants and electroconvulsive seizure (presumably animal equivalent of ECT) regulate distinct BDNF promoters in a brain-region- and disease-specific manner.[171–174] Furthermore, higher doses of one antidepressant (venlafaxine) were reported to have a suppressant effect on BDNF signaling compared with lower doses of the same agent.[175] While some of the studies reported a greater impact of serotonergic agents, others have given an advantage to noradrenergic antidepressants and their capacity to enhance BDNF signaling.[168,171,176] The timing of BDNF response may also differ. While noradrenergic agents, ECT, and exercise may elevate BDNF mRNA more rapidly, SSRIs may require a longer period to achieve the same goal.[174]

Regardless the differences, it appears that both SSRIs and NRIs rely on their ability to increase monoamine signaling to effect BDNF synthesis. In monoamine-depleted mice neither an NRI nor an SSRI was capable of elevating BDNF-TrkB–mediated signaling.[176] Furthermore, blocking NE transmission completely abolished the beneficial impact of exercise on the BDNF mRNA synthesis in the rodent hippocampus, while a 5HT antagonist still allowed for significant BDNF mRNA elevation. Authors of the study concluded that the ameliorative impact of exercise on BDNF synthesis may be predominantly mediated by the increase in NE transmission.[161] Intriguingly, antidepressants and exercise interact in an additive manner in their support of BDNF signaling and neuroplasticity.[161]

Most of the evidence substantiating the association between MDD and abnormalities in BDNF signaling originates from the studies involving peripheral blood levels of depressed patients. More direct support comes from the postmortem studies. One of these postmortem studies reported reduced expression of the pro-neuroplastic TrkB receptors, and elevated expression of pro-apoptotic p75NTR BDNF receptors in the PFC and hippocampus of suicide subjects (Major Depression was the most frequent diagnosis), relative to the control group.[177] Moreover, there may be an association between the CSF BDNF levels in depressed patients and suicidal ideation, assessed by a standardized scale.[178] Another study utilized peripheral blood samples to study the relationship between pro-BDNF, mature BDNF, and their primary receptors and depression scores on a standardized scale. Serum pro-BDNF and p75NTR levels were positively correlated, while mature BDNF and cognate TrkB receptor concentrations were negatively associated with the clinical measures of depression severity.[179] Furthermore, peripheral BDNF levels may be relevant indicators of the brain neurotrophin signaling since a correlation was found between the serum BDNF and the absolute cerebral concentration of *N*-acetylaspartate, a marker of neuronal integrity.[180] The relationship between peripheral BDNF levels and its brain function remains an open question.

Using a clever design, a group of investigators attempted to assess the proportion of brain-origin BDNF in the peripheral blood. Authors collected the blood directly from the jugular vein, reflecting the brain contribution to BDNF levels, and the arterial blood from the brachial artery. The venoarterial BDNF plasma concentration gradient represented an index of brain BDNF production. Significant correlation was noted between the suicide risk and the measure of brain-origin BDNF, but no relationship was found with the severity of depression.[181]

Moreover, previously non-psychiatrically ill individuals who have attempted suicide in response to psychosocial stress were found to have similarly decreased serum BDNF levels as depressed patients compared with the healthy controls.[182] Given that stress is also an established precipitant of depressive episodes and a trigger for inflammatory response, it is attractive to speculate about the relationship among stress, inflammation, and disruption in neurotrophic signaling as a potential trigger of suicidal ideations.

Numerous studies have explored the relationship between serum BDNF levels and various characteristics of MDD. Although the mechanism of serum BDNF regulation has not been fully elucidated, research indicates that it mostly originates from platelets.[183] Investigators have discovered an association between the serum BDNF levels and hippocampal volume in the first-episode, medication-free depressed patients.[184] One could speculate that disruption in the BDNF signaling may be linked with depression early in its course, but it might also explain some of the memory/learning deficits and endocrine perturbations, given the hippocampal role in these processes. Some of the studies have found a relationship between decreased serum BDNF levels and the severity of depression, as well as anxious/somatic symptomatology.[185] Diminished serum BDNF may also correlate with the duration of the previous depressive episode and persist even in the remitted state.[185]

Although most of the studies have found lower serum BDNF levels in MDD patients, relative to healthy controls, correlation with the severity of depression and disease recurrence has been inconsistent.[183,186–190] If we assume the changes in serum BDNF may reflect the severity of depression, one would anticipate lower neurotrophin levels in dysthymia than in MDD, and research data have borne out this expectation.[189] Additionally, while some researchers reported "normalization" of serum BDNF levels with successful treatment, other authors have noted treatment-related elevation of serum, but not to the level of healthy controls.[187,188] Even patients in sustained remission, lasting more than eight weeks, had a lower whole-blood BDNF level than did the healthy control group.[191]

The role of BDNF perturbations in MDD remission is further supported by TRP depletion studies. Healthy individuals respond to TRP depletion by elevating serum BDNF, but no such "compensatory" response takes place in MDD, possibly reflecting a flawed homeostatic mechanism.[192] If a peripheral increase in BDNF levels indeed reflects amelioration of depressive symptomatology, it stands to reason that it should correlate with antidepressant response. A study reported that increases in serum BDNF levels to 126 percent of the baseline after a week of antidepressant treatment, in concert with 50 percent reduction in their Hamilton Depression Rating Scale 17-item version (HAMD17) over the same time period, predicts the ultimate treatment response with 100 percent specificity.[193]

There may be some significant distinctions between plasma and serum BDNF levels in MDD. A group of researchers reported an association between clinical improvement following antidepressant treatment and elevation of plasma levels of BDNF; at the same time, serum levels of BDNF remained unchanged and consistently lower than in healthy controls.[194] The study authors speculated that plasma BDNF may be more of a state marker, while serum BDNF may be an indicator of trait. It may be premature to reach such a conclusion regarding serum BDNF as a trait marker, as many other studies have reported a correlation among antidepressant-induced clinical improvement, serum BDNF, and increased BDNF mRNA in the peripheral blood cells.[195] Lower plasma BDNF has been associated with childhood physical neglect and verbal memory impairment in the context of MDD, recurrence of depressive episodes, nonpsychotic depression, and suicidal behavior in MDD.[196,197] As the matter of fact, one study not only found no difference in plasma BDNF levels between nonsuicidal depressed patients and healthy controls but also reported that plasma BDNF levels beyond a certain specified point accurately classified suicidal depressed patients with 68.7 percent sensitivity and 78.1 percent specificity.[198]

Important gender differences may exist regarding BDNF regulation in MDD. Serum BDNF may be lower in depressed female patients than in males and is more likely to be correlated with the severity of depression as measured by the standardized scales.[186] Additionally, treatment response was reflected in serum BDNF increase in female but not male depressed individuals following a four-week course of antidepressant treatment.[199] Furthermore, women may have a greater reactivity of the BDNF regulatory mechanism in the face of adversity than do men. Researchers have discovered that women at high risk for developing depression who have experienced three or more stressful life events had significantly lower whole-blood BDNF levels compared with high-risk women who experienced only two or fewer stressful events.[200] There was no correlation between stressful life events and whole-blood BDNF levels in low-risk women or in men.[200] Overall, evidence suggests that women may have more sensitive BDNF regulatory mechanisms, manifested by a more pronounced decline in peripheral BDNF levels in face of adversity and ensuing depression, but also a more robust rebound following treatment intervention.

Due to wide variations in methodology and outcomes, it is difficult to draw overarching conclusions from individual studies exploring the relationship between peripheral BDNF levels and clinical characteristics of MDD. Results of meta-analyses may be more enlightening. A summary of data indicates that depressed individuals have lower plasma and serum BDNF—mature BDNF levels are particularly decreased—compared with healthy controls.[201-203] Moreover, peripheral BDNF levels tend to negatively correlate with the severity of depression (the lower the BDNF levels, the higher the depression scores on standardized scales).[201,202] Although successful antidepressant treatment is associated with elevation of peripheral BDNF levels, most often they still lag behind BDNF concentrations in healthy individuals.[201,202]

Several critical questions regarding the role of BDNF in the treatment of MDD have been raised. Is the BDNF-mediated support of neurogenesis and maturation of progenitor cells a crucial aspect of antidepressant treatment? How relevant is the BDNF-associated support of neuroplasticity and neural resilience in the treatment of MDD? Is the increase in BDNF a necessary feature of antidepressant therapies?

Let us begin with a review of the evidence supporting the importance of BDNF and neurogenesis in MDD etiology and treatment. MDD has been associated with a progressive volumetric decline in limbic (incorporating hippocampus), paralimbic (including ACC), and PFC areas, critical for unfettered stress response and emotional regulation.[204] Postmortem studies of mostly depressed suicide subjects have discovered compromised BDNF and TrkB expression in the hippocampus and PFC of these individuals compared with controls.[177,205] Peripheral studies have revealed reduced blood BDNF levels in depressed patients, which tend to normalize with antidepressant treatment.[161–163] Moreover, elderly depressed patients who experienced a clinical response to exercise also manifested a normalization of BDNF serum concentrations.[206] Several risk factors for depression, including extended sleep loss, chronic stress, and inflammation, are all capable of suppressing neurogenesis in the hippocampus and/or PFC.[207] BDNF is an influential trophic factor regulating NE and 5HT signaling in the brain.[161] Peripheral and direct CNS administration of BDNF enhances the survival of the newborn cells in the hippocampus.[161,163] Furthermore, chronic antidepressant treatment and exercise also propagate hippocampal neurogenesis.[161,163,208] Moreover, ablation of neurogenesis abrogates the behavioral benefits of antidepressant administration in rodents.[207]

In summary, evidence best supports a modified neurotrophic hypothesis of MDD, indicating the importance of antidepressant-mediated elevation of BDNF in neural plasticity, dendritic sprouting and remodeling, building and maintaining new synaptic contacts (especially regarding pyramidal glutamate neurons in the hippocampus),[163] and support of the new born cells.[163,209] Antidepressant-induced increase in BDNF signaling may be particularly relevant for activity dependent neuroplasticity and proper maintenance of neural connections.[210] However, neurogenesis may be important in some aspects of antidepressant action, such as improvement in cognition and decrease in anxious symptomatology.[207–209]

On the other hand, counterarguments highlight the fact that loss of hippocampal dentate gyrus granule neurons has not been established as an important etiological finding in MDD.[208] Additionally, adult neurogenesis contributes only 5 percent of the dentate gyrus cells, unlikely to adequately compensate for approximately 15 percent hippocampal gray matter volume loss in MDD.[208] Nor is reduction of hippocampal volume specific to MDD,[163,207] as it has also been observed in posttraumatic stress disorder, chronic stress, fibromyalgia, bipolar disorder, chronic insomnia, and schizophrenia. Additionally, pathological studies do not support neuronal loss as the primary finding in depression; it appears that decline in glial density and neuropil reduction take precedence.[3,163] Furthermore, disruption of neurogenesis has not been associated with depressive-like phenotype in the preclinical models.[207] Moreover, antidepressants, in clinically relevant doses, do not exert neurogenic effect on neural progenitor cells.[163] Finally, research has established that neurogenesis is not necessary for antidepressant activity of pharmacological agents, as they retained their behavioral benefits even when neurogenesis was chemically arrested.[209]

THE ROLE OF BDNF IN THE MEDICAL COMORBIDITIES OF MDD

BDNF dysregulation may have an important role in the etiology of medical comorbidities of MDD. Basic research has discovered that BDNF plays a role in the inhibition of the sympathetic response by promoting rapid ACh release mediated by its p75 receptor.[211] Dysfunction of BDNF signaling has been implicated in the aberrant sympathetic/parasympathetic balance, leading to perivascular inflammation and potentially increased risk of stroke.[212,213] Moreover, preclinical studies indicate that environmental activation of BDNF synthesis may regulate leptin production by adipocytes in a way that would induce cancer remission.[214] Hypothalamic interactions between BDNF, corticotropin-releasing factor (CRF), and histamine have an important role in the regulation of feeding behavior.[215] BDNF release is associated with increase in CRF and histamine signaling and subsequent suppression of feeding behavior.[215] Given its role in the regulation of sympathetic activity, inflammation, glucagon release, and weight regulation, it is of little surprise that BDNF dysregulation has been associated with type 2 diabetes and metabolic syndrome.[216–218]

Other Neurotrophic Factors in MDD

The role of several other neurotrophic factors, including GDNF, vascular endothelial growth factor (VEGF), insulin-like growth factor (IGF), and neurotrophin-3 (NT-3), has been researched in context of depression.

GLIAL-CELL-LINE–DERIVED NEUROTROPHIC FACTOR

GDNF, a member of the transforming growth factor (TGF) superfamily, is extensively distributed throughout the mammalian brain.[219,220] GDNF is an important modulator of monoamine synthesis. It plays a role in the development and survival of DA, 5HT, NE, and GABA neurons, as well as glial cells.[219–221] Furthermore, GDNF upregulates key synthetic enzymes and coenzymes (including tetrahydrobiopterin [BH4]) involved in monoamine synthesis.[221] Abolition of GDNF results in a demise of NE and DA neurons in their principal brainstem nuclei.[222] Stress is a known precipitant of depressive episodes and a trigger for an inflammatory response. Microglial activation acts as a transducer of peripheral inflammatory signals into a central oxidative stress and cytokine release.[87] Obviously, inhibition of microglial activation may ward off the detrimental effect of stress and prevent the initiation of depressive pathophysiology. Under the circumstances of excessive glutamate/NMDA signaling, ensuing excitotoxicity may precipitate neuronal apoptosis. In these circumstances astrocytes have been evidenced to respond by releasing GDNF, which prevents excitotoxicity via microglia modulation.[54] Furthermore, GDNF of astrocytic origin has a capacity to inhibit microglia activated by inflammatory stimuli.[223] Moreover, stress-precipitated methylation of the GDNF promoter, resulting in epigenetic silencing of neurotrophin production in the rodent nucleus accumbens, generates a depressive phenotype.[224] Thus, GDNF has emerged as an important regulator of neuronal and glial health and cognitive function, potentially reflecting an individual's ability to cope with stress.[224,225]

Several studies have reported decreased serum and whole-blood levels of GDNF in depressed patients compared with healthy controls.[219] Some studies have even noted a correlation between low serum levels of GDNF and the severity of depression.[226] Although eight weeks of antidepressant treatment produced significant elevation of serum GDNF in depressed patients,[227] even remitted patients may have lower whole-blood GDNF relative to healthy controls.[225] Other researchers have found lower peripheral blood cell levels of GDNF in actively depressed but not in remitted individuals.[228] Furthermore, a response to ECT in individuals with treatment-resistant depression was associated with an increase in serum GDNF levels; no significant elevation was observed in nonresponders.[229] Differences in the methodology and age of the study participants may account for some of the discrepancies, as age was reported to be associated with the reduction of peripheral GDNF levels in depressed patients.[219] Perhaps surprisingly, a postmortem study reveled elevated GDNF levels in the parietal cortices of depressed individuals compared with the control group. Authors of the study ascribed the GDNF elevation to a compensatory response related to neuronal and glial loss in MDD.[220]

VASCULAR ENDOTHELIAL GROWTH FACTOR

VEGF is a key regulator of angiogenesis, neurogenesis, neuroplasticity, and neural resilience. It is synthesized and released by multiple cell lines, including neural stem cells, astrocytes, endothelial, and ependymal cells.[230,231] Several signaling systems implicated in etiopathogenesis of MDD are also involved in regulation of VEGF release. Glutamate, NE, IL-4, IL-6, and 5HT via 5HT1A and 5HT2 receptors all induce VEGF release.[230,232,233] Additionally, DA and ACh also have a role in VEGF regulation.[233] On the other hand, stress-related molecules, such as CRF and cortisol, attenuate VEGF signaling overall while possibly increasing its levels in certain compartments.[230,231,233] In physiological circumstances VEGF provides important support to memory and learning-related processes.[230,233] Interestingly, VEGF genetic polymorphisms influence human hippocampal morphology.[234] Both acute and chronic stress has been shown to downregulate VEGF signaling.[230,233] Given the hippocampal role in memory and stress modulation, it is tempting to speculate whether its altered function and structure in MDD may be related to disruption in VEGF homeostasis.

The reports of changes in peripheral VEGF levels in MDD have been inconsistent. Several studies have found elevated plasma and serum VEGF levels, as well as increased VEGF mRNA, in peripheral blood cells; others have found no difference in VEGF levels between depressed patients and healthy controls.[230,231,233] Furthermore, there are a few reports of decreased serum and plasma levels in MDD patients compared with healthy controls. One of the studies discovered a correlation between decreased serum VEGF levels and suicidality in a depressed patient group.[230,231,233] Inconsistent reports may reflect the heterogeneity of MDD, different methodologies, dissimilar medication status, and different duration of depressive episodes.[230]

While preclinical data from animal models of depression unequivocally point to the ameliorating influence of antidepressant treatment, exercise, and ECT on peripheral and brain VEGF levels, accompanied by decrease in depressive phenotype, clinical reports are incongruent.[230,231] Several investigators found no change or even declines in the peripheral VEGF levels following antidepressant treatment.[230,231] A few studies have reported increases in serum and plasma levels in depressed patients relative to matched controls following antidepressant treatment, ECT, and sleep deprivation therapy.[230,231] In some instances elevation of peripheral VEGF levels correlated with clinical improvement measured by standardized depression rating scales.[230,231] One of the studies of SNRI treatment of depression had a remarkable outcome: early responders (>50 percent reduction in HAMD after six weeks of antidepressant therapy) had elevation of plasma VEGF levels, while early nonresponders (<50 percent improvement after six weeks of treatment) recorded a decline in their plasma VEGF levels.[233] Although overall data suggest that VEGF may play a role in the pathophysiology of depression and its treatment, further research is needed to clarify their association. Moreover, the relationship between peripheral and brain VEGF levels is uncertain.

INSULIN-LIKE GROWTH FACTOR-1

Research has not yet established a precise place for IGF-1 in the tapestry of intricate immune-endocrine-neurotrophic interactions that underpin the pathophysiology of MDD. In adulthood, IGF-1 is mostly produced by the liver and released into the bloodstream. While the developing brain produces significant amounts of IGF-1, in adulthood its CNS production is substantially reduced.[235] IGF-1 from the periphery does cross the BBB utilizing an active transport mechanism. Upon reaching the brain, IGF-1 engages densely distributed receptors, mediating nerve cell growth, development, and differentiation, as well as neurotransmitter synthesis and release.[235] IGF-1 has the ability to abrogate inflammation and oxidative stress-induced activation of microglia and suppress expression of inflammatory markers such as IL-1 and TNF while at the same time increasing expression of BDNF.[236,237] Furthermore, peripheral administration of IGF-1 in animal models has been shown to correct inflammation-induced glutamate/GABA imbalance, with subsequent improvement in cognition.[238] Unfortunately, interaction between the innate immune system and IGF-1 also flows in the opposite direction. Namely, proinflammatory cytokines such as TNF and IL-1 may induce a state of IGF-1 receptor resistance.[239]

In preclinical models of depression, peripheral and central administration of IGF-1 as well as induction of IGF-1 by exercise enhanced hippocampal neurogenesis and manifested antidepressant-like behavioral effects.[235,240] IGF-1 may play an especially important role in exercise-promoted neuroplasticity. Administration of anti-IGF-1 antibodies blocked behavioral antidepressant-like effects of exercise in the animal models.[241] Antidepressant administration has been associated with increased IGF-1 concentration in the rat brain and elevation of CSF concentration of IGF-1 in humans. Data from clinical studies are somewhat controversial and discrepant. While studies of MDD patients substantiated elevation of peripheral IGF-1 levels,[235,242] followed by decreases with antidepressant response,[243] CSF studies of depressed individuals reported reduction of IGF-1 subsequent to antidepressant therapy.[244] Better-designed studies are necessary before the role of IGF-1 in MDD can be properly determined.

The Role of Brain Inflammatory Signaling in MDD

Microglia-astroglia-oligodendroglia-neuronal "units" may be conceived as neural microsystems, which interface with peripheral macrosystems, such as autonomic, immune, and endocrine systems, providing a real-time integration of the peripheral regulatory signals with cerebral activity. Circumstances leading to neuroendocrine, autonomic, and neuroimmune dysregulation in MDD are described in some detail in Chapter 6. Elevation of peripheral proinflammatory cytokines, accompanied by perturbations in circulating corticosteroids, elevation of sympathetic, and decline of parasympathetic activity, exacts a destabilizing influence on the CNS function.

RELATIONSHIPS BETWEEN PERIPHERAL AND CENTRAL INFLAMMATION: ROLE OF THE BLOOD–BRAIN BARRIER

In the last three decades we have learned a lot about the propagation of the peripheral inflammatory signals and their influence on the brain, but many questions remain open. The previous concept of the brain as an "immuno-privileged" organ—not accessible to peripheral immune monitoring—separated from the peripheral circulation by the BBB, has largely been revised. As a consequence of more recent research, the BBB has been reconceptualized more as an active communication interface between the two compartments rather than an impermeable barrier separating the brain and the body.[245] Restrictive aspects of BBB are constantly modified in response to the changes in the physiological milieu of the brain and body. Peripheral inflammatory cytokines communicate with the CNS via several pathways. (a) Afferent neural fibers (i.e., vagal and, to a lesser extent, glossopharyngeal nerves), assisted by dendritic cells, are capable of detecting peripheral inflammatory status and conveying this information to the structures close to their CNS terminals, including barrier cells, blood vessels, other neurons, and circumventricular organs (e.g., area postrema, median eminence, and pineal gland). Vagal stimulation has a bidirectional effect: stimulation of efferent vagal fibers with TNF generates a peripheral anti-inflammatory effect, mediated by alpha-7 nAChRs.[246,247] (b) Stimulation of immune cells in the circumventricular organs leads to release of proinflammatory cytokines. Circumventricular organs are brain regions whose capillary beds are not endowed with a BBB. Inflammatory signals from the circumventricular organ immune cells are further propagated to neural elements, some of which project beyond the BBB.[246,247] (c) Peripheral immune signals may induce BBB cells (ependymal, endothelial, and choroid plexus cells) to release IL-1, IL-6, TNF, PGs, NO, and MCP-1 (see figure 7.3). (d) Saturable transport systems may transfer proinflammatory cytokines across the BBB.[247,248] IL-1, IL-6, and TNF are transported across the BBB by distinctive, unidirectional transport systems. In the case of TNF, transporters are identical with its p55 and p75 receptors. Furthermore, CNS cytokines can cross from CSF to blood with the reabsorption of CSF. Thus, the CSF contribution to blood cytokine levels can be quite meaningful.[245–247] (e) Disruption of the BBB due to CNS disease or peripheral infection may allow passage of inflammatory cells and mediators. (f) Although in physiological circumstances leukocytes cross into the CNS at a low rate, T lymphocytes appear to be more regular visitors. T cells gain access to the CNS via diapedesis (see figure 7.4), a "squeezing-through" process, facilitated by brain endothelial cell adhesion molecules. This is a rather slow and laborious process, as it may take T cells anywhere from 4 to 16 hours to complete this passage.[245]

FIGURE 7.3. **Response to dysregulated peripheral inflammatory signals. Microglia respond to derivatives of the peripheral inflammatory signals such as ones conveyed by perivascular macrophages, and propagate/transduce these signals to the central nervous system via release of ATP, cytokines, chemokines, RNS, and ROS (1). The inflammatory mediators released by microglia initiate a positive-feedback loop by inducing astrocytes to produce ATP and cytokines, which further facilitate microglial proinflammatory activity (2). Increased levels of ATP and inflammatory mediators lead to a cascade of events that result in destabilization and**

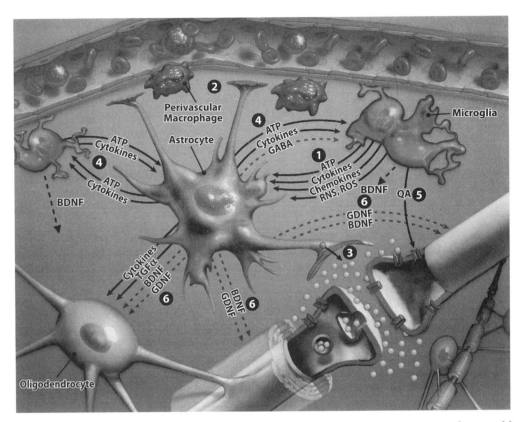

impairment of the normal functioning of both glia and neurons. Astrocytes are no longer able to maintain the integrity of the blood–brain barrier and optimal neurovascular coupling (3). Instead of removing excess glutamate from excitatory synapses, activated astrocytes release additional quantities of this neurotransmitter, producing an excess of glutamate that may impair synaptic communication (4) and lead to excitotoxicity via stimulation of extrasynaptic NMDA receptors. Activated astrocytes reduce GABA release (indicated by dashed lines) (5), which results in transformation of microglia such that they become amoeboid in shape and able to move throughout the brain while continuing to release inflammatory cytokines and ATP. Activated astroglia and microglia also reduce the release of neurotropic factors, such as BDNF and GDNF (6). The decline in BDNF and GDNF further perpetuates microglia activation, precipitating impairment in oligodendrocyte function and subsequent demyelination, as well as neuronal apoptosis. Activated microglia exhibit increased activity of the enzyme indoleamine 2,3-dioxygenase, which eventually converts tryptophan into quinolinic acid (QA). Increased tryptophan metabolism to quinolinic acid may diminish serotonin and melatonin signaling, while released quinolinic acid contributes to neurotoxicity via stimulation of extrasynaptic NMDA receptors (7). Abbreviations: RNS, reactive nitrogen species; ROS, reactive oxygen species; ATP, adenosine triphosphate; BDNF, brain-derived neurotrophic factor; GDNF, glial cell-derived neurotrophic factor; GABA, gamma aminobutyric acid; TGF-α, transforming growth factor-alpha.

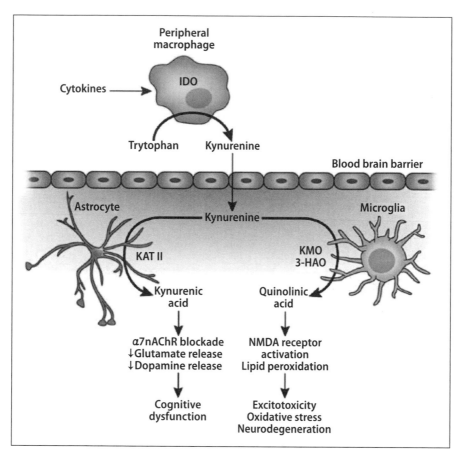

FIGURE 7.4. Inflammatory cytokines induce indoleamine 2,3-dioxygenase (IDO) activity in peripheral immune cells and brain cells, such as microglia, astrocytes, and neurons, precipitating the production of kynurenine, which is subsequently converted to kynurenic acid (KA) by kynurenine amino- transferase-II (KAT-II) in astrocytes, or quinolinic acid by kynurenine-3-monooxygenase (KMO) and 3-hydroxy-anthranilic acid oxygenase (3-HAO) in microglia or infiltrating macrophages. By antagonizing the alpha-7nAChRs, KA can reduce glutamate and dopamine, both of which can interfere with cognitive function. Quinolinic acid can activate NMDA receptors, precipitating increased glutamate release and lipid peroxidation, thereby advancing the excitotoxicity, oxidative stress, and possibly neural apoptosis.

THE ROLE OF INFLAMMATORY CYTOKINES REDEFINED

This is an opportune moment to dispense with the outdated concept regarding the "classical" role of the inflammatory molecules in the CNS. Although we have them labeled as such, "inflammatory" cytokines, including IL-1β, IL-6, and TNF, in physiological circumstances have a neuroplastic and neurotrophic-like role.[95,249] The boundary between the immune and neural system is much more blurry than we have been accustomed to believing. Not only do inflammatory cytokines support learning, memory, neural development, resilience, and differentiation in healthy circumstances,[95,249,250] but BDNF, a prototypical neurotrophic factor, has an important role in modulating the peripheral and central immune response.[251–254] There are even some functional similarities, as immune cells, much like neurons, utilize adhesion molecules to form synaptic junctions for the sake of information exchange.[255]

The impact of inflammatory cytokine levels in the CNS, including that of IL-1, on learning, memory, and cognition resembles an inverted-U curve. Physiological, constitutively expressed IL-1 is needed for LTP, memory formation, and learning, and possibly neurogenesis. Excessive IL-1 signaling, induced by enduring stress, social isolation, or somatic illness, has an opposite effect. Supraphysiological elevation of IL-1 in these circumstances impairs LTP, disrupts learning, and diminishes hippocampal neuroplasticity.[95,249,256]

Astroglia, microglia, and neurons are all capable of releasing IL-6.[120,249,257–259] In addition to supporting neuronal survival by induction of astroglial NGF release,[260] IL-6 protects the neurons from NMDA-mediated excitotoxicity by enhancing the expression of Bcl-2 mRNA (a neuroprotective factor) and suppressing caspase-3, also known as the "executioner protein" for its role in apoptosis (programmed cell death).[261]

Physiological levels of TNF are indispensable for normal brain development and homeostatic neuroplasticity. With new experiences and learning, the brain goes through a continuous stream of updates. At the cellular level these updates rely on the process of synaptic scaling. Astroglia release TNF in response to changes in neural activity. TNF subsequently regulates the cell-surface expression of AMPA and GABA-A receptors, and therefore NMDA-mediated synaptic strength and plasticity. Additionally, TNF mediates the release of neurotrophic factors NGF, BDNF, and GDNF from astrocytes and endocellular Ca^{2+} homeostasis.[95,256,262,263]

Furthermore, other immune cells, such as T lymphocytes and microglia, and immune signaling molecules, including IL-4, IL-10, and PGs, may play an important role in the regulation of learning memory, neuroplasticity, and neurogenesis.[249,264,265] Moreover, NFκB, a transcription factor that is both the main regulator of inflammatory cytokine synthesis and the primary endocellular target of cytokine signaling, also has a bivalent role in the regulation of memory and neuroplasticity. While physiological NFκB activity supports neuroplasticity, excessive, stress-activated NFκB signaling suppresses neurogenesis and produces a depressive-like phenotype in the preclinical models.[249,263,266]

Finally, inflammatory cytokines may influence brain plasticity, memory, and learning through an indirect, sleep-mediated path. Inflammatory cytokines, primarily IL-1 and TNF, are principal regulators of sleep, circadian rhythmicity, and sleep-related plasticity. The balance of neurotrophic factors and inflammatory cytokines during sleep is influential in synaptic pruning and proper memory formation.[267–269] The complex interaction among inflammation, sleep regulation, and neuroplasticity may have a particular relevance in MDD, given that both malfunction of inflammatory genes and an alteration in the circadian pattern of gene expression have been implicated in the etiopathogenesis of depression.[270,271] In conclusion, in physiological conditions, inflammatory cytokines in the CNS may be more aptly considered as neuromodulatory molecules.[262]

Regulation of Mood, Stress Response, and Immune Function at the Network Level: Roles of Neuroplasticity

There appears to be a reciprocal communication between the principal areas involved in mood regulation and stress response and the peripheral immune system. Some of the key limbic and paralimbic areas implicated in the pathophysiology of MDD, including the amygdala, insula, and ACC, have an important role in the regulation of autonomic and immune function.[87,272–274] Although direct data linking functional disturbance in these limbic/paralimbic areas to inflammation are not available, it is tempting to speculate that their aberrant activity may have a causal role in the ensuing immune dysregulation in MDD. Conversely, imaging studies have reported peripheral inflammation-related changes in the activity of several limbic and paralimbic areas, including sgACC, amygdala, insula, medial PFC, and basal ganglia/ventral striatum/nucleus accumbens.[275–278] One study used endotoxin to provoke peripheral inflammation, causing altered metabolism in the insula and ACC, accompanied by depression, fatigue, and loss of social interest.[278] Another group reported changed substantia nigra activity due to endotoxin administration, with concomitant psychomotor slowing.[279] The same stimulus, in separate studies, reduced ventral striatum activity, precipitating diminished response to reward cues[280] and enhanced amygdala response to socially threatening images.[275] Interestingly, a preclinical study revealed that a peripheral immune stimulus is capable of eliciting an amygdala response even in absence of central inflammatory cytokine induction.[281] Extending these findings, an imaging study reported an association between vaccination-induced peripheral inflammation and reduced connectivity among the sgACC, amygdala, mPFC, nucleus accumbens, and superior temporal gyrus.[276] Furthermore, an imaging study of women going through the bereavement process noted that peripheral inflammatory marker levels were correlated with sgACC and ventromedial PFC activity.[282] It is more than a coincidence that all of these limbic/paralimbic areas involved in regulation of mood and the stress response have also been implicated in the pathophysiology of MDD. An imaging study reported correlation between increased expression of inflammatory genes and a greater hemodynamic response to emotional stimuli in the ventromedial PFC, amygdala, and hippocampus of mood-disordered patients (predominantly MDD) relative to healthy controls. Moreover, in the same study, elevated expression of inflammatory genes was also linked with decreased thickness of the sgACC, hippocampus, and caudate in the mood-disordered group.[283]

Further extending these findings, a postmortem study detected an increased expression of transmembrane TNF in the dlPFC (BA 46) of MDD subjects relative to controls.[284] Enzymatic cleavage of transmembrane TNF generates soluble TNF. The two TNF receptors TNFR1 and TNFR2 have differential affinities for the two forms of the cytokine. TNFR2 predominantly expressed on microglia and endothelial cells has a preference for transmembrane TNF. Accumulating evidence points to a link between volumetric brain changes in MDD and elevation of inflammatory cytokines in the CNS. Hypothetically, elevation in inflammatory signaling, suppressed synthesis of neurotrophic factors (especially BDNF), and ensuing compromise in neuroplasticity are also associated with disturbances in glutamate and monoaminergic transmission.[277,285–291]

ELEVATION OF INFLAMMATORY CYTOKINES AND SYMPTOMS OF MDD

Preclinical studies have indicated that elevated levels of IL-6 in the CNS generate a depressive-like phenotype.[292] In contradistinction to proinflammatory IL-6, central anti-inflammatory IL-10 attenuated peripheral inflammation-induced fatigue and improved food intake.[293] Furthermore, activation of neuronal IL-10 receptors was associated with a greater expression of Bcl-2 (a resilience factor) and greater cell survival after glutamate-induced excitotoxicity.[293]

Several studies have explored the relationship between CSF cytokines and neuropsychiatric symptoms. Elevated CSF IL-8 has been linked with alexithymia,[294] while CSF IL-6 and TNF showed an association with postpartum depressed mood four days and six weeks after childbirth.[295] Furthermore, lower CSF IL-6 predicted future depression in a group of women prospectively studied for 17 years, possibly suggesting the inverse-U relationship between the IL-6 levels and CNS pathology.[296] Moreover, increased CSF IL-6 levels were detected in a group of MDD patients relative to healthy controls.[297] A study of CSF IL-6 levels in mostly MDD suicide attempters reported a correlation with scores on the Montgomery-Asberg Depression Rating Scale.[298] Another study found a correlation among pretreatment CSF IL-1 levels, posttreatment CSF IL-6 and TNF concentrations, and the intensity of suicidal ideation measured by a standardized scale.[178] Additionally, CSF IL-6 and TNF were associated with increased 5HT turnover (indicated by levels of its metabolite 5-hydroxyindoleacetic acid) and increased DA turnover (indicated by homovanillic acid levels).[298] Finally, a study involving unmedicated hospitalized MDD patients detected elevated CSF levels of IL-1 in the patient group compared with healthy matched controls.[299]

THE IMPACT OF INFLAMMATORY SIGNALING ON NEUROTRANSMISSION AND NEUROPLASTICITY

Microglia are the principal recipients of the inflammatory signals transmitted from the periphery of the body. Induced microglia undergo a phenotypical transformation and respond by augmenting the incoming signal by releasing the additional amounts of IL-1, IL-6, TNF, PGs, NO, and hydrogen peroxide. Mixture of these inflammatory molecules with ROS and RNS activates astroglia, causing them to release more of these inflammatory mediators. Once triggered, this positive feedback loop further propagates and amplifies cytokine signals from the periphery.[7,15,80,139,300,301] Several downstream effects are initiated by this feed-forward proinflammatory, pro-oxidant activity. For example, overexposure to ROS and RNS precipitates oxidative damage to oligodendroglia. Excessive TNF, released by microglia and astrocytes, combined with diminished neurotrophic support, produces oligodendroglia toxicity and subsequent impairment of myelination. Since oligodendroglia also have a role in glutamate uptake, their damage may compound the accumulation of this excitatory neurotransmitter.[61,62,89,302] As a reminder, microgliosis may be a proxy of a depressive "flare-up" and ensuing activation of neuropathology, as suggested by a postmortem study that found an elevation of microglia density in the dlPFC, ACC, and mediodorsal thalamus of mood-disordered patients who committed suicide, but not individuals carrying the same diagnosis who died from different causes.[139]

Oxidative stress, proinflammatory cytokines (e.g., IL-1, IL-6, TNF), and PGs (e.g., PGE2) in extrahepatic tissues synergistically induce indoleamine 2,3-dioxygenase (IDO), an enzyme that converts TRP to kynurenine (KYN), thereby diminishing its availability for 5HT and melatonin synthesis.[303–305] By contrast, anti-inflammatory cytokines, such as IL-4 and IL-10, preserve TRP by acting as IDO inhibitors.[303,306] Moreover, elevated glucocorticoids, due to either stress or MDD, may induce hepatic tryptophan 2,3-dioxygenase (TDO), which metabolizes TRP to KYN; further KYN metabolism mostly takes place extrahepatically.[303] To put things into proper perspective, only about 1 percent of TRP is converted into 5HT, while 99 percent of TRP is metabolized by TDO in the liver.[303] Peripheral KYN has the capacity to pass through the BBB. Once it has gained access to the CNS, it is further metabolized by microglia and astroglia. While astroglial metabolism of KYN usually terminates with kynurenic acid (KA), microglia usually metabolize KYN to QUIN.[307]

An imbalance of microglia–astroglia activity in MDD may result in a greater increase of QUIN than KA, with significant consequences for neurotransmission.[286,308] KA has antagonistic activity toward alpha-7 nAChRs and NMDA glutamate receptors.[309] As ACh also drives glutamate release from pyramidal neurons via alpha-7 nAChRs, its inhibition will produce a downstream reduction in glutamatergic afferent transmission to dopaminergic nuclei and consequently downgrade DA release in basal ganglia (figure 7.4).[310] Studies have correlated reduction of DA signaling in basal ganglia due to peripheral inflammatory cytokines with cognitive problems, anhedonia, and fatigue, all common symptoms of depression.[285,308,311]

The effect of QUIN on glutamatergic transmission is diametrically opposite of the KA influence. QUIN facilitates glutamate release and acts as an agonist at

NMDA receptors, possibly precipitating excitotoxicity directed at neurons and astrocytes. Indeed, studies have confirmed QUIN/KA imbalance in the CSF (see figure 7.4), both in depression induced by peripheral administration of interferon-gamma (IFN-γ) and in a group of mostly depressed suicidal patients.[285,286,308] Furthermore, a postmortem study of depressed suicidal subjects has discovered a significantly increased density of QUIN-positive microglial cells in the sgACC, perigenual ACC, and mid-ACC compared with matched controls.[119] A study investigating a relationship between peripheral, inflammation-induced KYN and suicidality in MDD patients found an increase of KYN only in suicidal patients, and not in nonsuicidal patients, compared with healthy controls.[312] Moreover, a different group of investigators discovered a correlation between peripheral blood concentration of KYN and a response to fluoxetine in a group of depressed patients.[313]

The presence of inflammatory mediators in the brain can have a complex and profound impact on monoamine signaling. Proinflammatory cytokines, such as IL-1 and TNF, may compromise serotonergic neurotransmission by increasing the expression of 5HT transporters on the cell membrane, consequently facilitating the reuptake of the neurotransmitter from the synaptic cleft.[285] Furthermore, mRNA expression of inflammatory cytokines was associated with elevated 5HT transporter activity in MDD patients.[314] While inflammation does reduce peripheral TRP levels by IDO and TDO activation, it does not appear to be a major depressogenic factor, as there was no concomitant reduction of TRP in the CSF.[285]

Inflammatory mediators in concert with ROS/RNS reversibly oxidize BH4, a key cofactor in the synthesis of monoamines, into a dihydrobiopterine or irreversibly into dihydroxanthopterin. Diminished availability of BH4 may interfere with DA, NE, 5HT, and melatonin synthesis.[132,285] Moreover, inflammation interferes with the function of vesicular monoamine transporter-2, which packages monoamines (DA, NE, 5HT) into vesicles in preparation for the synaptic release.[285] Additionally, preclinical studies provide evidence that inflammation may decrease the density of DA and NE transporters, thus disrupting catecholamine transmission.[285,315] Acute inflammation has also been shown to increase activity in the locus ceruleus (main NE nucleus in the CNS) and NE release in the hippocampus and hypothalamus.[285]

We have already mentioned that inflammation and IDO stimulation may directly contribute to depression as a result of the impact of KYN and its downstream metabolites on glutamatergic transmission. In addition to being a potent NMDA agonist, QUIN and inflammatory cytokines also stimulate glutamate release and interfere with its astroglial uptake.[285,316] In contrast to QUIN influence, KA downregulates the NMDA- and AMPA-mediated glutamate signaling[285,304,310,317,318] (see figure 7.4). We pointed out above that MDD tends to be associated with decreased astroglial density and increased microglial activity; this cellular imbalance may contribute to altered QUIN/KA ration and ensuing dysregulated glutamatergic activity. Since astrocytes also release GABA and provide an anti-inflammatory influence, their diminishing function in context of MDD may further augment inflammatory processes in the CNS.[39,303] Furthermore, NE via its beta and alpha-2 receptors, ACh via alpha-7 nAChRs, and 5HT via 5HT7 receptors regulate microglial proinflammatory cytokine release.[84,86,92] In concert with altered QUIN/KA ratio, inflammatory cytokines may self-perpetuate their own aberrant microglial release by altering monoamine transmission and alpha-7 nAChR-mediated cholinergic signaling.

Inflammation may also have a negative impact on neuroplasticity and neuro-trophic signaling. Administration of IFN-α has been associated with decreased systemic BDNF levels in humans, while peripheral IL-6 levels and BDNF had reciprocal values in a group of antidepressant-resistant MDD patients.[285,288] Pre-clinical studies have demonstrated that inflammatory cytokines phosphorylate the BDNF TrkB receptor and that IL-1 interferes with BDNF signaling by suppressing CREB.[285,287] We have already described an indirect influence of inflammation-induced extrasynaptic glutamate release from astrocytes, and subsequent binding to extrasynaptic NMDA receptors, as a suppressor of neuro-nal BDNF synthesis.[319]

An Integrated View of Immune, Neuroplastic, and Cellular Changes in MDD

Astrocytes have been found to be a major source of GABA in the CNS and may be important modulators of GABA activity in the hippocampus.[320] In the context of MDD, a shift in the microglia/astroglia balance, favoring microglial activity, may lead to excessive glutamate transmission relative to GABA output;[304,317,320] a domi-nance of T helper-1 (Th1) signaling (mostly proinflammatory) over Th2 activity (predominantly associated with release of the anti-inflammatory cytokines IL-4 and IL-10); and inadequate neurotrophic support for oligodendroglia, contributing to demyelination.[317,321]

The disturbance in sympathetic/parasympathetic balance associated with MDD may have significant repercussions on glia–neuron communication. Para-sympathetic activity has a stabilizing effect on microglia activity, while sympa-thetic input can play a dual role, either inhibiting or activating microglia.[85] In stressful situations it appears that sympathetic discharge induces microglial release of proinflammatory cytokines.[322] Consistent with this, a study that reported an increased NFκB activity in human volunteers after stress also indicated that alpha-1 receptor blockade obviated the stress-induced elevation of NFκB in ani-mals.[323] It appears that NFκB plays a pivotal role in catecholamine-induced synthe-sis of proinflammatory cytokines.[324] Proinflammatory cytokines and glucocorticoids have opposing effects on NFκB regulation.[325] Under usual circumstances gluco-corticoids have an immunosuppressant effect. However, MDD and sustained stress are accompanied by insufficient glucocorticoid signaling and glucocorti-coid receptor resistance.[291,326] Glucocorticoid resistance, in turn, may be associated with a "permissive" state, leading to an augmented inflammatory response.[291,326] Furthermore, in the context of aberrant stress responses, glucocorticoids have also been reported to increase NMDA activation in microglia and neurons.[97,327]

All in all, it appears that dysregulation of the hypothalamic-pituitary-adrenal, sympathetic, inflammatory systems in the context of chronic stress and MDD may be a self-perpetuating vicious cycle with a potential to disrupt adaptive glia–neuron signaling. Disturbed neuron–glia relationships in MDD may result in diminished neurotrophic support (involving, among others, BDNF and GDNF signaling), altered energy supply and oxidative regulation, massive releases of glutamate accompanied by compromised uptake, and accumulation of ROS and RNS, all of which may jointly contribute to neurotoxicity.[300,304,328]

Evidence suggests that neurotrophic factors, such as BDNF and GDNF, are synthesized within glia cells. Almost all classes of 5HT, NE, DA, cholinergic, GABA, glutamate, neurotrophin, and cytokine receptors are expressed on glial cell membranes. Additionally, astroglial membranes express transporters for monoamines (5HT, NE, DA) and glutamate. Probably about half of the monoamine uptake sites blocked by conventional antidepressants are located on glia cells.[2,15,87] However, unlike neurons, which release neurotransmitters in response to action potentials, glia cells discharge their transmitters in response to graded increases in cytoplasmic Ca^{2+}. This "analog" pattern of glial transmitter release, in contrast to the "binary" pattern of neuronal transmission, may have contributed to our long-standing neglect of the role of astroglia in neural signaling.[87]

Astroglia also have a role in regulating neuronal energy supply: at times of peak neuronal activity glia cells release lactate in response to increased energy needs. Positron emission tomography imaging studies reflecting glucose metabolism to a significant degree reflect glia activity. Cerebral perfusion is also significantly modulated by astroglia: on one end, astroglial extensions "sense" synaptic activity; on the other end, their distal processes, end feet, modulate vascular tone and capillary permeability. Therefore, functional MRI signals are substantially influenced by glial activity.[2,15,87]

Glial cell pathology has been reported in the sgACC, dlPFC, OFC, hippocampus, and amygdala of unmedicated MDD patients. It appears that both astroglia and oligodendroglia may be affected. Research has noted a prominent 19 percent reduction in oligodendroglia in the dlPFC of MDD patients. Considering the crucial role that the dlPFC plays in executive function and "top-down" limbic regulation, the implications of this finding are striking, because it may provide a neurobiological substrate for both the emotional dysregulation and cognitive dysfunction commonly observed in MDD.[87,98–100] A study using immunohistochemistry assessed microglia density in the dlPFC, ACC, thalamus, and hippocampus of depressed patients. The authors suggest that significant microgliosis (i.e., increased number of microglia) in depressed patients who committed suicide, relative to healthy controls, might be a marker of presuicidal stress.[139]

In contradistinction to widespread glial abnormalities, neuronal changes appear to be subtler and more discrete in MDD. For example, some authors have noted decreased pyramidal somal size in the hippocampus, ACC, dlPFC, and OFC in postmortem studies of MDD patients. The distribution of this cellular pathology overlaps remarkably with findings from structural and functional imaging studies. Therefore, MDD is more characterized by morphological and functional changes, rather than alterations in neuronal density.[2,87,98–100] In conclusion, Major Depression appears to be much more a "gliopathic" rather than "neurodegenerative" disease.

There is a continuous dance among GABA/glutamate transmission, immune modulation, and neurotrophic signaling in the brain.[249,261,317,329] Inflammatory cytokines, released by microglia (immune cells of the CNS) and astrocytes, are capable of triggering excessive glutamatergic transmission and causing damage to nerve and glia cells.[319] However, we should refrain from hastily defining inflammatory mediators as the "bad guys" in the CNS.

Emerging literature points to an essential role that the immune system plays in supporting learning and neuroplasticity.[249] An "inflammatory" cytokine IL-6 protects neurons from NMDA-induced apoptosis,[261] while TNF has a key role in regulating glutamatergic gliotransmission and synaptic scaling (an essential component in new learning).[329] T cells have an indispensable role in neuroprotection, neurogenesis, and memory formation,[249] while PGE2 pulls double duty by stimulating release of BDNF from astrocytes, thus supporting neuronal development and resilience.[330] T-cell–derived glutamate, IFN-γ, and IL-4 endow astrocytes with a neuroprotective phenotype.[331,332] Therefore, immune and neurotrophic signals seem to harmoniously blend in physiological circumstances, optimizing GABA and glutamate signaling.

So what brings trouble to this paradise? In one word, excess. Poorly regulated inflammatory signals contribute to diminished neurotrophic tone and glutamate-mediated excitotoxicity.[87,319,333] The scene of the crime is the glia–synaptic junction, composed of microglia, astroglia, oligodendroglia, and pre- and postsynaptic membranes. A combination of specific genetic and epigenetic vulnerabilities and environmental adversity most likely precipitates a homeostatic breakdown.[319] Reverberating chemical signaling between microglia and astroglia causes escalation in release of inflammatory cytokines, chemokines, PGs, and ROS and RNS. Activated astrocytes extrude copious amounts of glutamate and most likely inadequate amount of GABA and neurotrophic factors.[39,319,333] Along with KA, extrasynaptic glutamate and inflammatory cytokines may have a toxic impact on glia cells and neurons.[319,333]

In a groundbreaking study, Lee et al.[39] identified astrocytes as a major source of GABA transmission in the brain. Additionally, GABA of astrocytic origin has an important role in suppressing inflammatory cytokine release. In the presence of GABA, in a mixed culture of astrocyte and microglial cells, TNF and IL-6 concentrations were diminished by approximately 60 percent.[39]

After reading this chapter, a thoughtful and discerning reader may raise several questions. Will deeper understanding of pathophysiology underlying MDD symptoms advance our clinical practice, and if so, how? As we have previously mentioned, any specific pathophysiological mechanism has only probabilistic association with individual clinical symptoms. Therefore, anti-inflammatory strategies may benefit only a subset of depressed patients who have elevated inflammatory indicators. While several antidepressant treatments may elevate neurotrophic factors, these effects seem to be indirect, modest, and not always enduring benefits. Treatments focused on activation of intracellular cascades are still in development. Finally, improved insight into biological underpinning of MDD would indicate the need for phase-specific treatments for MDD, rather than the current one-size-fits-all approach.

References

1. Taber KII, Hurley RA. Astroglia: not just glue. *J Neuropsychiatry Clin Neurosci.* 2008; 20(2):124–129.
2. Rajkowska G, Miguel-Hidalgo JJ. Gliogenesis and glial pathology in depression. *CNS Neurol Disord Drug Targets.* 2007;6:219–233.
3. Rajkowska G, Stockmeier CA. Astrocyte pathology in major depressive disorder: insights from human postmortem brain tissue. *Curr Drug Targets.* 2013;14(11):1225–1236.
4. Kettenmann H, Verkhratsky A. Neuroglia: the 150 years after. *Trends Neurosci.* 2008;31:653–659.
5. Murai KK, Van Meyel DJ. Neuron glial communication at synapses: insights from vertebrates and invertebrates. *Neuroscientist.* 2007;13:657–666.
6. Halassa MM, Fellin T, Haydon PG. The tripartite synapse: roles for gliotransmission in health and disease. *Trends Mol Med.* 2007;13:54–63.
7. Volterra A, Meldolesi J. Astrocytes, from brain glue to communication elements: the revolution continues. *Nat Rev Neurosci.* 2005;6:626–640.
8. Haydon PG, Carmignoto G. Astrocyte control of synaptic transmission and neurovascular coupling. *Physiol Rev.* 2006;86:1009–1031.
9. Mangia S, Simpson IA, Vannucci SJ, Carruthers A. The in vivo neuron-to-astrocyte lactate shuttle in human brain: evidence from modeling of measured lactate levels during visual stimulation. *J Neurochem.* 2009;109(suppl 1):55–62.
10. Nehlig A, Coles JA. Cellular pathways of energy metabolism in the brain: is glucose used by neurons or astrocytes? *Glia.* 2007;55:1238–1250.
11. Rouach N, Koulakoff A, Abudara V, Willecke K, Giaume C. Astroglial metabolic networks sustain hippocampal synaptic transmission. *Science.* 2008;322:1551–1555.
12. Dinuzzo M, Mangia S, Maraviglia B, Giove F. The role of astrocytic glycogen in supporting the energetics of neuronal activity. *Neurochem Res.* 2012;37:2432–2438.
13. Takano T, Tian GF, Peng W, et al. Astrocyte-mediated control of cerebral blood flow. *Nat Neurosci.* 2006;9:260–267.
14. Gordon GR, Choi HB, Rungta RL, Ellis-Davies GC, MacVicar BA. Brain metabolism dictates the polarity of astrocyte control over arterioles. *Nature.* 2008;456:745–749.
15. Pav M, Kovaru H, Fiserova A, Havrdova E, Lisa V. Neurobiological aspects of depressive disorder and antidepressant treatment: role of glia. *Physiol Res.* 2008;57:151–164.

16. Verkhratsky A, Rodriguez JJ, Parpura V. Neurotransmitters and integration in neuronal-astroglial networks. *Neurochem Res.* 2012;37:2326–2338.

17. Porter JT, McCarthy KD. Astrocytic neurotransmitter receptors in situ and in vivo. *Prog Neurobiol.* 1997;51:439–455.

18. Li B, Zhang S, Li M, Hertz L, Peng L. Serotonin increases ERK1/2 phosphorylation in astrocytes by stimulation of 5-HT2B and 5-HT2C receptors. *Neurochem Int.* 2010;57:432–439.

19. Naganuma F, Yoshikawa T, Nakamura T, et al. Predominant role of plasma membrane monoamine transporters in monoamine transport in 1321N1, a human astrocytoma-derived cell line. *J Neurochem.* 2014;129:591–601.

20. Yoshikawa T, Naganuma F, Iida T, et al. Molecular mechanism of histamine clearance by primary human astrocytes. *Glia.* 2013;61:905–916.

21. Ramos AJ, Tagliaferro P, Lopez EM, Pecci Saavedra J, Brusco A. Neuroglial interactions in a model of para-chlorophenylalanine-induced serotonin depletion. *Brain Res.* 2000;883:1–14.

22. Zhang S, Li B, Lovatt D, et al. 5-HT2B receptors are expressed on astrocytes from brain and in culture and are a chronic target for all five conventional "serotonin-specific reuptake inhibitors." *Neuron Glia Biol.* 2010;6:113–125.

23. Peng L, Li B, Du T, et al. Astrocytic transactivation by alpha2A-adrenergic and 5-HT2B serotonergic signaling. *Neurochem Int.* 2010;57:421–431.

24. Yan M, Dai H, Ding T, et al. Effects of dexmedetomidine on the release of glial cell line-derived neurotrophic factor from rat astrocyte cells. *Neurochem Int.* 2011;58:549–557.

25. Gibbs ME, Bowser DN. Astrocytic adrenoceptors and learning: alpha1-adrenoceptors. *Neurochem Int.* 2010;57:404–410.

26. Christiansen SH, Selige J, Dunkern T, Rassov A, Leist M. Combined anti-inflammatory effects of beta2-adrenergic agonists and PDE4 inhibitors on astrocytes by upregulation of intracellular cAMP. *Neurochem Int.* 2011;59:837–846.

27. Gordon GR, Baimoukhametova DV, Hewitt SA, Rajapaksha WR, Fisher TE, Bains JS. Norepinephrine triggers release of glial ATP to increase postsynaptic efficacy. *Nat Neurosci.* 2005;8:1078–1086.

28. Mizuta I, Ohta M, Ohta K, Nishimura M, Mizuta E, Kuno S. Riluzole stimulates nerve growth factor, brain-derived neurotrophic factor and glial cell line-derived neurotrophic factor synthesis in cultured mouse astrocytes. *Neurosci Lett.* 2001;310:117–120.

29. Ohta K, Kuno S, Mizuta I, Fujinami A, Matsui H, Ohta M. Effects of dopamine agonists bromocriptine, pergolide, cabergoline, and SKF-38393 on GDNF, NGF, and BDNF synthesis in cultured mouse astrocytes. *Life Sci.* 2003;73:617–626.

30. Ohta K, Kuno S, Inoue S, Ikeda E, Fujinami A, Ohta M. The effect of dopamine agonists: the expression of GDNF, NGF, and BDNF in cultured mouse astrocytes. *J Neurol Sci.* 2010;291:12–16.

31. Kuric E, Wieloch T, Ruscher K. Dopamine receptor activation increases glial cell line-derived neurotrophic factor in experimental stroke. *Exp Neurol.* 2013;247C:202–208.

32. Vaarmann A, Gandhi S, Abramov AY. Dopamine induces Ca^{2+} signaling in astrocytes through reactive oxygen species generated by monoamine oxidase. *J Biol Chem.* 2010;285:25018–25023.

33. Todd KJ, Serrano A, Lacaille JC, Robitaille R. Glial cells in synaptic plasticity. *J Physiol (Paris).* 2006;99:75–83.

34. Rose CR, Blum R, Pichler B, Lepier A, Kafitz KW, Konnerth A. Truncated TrkB-T1 mediates neurotrophin-evoked calcium signalling in glia cells. *Nature.* 2003;426:74–78.

35. Stipursky J, Spohr TC, Sousa VO, Gomes FC. Neuron-astroglial interactions in cell-fate

commitment and maturation in the central nervous system. *Neurochem Res.* 2012;37: 2402–2418.

36. Sofroniew MV, Vinters HV. Astrocytes: biology and pathology. *Acta Neuropathol.* 2010; 119:7–35.

37. Hamilton NB, Attwell D. Do astrocytes really exocytose neurotransmitters? *Nat Rev Neurosci.* 2010;11:227–238.

38. Lee M, McGeer EG, McGeer PL. Mechanisms of GABA release from human astrocytes. *Glia.* 2011;59:1600–1611.

39. Lee M, Schwab C, McGeer PL. Astrocytes are GABAergic cells that modulate microglial activity. *Glia.* 2011;59:152–165.

40. Yoon BE, Woo J, Lee CJ. Astrocytes as GABA-ergic and GABA-ceptive cells. *Neurochem Res.* 2012;37:2474–2479.

41. Elmariah SB, Oh EJ, Hughes EG, Balice-Gordon RJ. Astrocytes regulate inhibitory synapse formation via Trk-mediated modulation of postsynaptic GABAA receptors. *J Neurosci.* 2005;25:3638–3650.

42. Liu YJ, Zhuang J, Zhu HY, Shen YX, Tan ZL, Zhou JN. Cultured rat cortical astrocytes synthesize melatonin: absence of a diurnal rhythm. *J Pineal Res.* 2007;43:232–238.

43. Clarke LE, Barres BA. Emerging roles of astrocytes in neural circuit development. *Nat Rev Neurosci.* 2013;14:311–321.

44. Stevens B. Neuron-astrocyte signaling in the development and plasticity of neural circuits. *Neurosignals.* 2008;16:278–288.

45. Tsai HH, Li H, Fuentealba LC, et al. Regional astrocyte allocation regulates CNS synaptogenesis and repair. *Science.* 2012;337:358–362.

46. Bains JS, Oliet SH. Glia: they make your memories stick. *Trends Neurosci.* 2007;30: 417–424.

47. Slezak M, Pfrieger FW, Soltys Z. Synaptic plasticity, astrocytes and morphological homeostasis. *J Physiol (Paris).* 2006;99:84–91.

48. Ashton RS, Conway A, Pangarkar C, et al. Astrocytes regulate adult hippocampal neurogenesis through ephrin-B signaling. *Nat Neurosci.* 2012;15:1399–1406.

49. Boehler MD, Wheeler BC, Brewer GJ. Added astroglia promote greater synapse density and higher activity in neuronal networks. *Neuron Glia Biol.* 2007;3:127–140.

50. Langle SL, Poulain DA, Theodosis DT. Neuronal-glial remodeling: a structural basis for neuronal-glial interactions in the adult hypothalamus. *J Physiol (Paris).* 2002;96:169–175.

51. Mitani H, Shirayama Y, Yamada T, Maeda K, Ashby CR Jr, Kawahara R. Correlation between plasma levels of glutamate, alanine and serine with severity of depression. *Prog Neuropsychopharmacol Biol Psychiatry.* 2006;30:1155–1158.

52. Allen NJ, Barres BA. Signaling between glia and neurons: focus on synaptic plasticity. *Curr Opin Neurobiol.* 2005;15:542–548.

53. Maruyama J, Miller JM, Ulfendahl M. Glial cell line-derived neurotrophic factor and antioxidants preserve the electrical responsiveness of the spiral ganglion neurons after experimentally induced deafness. *Neurobiol Dis.* 2008;29:14–21.

54. Boscia F, Esposito CL, Di Crisci A, de Franciscis V, Annunziato L, Cerchia L. GDNF selectively induces microglial activation and neuronal survival in CA1/CA3 hippocampal regions exposed to NMDA insult through Ret/ERK signalling. *PLoS ONE.* 2009;4: e6486.

55. Yu AC, Liu RY, Zhang Y, et al. Glial cell line-derived neurotrophic factor protects astrocytes from staurosporine- and ischemia- induced apoptosis. *J Neurosci Res.* 2007;85: 3457–3464.

56. Colton CA. Heterogeneity of microglial activation in the innate immune response in the brain. *J Neuroimmune Pharmacol.* 2009;4:399–418.

57. Nave KA, Trapp BD. Axon-glial signaling and the glial support of axon function. *Annu Rev Neurosci.* 2008;31:535–561.

58. Edgar N, Sibille E. A putative functional role for oligodendrocytes in mood regulation. *Translat Psychiatry.* 2012;2:e109.

59. Yamazaki Y, Hozumi Y, Kaneko K, Fujii S, Goto K, Kato H. Oligodendrocytes: facilitating axonal conduction by more than myelination. *Neuroscientist.* 2010;16:11–18.

60. Domercq M, Etxebarria E, Perez-Samartin A, Matute C. Excitotoxic oligodendrocyte death and axonal damage induced by glutamate transporter inhibition. *Glia.* 2005;52:36–46.

61. Pitt D, Nagelmeier IE, Wilson HC, Raine CS. Glutamate uptake by oligodendrocytes: implications for excitotoxicity in multiple sclerosis. *Neurology.* 2003;61:1113–1120.

62. Buntinx M, Moreels M, Vandenabeele F, et al. Cytokine-induced cell death in human oligodendroglial cell lines: I. Synergistic effects of IFN-gamma and TNF-alpha on apoptosis. *J Neurosci Res.* 2004;76:834–845.

63. Buntinx M, Gielen E, Van Hummelen P, et al. Cytokine-induced cell death in human oligodendroglial cell lines. II: Alterations in gene expression induced by interferon-gamma and tumor necrosis factor-alpha. *J Neurosci Res.* 2004;76:846–861.

64. Zhang YW, Denham J, Thies RS. Oligodendrocyte progenitor cells derived from human embryonic stem cells express neurotrophic factors. *Stem Cells Dev.* 2006;15:943–952.

65. Wong AW, Xiao J, Kemper D, Kilpatrick TJ, Murray SS. Oligodendroglial expression of TrkB independently regulates myelination and progenitor cell proliferation. *J Neurosci.* 2013;33:4947–4957.

66. Du Y, Fischer TZ, Clinton-Luke P, Lercher LD, Dreyfus CF. Distinct effects of p75 in mediating actions of neurotrophins on basal forebrain oligodendrocytes. *Mol Cell Neurosci.* 2006;31:366–375.

67. Du Y, Lercher LD, Zhou R, Dreyfus CF. Mitogen-activated protein kinase pathway mediates effects of brain-derived neurotrophic factor on differentiation of basal forebrain oligodendrocytes. *J Neurosci Res.* 2006;84:1692–1702.

68. Block ML, Zecca L, Hong JS. Microglia-mediated neurotoxicity: uncovering the molecular mechanisms. *Nat Rev Neurosci.* 2007;8:57–69.

69. Aguzzi A, Barres BA, Bennett ML. Microglia: scapegoat, saboteur, or something else? *Science.* 2013;339:156–161.

70. Yokoyama A, Yang L, Itoh S, Mori K, Tanaka J. Microglia, a potential source of neurons, astrocytes, and oligodendrocytes. *Glia.* 2004;45:96–104.

71. Carmen J, Magnus T, Cassiani-Ingoni R, Sherman L, Rao MS, Mattson MP. Revisiting the astrocyte-oligodendrocyte relationship in the adult CNS. *Prog Neurobiol.* 2007;82:151–162.

72. Kettenmann H, Kirchhoff F, Verkhratsky A. Microglia: new roles for the synaptic stripper. *Neuron.* 2013;77:10–18.

73. Wake H, Moorhouse AJ, Nabekura J. Functions of microglia in the central nervous system--beyond the immune response. *Neuron Glia Biol.* 2011;7:47–53.

74. Hanisch UK, Kettenmann H. Microglia: active sensor and versatile effector cells in the normal and pathologic brain. *Nat Neurosci.* 2007;10:1387–1394.

75. Bessis A, Bechade C, Bernard D, Roumier A. Microglial control of neuronal death and synaptic properties. *Glia.* 2007;55:233–238.

76. Parkhurst CN, Yang G, Ninan I, et al. Microglia promote learning-dependent synapse formation through brain-derived neurotrophic factor. *Cell.* 2013;155:1596–1609.

77. Li J, Ramenaden ER, Peng J, Koito H, Volpe JJ, Rosenberg PA. Tumor necrosis factor alpha mediates lipopolysaccharide-induced microglial toxicity to developing oligodendrocytes when astrocytes are present. *J Neurosci.* 2008;28:5321–5330.

78. Blank T, Prinz M. Microglia as modulators of cognition and neuropsychiatric disorders. *Glia.* 2013;61:62–70.

79. Deng Y, Lu J, Sivakumar V, Ling EA, Kaur C. Amoeboid microglia in the periventricular white matter induce oligodendrocyte damage through expression of proinflammatory cytokines via MAP kinase signaling pathway in hypoxic neonatal rats. *Brain Pathol.* 2008;18:387–400.

80. Frank MG, Baratta MV, Sprunger DB, Watkins LR, Maier SF. Microglia serve as a neuro-immune substrate for stress-induced potentiation of CNS pro-inflammatory cytokine responses. *Brain Behav Immun.* 2007;21:47–59.

81. Hanisch UK. Microglia as a source and target of cytokines. *Glia.* 2002;40:140–155.

82. Tanaka S, Ide M, Shibutani T, et al. Lipopolysaccharide-induced microglial activation induces learning and memory deficits without neuronal cell death in rats. *J Neurosci Res.* 2006;83:557–566.

83. Perry VH. Stress primes microglia to the presence of systemic inflammation: implications for environmental influences on the brain. *Brain Behav Immun.* 2007;21:45–46.

84. Carnevale D, De Simone R, Minghetti L. Microglia-neuron interaction in inflammatory and degenerative diseases: role of cholinergic and noradrenergic systems. *CNS Neurol Disord Drug Targets.* 2007;6:388–397.

85. Pocock JM, Kettenmann H. Neurotransmitter receptors on microglia. *Trends Neurosci.* 2007;30:527–535.

86. Kato TA, Yamauchi Y, Horikawa H, et al. Neurotransmitters, psychotropic drugs and microglia: clinical implications for psychiatry. *Curr Med Chem.* 2013;20:331–344.

87. Maletic V, Raison CL. Neurobiology of depression, fibromyalgia and neuropathic pain. *Front Biosci.* 2009;14:5291–5338.

88. Pascual O, Ben Achour S, Rostaing P, Triller A, Bessis A. Microglia activation triggers astrocyte-mediated modulation of excitatory neurotransmission. *Proc Natl Acad Sci U S A.* 2012;109:E197–E205.

89. Bezzi P, Domercq M, Brambilla L, et al. CXCR4-activated astrocyte glutamate release via TNFalpha: amplification by microglia triggers neurotoxicity. *Nat Neurosci.* 2001;4:702–710.

90. Wong WT, Wang M, Li W. Regulation of microglia by ionotropic glutamatergic and GAB-Aergic neurotransmission. *Neuron Glia Biol.* 2011;7:41–46.

91. Biber K, Neumann H, Inoue K, Boddeke HW. Neuronal "on" and "off" signals control microglia. *Trends Neurosci.* 2007;30:596–602.

92. Mahe C, Loetscher E, Dev KK, Bobirnac I, Otten U, Schoeffter P. Serotonin 5-HT7 receptors coupled to induction of interleukin-6 in human microglial MC-3 cells. *Neuropharmacology.* 2005;49:40–47.

93. Cardona AE, Pioro EP, Sasse ME, et al. Control of microglial neurotoxicity by the fractalkine receptor. *Nat Neurosci.* 2006;9:917–924.

94. Biber K, Pinto-Duarte A, Wittendorp MC, et al. Interleukin-6 upregulates neuronal adenosine A1 receptors: implications for neuromodulation and neuroprotection. *Neuropsychopharmacology.* 2008;33:2237–2250.

95. McAfoose J, Baune BT. Evidence for a cytokine model of cognitive function. *Neurosci Biobehav Rev.* 2009;33:355–366.

96. Heiman MG, Shaham S. Ancestral roles of glia suggested by the nervous system of *Caenorhabditis elegans*. *Neuron Glia Biol.* 2007;3:55–61.

97. Nair A, Bonneau RH. Stress-induced elevation of glucocorticoids increases microglia proliferation through NMDA receptor activation. *J Neuroimmunol.* 2006;171:72–85.

98. Rajkowska G, Miguel-Hidalgo JJ, Wei J, et al. Morphometric evidence for neuronal and glial prefrontal cell pathology in major depression. *Biol Psychiatry.* 1999;45:1085–1098.

99. Rajkowska G. Histopathology of the prefrontal cortex in major depression: what does it tell us about dysfunctional monoaminergic circuits? *Prog Brain Res.* 2000;126:397–412.

100. Uranova NA, Vostrikov VM, Orlovskaya DD, Rachmanova VI. Oligodendroglial density in the prefrontal cortex in schizophrenia and mood disorders: a study from the Stanley Neuropathology Consortium. *Schizophr Res.* 2004;67:269–275.

101. Bowley MP, Drevets WC, Ongur D, Price JL. Low glial numbers in the amygdala in major depressive disorder. *Biol Psychiatry.* 2002;52:404–412.

102. Cotter D, Mackay D, Chana G, Beasley C, Landau S, Everall IP. Reduced neuronal size and glial cell density in area 9 of the dorsolateral prefrontal cortex in subjects with major depressive disorder. *Cereb Cortex.* 2002;12:386–394.

103. Rajkowska G. Postmortem studies in mood disorders indicate altered numbers of neurons and glial cells. *Biol Psychiatry.* 2000;48:766–777.

104. Ongur D, Drevets WC, Price JL. Glial reduction in the subgenual prefrontal cortex in mood disorders. *Proc Natl Acad Sci U S A.* 1998;95:13290–13295.

105. Stockmeier CA, Mahajan GJ, Konick LC, et al. Cellular changes in the postmortem hippocampus in major depression. *Biol Psychiatry.* 2004;56:640–650.

106. Chana G, Landau S, Beasley C, Everall IP, Cotter D. Two-dimensional assessment of cytoarchitecture in the anterior cingulate cortex in major depressive disorder, bipolar disorder, and schizophrenia: evidence for decreased neuronal somal size and increased neuronal density. *Biol Psychiatry.* 2003;53:1086–1098.

107. Harrison PJ. The neuropathology of primary mood disorder. *Brain.* 2002;125:1428–1449.

108. Banasr M, Duman RS. Glial loss in the prefrontal cortex is sufficient to induce depressive-like behaviors. *Biol Psychiatry.* 2008;64:863–870.

109. Vostrikov VM, Uranova NA, Orlovskaya DD. Deficit of perineuronal oligodendrocytes in the prefrontal cortex in schizophrenia and mood disorders. *Schizophr Res.* 2007; 94:273–280.

110. Hamidi M, Drevets WC, Price JL. Glial reduction in amygdala in major depressive disorder is due to oligodendrocytes. *Biol Psychiatry.* 2004;55:563–569.

111. Regenold WT, Phatak P, Marano CM, Gearhart L, Viens CH, Hisley KC. Myelin staining of deep white matter in the dorsolateral prefrontal cortex in schizophrenia, bipolar disorder, and unipolar major depression. *Psychiatry Res.* 2007;151:179–188.

112. Huang H, Gundapuneedi T, Rao U. White matter disruptions in adolescents exposed to childhood maltreatment and vulnerability to psychopathology. *Neuropsychopharmacology.* 2012;37:2693–2701.

113. Aston C, Jiang L, Sokolov BP. Transcriptional profiling reveals evidence for signaling and oligodendroglial abnormalities in the temporal cortex from patients with major depressive disorder. *Mol Psychiatry.* 2005;10:309–322.

114. Sokolov BP. Oligodendroglial abnormalities in schizophrenia, mood disorders and substance abuse: comorbidity, shared traits, or molecular phenocopies? *Int J Neuropsychopharmacol.* 2007;10:547–555.

115. Barley K, Dracheva S, Byne W. Subcortical oligodendrocyte- and astrocyte-associated gene expression in subjects with schizophrenia, major depression and bipolar disorder. *Schizophr Res.* 2009;112:54–64.

116. Mosebach J, Keilhoff G, Gos T, et al. Increased nuclear Olig1-expression in the pre-genual anterior cingulate white matter of patients with major depression: a regen-erative attempt to compensate oligodendrocyte loss? *J Psychiatr Res.* 2013;47:1069–1079.

117. Miguel-Hidalgo JJ, Baucom C, Dilley G, et al. Glial fibrillary acidic protein immunore-activity in the prefrontal cortex distinguishes younger from older adults in major depressive disorder. *Biol Psychiatry.* 2000;48:861–873.

118. Si X, Miguel-Hidalgo JJ, O'Dwyer G, Stockmeier CA, Rajkowska G. Age-dependent reductions in the level of glial fibrillary acidic protein in the prefrontal cortex in major depression. *Neuropsychopharmacology.* 2004;29:2088–2096.

119. Steiner J, Walter M, Gos T, et al. Severe depression is associated with increased microg-lial quinolinic acid in subregions of the anterior cingulate gyrus: evidence for an immune-modulated glutamatergic neurotransmission? *J Neuroimflamm.* 2011;8:94.

120. Li Y, Barger SW, Liu L, Mrak RE, Griffin WS. S100beta induction of the proinflamma-tory cytokine interleukin-6 in neurons. *J Neurochem.* 2000;74:143–150.

121. Liu L, Li Y, Van Eldik LJ, Griffin WS, Barger SW. S100B-induced microglial and neuro-nal IL-1 expression is mediated by cell type-specific transcription factors. *J Neuro-chem.* 2005;92:546–553.

122. de Souza DF, Leite MC, Quincozes-Santos A, et al. S100B secretion is stimulated by IL-1beta in glial cultures and hippocampal slices of rats: likely involvement of MAPK pathway. *J Neuroimmunol.* 2009;206:52–57.

123. de Souza DF, Wartchow K, Hansen F, et al. Interleukin-6-induced S100B secretion is inhibited by haloperidol and risperidone. *Prog Neuropsychopharmacol Biol Psychia-try.* 2013;43:14–22.

124. Gos T, Schroeter ML, Lessel W, et al. S100B-immunopositive astrocytes and oligoden-drocytes in the hippocampus are differentially afflicted in unipolar and bipolar depression: a postmortem study. *J Psychiatr Res.* 2013;47(11):1694–1699.

125. Arolt V, Peters M, Erfurth A, et al. S100B and response to treatment in major depres-sion: a pilot study. *Eur Neuropsychopharmacol.* 2003;13:235–239.

126. Schroeter ML, Abdul-Khaliq H, Krebs M, Diefenbacher A, Blasig IE. Serum markers support disease-specific glial pathology in major depression. *J Affect Disord.* 2008;111:271–280.

127. Yang K, Xie GR, Hu YQ, Mao FQ, Su LY. The effects of gender and numbers of depres-sive episodes on serum S100B levels in patients with major depression. *J Neural Transm.* 2008;115:1687–1694.

128. Schroeter ML, Steiner J, Mueller K. Glial pathology is modified by age in mood disor-ders—a systematic meta-analysis of serum S100B in vivo studies. *J Affect Disord.* 2011;134:32–38.

129. Steiner J, Schiltz K, Walter M, et al. S100B serum levels are closely correlated with body mass index: an important caveat in neuropsychiatric research. *Psychoneuroen-docrinology.* 2010;35:321–324.

130. Michetti F, Corvino V, Geloso MC, et al. The S100B protein in biological fluids: more than a lifelong biomarker of brain distress. *J Neurochem.* 2012;120:644–659.

131. Shelton RC, Miller AH. Eating ourselves to death (and despair): the contribution of adiposity and inflammation to depression. *Prog Neurobiol.* 2010;91:275–299.

132. Haroon E, Raison CL, Miller AH. Psychoneuroimmunology meets neuropsychophar-macology: translational implications of the impact of inflammation on behavior. *Neu-ropsychopharmacology.* 2012;37:137–162.

133. Uher T, Bob P. Cerebrospinal fluid S100B levels reflect symptoms of depression in

patients with non-inflammatory neurological disorders. *Neurosci Lett.* 2012;529:139–143.

134. Hundal O. Major depressive disorder viewed as a dysfunction in astroglial bioenergetics. *Med Hypotheses.* 2007;68:370–377.

135. Gittins RA, Harrison PJ. A morphometric study of glia and neurons in the anterior cingulate cortex in mood disorder. *J Affect Disord.* 2011;133:328–332.

136. Bouhuys AL, Flentge F, Oldehinkel AJ, van den Berg MD. Potential psychosocial mechanisms linking depression to immune function in elderly subjects. *Psychiatry Res.* 2004;127:237–245.

137. Husarova V, Bittsansky M, Ondrejka I, Kerna V, Dobrota D. Hippocampal neurometabolite changes in depression treatment: a (1)H magnetic resonance spectroscopy study. *Psychiatry Res.* 2012;201:206–213.

138. Rajkowska G, Hughes J, Stockmeier CA, Javier Miguel-Hidalgo J, Maciag D. Coverage of blood vessels by astrocytic endfeet is reduced in major depressive disorder. *Biol Psychiatry.* 2013;73:613–621.

139. Steiner J, Bielau H, Brisch R, et al. Immunological aspects in the neurobiology of suicide: elevated microglial density in schizophrenia and depression is associated with suicide. *J Psychiatr Res.* 2008;42:151–157.

140. Rajkowska G, Miguel-Hidalgo JJ, Dubey P, Stockmeier CA, Krishnan KR. Prominent reduction in pyramidal neurons density in the orbitofrontal cortex of elderly depressed patients. *Biol Psychiatry.* 2005;58:297–306.

141. Sibille E, French B. Biological substrates underpinning diagnosis of major depression. *Int J Neuropsychopharmacol.* 2013;16:1893–1909.

142. Miguel-Hidalgo JJ, Dubey P, Shao Q, Stockmeier C, Rajkowska G. Unchanged packing density but altered size of neurofilament immunoreactive neurons in the prefrontal cortex in schizophrenia and major depression. *Schizophr Res.* 2005;76:159–171.

143. Rajkowska G, O'Dwyer G, Teleki Z, Stockmeier CA, Miguel-Hidalgo JJ. GABAergic neurons immunoreactive for calcium binding proteins are reduced in the prefrontal cortex in major depression. *Neuropsychopharmacology.* 2007;32:471–482.

144. Hercher C, Canetti L, Turecki G, Mechawar N. Anterior cingulate pyramidal neurons display altered dendritic branching in depressed suicides. *J Psychiatr Res.* 2010;44:286–293.

145. Kang HJ, Voleti B, Hajszan T, et al. Decreased expression of synapse-related genes and loss of synapses in major depressive disorder. *Nat Med.* 2012;18:1413–1417.

146. Duman RS, Monteggia LM. A neurotrophic model for stress-related mood disorders. *Biol Psychiatry.* 2006;59:1116–1127.

147. Linker R, Gold R, Luhder F. Function of neurotrophic factors beyond the nervous system: inflammation and autoimmune demyelination. *Crit Rev Immunol.* 2009;29:43–68.

148. Chen ZY, Bath K, McEwen B, Hempstead B, Lee F. Impact of genetic variant BDNF (Val66Met) on brain structure and function. *Novartis Found Symp.* 2008;289:180–195.

149. Segawa M, Morinobu S, Matsumoto T, Fuchikami M, Yamawaki S. Electroconvulsive seizure, but not imipramine, rapidly up-regulates pro-BDNF and t-PA, leading to mature BDNF production, in the rat hippocampus. *Int J Neuropsychopharmacol.* 2013;16:339–350.

150. Hashioka S, Klegeris A, Monji A, et al. Antidepressants inhibit interferon-gamma-induced microglial production of IL-6 and nitric oxide. *Exp Neurol.* 2007;206:33–42.

151. Shafer RA, Murphy S. Activated astrocytes induce nitric oxide synthase-2 in cerebral endothelium via tumor necrosis factor alpha. *Glia.* 1997;21:370–379.

152. Oliveira RM, Guimaraes FS, Deakin JF. Expression of neuronal nitric oxide synthase in the hippocampal formation in affective disorders. *Braz J Med Biol Res.* 2008; 41:333–341.

153. Xiong H, Yamada K, Han D, et al. Mutual regulation between the intercellular messengers nitric oxide and brain-derived neurotrophic factor in rodent neocortical neurons. *Eur J Neurosci.* 1999;11:1567–1576.

154. Schulte-Herbruggen O, Nassenstein C, Lommatzsch M, Quarcoo D, Renz H, Braun A. Tumor necrosis factor-alpha and interleukin-6 regulate secretion of brain-derived neurotrophic factor in human monocytes. *J Neuroimmunol.* 2005;160:204–209.

155. Furuno T, Nakanishi M. Neurotrophic factors increase tumor necrosis factor-α induced nuclear translocation of NF-kappaB in rat PC12 cells. *Neurosci Lett.* 2006;392: 240–244.

156. Hein AM, Stutzman DL, Bland ST, et al. Prostaglandins are necessary and sufficient to induce contextual fear learning impairments after interleukin-1 beta injections into the dorsal hippocampus. *Neuroscience.* 2007;150:754–763.

157. Madrigal JL, Garcia-Bueno B, Moro MA, Lizasoain I, Lorenzo P, Leza JC. Relationship between cyclooxygenase-2 and nitric oxide synthase-2 in rat cortex after stress. *Eur J Neurosci.* 2003;18:1701–1705.

158. Pinnock SB, Herbert J. Brain-derived neurotropic factor and neurogenesis in the adult rat dentate gyrus: interactions with corticosterone. *Eur J Neurosci.* 2008;27:2493–2500.

159. Juric DM, Miklic S, Carman-Krzan M. Monoaminergic neuronal activity up-regulates BDNF synthesis in cultured neonatal rat astrocytes. *Brain Res.* 2006;1108:54–62.

160. Hardingham GE, Fukunaga Y, Bading H. Extrasynaptic NMDARs oppose synaptic NMDARs by triggering CREB shut-off and cell death pathways. *Nat Neurosci.* 2002; 5:405–414.

161. Russo-Neustadt AA, Chen MJ. Brain-derived neurotrophic factor and antidepressant activity. *Curr Pharm Des.* 2005;11:1495–1510.

162. Hunsberger J, Austin DR, Henter ID, Chen G. The neurotrophic and neuroprotective effects of psychotropic agents. *Dialogues Clin Neurosci.* 2009;11:333–348.

163. Hanson ND, Owens MJ, Nemeroff CB. Depression, antidepressants, and neurogenesis: a critical reappraisal. *Neuropsychopharmacology.* 2011;36:2589–2602.

164. Garcia LS, Comim CM, Valvassori SS, et al. Acute administration of ketamine induces antidepressant-like effects in the forced swimming test and increases BDNF levels in the rat hippocampus. *Prog Neuropsychopharmacol Biol Psychiatry.* 2008;32:140–144.

165. Gomez-Pinilla F, Vaynman S, Ying Z. Brain-derived neurotrophic factor functions as a metabotrophin to mediate the effects of exercise on cognition. *Eur J Neurosci.* 2008;28:2278–2287.

166. Okamoto T, Yoshimura R, Ikenouchi-Sugita A, et al. Efficacy of electroconvulsive therapy is associated with changing blood levels of homovanillic acid and brain-derived neurotrophic factor (BDNF) in refractory depressed patients: a pilot study. *Prog Neuropsychopharmacol Biol Psychiatry.* 2008;32:1185–1190.

167. Siuciak JA, Lewis DR, Wiegand SJ, Lindsay RM. Antidepressant-like effect of brain-derived neurotrophic factor (BDNF). *Pharmacol Biochem Behav.* 1997;56:131–137.

168. Coppell AL, Pei Q, Zetterstrom TS. Bi-phasic change in BDNF gene expression following antidepressant drug treatment. *Neuropharmacology.* 2003;44:903–910.

169. Saarelainen T, Hendolin P, Lucas G, et al. Activation of the TrkB neurotrophin receptor is induced by antidepressant drugs and is required for antidepressant-induced behavioral effects. *J Neurosci.* 2003;23:349–357.

170. De Foubert G, Carney SL, Robinson CS, et al. Fluoxetine-induced change in rat brain expression of brain-derived neurotrophic factor varies depending on length of treatment. *Neuroscience.* 2004;128:597–604.

171. Dias BG, Banerjee SB, Duman RS, Vaidya VA. Differential regulation of brain derived neurotrophic factor transcripts by antidepressant treatments in the adult rat brain. *Neuropharmacology.* 2003;45:553–563.

172. Altar CA, Whitehead RE, Chen R, Wortwein G, Madsen TM. Effects of electroconvulsive seizures and antidepressant drugs on brain-derived neurotrophic factor protein in rat brain. *Biol Psychiatry.* 2003;54:703–709.

173. Chen B, Dowlatshahi D, MacQueen GM, Wang JF, Young LT. Increased hippocampal BDNF immunoreactivity in subjects treated with antidepressant medication. *Biol Psychiatry.* 2001;50:260–265.

174. Russo-Neustadt AA, Alejandre H, Garcia C, Ivy AS, Chen MJ. Hippocampal brain-derived neurotrophic factor expression following treatment with reboxetine, citalopram, and physical exercise. *Neuropsychopharmacology.* 2004;29:2189–2199.

175. Xu H, Steven Richardson J, Li XM. Dose-related effects of chronic antidepressants on neuroprotective proteins BDNF, Bcl-2 and Cu/Zn-SOD in rat hippocampus. *Neuropsychopharmacology.* 2003;28:53–62.

176. Rantamaki T, Hendolin P, Kankaanpaa A, et al. Pharmacologically diverse antidepressants rapidly activate brain-derived neurotrophic factor receptor TrkB and induce phospholipase-Cgamma signaling pathways in mouse brain. *Neuropsychopharmacology.* 2007;32:2152–2162.

177. Dwivedi Y, Rizavi HS, Zhang H, et al. Neurotrophin receptor activation and expression in human postmortem brain: effect of suicide. *Biol Psychiatry.* 2009;65:319–328.

178. Martinez JM, Garakani A, Yehuda R, Gorman JM. Proinflammatory and "resiliency" proteins in the CSF of patients with major depression. *Depress Anxiety.* 2012;29:32–38.

179. Zhou L, Xiong J, Lim Y, et al. Upregulation of blood proBDNF and its receptors in major depression. *J Affect Disord.* 2013;150:776–784.

180. Lang UE, Hellweg R, Seifert F, Schubert F, Gallinat J. Correlation between serum brain-derived neurotrophic factor level and an in vivo marker of cortical integrity. *Biol Psychiatry.* 2007;62:530–535.

181. Dawood T, Anderson J, Barton D, et al. Reduced overflow of BDNF from the brain is linked with suicide risk in depressive illness. *Mol Psychiatry.* 2007;12:981–983.

182. Deveci A, Aydemir O, Taskin O, Taneli F, Esen-Danaci A. Serum BDNF levels in suicide attempters related to psychosocial stressors: a comparative study with depression. *Neuropsychobiology.* 2007;56:93–97.

183. Karege F, Bondolfi G, Gervasoni N, Schwald M, Aubry JM, Bertschy G. Low brain-derived neurotrophic factor (BDNF) levels in serum of depressed patients probably results from lowered platelet BDNF release unrelated to platelet reactivity. *Biol Psychiatry.* 2005;57:1068–1072.

184. Eker C, Kitis O, Taneli F, et al. Correlation of serum BDNF levels with hippocampal volumes in first episode, medication-free depressed patients. *Eur Arch Psychiatry Clin Neurosci.* 2010;260:527–533.

185. Takebayashi N, Maeshima H, Baba H, et al. Duration of last depressive episode may influence serum BDNF levels in remitted patients with major depression. *Depress Anxiety.* 2012;29:775–779.

186. Karege F, Perret G, Bondolfi G, Schwald M, Bertschy G, Aubry JM. Decreased serum brain-derived neurotrophic factor levels in major depressed patients. *Psychiatry Res.* 2002;109:143–148.

187. Monteleone P, Serritella C, Martiadis V, Maj M. Decreased levels of serum brain-derived neurotrophic factor in both depressed and euthymic patients with unipolar depression and in euthymic patients with bipolar I and II disorders. *Bipolar Disord.* 2008;10:95–100.

188. Aydemir C, Yalcin ES, Aksaray S, et al. Brain-derived neurotrophic factor (BDNF) changes in the serum of depressed women. *Prog Neuropsychopharmacol Biol Psychiatry.* 2006;30:1256–1260.

189. Aydemir O, Deveci A, Taskin OE, Taneli F, Esen-Danaci A. Serum brain-derived neurotrophic factor level in dysthymia: a comparative study with major depressive disorder. *Prog Neuropsychopharmacol Biol Psychiatry.* 2007;31:1023–1026.

190. Molendijk ML, Bus BA, Spinhoven P, et al. Serum levels of brain-derived neurotrophic factor in major depressive disorder: state-trait issues, clinical features and pharmacological treatment. *Mol Psychiatry.* 2011;16:1088–1095.

191. Hasselbalch BJ, Knorr U, Bennike B, Hasselbalch SG, Sondergaard MH, Vedel Kessing L. Decreased levels of brain-derived neurotrophic factor in the remitted state of unipolar depressive disorder. *Acta Psychiatr Scand.* 2012;126:157–164.

192. Neumeister A, Yuan P, Young TA, et al. Effects of tryptophan depletion on serum levels of brain-derived neurotrophic factor in unmedicated patients with remitted depression and healthy subjects. *Am J Psychiatry.* 2005;162:805–807.

193. Dreimuller N, Schlicht KF, Wagner S, et al. Early reactions of brain-derived neurotrophic factor in plasma (plasma BDNF) and outcome to acute antidepressant treatment in patients with Major Depression. *Neuropharmacology.* 2012;62:264–269.

194. Piccinni A, Marazziti D, Catena M, et al. Plasma and serum brain-derived neurotrophic factor (BDNF) in depressed patients during 1 year of antidepressant treatments. *J Affect Disord.* 2008;105:279–283.

195. Cattaneo A, Bocchio-Chiavetto L, Zanardini R, Milanesi E, Placentino A, Gennarelli M. Reduced peripheral brain-derived neurotrophic factor mRNA levels are normalized by antidepressant treatment. *Int J Neuropsychopharmacol.* 2010;13:103–108.

196. Lee BH, Kim H, Park SH, Kim YK. Decreased plasma BDNF level in depressive patients. *J Affect Disord.* 2007;101:239–244.

197. Grassi-Oliveira R, Stein LM, Lopes RP, Teixeira AL, Bauer ME. Low plasma brain-derived neurotrophic factor and childhood physical neglect are associated with verbal memory impairment in major depression—a preliminary report. *Biol Psychiatry.* 2008;64:281–285.

198. Kim YK, Lee HP, Won SD, et al. Low plasma BDNF is associated with suicidal behavior in major depression. *Prog Neuropsychopharmacol Biol Psychiatry.* 2007;31:78–85.

199. Huang TL, Lee CT, Liu YL. Serum brain-derived neurotrophic factor levels in patients with major depression: effects of antidepressants. *J Psychiatr Res.* 2008;42:521–525.

200. Trajkovska V, Vinberg M, Aznar S, Knudsen GM, Kessing LV. Whole blood BDNF levels in healthy twins discordant for affective disorder: association to life events and neuroticism. *J Affect Disord.* 2008;108:165–169.

201. Sen S, Duman R, Sanacora G. Serum brain-derived neurotrophic factor, depression, and antidepressant medications: meta-analyses and implications. *Biol Psychiatry.* 2008;64:527–532.

202. Brunoni AR, Lopes M, Fregni F. A systematic review and meta-analysis of clinical

studies on major depression and BDNF levels: implications for the role of neuroplasticity in depression. *Int J Neuropsychopharmacol.* 2008;11:1169–1180.

203. Bocchio-Chiavetto L, Bagnardi V, Zanardini R, et al. Serum and plasma BDNF levels in major depression: a replication study and meta-analyses. *World J Biol Psychiatry.* 2010;11:763–773.

204. Frodl TS, Koutsouleris N, Bottlender R, et al. Depression-related variation in brain morphology over 3 years: effects of stress? *Arch Gen Psychiatry.* 2008;65:1156–1165.

205. Dwivedi Y, Rizavi HS, Conley RR, Roberts RC, Tamminga CA, Pandey GN. Altered gene expression of brain-derived neurotrophic factor and receptor tyrosine kinase B in postmortem brain of suicide subjects. *Arch Gen Psychiatry.* 2003;60:804–815.

206. Laske C, Banschbach S, Stransky E, et al. Exercise-induced normalization of decreased BDNF serum concentration in elderly women with remitted major depression. *Int J Neuropsychopharmacol.* 2010;13:595–602.

207. Lucassen PJ, Meerlo P, Naylor AS, et al. Regulation of adult neurogenesis by stress, sleep disruption, exercise and inflammation: implications for depression and antidepressant action. *Eur Neuropsychopharmacol.* 2010;20:1–17.

208. DeCarolis NA, Eisch AJ. Hippocampal neurogenesis as a target for the treatment of mental illness: a critical evaluation. *Neuropharmacology.* 2010;58:884–893.

209. Bessa JM, Ferreira D, Melo I, et al. The mood-improving actions of antidepressants do not depend on neurogenesis but are associated with neuronal remodeling. *Mol Psychiatry.* 2009;14:764–773, 739.

210. Kozisek ME, Middlemas D, Bylund DB. The differential regulation of BDNF and TrkB levels in juvenile rats after four days of escitalopram and desipramine treatment. *Neuropharmacology.* 2008;54:251–257.

211. Yang B, Slonimsky JD, Birren SJ. A rapid switch in sympathetic neurotransmitter release properties mediated by the p75 receptor. *Nat Neurosci.* 2002;5:539–545.

212. Kasselman LJ, Sideris A, Bruno C, et al. BDNF: a missing link between sympathetic dysfunction and inflammatory disease? *J Neuroimmunol.* 2006;175:118–127.

213. Kim JM, Stewart R, Kim SW, et al. BDNF genotype potentially modifying the association between incident stroke and depression. *Neurobiol Aging.* 2008;29:789–792.

214. Cao L, Liu X, Lin EJ, et al. Environmental and genetic activation of a brain-adipocyte BDNF/leptin axis causes cancer remission and inhibition. *Cell.* 2010;142:52–64.

215. Gotoh K, Masaki T, Chiba S, et al. Brain-derived neurotrophic factor, corticotropin-releasing factor, and hypothalamic neuronal histamine interact to regulate feeding behavior. *J Neurochem.* 2013;125:588–598.

216. Krabbe KS, Nielsen AR, Krogh-Madsen R, et al. Brain-derived neurotrophic factor (BDNF) and type 2 diabetes. *Diabetologia.* 2007;50:431–438.

217. Gotoh K, Masaki T, Chiba S, et al. Hypothalamic brain-derived neurotrophic factor regulates glucagon secretion mediated by pancreatic efferent nerves. *J Neuroendocrinol.* 2013;25:302–311.

218. Hristova M, Aloe L. Metabolic syndrome—neurotrophic hypothesis. *Med Hypotheses.* 2006;66:545–549.

219. Tseng PT, Lee Y, Lin PY. Age-associated decrease in serum glial cell line-derived neurotrophic factor levels in patients with major depressive disorder. *Prog Neuropsychopharmacol Biol Psychiatry.* 2013;40:334–339.

220. Michel TM, Frangou S, Camara S, et al. Altered glial cell line-derived neurotrophic factor (GDNF) concentrations in the brain of patients with depressive disorder: a comparative post-mortem study. *Eur Psychiatry.* 2008;23:413–420.

221. Bauer M, Suppmann S, Meyer M, et al. Glial cell line-derived neurotrophic factor up-

regulates GTP-cyclohydrolase I activity and tetrahydrobiopterin levels in primary dopaminergic neurones. *J Neurochem.* 2002;82:1300–1310.

222. Pascual A, Hidalgo-Figueroa M, Piruat JI, Pintado CO, Gomez-Diaz R, Lopez-Barneo J. Absolute requirement of GDNF for adult catecholaminergic neuron survival. *Nat Neurosci.* 2008;11:755–761.

223. Rocha SM, Cristovao AC, Campos FL, Fonseca CP, Baltazar G. Astrocyte-derived GDNF is a potent inhibitor of microglial activation. *Neurobiol Dis.* 2012;47:407–415.

224. Miller CA. Stressed and depressed? Check your GDNF for epigenetic repression. *Neuron.* 2011;69:188–190.

225. Takebayashi M, Hisaoka K, Nishida A, et al. Decreased levels of whole blood glial cell line-derived neurotrophic factor (GDNF) in remitted patients with mood disorders. *Int J Neuropsychopharmacol.* 2006;9:607–612.

226. Diniz BS, Teixeira AL, Miranda AS, Talib LL, Gattaz WF, Forlenza OV. Circulating Glial-derived neurotrophic factor is reduced in late-life depression. *J Psychiatr Res.* 2012;46:135–139.

227. Zhang X, Zhang Z, Xie C, et al. Effect of treatment on serum glial cell line-derived neurotrophic factor in depressed patients. *Prog Neuropsychopharmacol Biol Psychiatry.* 2008;32:886–890.

228. Otsuki K, Uchida S, Watanuki T, et al. Altered expression of neurotrophic factors in patients with major depression. *J Psychiatr Res.* 2008;42:1145–1153.

229. Zhang X, Zhang Z, Sha W, et al. Electroconvulsive therapy increases glial cell-line derived neurotrophic factor (GDNF) serum levels in patients with drug-resistant depression. *Psychiatry Res.* 2009;170:273–275.

230. Clark-Raymond A, Halaris A. VEGF and depression: a comprehensive assessment of clinical data. *J Psychiatr Res.* 2013;47:1080–1087.

231. Newton SS, Fournier NM, Duman RS. Vascular growth factors in neuropsychiatry. *Cell Mol Life Sci.* 2013;70:1739–1752.

232. Yang EV, Donovan EL, Benson DM, Glaser R. VEGF is differentially regulated in multiple myeloma-derived cell lines by norepinephrine. *Brain Behav Immun.* 2008;22: 318–323.

233. Fornaro M, Rocchi G, Escelsior A, et al. VEGF plasma level variations in duloxetine-treated patients with major depression. *J Affect Disord.* 2013;151(2):590–595.

234. Blumberg HP, Wang F, Chepenik LG, et al. Influence of vascular endothelial growth factor variation on human hippocampus morphology. *Biol Psychiatry.* 2008;64:901–903.

235. Schmidt HD, Shelton RC, Duman RS. Functional biomarkers of depression: diagnosis, treatment, and pathophysiology. *Neuropsychopharmacology.* 2011;36:2375–2394.

236. Grinberg YY, Dibbern ME, Levasseur VA, Kraig RP. Insulin-like growth factor-1 abrogates microglial oxidative stress and TNF-alpha responses to spreading depression. *J Neurochem.* 2013;126:662–672.

237. Park SE, Dantzer R, Kelley KW, McCusker RH. Central administration of insulin-like growth factor-I decreases depressive-like behavior and brain cytokine expression in mice. *J Neuroinflamm.* 2011;8:12.

238. Trejo JL, Piriz J, Llorens-Martin MV, et al. Central actions of liver-derived insulin-like growth factor I underlying its pro-cognitive effects. *Mol Psychiatry.* 2007;12:1118–1128.

239. O'Connor JC, McCusker RH, Strle K, Johnson RW, Dantzer R, Kelley KW. Regulation of IGF-I function by proinflammatory cytokines: at the interface of immunology and endocrinology. *Cell Immunol.* 2008;252:91–110.

240. Hoshaw BA, Malberg JE, Lucki I. Central administration of IGF-I and BDNF leads to long-lasting antidepressant-like effects. *Brain Res.* 2005;1037:204–208.

241. Duman CH, Schlesinger L, Terwilliger R, Russell DS, Newton SS, Duman RS. Peripheral insulin-like growth factor-I produces antidepressant-like behavior and contributes to the effect of exercise. *Behav Brain Res.* 2009;198:366–371.

242. Paslakis G, Blum WF, Deuschle M. Intranasal insulin-like growth factor I (IGF-I) as a plausible future treatment of depression. *Med Hypotheses.* 2012;79:222–225.

243. Weber-Hamann B, Blum WF, Kratzsch J, Gilles M, Heuser I, Deuschle M. Insulin-like growth factor-I (IGF-I) serum concentrations in depressed patients: relationship to saliva cortisol and changes during antidepressant treatment. *Pharmacopsychiatry.* 2009;42:23–28.

244. Schilling C, Blum WF, Heuser I, Paslakis G, Wudy SA, Deuschle M. Treatment with antidepressants increases insulin-like growth factor-I in cerebrospinal fluid. *J Clin Psychopharmacol.* 2011;31:390–392.

245. Erickson MA, Dohi K, Banks WA. Neuroinflammation: a common pathway in CNS diseases as mediated at the blood-brain barrier. *Neuroimmunomodulation.* 2012;19:121–130.

246. Banks WA. Blood-brain barrier transport of cytokines: a mechanism for neuropathology. *Curr Pharm Des.* 2005;11:973–984.

247. Quan N, Banks WA. Brain-immune communication pathways. *Brain Behav Immun.* 2007;21:727–735.

248. Vitkovic L, Konsman JP, Bockaert J, Dantzer R, Homburger V, Jacque C. Cytokine signals propagate through the brain. *Mol Psychiatry.* 2000;5:604–615.

249. Yirmiya R, Goshen I. Immune modulation of learning, memory, neural plasticity and neurogenesis. *Brain Behav Immun.* 2011;25:181–213.

250. Deverman BE, Patterson PH. Cytokines and CNS development. *Neuron.* 2009;64:61–78.

251. Asami T, Ito T, Fukumitsu H, Nomoto H, Furukawa Y, Furukawa S. Autocrine activation of cultured macrophages by brain-derived neurotrophic factor. *Biochem Biophys Res Commun.* 2006;344:941–947.

252. Kerschensteiner M, Gallmeier E, Behrens L, et al. Activated human T cells, B cells, and monocytes produce brain-derived neurotrophic factor in vitro and in inflammatory brain lesions: a neuroprotective role of inflammation? *J Exp Med.* 1999;189:865–870.

253. Linker RA, Lee DH, Demir S, et al. Functional role of brain-derived neurotrophic factor in neuroprotective autoimmunity: therapeutic implications in a model of multiple sclerosis. *Brain.* 2010;133:2248–2263.

254. Kerschensteiner M, Stadelmann C, Dechant G, Wekerle H, Hohlfeld R. Neurotrophic cross-talk between the nervous and immune systems: implications for neurological diseases. *Ann Neurol.* 2003;53:292–304.

255. Dustin ML, Colman DR. Neural and immunological synaptic relations. *Science.* 2002;298:785–789.

256. Khairova RA, Machado-Vieira R, Du J, Manji HK. A potential role for pro-inflammatory cytokines in regulating synaptic plasticity in major depressive disorder. *Int J Neuropsychopharmacol.* 2009;12:561–578.

257. Sallmann S, Juttler E, Prinz S, et al. Induction of interleukin-6 by depolarization of neurons. *J Neurosci.* 2000;20:8637–8642.

258. Schwaninger M, Petersen N, Prinz S, Sallmann S, Neher M, Spranger M. Adenosine-induced expression of interleukin-6 in astrocytes through protein kinase A and NF-IL-6. *Glia.* 2000;31:51–58.

259. Li Y, Liu L, Kang J, et al. Neuronal-glial interactions mediated by interleukin-1 enhance neuronal acetylcholinesterase activity and mRNA expression. *J Neurosci.* 2000;20: 149–155.

260. Otten U, Marz P, Heese K, Hock C, Kunz D, Rose-John S. Cytokines and neurotrophins interact in normal and diseased states. *Ann N Y Acad Sci.* 2000;917:322–330.

261. Liu Z, Qiu YH, Li B, Ma SH, Peng YP. Neuroprotection of interleukin-6 against NMDA-induced apoptosis and its signal-transduction mechanisms. *Neurotox Res.* 2011;19:484–495.

262. Vitkovic L, Bockaert J, Jacque C. "Inflammatory" cytokines: neuromodulators in normal brain? *J Neurochem.* 2000;74:457–471.

263. Figiel I. Pro-inflammatory cytokine TNF-alpha as a neuroprotective agent in the brain. *Acta Neurobiol Exp (Wars).* 2008;68:526–534.

264. Ziv Y, Schwartz M. Immune-based regulation of adult neurogenesis: implications for learning and memory. *Brain Behav Immun.* 2008;22:167–176.

265. Rook GA, Lowry CA, Raison CL. Lymphocytes in neuroprotection, cognition and emotion: is intolerance really the answer? *Brain Behav Immun.* 2011;25:591–601.

266. Koo JW, Russo SJ, Ferguson D, Nestler EJ, Duman RS. Nuclear factor-kappaB is a critical mediator of stress-impaired neurogenesis and depressive behavior. *Proc Natl Acad Sci U S A.* 2010;107:2669–2674.

267. Faraguna U, Vyazovskiy VV, Nelson AB, Tononi G, Cirelli C. A causal role for brain-derived neurotrophic factor in the homeostatic regulation of sleep. *J Neurosci.* 2008;28:4088–4095.

268. Tononi G, Cirelli C. Perchance to prune: during sleep, the brain weakens the connections among nerve cells, apparently conserving energy and, paradoxically, aiding memory. *Sci Am.* 2013;309:34–39.

269. Krueger JM. The role of cytokines in sleep regulation. *Curr Pharm Des.* 2008;14: 3408–3416.

270. Jia P, Kao CF, Kuo PH, Zhao Z. A comprehensive network and pathway analysis of candidate genes in major depressive disorder. *BMC Syst Biol.* 2011;5(suppl 3):S12.

271. Li JZ, Bunney BG, Meng F, et al. Circadian patterns of gene expression in the human brain and disruption in major depressive disorder. *Proc Natl Acad Sci U S A.* 2013; 110:9950–9955.

272. Ramirez-Amaya V, Bermudez-Rattoni F. Conditioned enhancement of antibody production is disrupted by insular cortex and amygdala but not hippocampal lesions. *Brain Behav Immun.* 1999;13:46–60.

273. Pacheco-Lopez G, Niemi MB, Kou W, Harting M, Fandrey J, Schedlowski M. Neural substrates for behaviorally conditioned immunosuppression in the rat. *J Neurosci.* 2005;25:2330–2337.

274. Irwin MR, Cole SW. Reciprocal regulation of the neural and innate immune systems. *Nat Rev Immunol.* 2011;11:625–632.

275. Inagaki TK, Muscatell KA, Irwin MR, Cole SW, Eisenberger NI. Inflammation selectively enhances amygdala activity to socially threatening images. *Neuroimage.* 2012;59:3222–3226.

276. Harrison NA, Brydon L, Walker C, Gray MA, Steptoe A, Critchley HD. Inflammation causes mood changes through alterations in subgenual cingulate activity and meso-limbic connectivity. *Biol Psychiatry.* 2009;66:407–414.

277. Felger JC, Miller AH. Cytokine effects on the basal ganglia and dopamine function: the subcortical source of inflammatory malaise. *Front Neuroendocrinol.* 2012;33:315–327.

278. Hannestad J, Subramanyam K, Dellagioia N, et al. Glucose metabolism in the insula

and cingulate is affected by systemic inflammation in humans. *J Nucl Med.* 2012;53: 601–607.

279. Brydon L, Harrison NA, Walker C, Steptoe A, Critchley HD. Peripheral inflammation is associated with altered substantia nigra activity and psychomotor slowing in humans. *Biol Psychiatry.* 2008;63:1022–1029.

280. Eisenberger NI, Berkman ET, Inagaki TK, Rameson LT, Mashal NM, Irwin MR. Inflammation-induced anhedonia: endotoxin reduces ventral striatum responses to reward. *Biol Psychiatry.* 2010;68:748–754.

281. Prager G, Hadamitzky M, Engler A, et al. Amygdaloid signature of peripheral immune activation by bacterial lipopolysaccharide or staphylococcal enterotoxin B. *J Neuroimmune Pharmacol.* 2013;8:42–50.

282. O'Connor MF, Irwin MR, Wellisch DK. When grief heats up: pro-inflammatory cytokines predict regional brain activation. *Neuroimage.* 2009;47:891–896.

283. Savitz J, Frank MB, Victor T, et al. Inflammation and neurological disease-related genes are differentially expressed in depressed patients with mood disorders and correlate with morphometric and functional imaging abnormalities. *Brain Behav Immun.* 2013;31:161–171.

284. Dean B, Tawadros N, Scarr E, Gibbons AS. Regionally-specific changes in levels of tumour necrosis factor in the dorsolateral prefrontal cortex obtained postmortem from subjects with major depressive disorder. *J Affect Disord.* 2010;120:245–248.

285. Felger JC, Lotrich FE. Inflammatory cytokines in depression: neurobiological mechanisms and therapeutic implications. *Neuroscience.* 2013;246:199–229.

286. Erhardt S, Lim CK, Linderholm KR, et al. Connecting inflammation with glutamate agonism in suicidality. *Neuropsychopharmacology.* 2013;38:743–752.

287. Tong L, Balazs R, Soiampornkul R, Thangnipon W, Cotman CW. Interleukin-1 beta impairs brain derived neurotrophic factor-induced signal transduction. *Neurobiol Aging.* 2008;29:1380–1393.

288. Yoshimura R, Hori H, Ikenouchi-Sugita A, Umene-Nakano W, Ueda N, Nakamura J. Higher plasma interleukin-6 (IL-6) level is associated with SSRI- or SNRI-refractory depression. *Prog Neuropsychopharmacol Biol Psychiatry.* 2009;33:722–726.

289. Goshen I, Kreisel T, Ben-Menachem-Zidon O, et al. Brain interleukin-1 mediates chronic stress-induced depression in mice via adrenocortical activation and hippocampal neurogenesis suppression. *Mol Psychiatry.* 2008;13:717–728.

290. Felger JC, Li L, Marvar PJ, et al. Tyrosine metabolism during interferon-alpha administration: association with fatigue and CSF dopamine concentrations. *Brain Behav Immun.* 2013;31:153–160.

291. Raison CL, Capuron L, Miller AH. Cytokines sing the blues: inflammation and the pathogenesis of depression. *Trends Immunol.* 2006;27:24–31.

292. Sukoff Rizzo SJ, Neal SJ, Hughes ZA, et al. Evidence for sustained elevation of IL-6 in the CNS as a key contributor of depressive-like phenotypes. *Translat Psychiatry.* 2012; 2:e199.

293. Zhou Z, Peng X, Insolera R, Fink DJ, Mata M. Interleukin-10 provides direct trophic support to neurons. *J Neurochem.* 2009;110:1617–1627.

294. Uher T, Bob P. Cerebrospinal fluid IL-8 levels reflect symptoms of alexithymia in patients with non-inflammatory neurological disorders. *Psychoneuroendocrinology.* 2011;36:1148–1153.

295. Boufidou F, Lambrinoudaki I, Argeitis J, et al. CSF and plasma cytokines at delivery and postpartum mood disturbances. *J Affect Disord.* 2009;115:287–292.

296. Kern S, Skoog I, Borjesson-Hanson A, et al. Lower CSF interleukin-6 predicts future

depression in a population-based sample of older women followed for 17 years. *Brain Behav Immun.* 2013;32:153–158.

297. Sasayama D, Hattori K, Wakabayashi C, et al. Increased cerebrospinal fluid interleukin-6 levels in patients with schizophrenia and those with major depressive disorder. *J Psychiatr Res.* 2013;47:401–406.

298. Lindqvist D, Janelidze S, Hagell P, et al. Interleukin-6 is elevated in the cerebrospinal fluid of suicide attempters and related to symptom severity. *Biol Psychiatry.* 2009;66: 287–292.

299. Levine J, Barak Y, Chengappa KN, Rapoport A, Rebey M, Barak V. Cerebrospinal cytokine levels in patients with acute depression. *Neuropsychobiology.* 1999;40:171–176.

300. Gavillet M, Allaman I, Magistretti PJ. Modulation of astrocytic metabolic phenotype by proinflammatory cytokines. *Glia.* 2008;56:975–989.

301. Carson MJ, Doose JM, Melchior B, Schmid CD, Ploix CC. CNS immune privilege: hiding in plain sight. *Immunol Rev.* 2006;213:48–65.

302. Xiao Y, Yang XF, Xu MY. Effect of acetylcholine on pain-related electric activities in hippocampal CA1 area of normal and morphinistic rats. *Neurosci Bull.* 2007;23: 323–328.

303. Myint AM, Schwarz MJ, Muller N. The role of the kynurenine metabolism in major depression. *J Neural Transm.* 2012;119:245–251.

304. McNally L, Bhagwagar Z, Hannestad J. Inflammation, glutamate, and glia in depression: a literature review. *CNS Spectr.* 2008;13:501–510.

305. Myint AM, Kim YK. Cytokine-serotonin interaction through IDO: a neurodegeneration hypothesis of depression. *Med Hypotheses.* 2003;61:519–525.

306. Sublette ME, Postolache TT. Neuroinflammation and depression: the role of indoleamine 2,3-dioxygenase (IDO) as a molecular pathway. *Psychosom Med.* 2012;74:668–672.

307. Myint AM. Kynurenines: from the perspective of major psychiatric disorders. *FEBS J.* 2012;279:1375–1385.

308. Raison CL, Dantzer R, Kelley KW, et al. CSF concentrations of brain tryptophan and kynurenines during immune stimulation with IFN-alpha: relationship to CNS immune responses and depression. *Mol Psychiatry.* 2010;15:393–403.

309. Yoshida J, Shigemura A, Ogino Y, Denbow DM, Furuse M. Two receptors are involved in the central functions of kynurenic acid under an acute stress in neonatal chicks. *Neuroscience.* 2013;248C:194–200.

310. Wu HQ, Rassoulpour A, Schwarcz R. Kynurenic acid leads, dopamine follows: a new case of volume transmission in the brain? *J Neural Transm.* 2007;114:33–41.

311. Miller AH, Haroon E, Raison CL, Felger JC. Cytokine targets in the brain: impact on neurotransmitters and neurocircuits. *Depress Anxiety.* 2013;30(4):297–306.

312. Sublette ME, Galfalvy HC, Fuchs D, et al. Plasma kynurenine levels are elevated in suicide attempters with major depressive disorder. *Brain Behav Immun.* 2011;25:1272–1278.

313. Mackay GM, Forrest CM, Christofides J, et al. Kynurenine metabolites and inflammation markers in depressed patients treated with fluoxetine or counselling. *Clin Exp Pharmacol Physiol.* 2009;36(4):425–435.

314. Tsao CW, Lin YS, Chen CC, Bai CH, Wu SR. Cytokines and serotonin transporter in patients with major depression. *Prog Neuropsychopharmacol Biol Psychiatry.* 2006;30: 899–905.

315. Clements JD, Jamali F. Norepinephrine transporter is involved in down-regulation of

beta1-adrenergic receptors caused by adjuvant arthritis. *J Pharm Pharmaceut Sci.* 2009;12:337–345.

316. Ida T, Hara M, Nakamura Y, Kozaki S, Tsunoda S, Ihara H. Cytokine-induced enhancement of calcium-dependent glutamate release from astrocytes mediated by nitric oxide. *Neurosci Lett.* 2008;432:232–236.

317. Muller N, Schwarz MJ. The immune-mediated alteration of serotonin and glutamate: towards an integrated view of depression. *Mol Psychiatry.* 2007;12:988–1000.

318. Dantzer R, O'Connor JC, Freund GG, Johnson RW, Kelley KW. From inflammation to sickness and depression: when the immune system subjugates the brain. *Nat Rev Neurosci.* 2008;9:46–56.

319. Miller AH, Maletic V, Raison CL. Inflammation and its discontents: the role of cytokines in the pathophysiology of major depression. *Biol Psychiatry.* 2009;65:732–741.

320. Jow F, Chiu D, Lim HK, Novak T, Lin S. Production of GABA by cultured hippocampal glial cells. *Neurochem Int.* 2004;45:273–283.

321. Xiao BG, Link H. Is there a balance between microglia and astrocytes in regulating Th1/Th2-cell responses and neuropathologies? *Immunol Today.* 1999;20:477–479.

322. Garcia-Bueno B, Caso JR, Leza JC. Stress as a neuroinflammatory condition in brain: damaging and protective mechanisms. *Neurosci Biobehav Rev.* 2008;32:1136–1151.

323. Bierhaus A, Wolf J, Andrassy M, et al. A mechanism converting psychosocial stress into mononuclear cell activation. *Proc Natl Acad Sci U S A.* 2003;100:1920–1925.

324. Szelenyi J, Vizi ES. The catecholamine cytokine balance: interaction between the brain and the immune system. *Ann N Y Acad Sci.* 2007;1113:311–324.

325. Pace TW, Hu F, Miller AH. Cytokine-effects on glucocorticoid receptor function: relevance to glucocorticoid resistance and the pathophysiology and treatment of major depression. *Brain Behav Immun.* 2007;21:9–19.

326. Raison CL, Miller AH. When not enough is too much: the role of insufficient glucocorticoid signaling in the pathophysiology of stress-related disorders. *Am J Psychiatry.* 2003;160:1554–1565.

327. Takahashi T, Kimoto T, Tanabe N, Hattori TA, Yasumatsu N, Kawato S. Corticosterone acutely prolonged N-methyl-DS-aspartate receptor-mediated Ca2+ elevation in cultured rat hippocampal neurons. *J Neurochem.* 2002;83:1441–1451.

328. Hayley S, Poulter MO, Merali Z, Anisman H. The pathogenesis of clinical depression: stressor- and cytokine-induced alterations of neuroplasticity. *Neuroscience.* 2005;135: 659–678.

329. Santello M, Bezzi P, Volterra A. TNFalpha controls glutamatergic gliotransmission in the hippocampal dentate gyrus. *Neuron.* 2011;69:988–1001.

330. Hutchinson AJ, Chou CL, Israel DD, Xu W, Regan JW. Activation of EP2 prostanoid receptors in human glial cell lines stimulates the secretion of BDNF. *Neurochem Int.* 2009;54:439–446.

331. Garg SK, Banerjee R, Kipnis J. Neuroprotective immunity: T cell-derived glutamate endows astrocytes with a neuroprotective phenotype. *J Immunol.* 2008;180:3866–3873.

332. Garg SK, Kipnis J, Banerjee R. IFN-gamma and IL-4 differentially shape metabolic responses and neuroprotective phenotype of astrocytes. *J Neurochem.* 2009;108:1155–1166.

333. Brown GC, Neher JJ. Inflammatory neurodegeneration and mechanisms of microglial killing of neurons. *Mol Neurobiol.* 2010;41:242–247.

CHAPTER 8

Functional and Structural
Brain Changes in Depression

When discussing changes in brain function or structure that are characteristic of depression, we face the same challenge as a painter staring at an empty canvas pondering how to accurately depict the flight of a bird. First he has to choose which bird he wishes to paint. Although it is not an easy choice, the form and color of the bird need to match his overall idea and the sensibility of the painting. The task in front of us is infinitely more complex. Accumulated scientific data suggest that the diagnosis of major depressive disorder (MDD) does not reflect a single biological entity. Therefore, we are making a choice among a multitude of depressions—which one is the most representative? The limitations of language will require that we speak of MDD as if it is a single entity, but in truth any statement we make in discussing this topic is by necessity reductionistic, probabilistic, and relative. Painting is not a dynamic medium; therefore, the flight of a bird on the canvas will be a frozen frame, an offering to be elaborated by our imagination. Like the flight of a bird, depression is not a static phenomenon but, rather, a dynamic struggle between the pathophysiological processes of the disease state and the healing homeostatic activities each individual brain and body bring to this painful condition. Gender, age, personality organization, resilience factors, wellness practices, and the existential context, as well as the presence of medical and psychiatric comorbidities, all have a role in continuously defining the activity patterns and structural brain changes that occur in depressed individuals. Because of these complexities, what we see when we examine MDD will be to a large extent influenced by our choice of the window of observation.

Our emotional reality appears to be actively construed rather than passively experienced.[1] Indeed, an individual's emotional experience of the world is a synthetic process, perpetually infusing perceived elements of internal and external reality, assigning them meaning and merging them with the flow of ongoing mental activity. This process of fusion is an elaborative one—the quality of "incoming" emotions can dramatically alter the priorities of our current mental state and activate a repertoire of adaptive responses. Think for a moment about the last time when you were running late for an important meeting. Much to your relief, that morning the traffic was flowing well and it looked like you were going to make it to the meeting after all. But then a mile before your exit you saw flashing red and blue lights in the rearview mirror, accompanied by a shrill siren. This simple sensory experience and the associated emotions are likely to evoke a somatic response, such as a wave of nausea. With this feeling comes a radical rearrangement of your priorities. The converse is also true. In the midst of a depressive episode, although one is sharing a meal and a glass of wine with good friends, there may be an unbridgeable gap of emotional distance. Good humor is unable to penetrate the shell of despair and morose ruminations. Bitter self-reproach about feeling like a wet towel is dissonant with the general cheerfulness of your colleagues, but inescapably lowers your mood even further. It is safe to assume that, as with the unwelcome encounter with the police, the flow of emotions amidst one's friends is reflected in an underlying change of brain functioning.

To classify emotions, one can imagine a coordinate system defined by axes of emotional valence and arousal. Positive emotions such as happiness, joy, contentment, and ecstasy are clearly accompanied by different levels of arousal. The same is true of negative emotions, including sadness, fear, anger, and pain. Negative emotions associated with heightened arousal tend to produce a suite of bodily responses. Fear and anger can both be induced by threatening stimuli. Emotional pain and sadness occur in response to a loss or disruption of bodily integrity. In all these circumstances it may be advantageous to prepare our bodies for an adaptive response, even if such a response feels uncomfortable. Autonomic activation suspends nonessential activities, such as digestion or skin perfusion, in favor of redistributing blood to critical organs such as brain, heart, and muscles. Additionally, activation of the hypothalamic-pituitary-adrenal (HPA) axis ensures that glucose is mobilized from the tissues to provide an uninterrupted supply of energy for emergency responses. Finally, immune activation prepares us for the possibility of bodily injury. See Table 8.1 for a list of abbreviations relevant to this chapter.

As these examples suggest, it is clear from an evolutionary perspective that an integrated, parsimonious, emergency repertoire in response to negative emotions may lead to an adaptive advantage. One can therefore postulate that emotions are adaptive cues, essential for integrated homeostatic responses to changes in our internal and external environment that have been especially relevant to reproductive fitness across human evolution. In this chapter we endeavor to show, however, that emotions and thoughts that are common in the context of depression may have lost their adaptive quality. To put this discussion into a depression-

TABLE 8.1. Commonly used abbreviations in this chapter

ACC	anterior cingulate cortex
CSF	cerebrospinal fluid
CSPT	cortico-striato-pallido-thalamic
dACC	dorsal anterior cingulate cortex
dlPFC	dorsolateral prefrontal cortex
DMN	default mode network
dmPFC	dorsomedial prefrontal cortex
EN	executive network
fMRI	functional magnetic resonance imaging
HPA axis	hypothalamic-pituitary-adrenal axis
LOPFC	lateral orbital prefrontal cortex
mACC	medial anterior cingulate cortex
MCC	mid-cingulate cortex
mPFC	medial prefrontal cortex
NAcc	nucleus accumbens
OFC	orbitofrontal cortex
OPFC	orbital prefrontal cortex
PCC	posterior cingulate cortex
PFC	prefrontal cortex
rACC	rostral anterior cingulate cortex
sgACC	subgenual anterior cingulate cortex
SN	salience network
vlPFC	ventrolateral prefrontal cortex
vmPFC	ventromedial prefrontal cortex
vPFC	ventral prefrontal cortex

relevant biological context, we focus on abnormalities in central nervous system (CNS) structure and function as they relate to these depressive thoughts, emotions, and symptoms.

Structural and Functional Brain Changes in Depression

In 1905 Alfred Walter Campbell, an Australian neurologist, published a seminal paper focusing on the localization of neural function. He postulated that neural functions map onto a network of interconnected neural structures. Although such a statement might now be considered obvious and perfunctory in neuroscience circles, at the beginning of the twentieth century it was prophetic. To place it in a proper historical perspective, Campbell's work was published just four years after Sigmund Freud's update of psychoanalytic theory in "The Psychopathology of Everyday Life" and a year after Emil Kraepelin's "Comparative Psychiatry" delineating dementia praecox from manic-depressive insanity. Campbell named his integrative functional anatomical approach "hodology." A contemporary term, the *connectome*, is a modern derivative of the same principle, based on a sophisticated computerized analysis of the pattern of coactivation of brain structures, known anatomical connections, computerized tractography, and diffusion tensor imaging, a modern technique that evaluates white matter tracts connecting functionally related brain areas.

Although there is a significant overlap between the structure and function of neural networks, it would be wrong to conclude that they have a simple linear relationship. While there cannot be functional connectivity without a structural substrate (trains cannot run without tracks), in contrast to structural connections, which are relatively static (development, genetics, and frequent usage can influence the "strength" of connections), functional connections are very dynamic. Their purpose is to instantiate and coordinate adaptive processes of the highest priority to conditions as they change on a moment-by-moment and day-by-day basis.

As an illustration, consider an air traffic map of the North America or a subway map of a major metropolitan area. A few brief moments of observation will reveal that some locations are hubs or nodes, receiving much more traffic than others. If we have an opportunity to study traffic over a longer period of time, other patterns of activity will become apparent and another level of understanding will emerge. We will start recognizing that some of the nodes and their connections belong to the same functional units, such as airlines or subway lines. We will also notice that some nodes/hubs are shared by several lines, providing opportunities for "switches."

In an infinitely more complex way, something similar takes place in the brain. Specific neural functions are subserved by temporal and spatial organizational units, or networks. Networks share elements, or nodes, and are mutually interdependent in their activity patterns. Connections between nodes are referred to as edges. Either a structural or a functional failure in one of the major hubs or edges may disrupt the functioning of several networks. If you have been marooned at an airport because a major winter storm has closed several hubs, you will have a full appreciation of this analogy. Much as with air traffic or subway maps, connections in the human brain change with time and increase in complexity. Therefore, maintaining a developmental perspective is essential for proper understanding of neural phenomena.

In the discussion that follows we first focus on depression-related functional and structural changes in limbic formations, including the amygdala, hippocampus, ventral striatum/nucleus accumbens (NAcc), and hypothalamus, and their basic functions and the nodes in which they participate. We then discuss their organization in networks, and finally the role of networks in MDD. Because the limbic system shares several components with the so-called salience network (SN),[2–4] it may be parsimonious to discuss them in an integrated fashion. The SN includes interconnected limbic areas such as amygdala, ventral striatum/NAcc, hypothalamus, and related subcortical areas encompassing the dorsomedial thalamus, periaqueductal gray, and substantia nigra/ventral tegmental area. The dorsomedial thalamus appears to be the key link between paralimbic cortical areas and subcortical structures. Additionally, the SN has rich connections with paralimbic areas, including the frontoinsular cortex, which is composed of anterior insula, dorsal anterior cingulate cortex (dACC), and superior temporal lobe, but also the supplementary motor area and dorsolateral prefrontal cortex (dlPFC).[2–4]

Highly integrated sensory signals that reflect changes in the internal or external environment are funneled into the SN. The resulting emotional information serves as an impetus that mobilizes a repertoire of adaptive responses. Fear, pleasurable touch, the face of a loved one, the enjoyment of music, emotional and empathetic pain, social rejection, craving for drugs of abuse, hunger, and visceral sensations are all associated with activation of the SN.[2,4] Since the SN, the central executive network (EN), and the default-mode network (DMN), discussed later in this chapter, have shared nodes, dysfunction in one of the networks has repercussions for the activity of the other circuits. Said simply, a decision to act or not to act, and what action to take in response to environmental change, is largely mediated by the function of the limbic system and the SN.

Changes in Limbic Formations and the Salience Network in MDD

THE ALMOND

The amygdala is an almond-shaped (hence the name) formation located in the middle temporal lobe that specializes in novelty detection. Although the amygdala reacts to both positive and negative novelty, it seems to be equipped to preferentially respond to ambiguous and unusual stimuli. For example, one study found stronger amygdala responses and heightened arousal in response to photo presentations of complex graphic art, unusual skyscrapers, and leafy sea dragons (a type of a seahorse) than to photographs of flowers, shoes, and mushrooms.[5] Which aspect of novelty does the amygdala register? Is it activated by unusual shapes, smells, or rattling sounds? Is it really the sensory aspect of the stimulus or its relevance for our adaptation and survival that matters most? Science is beginning to provide some answers to these questions.

The amygdala (see figure 8.1) is not an anatomically singular entity; it is composed of functionally and anatomically distinct subunits, or nuclei. The basolateral nucleus processes emotional events focusing on their sensory aspects, while the central nucleus encodes their motivational and affective relevance. In other words, the taste and aroma of hot chocolate would be evaluated by the basolateral nucleus of the amygdala, while the central nucleus would capture the drink's appeal on a blustery winter day.[6] The amygdala appears to play a key role in guiding behavioral choices in unpredictable and ambiguous circumstances.

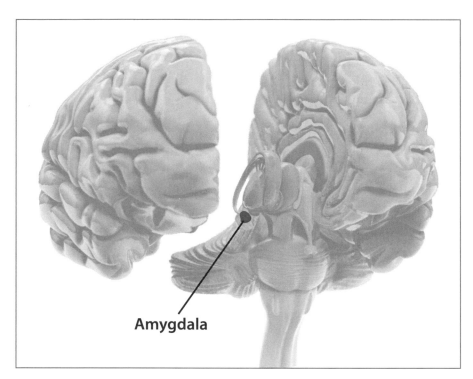

FIGURE 8.1. Amygdala.

Although dozens of publications have highlighted the cardinal role played by the amygdala in aversive conditioning and emotional learning, some key questions have remained unanswered until recently. For example, is it the quality of emotion (valence) or its intensity and the accompanying arousal that necessitates amygdala participation in the learning process? The answer to this question is very important, given studies showing that the amount of amygdala activity involved in the encoding of events into our memory determines our subsequent likelihood of recall.[7] Let's illustrate this with a thought experiment. Suppose that last January your car hit an ice patch on the highway and after a terrifying skid ended up in the ditch. Since then, every time you have driven by that section of road it induces anxiety and unpleasant visceral sensations. Is it the negative quality of the experience, the level of arousal, or both that stimulated your amygdala and cemented this unfortunate event into your memory?

A series of astutely designed studies found that it is primarily the arousal level that engages the amygdala–hippocampal loop and ensures encoding of these memories important for our survival. Another circuit that includes the dorsomedial PFC (dmPFC), ventrolateral PFC (vlPFC), and hippocampus is more involved in encoding memories based on the valence of experienced emotions. While the dmPFC seems to be more active in the memorization of positive experiences, the vlPFC is preferentially activated in the processing of negative ones.[7,8]

Emotional responses are often initiated outside our consciousness. Many times our depressed patients have mentioned feeling uneasy or intimidated in the presence of their acquaintances without fully understanding why. Imaging studies have identified robust amygdala activation in response to visual and auditory stimuli, even when they are presented for such a brief period of time that only subcortical processing takes place without any conscious awareness—what we don't see can frighten us.[9] In summary we find that the amygdala is a part of a rapid-response system that either consciously or unconsciously evaluates novelty, regardless of its emotional valence, with some preference for ambiguous, uncertain, and threatening events. If the experience is associated with a heightened arousal, presumably indicating a greater survival value, the amygdala, assisted by the hippocampus, will make sure that such an occurrence is properly stored and cataloged in our memory bank.

Neuroimaging studies suggest that functional abnormalities of the amygdala may play a significant role in the development of depressive symptoms and that pathophysiological processes inherent to depression may in turn damage this extremely important brain structure. Functional neuroimaging studies have for the most part found increased activity in the amygdala of depressed individuals.[10] As we have already mentioned, the amygdala plays an important role in rapidly assessing and assigning emotional value to surprising and ambiguous stimuli, so it is no wonder that patients with MDD react to angry and fearful faces with an increased amygdala reactivity, even when these faces are presented for such a brief period of time that they remain below the level of conscious awareness.[10–12]

In some instances negative and positive visual stimuli are "masked." For example, pictures of intensely emotional (angry, frightened, sad) or neutral facial expressions are presented to subjects for a very brief time (~35–40 msec), insufficient for the image to be registered in the visual occipital cortex. This presentation is followed by an emotionally neutral task, such as viewing images of inanimate objects, plants, and nonthreatening animals, or comparing the facades of houses to determine if they are alike. Researchers found that increased amygdala activity in depressed individuals, elicited by ultrabrief, unconscious viewing of the affectively loaded negative images, tended to bleed into the emotional impression of otherwise neutral content.[13] This type of amygdala overactivity and its "infectious" tendency may be conducive to excessive worries, anxiety, and emotional misattribution, all of which are commonly observed in patients with MDD.[14,15] Unfortunately not all types of emotional experiences are equally influential in depressed patients: amygdala activity evoked by hearing negative words was sustained, while activation precipitated by positive words decayed rapidly, based on the study by Siegle et al.[16] Excessive or extended amygdala activity in response to negative cues has been identified either as a risk for a new-onset depressive episode or a prognosticator of relapse in established MDD patients.[17,18]

We have previously suggested that the pathophysiological processes underlying depression may have a deleterious effect on the integrity of the amygdala. Indeed, structural neuroimaging studies have confirmed this expectation. The early course of depression and its initial severity tend to be associated with amygdala enlargement.[19–21] It is tempting to speculate that early MDD-associated amygdala enlargement may be a "hypertrophy" related to excessive activity. Subsequent volumetric imaging studies and meta-analyses have left us with equivocal findings. According to some authors amygdala size appears unaffected by the course of depression, while others have found a decrease in the volume of core nuclei of the amygdala in patients with recurrent depressive episodes.[22–24] A meta-analysis offers some clarification—it appears that the medication status of the depressed study subjects has a significant bearing on amygdala size.[25] While depressed patients treated with antidepressants had either no decline or even amygdala enlargement, unmedicated patients suffered a significant decrease in volume, presumably related to the course of the illness. Unfortunately meta-analytical studies share with cross-sectional studies the significant limitation that they are unable to unambiguously determine the causal directions behind observed associations.

Do depressed unmedicated individuals experience a decline in amygdala volume due to the disease process, or is the recurrence of depression a consequence of having a smaller amygdala? Fortunately, a longitudinal study has shed some light on the nature of association between ongoing depression and loss of brain volume. A three-year prospective study noted a decline in amygdala gray matter (especially on the left side) over time in MDD patients compared with control subjects, indicating that the association between MDD and reduced amygdala volume results, to some degree at least, from a corrosive effect of the disease process itself on the brain.[26]

Because the amygdala and other limbic structures have significant bidirectional connections with the hypothalamus and autonomic nervous system, it is no surprise that sympathetic and neuroendocrine dysregulation frequently accompanies mood disorders.[27,28] Autonomic, endocrine, and amygdala-related repercussions on the workings of other major neural networks in MDD are discussed later in this chapter.

THE RECLINING NUCLEUS

Named for its appearance when viewed in cross-sectional brain slices—the nucleus accumbens vaguely resembles a person comfortably reclining in a hammock—the NAcc is one of the principal subcortical areas associated with the processing of rewarding stimuli. Similar to the amygdala, the NAcc also has bivalent effects relevant to depression. Imaging studies have shown that both positively and negatively loaded emotionally novel stimuli activate the NAcc. This brain area receives rich innervation from the amygdala, insula, thalamus, cingulate cortex, and PFC. Due to this diversity of inputs, the NAcc is ideally positioned to integrate sensory, emotional, and cognitive information and participate in the selection and initiation of adaptive responses to environmental challenges and opportunities. Once complex information related to the novelty is processed, the NAcc may then convert it into a neurobiological equivalent of motivation, especially in response to events of positive valence (associated with pleasure or reward). The pursuit of food and sexual activity is mediated by the NAcc, as is the misguided pursuit for drugs of abuse.[29] In its function as a neural link between motivation and action, the NAcc is capable of orchestrating a body-wide adaptive response via its motoric efferents that project to the substantia nigra and globus pallidus and via outputs to autonomic and endocrine areas of the brain, such as the lateral hypothalamus.[30] The NAcc responds to both valence and arousal-related aspects of the incoming information. Interestingly, if the elicited emotion is negative both the amygdala and NAcc respond with increased activity, whereas only the NAcc is recruited if the emotional stimulus is of positive valence.[30]

The evolutionary benefit of having a prompt and effective association between positive motivation and adaptive activity is obvious. But consider an equally obvious follow-up question. Wouldn't it be beneficial to have this gestalt of positive motivation and rewarding activity filed into memory banks for future use? Wouldn't it be good to be able to find that cozy restaurant, serving delicious, steaming French onion soup the next time we get chilled during a walk on a snowy evening? The NAcc has evolved to provide us with exactly this service. A functional loop that connects the NAcc (reward detection), ventral pallidum, dopaminergic ventral tegmental area (signaling relevance), and hippocampus (access to memory banks) does just this. This loop ensures that information related to substantially rewarding novelty is safely stored in the hippocampus for future use.[31]

We have already mentioned that our perception of reality is not a passive phenomenon but, rather, is an active process that sometimes involves quite a bit of editing. Let's imagine a golfer who hits a hard drive, only to see the ball disappear into the middle of a water feature, generating a distant "plop." One way that he can deal with this heartburn-inducing mixture of humiliation, self-anger, and disappointment is to remind himself that he is enjoying a gorgeous day in the fresh air, combined with plenty of healthy exercise, soon to be followed by a beer with old friends. The ensuing improvement in the golfer's emotional tone is a likely consequence of a neural process called reappraisal. The amygdala, NAcc, and vlPFC are the principal components of the reappraisal loop. Imaging studies have found that, following a reappraisal attempt, increased amygdala activity correlates with a more negative residual emotional response, whereas increased vlPFC and NAcc activation predicts a successful reappraisal, resulting in diminished negative emotion or even a new positive feeling.[32]

An imaging study utilized an incentive task in which the presentation of a visual cue required a subsequent appropriate response that was accompanied by a delayed monetary reward. Thirty unmedicated depressed patients were compared with 31 healthy subjects. Relative to the healthy subjects, the depressed patients showed much weaker activation on functional MRI (fMRI) in the NAcc and the caudate nucleus bilaterally while awaiting the reward. Does this mean that the principal pleasure zone is less responsive to reward in depression? Anhedonic symptoms and the severity of depression were also associated with a lesser caudate volume in depressed patients compared with the healthy control group.[33] A separate study by the same group found a correlation between the intensity of anhedonia in depressed patients and diminished volume and activation of the NAcc in response to a monetary reward.[34] Yet another fMRI study used positive verbal cues such as "heroic" and "admired," negative ones like "worthless" or "burden," and neutral words to compare brain activation in 10 unmedicated depressed patients and 12 healthy comparison subjects. Researchers found that the depressed group showed less activation in the ventral striatum/NAcc in response to positive words compared with healthy controls. On the other hand, there was no difference between the groups in neural responses to negative or neutral verbal cues.

Taken together, these findings suggest that MDD is characterized by compromised function of motivational/reward pathways in the brain and that this dysfunction provides a neural substrate for the reduced ability to experience joy and pleasure so often reported by individuals suffering from MDD.[35] Sadly, this pattern of neural functioning appears to be heritable, given findings from an fMRI study comparing 17 adolescents from families in which one of the parents suffered from depression with 22 offspring of parents who had no history of depression.[36] In a condition of unconstrained attention, the adolescents at high risk for MDD had greater activation in the amygdala and NAcc while viewing fearful faces and lower activity in the NAcc in response to happy faces. Thus, it appears, unfortunately, that propensity to see "the glass as half-empty" may be hardwired into the minds of at least some children of depressed parents.

In summary, the NAcc can be profitably thought of as a hub within the brain's reward circuitry that tends to operate suboptimally in depressed individuals. As a result, depression is associated with a compromised ability to feel pleasure while anticipating an activity and an incapacity to experience joy once happy events have occurred.

THE SEAHORSE

The hippocampus is a key limbic area that resides deep in the mid-temporal lobe. When viewed in cross section, it reminded early observers of a seahorse, hence its fanciful name. The hippocampus is involved in a striking array of brain functions.

It is located at the "crossroads" of circuitry that regulates the activity of the HPA axis and, by extension, the stress response more generally. It also modulates mood and actively participates in the consolidation of memory, especially contextual, declarative, and spatial memories.[28,37] Thus, when depressed patients complain of not being able to find their glasses and keys or frequently pause, searching for the right word to express themselves, they may be manifesting signs of hippocampal malfunction.

Yet it would be an error to conclude that the hippocampus is functionally homogeneous. In fact, the anterior part of hippocampus is involved in indexing and processing novelty-related information, whereas the posterior hippocampus responds more to recognition of familiarity.[38] Both areas are presumably engaged in the process of generalization, however. By this we mean the process whereby novel information is first evaluated and then compared with past experiences. If the similarity between current conditions and past experiences is sufficiently relevant, information about current conditions is properly labeled and committed to memory. This process of generalization also involves dopaminergic midbrain areas that also contribute to assigning relevance to sensory signals.[39]

Given its proficiency in sorting out new information and recognizing similarity with past experiences, it is not surprising that the hippocampus has an important role in cognitive set shifting, because to shift sets we need to evaluate a new entity and detect if it is similar or different from previous experiences. Let us say that we are playing a simple stacking card game with our children. Cards of the same suit or bearing a same number can be placed on top of each other. On the top of the deck is a seven of clubs, which has followed several other cards in the same suit. One of the players now places a seven of hearts on the top. The rule has changed, and now sorting needs to proceed not by suit but by number. An imaging study has found that the caudate nucleus was active while the new rule was unknown. However, the recognition of the new rule increased hippocampal activity, presumably reflecting its role in the storage of new association into the memory. Periods of hypothesis testing and "unlearning" of the old (now obsolete) rule were associated with decreased hippocampal activity.[40] It is as if following the recognition of a new rule and its storage, the hippocampus placed itself in a standby mode, awaiting new information that either supports or invalidates the existing hypothesis.

In addition to the areas mentioned thus far, the hippocampus (figure 8.2) can also be functionally partitioned into a dorsal area, which has a greater competency in cognitive processes, and a ventral region, which is more involved in modulating emotions and the stress response.[41] Consistent with this dorsal/ventral portioning, gene expression patterns in the dorsal hippocampus parallel those of cortical areas involved in information processing, whereas gene expression patterns within the ventral region are similar to those observed in the amygdala and hypothalamus (both of which are involved in regulation of emotions

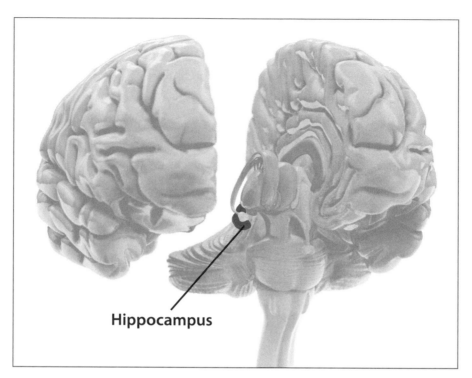

FIGURE 8.2. **Hippocampus.**

and stress response). Despite these functional divisions, however, it would be wrong not to recognize that there is robust collaboration between the dorsal and ventral components of the hippocampus, consistent with the obvious truth that learning from stressful situations is of paramount importance for our survival. In support of this idea, preclinical findings suggest that hippocampal damage disrupts adaptive learning processes that follow a stressful experience.[42]

The hippocampus has a principal role in helping individuals adapt to the ever-changing environment. However, its central location may render it vulnerable to functional perturbations that accompany extreme stress and mood disorders.[28] For example, a prospective study monitored stress levels and changes in hippocampal volume over a 20-year period in 48 healthy, postmenopausal women. Voxel-based morphometry, a radiological technique utilized to estimate structural changes in the brain, established that chronic life stress predicted a decline in hippocampal volume.[43]

Consistent with the intimate relationship between chronic stress and MDD, similar hippocampal changes have been recognized in depressed individuals. In fact, alterations in hippocampal volume are among the most common radiological findings in patients with MDD.[37] Data provide a likely explanation for this association, by strongly suggesting that pathophysiological processes inherent to depression may be the cause of reduction in hippocampal volume. Indeed, an imaging study made volumetric comparisons among 20 never-treated first-episode depressed patients, 17 subjects who had suffered from multiple depressive episodes, and healthy controls. Both groups of depressed patients had impaired performance on memory tests, but only the patients with multiple episodes manifested a significant reduction in hippocampal volume. Illness duration and hippocampal volume were inversely correlated, indicating that MDD may have a "toxic" impact on both hippocampal function and structure.[44] Similarly, another study found an inverse relationship between days of untreated depression and hippocampal volume,[45] and yet another reported a negative correlation between duration of depression and hippocampal volume, corrected for age and intracranial volume.[46] Furthermore, a prospective three-year study found a significant decline in hippocampal gray matter volume in MDD patients compared with healthy controls.[26]

Research provides an intriguing perspective on the relationship between MDD and hippocampal volume. Many patients who suffer from MDD have experienced an early trauma or major adversity. A group of authors discovered that childhood maltreatment had an independent effect on hippocampal volume in a group of depressed patients. Patients, who, in addition to MDD, had a history of childhood trauma had significantly reduced hippocampal volumes compared with subjects who were depressed but had no prior history of early-life adversity. As the matter of fact, depressed patients without a maltreatment history had hippocampal volumes indistinguishable from those of the healthy controls.[47] A different group replicated these findings and further extended them by noting that even maltreated nondepressed individuals had diminished hippocampal volume relative to other healthy controls. Furthermore, hippocampal volume in the entire sample was inversely correlated with the score on the Childhood Trauma Questionnaire.[48]

Successful antidepressant treatment appears to have a protective effect, given that initially depressed patients who remitted with treatment lost significantly less hippocampal volume over a three-year period compared with those who continued to experience depressive symptoms over that period.[26] Consistent with these findings, one post hoc analysis has found a significant increase in hippocampal volume (21 percent, $p = 0.004$) after six to seven months of antidepressant treatment in a small subset of patients suffering from atypical depression.[37] Additional treatment benefits are implied by a magnetic resonance spectroscopy study, which noted a significant association between hippocampal elevation of N-acetylaspartate (a marker of neuronal density, function, and myelination), choline compounds (a marker of membrane integrity, and metabolism) and treatment response and detected reduced glutamine in depressed subjects.[49] Glutamate is the principal excitatory neurotransmitter, eventually metabolized into glutamine after being taken up by astrocytes. The ratio of glutamine to glutamate is an indicator of appropriate astroglial function (more about the role of astroglia in following chapters). Decreased glutamine may speak of compromised glial ability to maintain glutamate/gamma-aminobutyric acid (GABA) balance and therefore equilibrium between excitatory and inhibitory signaling. To our knowledge, this was the first study to provide evidence that successful treatment with two different antidepressants, a predominantly noradrenergic one and another that is mostly serotonergic, may lead to functional and structural restitution of hippocampal neuron and astroglia function.[49]

In summary, cumulative evidence points to the detrimental impact of disease-related processes on the hippocampus at multiple levels. Neurotransmission and neuron glia relationships are disrupted, and there are alterations in structural integrity that manifest in impaired hippocampal function. Given the diverse roles played by the hippocampus, it is not surprising that abnormal hippocampal function results in complex symptomatic manifestations. The good news, on the other hand, is that successful treatment may arrest or even partially reverse the patterns of hippocampal deterioration seen in depression.

The centrality of the hippocampus frames its role in MDD as an alpha-and-omega brain structure. It regulates the storage of information into contextual memory, thereby providing emotional coloring to our experiences, thus influencing our future adaptive responses. Additionally, the hippocampus participates in cognitive processes and declarative memory (enabling us to name persons and objects), greatly influencing our social communication preferences and abilities. Finally, it is a key component of the stress-response system, allowing negative emotions to mobilize bodily resources (circulatory, endocrine, and immune) in preparation for an adaptive response to adversity. It is no surprise, then, that disruption in hippocampal structural and functional integrity readily translates into the cognitive, emotional, and somatic symptoms of depression.

THE HYPOTHALAMUS (SEE FIGURE 8.3)

Dysfunction of PFC–limbic circuitry is one of the cardinal features of depression. The resultant poorly modulated functioning of limbic areas, such as the amygdala and hippocampus, is "funneled" into abnormalities in hypothalamic activity.[50] We do not further elaborate on the disturbance of the HPA axis in depression as it is exhaustively discussed in Chapters 5 and 6.

The Role of Paralimbic Cortical Structures in MDD

THE ISLAND

The insular cortex, imagined as an island-like shape, has emerged as a paralimbic structure of tremendous relevance to sensory-emotional-motor integration and regulation. The insula is a pyramid-shaped structure concealed under the folds of the temporal, fronto-orbital, and parietal opercula ("lids"). The insula is distin-

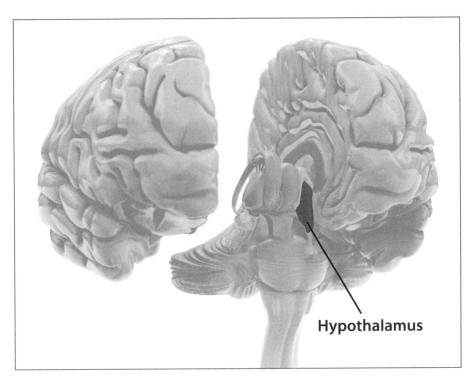

FIGURE 8.3. Hypothalamus.

guished from surrounding cortical areas by its vast heterogeneity of architecture.[51,52] It has rich direct and indirect connections with other limbic (e.g., amygdala, NAcc/ventral striatum, and hippocampus) and paralimbic cortical areas (ACC and lateral-orbital [LOPFC]). Because of its information-processing and communication potential, the insula is widely considered to be the primary target of thalamocortical projections. Moreover, a functional unit composed of the anterior insular cortex and ACC is believed to be the fundamental source of bodily and emotional self-awareness.[53] As such, the insula plays an essential role in sensory-affective integration. Without "translation" into their emotional counterparts, our sensory experiences might be "stranded," devoid of meaning. Were this to happen, our capacity to generate adaptive responses to changing environmental conditions would be significantly impaired.

The insula (figure 8.4) appears to have a horizontal organization. The posterior insula is the receptive end. It is a recipient of multimodal sensory information, and its activation appears to be in proportion to the "objective" intensity of the sensory stimuli. The middle insula has an evaluative role. It "contextualizes" the flow of sensory information by incorporating it into our current stream of emotions. The anterior pole of insular cortex has a role in providing an emotional echo of the sensory experiences by assigning it a personal meaning (subjective salience).[53,54]

Thirst, itch, "air hunger," bowel and bladder distention, penile stimulation,

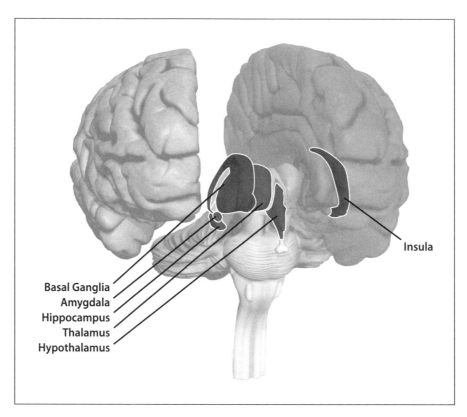

FIGURE 8.4. Insula.

sexual arousal, and cold and warm sensations are all accompanied by insular activation.[53] The ascending tactile nerve fibers project to the insula, providing it with an opportunity to process the quality of human touch. When skin is stroked at the speed of approximately 3 cm/sec, it is accompanied by a robust posterior insula activity, resulting in an intense hedonic (pleasurable) experience. Beyond simple somatic sensations, the insula plays a role in complex sensory–affective integration. An intriguing imaging study reports that the quality of female orgasm correlates with the degree of insular activation.[55] Moreover, even observed caresses will induce a similar change in insular activity.[56]

The insula also plays a key role in the experience and modulation of pain. The insula, ACC, and somatosensory cortices I and II are often described as comprising the key components of the "pain matrix," which is the brain circuit responsible for processing pain stimuli. The degree of insular activity reflects the subjective intensity of pain. Although both the insula and ACC respond to pain with increased activation, under heavy sedation ACC involvement ceases while insula and somatosensory cortex I and II responses survive, suggesting their involvement with processing fundamental aspects of pain. After insular injury we can still identify the sensory aspect of pain, but it becomes devoid of any unpleasant quality. Further substantiating insular involvement in the integration of sensory and emotional experience, research has found that "catastrophizing" responses to pain were associated with ruminative thoughts and augmentation of insular activity.[57] Fear, anxiety, depression, and attention focused on pain can all increase subjective pain intensity, and are all associated with a greater insular activation. Distraction from pain has an opposite effect.[58,59] The anterior insula is also activated in anticipation of pain and during empathic response to another person's pain.[57]

An intriguing study investigated the influence of our anticipatory bias on experienced intensity of pain. Identical stimuli were administered under two conditions: when subjects assumed that the stimulus was entirely safe (low threat), and when they expected that it was potentially harmful (high threat). As you have probably anticipated, stimulation under the high-threat condition was more frequently associated with the experience of pain, compared with the low-threat condition. Moreover, an increased bias toward rating the experience as painful under the high-threat condition was associated with greater functional coupling of the ACC and mid-cingulate cortex (MCC), providing a potential neural substrate for the contextual modulation of pain.[60]

Robust, pain-induced, insular activation was also associated with increased sympathetic nervous system response, indicating its role in orchestrating the body's pain response.[61,62] In fact, a comprehensive review has concluded that the "pain matrix" may be a misnomer, because the same brain areas tend to be responsive to a variety of threatening and noxious sensory signals. The same circuit, inclusive of the insula, may be better conceptualized as a defensive salience-detection system.[57]

More complex forms of sensory–emotional coupling also take place in the insula. For example, the experience of our body in motion during physical exercise is purportedly mediated by insular function. Anosognosia, a mistaken notion that our limbs function normally when that is unfortunately not the case, is a known consequence of a stroke or an anatomical injury to the posterior insula. Perplexed and distraught patients affected by this malady may be seen manipulating and pushing their own limbs, because they may feel odd, or like they do not belong to them.[63]

Other functions attributed, at least in part, to the insula include sensing the passage of time, sensing rhythm, experiencing a "feeling of knowing," recognizing familiar persons, situations and objects, recognizing oneself, being aware of one's heartbeat, recognizing when one has made an error, and experiencing an emotional response to hearing laughter, crying, and the affective tone of speech.[64] Moreover, the insula has a very intricate role in speech. Both sensory processing of spoken language and a motoric preparation for an utterance have been linked with insula activity. More generally, the anterior insula often appears to be a brain area crucial for commencing behavior. It has been implicated in speech planning and articulation.[65] The adjustment of the autonomic system to the respiratory needs of speech may also be orchestrated by the insula.[66] (We discuss the role of insula in response initiation later in this chapter as we discuss insular participation in neural networks.)

One can even conceptualize the insula as one of the key brain areas involved with affiliation and social interactions. Consistent with this, viewing one's own versus other familiar children has been associated with increased insula activation. Furthermore, social rejection tends to precipitate a significant change in insula function.[64,67] Based on the cumulative evidence, some authors have even concluded that the insula is the key neural structure mediating awareness not only of ourselves but also of our physical and social milieu.[53]

Moreover, the insula has an intriguing role in complex mind-body interactions. Incoming immune signals, conveyed by inflammatory cytokines, activate ascending vagal nerve projections leading to the nucleus of the solitary tract and are ultimately received by the insula.[53,68,69] In this respect, there is a remarkable parallel to peripheral pain fibers projecting to the insula. Much as it does with pain, the insula also provides an emotional and cognitive response to incoming immune signals.[70] One might conclude from this that the insula is home to higher-order representations of the visceral states.[69] Together with the MCC, the insula may be involved in generating a sense of fatigue, confusion, and even disgust in response to peripheral inflammatory signals.[70,71] Also paralleling its role in pain regulation, where it is the origin of the descending pain-modulatory pathways, the insula has an analogous role in immune modulation.[72,73] Due to its connections to the nucleus of the solitary tract, the parabrachial pontine nucleus, and indirectly, via the amygdala, the bed nucleus of stria terminalis, the insula has its hands on the reins of the principal autonomic, immunosensitive, and immunoregulatory brain areas.[72,74] As one might predict, insular injury disrupts both conditioned immunosuppression and immune stimulation.[73,74]

One could summarize insular function by framing it as a brain area involved in monitoring the continuous flow of sensory information, identifying the relevant inputs, and "labeling" them as attention-worthy, subsequently directing them toward the brain structures involved in higher cognitive processes, such as working memory and attention, while at the same time disconnecting the DMN. Thus, the insula-ACC unit becomes the central switch regulating relationships among the SN, DMN, and EN (see figure 8.5). The ultrarapid rapid transfer of information between the insula and ACC is conducted by von Economo, or spindle, neurons, whose uniquely large axons accommodate greater signaling speeds.[75] It appears that insula and dACC SN/DMN/EN switching activity is aided by the ventrolateral PFC (vlPFC). The insula–vlPFC connection exercises a dual role: either engaging in top-down emotional regulation, mediating between EN-related cortical structures (e.g., the dlPFC) and limbic SN areas, or coupling EN with SN in response to ascending emotional signals.[76]

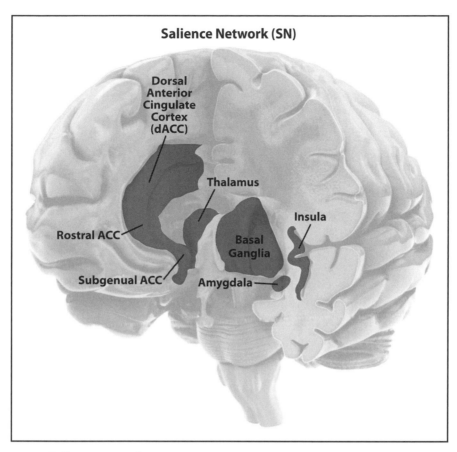

FIGURE 8.5. Salience network.

Several imaging studies have found alterations in insula function and structure in MDD. One of these studies found an inverse correlation between the severity of insomnia in MDD patients and insula activity.[77] Imaging studies have also found altered brain responses in MDD patients "challenged" by photographs of emotionally expressive faces, most likely due to dysfunction of frontolimbic circuitry in which the insula is a central component. Specifically, while depressed patients manifested diminished insula activity in response to positive facial expressions, negative images elicited an exaggerated insular response, which correlated with the severity of MDD symptomatology.[78]

Furthermore, "neuroticism," a personality trait that reflects a negative emotional bias in an individual's interactions with the environment, is associated with an augmented insula activity during any decision-making process, but particularly when the most probable outcome is obvious.[79] It is as if even obvious choices elicit caution associated with negative emotionality in people who are depressed. This result sheds new light on the established relationship between neuroticism and vulnerability for depression.

Insula hypoactivation was noted in the resting state but also during homeostatic shifts in MDD patients compared with healthy controls.[80–82] Even first-degree relatives of MDD patients tend to manifest attenuated resting-state insula activity relative to healthy individuals, suggesting that it may also be a vulnerability marker for the condition.[83] Could this mean that the predilection for depression may be associated with an aberrant sensory-affective coupling that alters the quality of one's interaction with the environment?

Sleep deprivation, which is unfortunately quite common in mood-disordered patients, has a profound influence on insula function. Individuals who are short on sleep tend to manifest diminished insula activation during decision making, accompanied by less defense against losses and a greater pursuit of gains (also accompanied by NAcc activation).[51] This may mean that the lower insula activity in sleep-deprived individuals is a neurobiological basis for the type of risk-taking behaviors that are known to increase the risk for depression.

In general, MDD patients appear to have decreased activity of the insula, which tends to improve with antidepressant treatment.[84,85] Neuroimaging studies, utilizing labeling of serotonin 5HT2 receptors, have also characterized altered serotonergic transmission in the insula in MDD subjects.[86] Beyond functional changes, MDD also appears to be associated with structural alterations of the insula. Both current and remitted MDD patients have been shown to manifest reductions in insular volume compared with healthy individuals.[87]

A remarkable study has placed insular pathology center stage in our discussion of brain changes in depression. In response to photographs depicting facial expressions of disgust, a known "challenge" for evaluation of insular function, depressed patients relative to healthy controls had reduced insula activation. Moreover, volumetric analysis found a direct correlation between insular gray matter volume and severity of depression, measured by the Hamilton Depression Rating Scale, Beck Depression Inventory, and Snaith-Hamilton Pleasure Scale. Key symptom domains of depression, including impaired ability to experience pleasure, were inversely correlated with insular and ACC gray matter volumes.[64] In summary, cumulative evidence implicates insular dysfunction as one of the central and defining features of MDD.

THE BELT

The cingulate ("belt-like") cortex is a band of gray matter interposed between limbic formations and cortical structures. The cingulate has been parceled into discrete substructures via cytoarchitectural and sophisticated imaging techniques.[88–91] In spite of significant gains, scientific consensus remains elusive both in terms of arriving at a common nomenclature for different cingulate regions and in assigning unambiguous function to these areas. With this limitation in mind, we have done our best to accurately represent extant, at times controversial, scientific evidence related to the cingulate.

Anterior Cingulate Cortex

The subgenual ACC (sgACC; Brodmann area [BA] 25) and subcallosal ACC (alternatively called the pregenual anterior cingulate cortex; BAs 24a and b) are sometimes jointly referred to as the ventral ACC. The rostral ACC (rACC, BA 24c) and dACC (BA 32) are often identified simply as the dACC or, more recently, as the MCC.[88–91] Located behind the ACC, as one might anticipate, is the posterior cingulate cortex (PCC; BAs 23 and 31).[92] See figure 8.6.

The sgACC has anatomical connections with the dopaminergic ventral tegmental area, periaqueductal gray, hypothalamus, and dorsal medulla, all of which highlights the importance of the ACC for states related to arousal and drive.[88–91] Autonomic projections from the sgACC to the amygdala, periaqueductal gray, and nucleus of the solitary tract in the medulla provide this "limbic" portion of the ACC an opportunity to instigate an adaptive response to negative emotional events.[89] Reciprocal connections between the rACC and amygdala allow the alarm signal to be propagated into the body to more effectively mobilize the response systems. Conversely, stress-activated HPA axis (re)activity predicts the degree of connectedness between the sgACC and SN-affiliated insula–dACC complex, thus effecting the SN/EN/DMN switch. In plain language, sgACC

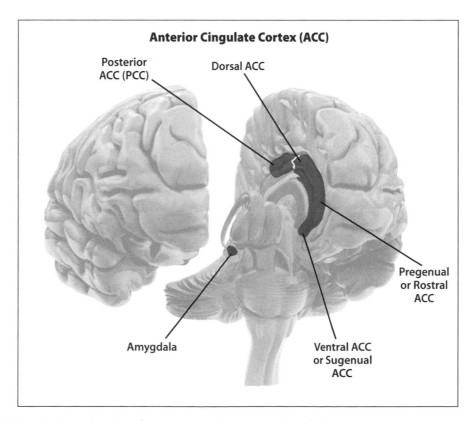

FIGURE 8.6. Anterior cingulate cortex and posterior cingulate cortex.

appears to act as a bidirectional neuroendocrine switch either engaging bodily fight-or-flight responses or enhancing the connection between SN and EN in response to bodily distress signals.[93]

Pregenual ACC and anterior MCC are recipients of integrated intero- and exteroceptive information from the anterior insula and signals from the amygdala.[54,94] Due to the mediating role of the insula and amygdala, sensory influx is fused with an emotional valuation of novel events and their corresponding personal meaning. These integrative processes help promote our homeostatic efforts by maintaining a dynamic subjective image of our bodily state and the surrounding environment.[54] Hunger pangs, a melancholy tune, or sunburned skin share an ability to elicit a reaction from the lower portion of the ACC, summoning an adaptive response.

The rACC and anterior MCC ought not to be conceptualized as a passive recipient of information from other brain areas. Rather, it is an integration hub capable of orchestrating adaptive responses. In addition to receiving inputs related to pain (it is the primary target of the spinothalamic tract), it also receives dopaminergic fibers from the substantia nigra and the ventral striatum communicating information about various types of reinforcers.[95] If prompt action is required, the rACC/anterior MCC can communicate with the spinal cord and primary motor, premotor, and supplemental motor areas in the brain, as well as facial nucleus, coordinating a range of motor responses, from a change of facial expression to yanking our hand away from a hot plate.

The posterior MCC is a target for projections from the mid- and posterior insula, a brain area that assists the cingulate in its numerous and diverse tasks, including error detection, anticipation, focusing attention on relevant stimuli, bodily orientation, decision making, and response selection.[54,69] In summary one can conceive of the ACC as a hub for processing integrated sensory and emotional information, detecting relevant changes in internal and external environment, and based on contingencies, selecting the most appropriate adaptive responses.[54,69,89,90,95] In this role the ACC is adept at generating a full repertoire of adaptive activities, from the valuation of incoming stimuli, to the selection of the goal and the most appropriate course of action, concluding with outcome evaluation.[96]

Posterior Cingulate Cortex and the Default-Mode Network

The PCC is a portion of cingulate cortex that extends posterior to the central sulcus. It has extensive direct and indirect connections with parietal and prefrontal areas involved with attention, as well as with brain regions involved in motivation and learning, such as the thalamus, caudate, amygdala, parahippocampal gyrus, ACC, and orbitofrontal cortex (OFC).[97] Due to its central location and rich connections, the PCC is involved in gathering detailed information about the consequences of our current behaviors. If undesirable environmental outcomes are detected, the PCC will initiate a strategy shift. The PCC is a structure capable of computing variations, probabilities, and uncertainty, thanks to its relationship with memory banks and contingency monitoring brain areas. Hence, when unexpected events take place, the PCC fosters flexibility and exploration in the service of discovering novel adaptive solutions.[92,97–100] While fear, loneliness, and pain activate the MCC, happiness and contentment tend to coincide with increased PCC activity.[89,101] It would be very difficult to manage contingencies required to pilot a plane or enjoy skiing on a snowy slope without effective PCC involvement.

The PCC is a functional anchor of the DMN (figure 8.7), which shows increased activity when the brain is at rest or involved in a social communication and diminished activation during cognitively demanding tasks.[2,3] In addition to the PCC, the DMN incorporates other midline cortical structures such as the ventromedial PFC (vmPFC), dmPFC, inferior parietal lobule, lateral temporal cortex, medial temporal lobe (MTL; including the hippocampal formation), and angular gyrus.[2,102,103] Some authors have also included the rACC as an important DMN component, as opposed to its more conventional SN designation.[104] Despite forming a coherent network, not all components of the DMN are activated to an equal

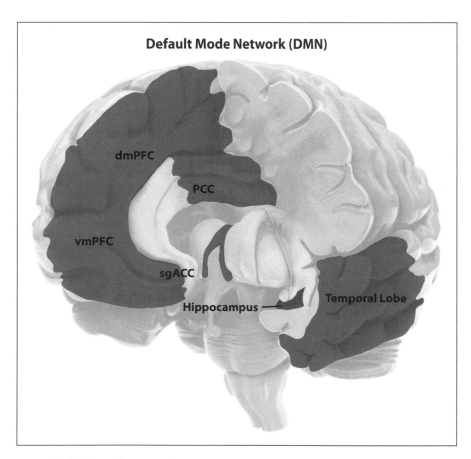

FIGURE 8.7. Default-mode network.

degree by any particular task. If one is going through a box of old photographs, reminiscing about childhood trips to the beach, or agonizing on the drive home about the mistakes made during the morning presentation, increased PCC activity combined with hippocampal activation is a likely corollary. Trying to explain why we like the book that we are reading to the airline passenger seated next to us is likely to involve medial PFC activity. Episodic memory engages MTL, while remembering the meaning of a television debate requires angular gyrus mediation.[2,3] In short, the DMN goes off-line when we are involved in task-oriented behaviors or problem solving but shows greater engagement during self-referential processes, episodic, semantic, and autobiographical memory retrieval, value-based decision making, social cognition, and emotional regulation.[2,3] Moreover an fMRI study of healthy subjects discovered increased at-rest activity in the PCC, vmPFC, and dmPFC that correlated with measures of emotions. Because the same DMN areas have a role in extero- and interoception, it has been a challenge to prove that the change of the fMRI signal in DMN areas truly reflected emotions in the resting state. In contrast to elevated DMN activity corresponding to emotional intensity during rest, there was no correlation between the activation in these same brain areas and involvement in intero- or exteroception. Could this pattern of DMN activity correlate with mind wandering and hopelessness, so often described by depressed patients[102]?

Imaging studies have implicated the ACC in the pathophysiology of MDD more often than any other brain area. Most of this research emphasis has focused on the role of the sgACC in depression (see figure 8.6). The sgACC participates in assessing the salience of emotional and motivational information and thus guides necessary behavioral adjustments in response to changing environmental conditions. It is also involved in the modulation of sympathetic and neuroendocrine responses. Typically, functional imaging studies report increased metabolism in the sgACC in MDD (especially when corrections are made for its reduced volume in depression).[105] Moreover, the intensity of sadness in MDD has been associated with increased blood flow into the sgACC and anterior insula.[106] One study found that the strength of the connection between the sgACC and hippocampus in MDD predicts subsequent decline in dlPFC activity. Activity in sgACC and vmPFC was found to be mutually reinforcing.[107] This finding can be extended to mean that aberrant connectedness between sgACC and paralimbic areas may be a key event in strengthening SN–DMN connection in MDD at the expense of cortical EN involvement. Thus, abnormal sgACC activity and connections with limbic and paralimbic structures may have primacy in defining MDD pathophysiology.[107] In contrast, structural studies have noted a significantly diminished volume of sgACC in MDD subjects. For example, in one study the sgACC had a 48 percent smaller volume in individuals with familial depression compared with healthy controls.[105] Furthermore, the extent of anomalous sgACC connectivity also correlates with duration of depressive illness.[2] These sgACC structural and functional differences likely contribute to the disturbances of motivation, limbic (especially amygdala) regulation, and neuroendocrine function so commonly exhibited by MDD patients.[105,108]

Although lower and anterior areas of the ACC have been the primary focus of research, more dorsal areas of the ACC are now attracting greater attention for their putative role in MDD. For example, a study of MDD patients reported an association between gray matter volume reductions of the dACC and dlPFC and increased symptom severity in patients suffering from MDD.[109] Even unaffected relatives of MDD patients have more difficulty inhibiting negative emotions, which is associated with greater MCC activity relative to a healthy control group.[110] These findings resonate with those of another study, which described aberrant reciprocal connectivity between the supragenual ACC and amygdala in unmedicated depressed patients.[108] In summary, research supports the hypothesis that paralimbic and cognitive regions have a role in "top-down" modulation of limbic areas and that depression is likely a manifestation of functional impairments of this modulatory capacity.[111,112]

Finally, convergent lines of evidence suggest that functional anomalies in the ACC are associated with a compromised treatment response. A study noted that normalized sgACC activity accompanies a good response to either an active antidepressant or placebo.[113] Moreover, greater pretreatment rACC activity may be a positive predictor of a favorable treatment response following antidepressants, sleep deprivation, and repetitive transcranial magnetic stimulation, but not placebo.[104] Increased pretreatment rACC activity may be a neural correlate of preserved adaptive self-reflection, which may provide depressed patients with an adaptive advantage.[104] In contrast, decreased function and volume of the pregenual ACC has been associated with delayed benefits of the antidepressant treatment.[109]

Research into the role of the PCC in MDD has brought to surface some very exciting evidence. Ever since the PCC became identified as a prominent node in the DMN, its role in MDD has become a focus of intensive research. If activity in the PCC and dmPFC is indeed associated with self-reflection and a "wandering mind," especially if one is not engaged in any particular task, shouldn't we expect altered function in these areas in the context of depression? Contemporary research has confirmed these suspicions. We described earlier in this chapter how the sgACC funnels information from limbic areas to PFC areas, which alerts them to relevant environmental changes and mobilizes them to engage in an adaptive response. When sgACC/anterior insula signals (key components of the SN) reach the PFC, directing attention to a situation that needs to be addressed right away, it should be all business. The DMN, likely to be involved in such things as making plans for the weekend or reminiscing about the delicious taste of the roasted duck last night, ought to go off-line, to be promptly replaced by activation of the EN.

Unfortunately this seamless, harmonious handoff does not occur in the context of depression. Signals from the sgACC, presumably conveying negative emotions (sadness, dejection, anxiety), enter a short circuit with the DMN, becoming a subject for rumination. One study noted an sgACC "intrusion"—hyperconnectedness between the sgACC and the most prominent components of the DMN (the dmPFC and PCC) in depressed individuals.[114] Furthermore, a quantified resting state connectivity between the sgACC and the members of the DMN network was significantly correlated with the duration of an MDD episode, possibly qualifying resting-state connectivity between these brain areas as a measure of "refractoriness" of depression.[114]

Another group made a very intriguing observation by combining a ruminative response scale (a self-report measure of rumination), Beck Depression Inventory–II, and fMRI findings. These researchers concluded that depressed individuals had greater activation of the PCC and dmPFC, which coincided with high levels of maladaptive rumination, such as recall of miserable autobiographical memories and mind wandering, and lower levels of adaptive self-reflection, relative to healthy control subjects.[115] By contrast, neuroimaging studies have associated adaptive self-reflection with rACC activation. Unfortunately, rACC function, crucially important to both SN and DMN, tends to be disrupted in MDD.[104] In other words, abnormally fused DMN and SN activity is emerging as a neural substrate for depressive ruminations.

Further extending these findings, another group noted increased connectivity between the sgACC and PCC in a resting state but not during task engagement in patients with MDD, which was significantly correlated with brooding and ruminations, as assessed by the ruminative response scale.[116,117] Several other studies provide supportive findings. One reported increased depressive ruminations associated with altered PCC connectivity in the first episode of MDD compared with healthy controls,[118] and another one noted altered PCC and vmPFC function in depressed individuals, which correlated with the severity of depression and feelings of hopelessness.[119] Extending these findings regarding rumination in MDD, aberrant PCC activity was even observed in individuals who are unhappy in love compared with individuals with happy romantic attachments.[120]

In summary, the changes in PCC activity, in the context of depression, appear to reflect a general "inward" orientation with a propensity toward morose, depressive ruminations, brooding, and preoccupation with gloomy autobiographical memories, leading frequently to hopelessness. At the end of this chapter we provide a more in-depth analysis of the functional imbalance between neural networks that characterizes MDD, and how it may be responsible for the myriad symptoms of depression.

Prefrontal Cortical Changes in Depression

Alterations in PFC function and structure are common findings in MDD. However, because individual subregions of the PFC have substantially different functions, a detailed description of their respective roles is required to fully understand how malfunctioning of these brain areas contributes to MDD. We focus on the four subregions that have been most often implicated in MDD: the dmPFC, vmPFC, vlPFC, and dlPFC. Since the vlPFC and dlPFC are also key components of the EN, we also describe this important neural circuit.

DORSOMEDIAL PREFRONTAL CORTEX

The dmPFC (figure 8.8) has been previously mentioned, along with the PCC, as a principal component of the DMN. The dmPFC incorporates medial components of BAs 8, 9, and 10. Although this prefrontal structure participates in a variety of complex cognitive and emotional processes, it is best known for its "self-referential" function.[121] Relevant to this, imaging studies have noted a curious pattern of activity in the dmPFC. When an individual is involved in a cognitive task, such as solving problems, the dmPFC has attenuated activity, in contrast to a resting state, when it manifests its greatest metabolic activity. Whether one is carefully rehearsing a marriage proposal or reminiscing about a first date, the odds are that these processes will be associated with a greater dmPFC engagement. Imaging studies have provided evidence that the dmPFC participates in a range of such self-related processes, including free association, self-initiated thinking, task-unrelated imag-

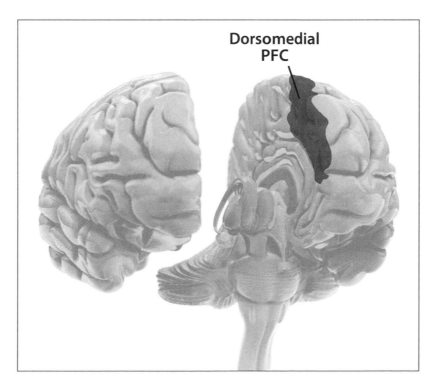

FIGURE 8.8. Dorsomedial prefrontal cortex.

ery, inner rehearsal and speech, entertaining hopes and aspirations, autobiographical musings, and monitoring and reporting one's own mental states.

Interestingly, these capacities appear to have made the dmPFC ideally suited for involvement in attributing similar mental states to other people. Not surprisingly, therefore, imaging studies attempting to locate the neural correlates of empathy and theory of mind (the ability to attribute intention, desires, and beliefs to others) have repeatedly identified the dmPFC (BA 8), along with the superior temporal gyrus, temporoparietal junction, and OFC, as the principal mediators of this faculty.[122] Moreover, the dmPFC has been associated with automatic emotional control and self-appraisal.[123] Some authors have gone as far as proclaiming this introspectively preoccupied neural hub as the seat of selfhood.[121,124–126]

Neuroimaging research has shown that patients suffering from MDD demonstrate aberrant patterns of activity in the dmPFC.[114,115,127–129] Excessive dmPFC activity in MDD may be associated with excessive self-focus, rumination about negative past events, and drudging up self-recriminating, disturbing, and humiliating autobiographical material, at the expense of more realistic self-reflection, positively valenced thoughts, and adaptive problem solving.[114,115,124,127–130] One group emphasizes the centrality of the dmPFC in generating varied depressive symptoms, dubbing it "the dorsal nexus."[114]

Does aberrant activity in the dmPFC in the context of depression coincide with structural changes in this brain region? Probably the best answer currently available comes from a three-year longitudinal study using volumetric imaging techniques to evaluate structural brain changes in MDD. Over time, MDD patients suffered a greater gray matter volume decline in the dmPFC than did healthy controls.[26] These findings indicate that previously described functional changes in the dmPFC may also be accompanied by volumetric alterations over the course of the disorder. Thus, it appears that the structural decline in this key brain region may be, at least in part, a consequence of the disease process itself.

VENTROMEDIAL PREFRONTAL CORTEX AND THE DEFAULT-MODE NETWORK

The vmPFC has rich reciprocal connections with limbic formations, the hypothalamus, periaqueductal gray, brainstem, and spinal autonomic centers.[28,131–133] These connections enable it to modulate parasympathetic/sympathetic balance and endocrine responses to environmental challenges, as well as to accommodate changes in emotional tone.[134,135] Furthermore, based on animal studies, medial PFC pyramidal neuron projections appear to exert a regulatory influence over the primary serotonergic (dorsal nuclei raphae) and dopaminergic nuclei (ventral tegmental area).[136,137] However, many of the potentially significant consequences of altered vmPFC function and structure for dopamine and serotonin signaling in MDD remain to be fully researched.

Intricate bidirectional connections between the vmPFC and vlPFC and the ACC provide for the vmPFC's dual role in top-down emotional modulation and bottom-up response selection.[96] Thus, the vmPFC is not only a major target for ascending limbic projections but also modulates amygdala and hippocampal activity through a complex circuit of feedback connections.[27,132] Most likely, vmPFC "top-down" modulation of the amygdala is mediated by GABA interneurons.[138] The vmPFC is uniquely positioned to receive information from the insula, amygdala, and ventral striatum, which provide salience values for incoming signals from the internal or external environment, whereupon these values can be scaled to differentially guide our behaviors. Let's illustrate this idea with a story. Imagine a scenario where at the end of a long ski day we crave a steaming mug of hot chocolate, while at the same time we struggle with the appeal of getting our uncomfortable ski boots off as soon as possible. Along with assigning the reward value to both options, the vmPFC can also attribute the intrinsic costs (the "hassle" factor), and then assist us with selecting the most adaptive or subjectively preferred behavior.[96] It is no great surprise that the vmPFC plays a key role in regulating both appetitive drives and pain responses.[139] The vmPFC also appears to be preferentially involved in emotional decision making ("hot reasoning") as opposed to more cognitively based determinations, which rely more on the dlPFC and vlPFC.[140] Thus, learning how to like and enjoy things, but also unlearning the fear associated with certain circumstances, is mediated by the vmPFC.[141,142]

While the vmPFC acts as a gatekeeper, presumably by tagging relevant events and their emotional correlates for further cortical processing and eventual selection of adaptive responses, it also plays an important role in the so called top-down regulation of emotion. We have previously indicated that emotions are not passively generated echoes of internal and external events but, rather, are actively construed and edited creations. When circumstances demand it, we can volitionally alter and suppress emotions that might otherwise interfere with a high-priority cognitive process. This is so because an arch originating from dlPFC, extending through vlPFC and subsequently projecting to the vmPFC, ACC, and the limbic and brainstem areas, can censor, modify, or completely abolish our maladaptive feelings and their autonomic and endocrine derivatives.[111,143–146] Furthermore, higher endogenous cortisol, an indirect biomarker of the stress response, is associated with greater inverse vmPFC–amygdala coupling, presumably in attempt to downregulate excessive negative emotion.[147]

Unfortunately, a pathway moving in the opposite direction can also be activated. Anxiety, sadness, anger, stress (especially social stress), morose ruminations, and other emotional distractors can travel in a reverse direction, engaging the amygdala, sgACC, vmPFC, and eventually the dlPFC, creating a disruption in executive functioning.[144,148–153] This was shown strikingly in a study in which subjects experiencing negative emotions, induced by inhaling an odor of rotten yeast, exhibited impaired performance on a task involving working memory and dlPFC engagement.[154] Notably, even peripheral inflammation, induced by receiving an injection of typhoid vaccine, resulted in greater activity in the vmPFC and PCC, both of which are key DMN components. Concomitantly, the dlPFC (the EN hub) demonstrated greater "strain," reflected in augmented perfusion rates during performance of a cognitive task associated with emotional interference.[70] In addition, increased peripheral inflammation was associated with greater activation in the two SN hubs—the insula and ACC—which was in turn highly correlated with the degree of fatigue and confusion experienced by the subjects. It is truly remarkable how the pattern of aberrant interactions between the principal networks involved in mood regulation caused by inflammation resembles those induced by MDD (see figure 8.9).

Now that we have shed some light on the role of the vmPFC in directing not only upward-bound emotional traffic but also top-down regulation of affect and its neuroendocrine and autonomic companions, let's more closely examine functional changes observed in the vmPFC in the context of MDD. Given the evolutionary advantage of linking negative affect, normally associated with a threat, danger, or loss, with bodily defensive apparatus, represented by neuroendocrine, autonomic, and immune systems, and the key regulatory role fulfilled by the vmPFC, one would anticipate major perturbations in this anatomical structure in the context of MDD. As we've discussed, under normal physiological circumstances excessive or aberrant limbic activity elicits a top-down regulatory response engaging the vmPFC. Increased vmPFC activity is associated with a decline in amygdala firing, effectively dampening the inappropriate alarm signal.

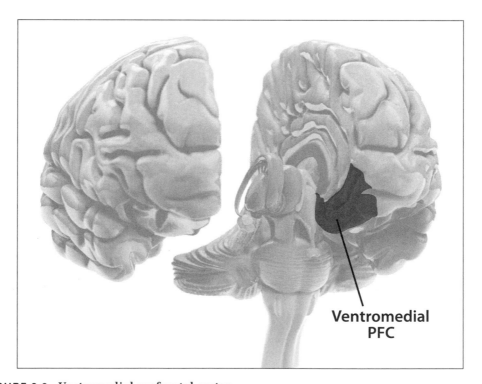

Ventromedial PFC

FIGURE 8.9. Ventromedial prefrontal cortex.

In MDD something unusual happens: activation of the top-down regulatory arc and increased vmPFC activity are paradoxically associated with a greater, rather than lesser, amygdala firing.[145,146,155] Instead of being attenuated, the alarm is amplified, generating perpetually abnormal HPA and autonomic activity. Why would this be so? A plausible explanation stems from research linking stress with reversed plasticity in the vmPFC–amygdala connection.[156] This preclinical study found that animals exposed to inescapable stress develop anomalous neuroplasticity in the pathway connecting the vmPFC and amygdala, potentiating their joint activation, contrary to the normal circumstances when an increase in vmPFC activity leads to suppression of amygdala firing.[156] It is as if the brain has become sensitized by unpredictable and unavoidable adversity and has adapted by perpetuating vigilance and increased sensitivity to environmental danger signals.

Like other DMN areas, the vmPFC tends to manifest greater activity in individuals with MDD than in normal controls.[84,155,157] Not surprisingly, given its role in the DMN, elevated vmPFC activity in MDD patients has been linked with melancholy ruminations, hopelessness, intensity of negative affect, and overall severity of depression.[119,158,159] One study even found a correlation between vmPFC activity and trait anhedonia, or diminished capacity to experience pleasure, in a nonclinical sample.[160] Furthermore, a study of healthy children and adolescents never treated for depression demonstrated increased vmPFC fMRI activity while viewing pictures of fearful facial expressions. Intriguingly, the degree of increased vmPFC activity correlated with depressed mood, as measured by the Beck Depression Inventory, possibly indicating that vmPFC activation may be a neurophysiological correlate of negative mood induced by an emotionally laden stimulus.[161]

Some authors posit that neuroticism, a personality trait associated with more frequent negative mood states, heightened sensitivity to negative information, and negative appraisal (including self-appraisal), may confer vulnerability toward MDD. In one study, higher neuroticism scores were correlated with elevated vmPFC activity in subjects viewing pictures of sad faces, but not happy or fearful expressions.[162] Aberrant vmPFC activity may even be a trait marker for MDD, embodying a biological predilection toward depression and automatic negative self-referential processes.[127] Moreover, depressed mood scores tend to correlate with elevated vmPFC activity.[161] Altered vmPFC activity in MDD has also been associated with compromised ability to spontaneously engage in positive or hopeful thinking,[124] as well as anticipation and selection of rewards.[163]

Hyperreactivity of the vmPFC, combined with reduced activation in the ventral striatum and other reward-related brain regions during reward selection and anticipation may be a consequence of an altered reward/risk bias in MDD, whereby depressed individuals minimize the benefits while exaggerating the possible risks of their actions.[163] As we would have assumed, excessive vmPFC activation in response to emotional stimuli tends to interfere with cognitive performance in MDD subjects.[164] In addition to functional changes, several authors have found significant reductions in vmPFC volume (up to 32 percent) in MDD patients compared with healthy controls.[165–167]

VENTROLATERAL PREFRONTAL CORTEX

The vlPFC (figure 8.10) plays a major role in suppressing maladaptive and perseverative emotional responses. As we have already mentioned, the vlPFC participates in the volitional regulation of emotion and cognitive reappraisal.[1,111] To better understand this, let's use an example from the literature. If one looks at a photo of a group of crying women in front of a church, one may come to an automatic assumption that we are looking at a funeral scene. We can then ask ourselves to reconceptualize the picture as a happy wedding scene in which the women are overwhelmed with joy for the young couple. To succeed in this contextual switch, one has to volitionally override the previous sad feelings to replace them with the happy ones. Imaging studies have provided evidence that this type of cognitive reappraisal is associated with dlPFC and vlPFC activation and concomitant decrease in amygdala and insular activity that is proportional to subjective measures of reduced sadness.[144,168]

Successful reappraisal is associated not only with increased vlPFC activity

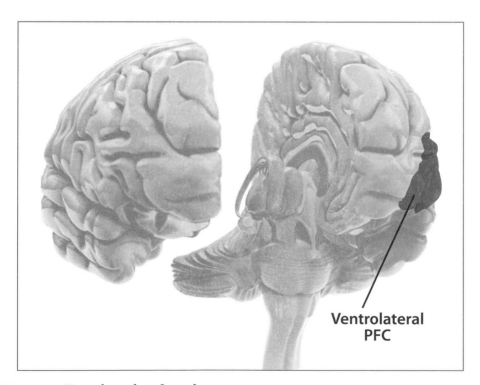

Ventrolateral PFC

FIGURE 8.10. Ventrolateral prefrontal cortex.

accompanied by reduced amygdala firing but also with an increase in ventral striatum and NAcc activity (the brain areas associated with reward and positive affect), which contributes to effective emotional modulation.[1] Furthermore, vlPFC activity has been associated with reduced self-reported distress in studies of social exclusion.[67] Imaging research has also identified the vlPFC as a central component in the PFC circuitry involved in moral and social judgment.[169] Expanding its already varied repertoire even further, the vlPFC has been found to be involved in many highly intricate cognitive processes, such as extracting and temporarily maintaining the information about the nature and type of the relationship between items.[170] Next time you are working on a complicated word puzzle, you would do well to thank your vlPFC for assisting you in that task.

Increased vlPFC activity is one of the most frequently replicated imaging findings in MDD.[84,171,172] Although total consensus is lacking, greater vlPFC activity in depression is most likely an unsuccessful compensatory attempt at top-down regulation of the excessive limbic activity reflected in the maladaptive feelings of sadness, despair, and dejection.[84] A resting-state fMRI study noted that the degree of vlPFC activation correlated with MDD patients' Hamilton Depression Rating Scale scores (administered immediately before scanning) and the duration of their depressive episodes.[129] Based on what we know about the role of the vlPFC in warding off emotional interference with cognitive processes, we would suppose that this function is compromised in the context of MDD. In support of this hypothesis, one study noted attenuated activity in depressed patients' executive brain areas, including the dlPFC and vlPFC, in the presence of the emotional distractors.[85] A standard "challenge" test of top-down volitional emotional modulation involves subjects who are instructed to enhance or suppress emotions provoked by the negative and positive pictures. Hypothetically this paradigm evaluates the ability of dlPFC–vlPFC–vmPFC–sgACC axis to regulate amygdala, insula, and thalamus responses to the emotionally valenced images. In healthy volunteers viewing negative pictures, increased vlPFC activity was associated with decreased amygdala firing rate, while the reverse was true in depressed individuals.[146] This volitional emotion-modulating system not only did not function properly in depressed patients but backfired.

Several meta-analyses have reported a significant reduction in vlPFC gray matter volume of MDD patients relative to healthy subjects.[166,167,173] Moreover, the patients' age was inversely associated with vlPFC gray matter volume, possibly suggesting accelerated age-related involution of this brain region in individuals afflicted by MDD.[167] Reduction in vlPFC gray matter volume was also associated with greater severity of depression as measured by the Montgomery-Asberg Depression Rating Scale and impaired performance on the Wisconsin Card Sorting Test, a commonly used test of executive function.[174]

In summary, it appears that depression is associated with detrimental changes in vlPFC function and structure. Indeed, depression negatively impacts the ability of the vlPFC to carry out its varied roles, including volitional regulation of emotion, suppression of maladaptive feelings and impulses, containing the upward flow of sensory and affective information that threatens to disrupt the higher cognitive processes, and even indirect (via its connections with vmPFC) modulation of endocrine and autonomic correlates of negative emotions.

DORSOLATERAL PREFRONTAL CORTEX AND THE EXECUTIVE COGNITIVE NETWORK

The dlPFC is a principal component of the EN (figure 8.11), which also includes the dACC and parts of the parietal cortex.[90,111,158] Unlike the vmPFC and OFC, which seem to have evolved from limbic and subcortical areas, the dlPFC is an evolutionary expansion of motor, premotor, and supplementary motor cortices and the basal ganglia.[169] Evidence suggests that the dlPFC exercises a "top-down" regulatory influence over limbic structures to optimally allocate our neural resources by refocusing them on matters of the highest priority.[111,113,175]

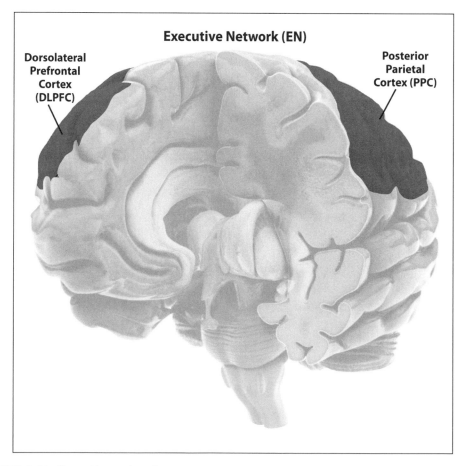

FIGURE 8.11. Executive network.

Let's illustrate this with an example. Suppose we are driving through the mountains engaged in a lively discussion with our friend about the outcome of the recent college basketball tournament. Midway through our impassioned conversation a thunderstorm accompanied by torrential rain starts. It may be a good idea, once the downpour is upon us, to calm the emotions and shift the focus from the tournament to the road and the task of driving. We have already described the two pathways through which dlPFC can accomplish this goal: either an indirect path—dlPFC to vlPFC to vmPFC to sgACC and rACC, ending with the limbic areas (amygdala and or ventral striatum), or a more immediate connection going directly from the posterior vlPFC to the amygdala.[175] Using either pathway, the dlPFC can instantiate top-down affective regulation to fight off the distraction or to reappraise our emotional state when circumstances demand this.

Most often limbic inhibition by the dlPFC and other cortical areas is not continuous; it tends to be task specific. As we all know from personal experience, stress and other strong emotions can sometimes interfere with our cognitive processes. When this happens, the dlPFC steps in and tamps down these unwelcome distractions. On the other hand, we do not want to disregard potentially crucial incoming emotional signals warning us about important environmental changes. Although we want to ignore an annoying toothache so that we can focus on our reading, it would not be a good idea to disregard a fire alarm. The dlPFC cooperates with the ACC in identifying these types of conflicting agendas. When the circumstances demand it, the dlPFC can divide our attention so that we can multitask.[176–178]

Sometimes we need to inhibit our usual routines to adapt to an environmental change. Let's say a European or a US citizen is vacationing in a Caribbean country where the traffic rules require that one drives on the left side of the road. After pulling out from a parking space, one engages in firmly established routine: driving in the right-hand lane. Once we've done this, the specter of traffic coming straight at us is likely going to generate anxiety, signaling a conflict. If we are lucky, the dlPFC should assume its critical role by enabling us to inhibit a prior routine, which will shift our driving strategy in a timely manner, such that we avoid a head-on collision by quickly steering into the left lane, thereby successfully negotiating a novel demand.[177,179] This little vignette also highlights the fact that the dlPFC plays a role in decision making and initiation of voluntary action, in concert with the presupplementary motor area and the parietal cortex.[180]

Working memory involves active maintenance and manipulation of information in the service of task completion, and it is one of the key functions of the dlPFC.[178] Working memory allows for important information to be retained online for further elaboration, prioritization, and processing. Beyond the simple retention of information and attention, the dlPFC also registers the passage of time and keeps our information stores updated.[177,178] Maintaining information in working memory is necessary for our ability to form mental representations of the relationships between the various entities we encounter in the world around us.

Information about these relationships is organized hierarchically in the dlPFC, with progressively more abstract information stored toward the anterior pole of this region of the PFC.[178] So, for example, if we were examining a large collection of photographs, first attempting to differentiate female from male faces, next looking for males with beards, and finally trying to detect Sigmund Freud look-alikes, we would likely be engaging progressively more rostral (anterior) portions of the dlPFC. When we are "stretching" our working memory with increased load, this is reflected in greater dlPFC activation in imaging studies.[175] Of course, dealing with pesky incoming stimuli while attempting to store and maintain information in the dlPFC can sometimes be a challenge. The maintenance of effortful sustained attention in these trying circumstances seems to be a dlPFC specialty.[181]

The quality of "incoming" emotion may have a differential influence on dlPFC functioning. It appears that the dlPFC preferentially handles positive, rewarding cues, while increased vlPFC activation coincides with an influx of negative stimuli.[175] There is even some limited, albeit controversial, evidence suggesting that positively valenced emotions can enhance dlPFC manipulation of data in working memory.[175] Therefore, positive emotions may facilitate the storage of information in dlPFC-related working memory, while negative emotions may engage vlPFC-related processes, initiating the elimination of the unwelcome intrusion. Furthermore, the dlPFC appears to be more engaged by a change of "rules" than by the quality of feedback (positive or negative) resulting from one's actions.[182]

More complex decision making involving the evaluation of contingencies also relies on the dlPFC and its capacity to maintain the relevant information online. A network that includes the dlPFC, OFC, and putamen identifies the "rules" in any given situation based on extant contingencies. Upon completion of the task at hand, the system usually goes offline. If the observed contingencies do not fit any identifiable pattern, the circumstances are labeled as uncertain, and the network remains active in a vigilant state.[183,184] Moreover, in a stressful situation, which is identified as controllable, this network (most likely via its vmPFC and ACC connections) will activate endocrine, sympathetic, and immune responses. On the other hand, if the stressor is deemed to be uncontrollable, the dlPFC's connections with the ACC and dorsal striatum will have an upper hand, vagal parasympathetic activation will prevail, and the immune response will be suppressed. Thus, our dlPFC-based evaluation of the perceived level of control over stressful events will influence selection and allocation of our autonomic, endocrine, and immune resources.[183,184]

Given what we've discussed so far, it is clear that the dlPFC (figure 8.12) plays a primary role in the top-down regulation of emotion, effortful sustained attention, working memory, strategy shifting, inhibition of routine but inappropriate responses, and the representation of abstract relationships. In addition to these roles, the dlPFC is important for social cognition and moral judgment.[169,104] Fur-

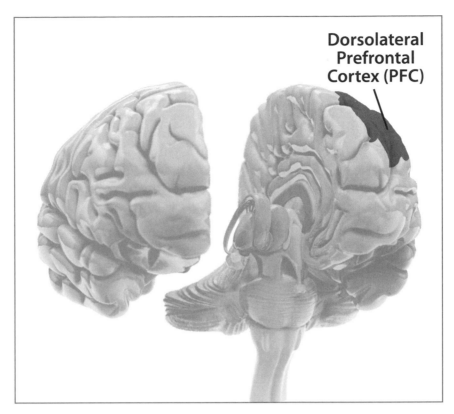

**Dorsolateral
Prefrontal
Cortex (PFC)**

FIGURE 8.12. Dorsolateral prefrontal cortex.

thermore, the gray matter volume of the dlPFC, and especially its anterior portion (BA 10), along with white matter tracts originating from this brain segment, correlates with an individual's ability to introspect. Sophisticated imaging studies have linked this anterior PFC structure with metacognitive ability, which includes a capacity to discriminate correct from erroneous decisions over time.[185]

Decreased activity in the dlPFC in MDD may contribute to number of notable symptoms and signs of the disorder, including compromised working memory, impaired sustained attention, and executive dysfunction.[113] Not surprisingly, then, studies have associated cognitive impairment in depressed patients with altered dlPFC function.[171] Diminished dlPFC activity has been correlated with duration of depression and with its severity, as measured by Hamilton Depression Rating Scale.[129] Decreased dlPFC activity in depressed individual has also been found to correlate with the intensity of one's sadness,[106] poor planning,[84] inadequate and delayed responses to negative emotional stimuli,[84,85] increased amygdala reactivity following an emotional challenge,[11] compromised performance on executive function (n-back task) and memory tests,[186–188] and psychomotor slowing.[189,190]

One might suspect based on our earlier discussion that dlPFC dysfunction would likely be associated with inadequate coping with emotional and cognitive distractors. Imaging studies have confirmed this by revealing dlPFC hyperactivity in depressed patients trying to ward off either emotional (fearful and sad stimuli) or cognitive interference, most likely reflecting a "strain" due to heightened load and functional insufficiency of this PFC area.[191–193] Other research further extended these conclusions. When depressed subjects were asked to judge the intensity of negatively valenced facial expressions, their responses were associated with increased dlPFC activity compared with healthy controls. Hyperactivity of the dlPFC during performance of this task requiring emotional regulation correlated with the severity of depression,[194] suggesting that a compromised ability of the dlPFC to filter out emotional and cognitive distractors may be the biological underpinning of several depressive symptoms.

An important duty of the dlPFC is to engage in problem solving once the ACC has detected an error, typically a consequence of our actions not producing the desired/expected outcome. In depressed patients, despite intense ACC signaling communicating that an error has occurred, the dlPFC fails to engage.[195] This finding may reflect an impaired ability to impose executive control in circumstances when the initial adaptive response has failed. Could this be one of the reasons for the reluctance and indecisiveness that depressed patients often demonstrate when needing to make significant changes in their lives? Disturbances in dlPFC function may be present very early in the course of MDD. A study reported diminished markers of glial function, myelination, and cell growth in the dlPFC of depressed children and adolescents relative to the healthy controls.[196] There have been many attempts through the years to identify neuroimaging fingerprint(s) of depression. One of these studies identified a pattern of aberrant brain activity that appears to readily differentiate depressed patients from a healthy cohort. A combination of altered amygdala, ACC, superior temporal gyrus, and dlPFC activity correctly classified depressed patients with 84 percent sensitivity and 89 percent specificity.[12]

In addition to functional abnormalities in MDD, a three-year prospective study reported significantly greater dlPFC gray matter decline in unremitted MDD patients compared with control subjects and with MDD subjects who attained remission during the study.[26] Similarly, meta-analyses of gray matter changes in depression have identified diminished dlPFC volume as one of the more common findings.[197] Decreased dlPFC volume in depressed patients relative to healthy controls has been associated with cognitive deficits in elderly individuals with remitted depression[194] and with worse performance on tests of executive function in younger patients.[174] Reductions in dlPFC gray matter volume also appear to correlate with a greater depression severity.[174] Finally, thinning of PFC areas, including the dlPFC, has been reported in individuals with increased familial risk for depression, indicating that functional and structural aberrations in this brain area may be a part of a genetically or epigenetically conferred risk for depressive diathesis.[198] Taking the available data as a whole, it appears that reduced dlPFC volume is both a risk factor for the development of depression and an outcome of the disease state itself. The relative importance of these two causal relationships in depression, however, remains an unanswered question.

Subcortical Regions: Thalamus and Basal Ganglia

THE THALAMUS AND THE CORTICO–STRIATAL–PALLIDO–THALAMIC CIRCUIT

Although subcortical regions have not been the focus of imaging research to the same degree as cortical and limbic regions, functional and structural changes in the basal ganglia and thalamus have been reported in patients suffering from Major Depression.[199] Even though the thalamus is best known as a relay station that provides rapid and efficient sensory-motor integration for the pathways leading to and from higher cortical areas, its role in CNS functioning is far more intricate and extensive than any simple relay station metaphor would suggest.[200]

The thalamus (figure 8.13) is a key node in the networks that connect cortical regions with limbic structures and the basal ganglia. The cortico-striato-pallido-thalamic (CSPT) pathway projects from the cortex to the basal ganglia (striatum and globus pallidus, see figure 8.14) and then on to the thalamus before looping back to the cortex.[201] The cortex can exert both activating and inhibitory influ-

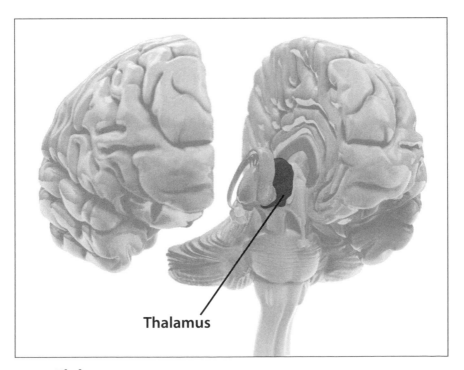

Thalamus

FIGURE 8.13. Thalamus.

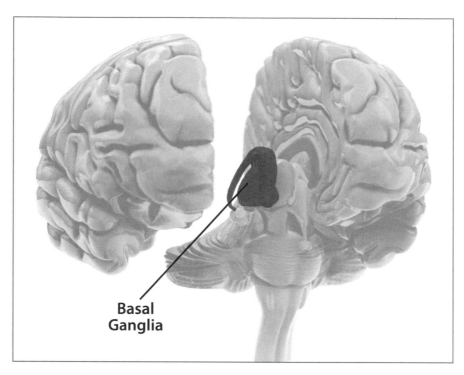

FIGURE 8.14. Basal ganglia.

ences over the thalamus through distinct paths. A loop that originates from the medial PFC connects with the mediodorsal thalamic nucleus via limbic areas, such as the amygdala, parahippocampus, entorhinal cortex, and subiculum, and utilizes glutamate, the main excitatory neurotransmitter. In contrast, pathways that originate from the cortex and synapse in the basal ganglia before projecting to the thalamus are GABAergic and therefore inhibitory.[201] Adjustments via these parallel but opposed corticothalamic pathways are somewhat analogous to manually adjusting the focal length of the camera lens by rotating the rings clockwise and counterclockwise until the object of our interest is in focus. In a similar fashion the cortex fine-tunes sensory input and motor responses to best serve selected attentional needs. In other words, the cortex has the ability to either facilitate or impede the flow of sensory and motor information through the thalamus, which in turn typically either supports or interrupts ongoing behavior. Thus, the thalamus can be conceptualized as a "behavioral clutch" that supports an adaptive shift in behavioral patterns in response to ever-changing environmental conditions.[201]

The CSPT circuit has three topographically distinct divisions.[202] Motor and premotor cortices project directly to caudal putamen, forming the motor division, charged with regulating goal directed motor behavior. The dlPFC and dorsal caudate are the components of the executive/cognitive division, involved in focusing attention and updating working memory. The affective/limbic division is composed of the vmPFC, ACC, and ventral striatum/NAcc complex; its principal role is regulation of emotional behavior, particularly related to reward and motivation.

Imaging studies have identified the thalamus as a hot spot in CSPT loops that integrates multiple signals reflecting motivation, emotional drive, planning, and cognition.[203] Expected gains, difficulties, and necessary attentional resources are processed in CSPT circuits in coordination with the mesencephalic monoaminergic (especially dopaminergic) nuclei.[204] When difficult tasks are also associated with considerable rewards, CSPT loops can engage cortical centers to more precisely manage resource allocation in pursuit of the adaptive goals. In plain language, in preparation for future action, we assess potential gains, difficulties, and our own abilities. If we sense that success of a given endeavor will be a "close call," cortical resources are engaged for further elaboration.

Additionally, pathways leading from the cortex to thalamus and on to the cerebellum are involved in generating automatic emotional and cognitive responses.[205] Disruptions in the proper functioning of these cortico–thalamic–cerebellar loops may result in cognitive and emotional disturbances, dubbed by some authors as cognitive and affective dysmetria (clumsiness, lack of coordination).[206] Furthermore, hippocampus–thalamus pathways play an important role in relational and nonrelational memory processes.[207,208]

Depressed patients often avoid social events because they do not believe that they are likely to have a good time, and they "don't want to be a drag." It is not uncommon for depressed individuals to complain of feeling emotionally distant and out of sync with their loved ones. Their reasoning and decision making appear to be entirely internally driven, discounting relevant social and environmental information. Could these depressive behavioral patterns be influenced by abnormal corticothalamic regulation? If we conceive of depressive affect as a form of emotional behavior, we can entertain a hypothesis that corticothalamic dysfunction results in the lack of adaptive flexibility, impeding the transition from sadness and dejection to a more environmentally congruent mood state.

In general, functional imaging studies have reported increased thalamic activity in depressed individuals. Resting state functional connectivity imaging has shed more light on the important role that the thalamus may play in the pathophysiology of depression. One study found attenuated connectivity between the emotional components of the CSPT network—the vmPFC, sgACC, and ventral striatum—in depressed individuals compared with healthy controls. Compromised connectivity between the components of the affective division was predictably associated with diminished motivation and more pronounced depression. On the other hand, reduced connectivity between the medial PFC and dorsal caudate, the key components of the executive division, in depressed subjects relative to healthy controls was linked to psychomotor retardation and difficulty initiating activities.[202] The study also revealed increased connectivity between the ventral striatum and PCC in MDD patients compared with controls. This finding is of particular interest since in physiological circumstances the ventral striatum acts as a switch disengaging the DMN and mobilizing the EN in response to relevant ascending sensory information. This aberrant connectivity between the ventral striatum and the components of the DMN and the EN may underpin the tendency toward self-referential ruminative preoccupation and away from externally directed processing, notoriously associated with the severity of depression.

Another aspect of depression-associated thalamic dysfunction has captured researchers' interest. Along with recurring negative ruminative preoccupation, due to excessive DMN activation, and impaired motivational regulation, ostensibly related to malfunction of the affective division of the CSPT circuit, another cardinal feature of depression, attentional bias toward negative information, may also be based on a glitch involving thalamic processing. The pulvinar (literally, a cushion or an empty throne to be occupied by a deity) is a key thalamic area endowed with direct monosynaptic connections with principal limbic/SN regions: amygdala, insula, and dACC. Connections between the pulvinar and SN subserve its main function: emotional attention and awareness. Greater baseline activity in the pulvinar in MDD may be the foundation for augmented awareness and attention to negative emotions generated by the amygdala, insula, and other SN areas.[209] As a matter of fact, a meta-analysis of the functional neuroimaging studies of MDD highlights the role of resting-state overactivity of the pulvinar and incorporates it into an elegant neurophysiological explanation of depressive phenomena. This two-step explanatory model first emphasizes increased attention to negatively valenced information due to elevated pulvinar activity, followed by failure of this information to ascend along the CSPT circuit to its final destination in the dlPFC and related EN areas. Thus, exaggerated negative emotions are not subjected to adaptive cortical scrutiny, contextual processing, and critical reappraisal.[210] In plain English, the depressed person is immersed in dark and morose self-preoccupation, which builds on already negatively biased experience of reality while escaping the critical review and adaptive correction commonly supplied by the cortex in healthy circumstances.

Furthermore, imaging studies have discovered that thalamic hypermetabolism tends to be associated with increased activity in the sgACC and decreased metabolic activity in the dACC,[211] both of which have been previously reported in MDD. Some investigators have postulated that aberrant thalamic activity in depressed patients may be the precipitant of excessive SN response to negative stimuli.[209] In contrast, even remitted depressed patients displayed an attenuated thalamic response to rewarding stimuli.[212] The preponderance of data point in the same direction, implicating thalamic dysfunction in the imbalance among major resting-state networks observed in MDD. Poor thalamic modulation may contribute to excessive activity in several components of the SN associated with negative emotionality, including the amygdala, insula, and sgACC, as well as diminished activity in the ventral striatum/NAcc response to rewarding stimuli. In the context of normal neural network function, one would not expect SN and

DMN activities to be simultaneously increased, but in depression they are. Abnormal thalamic and sgACC coupling with the DMN is believed to be the primary culprit for this odd coupling.[211] This aberrant connectedness between limbic areas and DMN promotes the inappropriate bleeding of negative emotionality into the DMN network. The usual role of the DMN involving self-reflection and manipulation of autobiographical memories is converted into vulnerability toward perpetual morose ruminations, brooding, and dejection, all of which are notorious manifestations of depressed mood.

Moreover, researchers have reported a correlation between the severity of depression and increased thalamic activity in unmedicated patients.[213] Further extending these findings, an imaging study has established a relationship between treatment-resistant depression and thalamic activity. At the onset of the study all the depressed patients manifested reduced connectivity among prefrontal–limbic–thalamic areas, as assessed by advanced fMRI imaging. This pattern of cerebral activity could be interpreted as inadequate cortical/EN regulation of thalamic and other SN-related structures. Subsequently, patients were treated for a minimum of six weeks with one of three antidepressant regimens: selective serotonin reuptake inhibitors, serotonin-norepinephrine reuptake inhibitors, or tricyclics. If patients had less than a 50 percent reduction on the Hamilton Depression Rating Scale (HAM-D) scale scores after six weeks of treatment, they were identified as poor responders. Patients who had a poor response to two different treatment regimens were labeled treatment refractory. Depressed individuals who responded to conventional antidepressant therapy had a disturbance in ACC, amygdala, hippocampal, and insular connectivity on the initial scan. Intriguingly, treatment-refractory patients manifested aberrant connectivity between prefrontal areas and the thalamus.[214]

These findings raise very important questions. Is the subtype of depression that responds to conventional antidepressant treatment physiologically different from treatment-refractory depression? Alternatively, is treatment-refractory depression an evolution of a more common form, associated with a greater disturbance in corticothalamic circuitry? Are there specific symptoms or biological manifestations (aside from the imaging findings) of this treatment-refractory, subcortical type of depression, which would help clinicians identify it? In addition to already described functional alterations, several meta-analyses of volumetric studies and postmortem reports have noted decreased thalamic size in patients suffering from depression compared with unaffected controls.[166,215,216]

CEREBELLUM

Some, but not all, studies, have found alterations in cerebellar function in patients with MDD.[84,199] This is of particular interest because the vermis of the cerebellum has been implicated in generating automatic emotional responses, including empathy, to facial expressions.[217–219]

Abnormal Connections Among the Brain Regions in MDD

Earlier in this chapter we described patterns of functional connectivity between brain regions most frequently implicated as abnormal in MDD. It is now a good time to extend this discussion by reviewing two different scenarios underlying functional connectivity. In the first scenario connectivity is identified as a pattern of coactivation in imaging studies, based on whether mathematical formulas determine if connectivity between anatomical regions is statistically significant or not. The pattern of coupling identified by this approach does not always coincide with known anatomical connections within the human brain. One can imagine a situation in which two distant brain areas belong to two distinct but interconnected networks. Activation of one of the networks, or its components, will likely spread to the constituents of the other network. Therefore, two areas that have no direct anatomical connections may still be activated in a close temporal proximity and hence be identified as having functional connectivity.

In the other scenario, in a more orthodox sense functional coupling is a consequence of the anatomical connections between two brain regions. White matter tracts are the neurological underpinning of the aforementioned anatomical connections. White matter is a product of myelination of the long neural axons by the oligodendroglia. Oligidendrocytes myelinate nerve fibers by wrapping up to 150 layers of tightly compressed cell membrane around axons. Myelination is a feature of vertebrate neurons that allows for rapid and powerful transmission of electrochemical signals along the lengthy axons. Its evolutionary importance may be reflected in the fact that white matter constitutes more than half of the mass of the human brain, a far greater proportion than in any other mammal.[220,221]

It would be erroneous to believe that, once established, white matter tracts remain static. Contrary to common belief, myelination of white matter tracts in the human brain is not complete until the third decade of life. Our life experiences and skill acquisition continuously shape the evolution and expansion of white matter within the brain. For example, imaging studies have discovered that structural white matter changes correlate with the number of hours that professional musicians spend practicing their instrument.[221] If learning new skills through repetition is capable of inducing white matter changes in adulthood, what would happen in the context of persistently altered brain activity pattern that accompanies the lengthy, recurrent depressive episodes?

White matter changes in MDD do not appear to be particularly age related; rather, they are present during the earliest stages of the illness and may even precede it. Several imaging studies comparing depressed patients with healthy controls have found white matter abnormalities in MDD, especially in elderly patients, even when corrections were made for age and vascular status.[222] However, changes in corticosubcortical white matter tracts have also been observed in treatment-naïve younger populations suffering from their first depressive episode. These results suggest that disrupted white matter connections may be a part of the fundamental pathophysiology of depression, present from the very beginning of the illness, possibly even predating it and advancing with the progression of the disease.[223] Extending these findings, a magnetic resonance spectroscopy study noted a decrease in biochemical indicators of oligodendroglia and white matter integrity in the dlPFC of first-episode depressed patients,[224] while another research group reported altered ACC white matter microstructure in adolescents suffering from depression.[225]

Emerging evidence suggests that there may be a relationship between white matter alterations and treatment response in depression. Several studies have reported compromised integrity of cortico–basal ganglia–thalamic and PFC–limbic circuits in depression.[108,226,227] We mentioned earlier in this chapter that disruption in corticothalamic circuitry tends to result in a lack of response to antidepressant treatment. Another study has found that disrupted subcortical white matter circuitry combined with low folate levels predicted a lesser response to antidepressant treatment.[228]

Several imaging studies have established a relationship between white matter changes and specific symptom domains in MDD. Abnormal white matter microstructure in the ventral tegmental area/nigrostriatal circuitry (involved with reward and aversion signaling) resulted in greater trait anxiety in a subgroup of depressed patients.[229] Moreover, disruption of frontal lobe, insula, and adjacent basal ganglia white matter in depressed individuals has been correlated with cognitive disturbance, as reflected by impaired performance on the Stroop test.[230] Another study reported that whole-brain white matter in depressed subjects correlated with episodic memory, processing speed, and executive function.[222] In aggregate, imaging evidence confirms our assumption about the importance of proper white matter tract function for correct information processing in the primary brain networks involved in cognition and emotional regulation.

Aberrant connectivity between limbic and paralimbic prefrontal areas has also been reported in MDD patients.[11,222,226,227] A review highlights the fact that white matter pathology in MDD patients involves the principal cortical and limbic areas, including the dlPFC, vmPFC, amygdala, insula, and hippocampus, the same ones that have previously been implicated by functional imaging studies. Furthermore, imaging findings of white matter alterations were consistent with the reported genetic abnormalities in depressed patients, affecting myelination, axonal growth, and synaptic function.[231] Additionally, the degree of microstructural abnormalities in the uncinate fasciculus, a white matter bundle connecting the amygdala and hippocampus with the vlPFC and vmPFC, was found to directly correlate with the severity of depression.[232] White matter abnormalities in the fronto–cerebellar–thalamic circuitry have also been reported in the context of depression.[233]

In summary, functional networks, which are probabilistic constructs based on the likelihood of coactivation of particular brain regions, have a material underpinning substantiated by anatomical neural networks. Brain networks are composed of distributed, sometimes relatively distant interconnected neural structures. Therefore, reliable and rapid information transfer is necessary for proper brain function. Thousands of myelinated axons, entwined into white matter tracts, provide for smooth communication within and between these networks. Multidisciplinary evidence suggests that genes involved in the regulation of white matter formation are altered in depressed patients. Possibly due to interaction between genetic and epigenetic vulnerabilities with other pathophysiological mechanisms of depression, oligodendroglia cells involved in the production of myelin are also dysfunctional and reduced in numbers in MDD sufferers. Hence, cumulative evidence suggests that disruption in the functional connectivity of the networks that provide cognitive-emotional integration and the control of mood and stress responses may be responsible for some of the complex manifestations of MDD.

Synthesis

We now attempt a cogent summary of the relationship between functional and structural brain changes and the symptoms of depression, or perhaps we should say "depressions." The task of establishing a consistent pattern of functional and structural brain changes associated with MDD is a bit akin to solving a Magic Eye puzzle. For those of you not acquainted with the Magic Eye, this has become a generic name for autostereograms, which are two-dimensional dot puzzles that allow viewers to "discover" a "hidden" three-dimensional image by adjusting the focal length and divergence of their eyes. Focusing each eye on a different part of the puzzle creates an illusion of depth. If we shift our gaze ever so slightly, or move the puzzle farther away from our eyes, the image will disappear.

MDD is a descriptive diagnostic entity, which does not appear to have a clearly definable and precisely matching pathophysiology. No matter which biological marker(s) of depression we choose, be it increased amygdala and sgACC activity, diminished hippocampal volume, cortisol receptor insensitivity, or increased inflammatory cytokines, we will find a distribution of these markers within the population of depressed patients. Some patients will manifest the given biological marker to a greater extent, others to a lesser extent, and in yet other patients it will be indistinguishable from the average values observed in healthy controls. In other words, we are dealing with a probabilistic clinical entity, which appears to have a solid core and tends to fray around the edges, blending into the spectrum of normalcy. It is also safe to assume that when we confront MDD, we are in fact dealing with multiple pathophysiological entities that share phenotypical manifestations. Unless we look at depression in just the right way, it starts blending into the background. We believe that it is more correct to conceptualize this clinical phenomenon as the plural *depressions*, yet for the sake of custom and simplicity we will continue to refer to it in a singular form.

Where do depressive symptoms originate? Based on our reading of the literature they have multiple sources distributed within the brain and the rest of the body. The symptomatic manifestations of depression most likely reflect a blend of "normal," adaptive mind-body responses to changes in our environment, specific changes in body and brain functioning related more specifically to depression, alterations in brain connectivity and structure caused by the disease chronicity, and our organism's compensatory responses elicited by the disease state.[72,234–237] Initial hopes that neuroimaging techniques might lead to the discovery of patterns of dysfunction in certain brain area(s) that would be reflected in the specific depressive symptom(s) now seems implausible. Rather, a single symptom, or several related symptoms, tends to map more accurately onto dysfunction of neural circuits, which are composed of several distributed yet interconnected brain areas.

The first wave of functional imaging studies (single-photon emission computed tomography, positron emission tomography, fMRI) identified a relatively consistent pattern of altered activity in the limbic and cortical areas of patients suffering from depression. Increased activity in limbic and paralimbic areas (amygdala, sgACC, insula, vmPFC) was usually accompanied by decreased perfusion/metabolic rates in dorsal "executive" cortical areas (dACC, dlPFC). These findings were most often interpreted as evidence of either excessive limbic activity interfering with the functioning of cognitive/executive cortical areas, or inadequate "top-down" cortical modulation of limbic circuitry. Frequently, explanations for the varied emotional and cognitive symptoms of depression evoked a combination of these two mechanisms. Furthermore, cytoarchitectural changes, involving neurons, glia, and the white mater tracts, tracked well with the pattern of abnormalities in the corticolimbic functions and structures typically detected by the imaging studies.[28,84,157,238–242]

More recent imaging studies have elaborated on this prior perspective by shedding light on an aberrant communication dynamic among the three major neural networks in depressed patients. We have already extensively discussed the compositions of the DMN, SN, and EN cortical networks, so we now focus on their interactions in the context of MDD. Under normal physiological conditions, the DMN is involved in contemplation, reminiscing, social interactions, self-reflection, and planning of future endeavors. One can conceive of the DMN as a bridge between the past and the future in that it allows us to use past contingencies to construe, enrich, and explore various scenarios to construct the best possible predictions about the future.[104] At times the DMN collaborates with other networks. When our thoughts are unbidden, internally generated, unburdened by the need to address issues imposed by the external environment, the DMN connects with EN-related frontoparietal cortical areas. The connection between the

DMN and EN helps mobilize our attention and working memory resources to support the internal stream of thought. If we are involved in the planning of future actions or reminiscing about the past, the MTL will join in, providing access to our library of the autobiographical memories. In these circumstances, input from SN-related sensory/emotional areas will be muted, so as not to disrupt our train of thought.[243–247] Creative thinking utilizes similar connections among the DMN, EN, and MTL. Generating creative ideas is associated with the DMN–MTL link (presumably drawing on memory resources), while the evaluation of the novel ideas relies on DMN–EN collaboration.[248]

Meditation provides a very specific scenario for DMN–EN coupling. The burgeoning imaging literature has explored different forms of meditation. It is beyond the scope of this chapter to provide a comprehensive review of all the diverse modalities, so we focus on their most prominent common characteristics. Several Eastern meditation traditions, including Zen and Vipassana, can be characterized as combinations of focused attention and open monitoring styles. The focused attention style, as the name suggests, is based on sustained focus on a chosen object. By contrast, open monitoring meditation entails a moment-to-moment monitoring of one's experience.[249] Increased connectivity between DMN areas (PCC, medial PFC) and EN-related areas (the dlPFC and the parietal cortex) has been noted in several studies.[250–253] More efficient EN engagement may translate into a more adaptive attentional disengagement from self-reflective, rumination-prone DMN activity. Consistent with this possibility, altered connectivity between components of the DMN has been described in several studies.[250,253] More experienced meditators using the mindfulness method, compared with less experienced ones, exhibited a greater uncoupling of the dmPFC and vmPFC while meditating, possibly reflecting a diminished propensity toward self-referential emotional judgments. Lastly, imaging studies indicate that meditators have reduced functional connectivity between SN areas (insula, ACC) and DMN areas (dmPFC, PCC) and a greater functional connectivity between SN and EN brain areas (dlPFC, parietal cortex).[251–255]

These changes in functional connectivity between the principal components of the three major networks (SN, EN, and DMN) can alternatively be interpreted as a neural correlate of greater awareness of the momentary sensory experiences or *disidentification*, a term from mindfulness meditation literature, designating intentional avoidance of elaboration of the sensory experiences. Focus on "pure" unprocessed sensory experience may result in more effective shifting between the networks, improved cognitive-attentional engagement, and decreased propensity toward ruminations, self-referential thinking, and mind wandering.[249–252,254–257] Several functional imaging studies have reported an association between the amount of meditation experience and changes in functional connectivity between relevant brain areas, while one volumetric study indicated that experienced meditators, compared with a group of demographically matched nonmeditators, had greater gray matter volume of the insula, hippocampus, and inferior temporal gyrus.[250,251,253,256,258] The cumulative implication of these imaging studies is that meditation experience may translate into neuroplastic changes in various brain networks, thus altering their functional dynamics.

Although a burst of activity in SN structures (thalamus, insula, ventral striatum, amygdala, and dACC) usually signals that some important change in the environment has taken place and it is time to snap out of DMN mode and engage in active coping, sometimes the SN and DMN can form a more enduring functional coupling. Stronger, longer-lasting SN–DMN coupling may act as an emotional amplifier aimed at more robust recruitment of attentional resources. This coupling can occur in several substantially different emotional situations. Extended activation of SN areas (amygdala and ACC), coincident with greater activity in the DMN-related PCC and dmPFC, is the most likely neural basis for optimism.[259] Successful integration of autobiographical and self-referential information with emotional flow allows us to project an optimistic bias toward future events. An imaging study has identified neural processes that may underpin the experience of optimism. Radiological images in this study were acquired while subjects thought of a pleasant autobiographical event that might occur in the future. A psychological scale was used to evaluate each subject's trait optimism. Coupling between the rACC and amygdala was strongly correlated with the measures of optimism.[259] Another intriguing implication of this study is based on evidence that the relationship between the DMN and SN may be bidirectional. In one study, projected future experience, coincident with activation of DMN areas (dmPFC and PCC). instantiated a robust limbic response in the amygdala (SN). Another study confirmed that activation of DMN regions at rest (vmPFC, dmPFC, and PCC) can induce an emotional change.[102] In other words, our own spontaneous creative and optimistic thoughts can generate an emotional change.

Unfortunately, negative experiences cam engender a similar coupling between the SN and DMN. An imaging study focused on the neural consequences of social stress. Researchers utilized the Trier Social Stress Test paradigm. Subjects were asked to give a five-minute free speech about their positive and negative characteristics while being scrutinized by a selection committee of "mental health experts." An hour later a resting-state fMRI imaging study was conducted. The outcome demonstrated robustly increased coactivation of the SN (amygdala) and DMN (PCC and medial PFC). This enduring coupling of DMN areas, involved in generating autobiographical memories, and the amygdala (SN) is believed to facilitate the maintenance, storage, and consolidation of self-relevant information into memory banks.[149] Coupling between the amygdala and vmPFC was supported by an increase of endogenous cortisol.[147]

A study noted that in healthy individuals a laboratory-based social-evaluative threat triggered ruminative thoughts that persisted for three to five days.[260] Furthermore, another imaging study described a relationship between the degree of negative affectivity, a measure of harm avoidance, and self-referential processing in several key DMN areas (vmPFC, dmPFC, and PCC).[128] Greater negative affectivity was associated with a more pronounced propensity toward DMN-related self-reflective thought. Recognition of social inequality and social pain, caused by social exclusion, also activated the insula–ACC circuit (SN) coupled with the medial PFC or PCC (DMN) activity.[261,262]

In an interesting turn of events, one study attempted to treat pain associated with social rejection with acetaminophen, a common physical pain reliever that is the active ingredient in Tylenol.[263] Much to everyone's surprise, 1000 mg acetaminophen, taken daily for three weeks, substantially reduced reports of social pain. Moreover, fMRI imaging discovered a correlation between the decline in social pain and reduction in dACC and insula activity (the principal components of EN and SN) in response to a social exclusion paradigm.[263] It appears that the insula–ACC unit (SN) is capable of detecting not only a spectrum of somatic and external stimuli (pain, inflammation, sounds, facial expressions, social inequality) but also subtle changes in neural states such as distress, depression, and pain associated with social rejection.[70,53,261]

Interestingly, it was exactly this increase in activity of coupled SN and DMN areas that predicted self-sacrificing, egalitarian, and empathizing prosocial behaviors in other studies.[261,262] A different group, also using fMRI imaging, found that narratives, based on true stories, that inspired admiration or compassion elicited increased activity in the very same SN (insula, ACC) and DMN (precuneus, PCC) brain areas.[264] Given that we are social beings, it is tempting to speculate that a sustained SN–DMN connection, following an unsettling social event or a stressful interruption, may act as a "mental capacitor," amplifying and maintaining survival-relevant information. Therefore, rumination may be a mental correlate of an important neural process tasked with emphasizing and storing self-relevant social information, a form of "mental digestion." While self-reflection and ruminative mulling over of recent events may bolster the pursuit of a new social compass, in the face of a dramatic change it also acts as a springboard for prosocial behaviors, providing us with an adaptive advantage.

Among normally occurring emotional states, grief is probably the closest to depression. An imaging study compared 12 women who had lost an unborn child due to malformations and 12 women who delivered healthy babies.[265] The viewing of happy baby faces by the grieving women was associated with an increased activation of DMN-related areas (PCC and vmPFC), as well as brain regions associated with the SN (ACC and thalamus).[265] A similar activation pattern was observed in an older fMRI study of women grieving the loss of a loved one. When viewing photographs of the deceased person or listening to words specific to the death event, bereaved women experienced increased activity in the PCC, vmPFC, and dmPFC (DMN areas), as well as in the ACC and insula (SN hubs).[266]

It is interesting, that in addition to partly replicating imaging findings characteristic of depression, grief may also activate similar somatic responses. Studies found that sgACC (SN)–DMN coupling in grief states was associated with a decline in parasympathetic tone[267] and an increase in salivary inflammatory markers,[268] much like the changes that we would encounter in the context of depression.[269] Unlike depression, however, grieving individuals may utilize dlPFC (EN)–amygdala (SN) coupling to intentionally suppress feelings of grief.[270] Uncomplicated grief, much like social rejection, may resort to increased SN–DMN coupling as an adaptive maneuver to allow an individual time to grieve, process the catastrophic loss, and prepare for a life after this drastic social change.

Paradoxically, it may very well be that an aberration of this adaptive collaboration among the brain's major neural networks gives rise to the symptoms of depression. Depression may be borne out of the neural mechanisms intended to cope with grief, social distress, and illness or to maintain optimism in the face of life's challenges. Under normal circumstances, components of the extended SN network are supposed to monitor the flow of sensory information, translate it into appropriate emotional correlates, and then smoothly integrate these bits of information with our affective and cognitive states. Sensory information is initially processed in the thalamus and subsequently forwarded for further elaboration and emotional translation to the insula. Sensations reflecting important changes in our internal and external environment, such as threat to our bodily integrity, danger, or impending loss, are appropriately translated in the insula into the emotions of fear, anger, or sadness and given the corresponding priority labels. Subsequently, these emotions are forwarded to limbic areas, such as the amygdala and NAcc/ventral striatum, where their quality, intensity, and priority are further elaborated. In the hippocampus, emotions that have a significant adaptive value are linked with the circumstances that have precipitated them in the past.

Both limbic circuits and the thalamus have an ability to trigger a rough but rapid motoric, endocrine, autonomic and immune response. Let's say, by way of example, that we have just had a falling out with our best friend or a romantic partner. Our emotions are intense but not reflective of an urgent situation. In this situation, the ensuing mix of anger, anxiety, frustration, and sadness is conveyed to the "SN terminal," the point of interface between the insula–ACC duo, and the EN and DMN, where information is conveyed for more sophisticated elaboration. While the DMN is engaged in rumination and self-reflection and is accessing autobiographical memory banks in the MTL, the EN is utilizing working memory, focused attention and problem-solving capacities to find a solution. During these coping activities, the EN has the top-down capacity to attenuate (or accentuate) the flow of sensory information from the thalamus and to mitigate emotional processing in limbic and paralimbic areas (e.g., the amygdala, insula, ventral striatum, sgACC), allowing only the most relevant information to ascend for full cortical processing. In other words, the EN and DMN have hung up a Do Not Disturb sign, allowing only the highest-priority sensory and emotional signals to intrude on its work. Once the solution has been found, be it a plan for a conversation laced with apologies that might help resolve the difference or an acceptance of the inevitable end of the relationship, DMN-mediated rumination is concluded, while the EN, via top-down modulation, calms limbic areas, leaving all the networks reset and ready for the next chapter of life.

In contrast, in the context of depression just about everything that can go wrong does go wrong. Sensory information from the thalamus has a facilitated path to the insula, where it is converted to an emotional signal with a negative bias and subsequently conveyed to the amygdala and hippocampus for further processing. Support for this scenario comes from imaging studies reporting greater connectivity among the thalamus, insula, and amygdala of depressed subjects compared with healthy controls.[146,226] Input from SN components, bearing negatively charged affective information, has facilitated access to contextual memory stored in the hippocampus of depressed individuals.[271,272]

Several imaging studies have reported aberrant connectivity between components of the SN, such as the thalamus, amygdala, hippocampus, and sgACC, and DMN structures.[211,272,273] This "short-circuiting" between the SN and DMN allows negatively valenced emotions to enter a reverberating ruminative loop.[114,124,127,155,211] Once engaged, DMN components, including the vmPFC, dmPFC, PCC, and MTL, continue to elaborate the negative emotions, readily supplying depressive self references, and via the PCC–hippocampus connection, resurrecting autobiographical memories of past failings and disappointments.[115,127,271,274] Consistent with this, the intensity of coupling between the SN-related sgACC and the PCC (a DMN area) was found to be highly correlated with behavioral measures of rumination and brooding but not adaptive self-reflection in patients with MDD.[115,116] Extending these findings, a separate imaging study reported an association between the degree of DMN activation and feelings of helplessness, as well as overall depression severity.[119] In contrast, rACC activity (another major DMN hub) actually predicts adaptive self-reflection, dACC-mediated recruitment of dlPFC and other EN areas in problem solving, and top-down emotional regulation.[104]

Excessive activation of the DMN is not unique to depression. In fact, a similar engagement of DMN regions, resulting in ruminations, can be elicited by social distress, posttraumatic stress disorder or even inflammatory activation.[70,149,274,275] Unfortunately, even EN structures can become caught up in this vicious circle. Instead of allocating attentional and working memory resources to problem solving and top-down suppression of maladaptive depressive feelings, EN components now serve as a stand-in for ineffective implicit (usually unconscious) emotion-modulating circuitry. Under normal physiological circumstances, midline structures, such as the vmPFC and ventral ACC will automatically regulate the ascending flow of emotion mediated by the insula and amygdala, but this is not the case in depression.[117,235] Instead executive areas are forced into a "job-sharing" situation where they need to process information in working memory, manage attentional resources, while at the same time trying to extricate the DMN from its ruminative cycle.[114,115,117,129,274,276]

Unfortunately, overworking the EN often leads to a drop-off in cognitive functioning. Imaging research has put forth an intriguing hypothesis. Aberrant interplay between DMN regions (also referred to as a task-negative network) and the EN (often labeled as a task-positive network) may produce cognitive dysfunction manifested in impaired attention, cognitive reactivity, and propensity toward rumination. These cognitive impediments may in turn represent risk factors for recurrence of MDD.[277] Current research indicates that cognitive impairments in MDD tend to be persistent, nonspecific, and progressive, with a greater number of episodes leading to an increased cognitive burden.[278,279]

Imaging studies have demonstrated a central role of the dmPFC and adjacent areas (DMN components) in "hot-wiring" together the EN, DMN, and SN,[114] creating what some have dubbed the "dorsal nexus."[114] Is this pattern of aberrant connectivity a state-dependent feature of MDD, or is it an enduring feature of the disease state? Unfortunately contemporary imaging research does not encourage optimism. A multimodal MRI study combining structural and functional evaluation compared 20 recovered MDD patients with matched healthy controls.[280] This study provided direct evidence of DMN hyperconnectivity even in recovered MDD patients. Ongoing DMN hyperconnectivity in remitted MDD sufferers may underpin the previously described psychological propensity toward rumination and preferential focus on internal experiences, at the expense of maintaining adaptive communication with the external environment. Imaging evidence implicates hypofunction of the dorsal nexus right dmPFC (BA 9) in ineffectual switching between DMN and adaptive task-positive, goal-oriented EN activity.[280] DMN hyperconnectivity has been associated with a structural anomaly of a key DMN hub, the precuneus/PCC complex.

Structural studies have confirmed that the PCC/precuneus hypogyrification (abnormal cortical folding) may be associated with anomalous hyperconnectivity between precuneus/PCC and the dorsal nexus dmPFC. Conversely, hypergyrification of the ACC may be reflected in decreased connectivity between this SN hub and the EN regions. Therefore, diminished connection between SN (ACC) and temporoparietal regions, involved in processing external cues (including spoken language), may interfere with social communication and active coping.[280] These results raise a daunting possibility that interaction between biological vulnerability and early-life adversity may have altered neural development, which resulted in aberrant gyrification and ensuing altered connectivity among the dmPFC, EN, and SN, manifested by preferentially inward orientation at the expense of adaptive communications with the external environment.[280] In other words, hard-wired structural changes in MDD may in some patients be an enduring liability toward recurrence of depression, manifesting in maladaptive psychological tendencies.

Neither corticolimbic nor corticothalamic pathways are capable of effectively stemming the tide of invasive sensations and distressing emotions flowing from the SN into the DMN.[114,209,211,213] Instead of the orderly and harmonious collaboration between the major neural network seen in healthy euthymic individuals, imaging studies of depressed subjects have identified random activity, centralized around network nodes, accompanied by disintegration of adaptive network connectedness.[129,272] A simple analogy may help clarify this complex scenario. Let's say that a freeway is the main thoroughfare connecting two major cities. Under usual circumstances the freeway traffic is rather heavy, since relatively few vehicles use the multiple country roads that provide alternative connections between these cities. Smaller towns along these country roads enjoy a comfortable traffic pattern. However, if the freeway falls into a state of disrepair, and two lanes are closed for roadwork, traffic pattern will shift. All of a sudden the narrow country roads will have to handle a significant increase in traffic volume due to detours on the freeway. Bottlenecks will emerge: intersections in the smaller towns will be jammed with vehicles, resulting in lengthy delays and an overall decrease in driving efficiency. One will likely see an increase in local "connectedness," combined with an overall decline in the efficiency of long-distance commutes.

Instead of normal homeostatic coupling of sensorimotor SN areas with cognitive (EN) and linguistic resources, in depression sensorimotor and affective regions are functionally fused. Perpetual ruminative activity in the DMN appears to be detected by the insula, eliciting an amplified negative emotional response from SN structures.[127,209] Imaging studies have revealed that in depression EN-related structures (e.g., dlPFC and vlPFC) are not effective in engaging DMN-related structures (e.g., vmPFC) in their attempt to suppress excessive amygdala activation, which is likely a neural correlate of the negative emotionality that is so rampant in MDD. Typically, elevation of vmPFC activity leads to diminished sgACC and amygdala activation; however, in depression the opposite is true. Furthermore, inadequate frontocingulate communication leaves the rACC "stranded," unable to recruit the dACC and dlPFC (EN formations) in problem solving and top-down emotional regulation.[104] Translated into layman's terms, the brain detects that it is stuck in the wrong loop and responds with an amplification of distress.

It is this state of distress that most likely triggers bodily response systems in ways that are commonly seen in MDD, including HPA axis activation, increased sympathetic tone, attenuated parasympathetic activity, and the mobilization of innate immunity.[269] This degree of distress may even affect our vision. Activation of sympathetic tone, combined with the withdrawal of parasympathetic signaling, produces a dilatation of the pupil. There is a trade-off involved here: we will benefit from a finer-grade image of the threat that we are facing at the expense of the broader field of vision. Excessive coupling of the SN and DMN in depression, combined with maladaptive EN activity, may be an attempt of internal reconstitution that has gone awry. Our psychological "eye" is constricted, focused inward, endlessly dwelling on the causes of our misfortune, connecting them with painful autobiographical memories, while simultaneously excluding potentially distracting divergent associations, creative thinking, future planning, and social interests.[274]

This pattern of allocation of attentional resources in depression is patently maladaptive. Depressed persons are nonproductively focused on everything that makes them unhappy while ignoring all potential sources of joy. In this situation, emotional and cognitive horizons have collapsed. Harmonious, fluid attendance to the external and internal environment is disrupted. The depressed individual is trapped, all alone in his or her world, suffused with grief, dejection, and grim memories and devoid of hope.

As an intriguing tangent, we have previously mentioned that the consistent practice of meditation alters the patterns of communication between the main brain networks. Meditation increases the functional connectivity between some of the network components while reducing the connection between others. These functional changes are underpinned by demonstrable structural alterations in gray and white matter of the brain.[258,281] Educated speculation would suggest that the persistent rerouting of brain activity might induce neuroplastic processes. In terms of its impact on the function of the main brain networks, meditation could be perceived as "antidepression." We are not alluding to the use of meditation as a treatment for depression (this topic is addressed. Our focus here is on the patterns of brain activity created by the extensive practice of meditation, which represents a striking contrast to the functional configuration present in depression.

Depression is characterized by the excessive coupling of the SN with the DMN, producing ruminations and attention to negative autobiographical memories, accompanied by joint DMN and SN interference with proper EN function. Meditation, in contrast, produces an opposite pattern of activity, including a weakening of the connection between the SN and DMN. This uncoupling is possibly due to the meditator's emphasis on avoiding the evaluation of sensory experiences and emotional states. Also in contrast to depressed individuals, meditators manifest improved connectedness between the SN and EN, possibly indicating a more efficient switching process from off-task DMN activity to on-task EN activity whenever circumstances require. The big question is, if the diligent practice of meditation can induce neuroplasticity-based functional and structural brain changes, can depression and the conditions leading to depression do the same, albeit in the opposite direction?

We have already mentioned that medical illness,[282] chronic inflammation,[283,284] childhood adversity,[285] insecure attachment,[275,286] and stress,[287,288] especially stress due to social disruption, can all precipitate depression. It is intriguing that stress and inflammation are accompanied by a similar pattern of functional brain changes as depression.[70,72,236,269,289] Chronic exposure to stress can also be associated with gray and white matter changes in the brain resembling the ones reported in depression.[43,290] Could pathophysiological pathways shared by stress, inflammation, somatic illness, and social distress have access to the mechanisms regulating neuroplasticity because of their evolutionary importance? If so, can depression be conceived as an adaptive learning process gone awry? Could we have become "sensitized" by factors such as early-life adversity such that our minds and bodies engage in an exaggerated defensive repertoire when things that remind us of our old woes strike again?

Researchers have reported that even in nonclinical populations, perseverative cognitions, persistent worries, and ruminations (including unconscious ones) have all been associated with HPA activation, decreased vagal tone, increased sympathetic activity, and aberrant immune activation (lympho- and leukocytosis, combined with the natural killer cell dysfunction). In all likelihood, this state of affairs has led to not only an increase in negative affect but also a greater risk of chronic pain and sleep disorders, as well as cardiovascular, respiratory, and gastrointestinal disease.[291–294] Altered connectedness between the vlPFC (an EN structure), dmPFC (a DMN hub), and the temporal pole (functionally associated with socially relevant semantic knowledge) is associated with an attributional bias in MDD patients. While emotionally healthy individuals readily accept responsibility for positive events, negative events tend to be ascribed to external factors. Depressed patients manifest the opposite tendency. They are inwardly focused and pessimistic and eagerly accept responsibility for negative incidents, a propensity that has been labeled "depressive realism."[295]

Could ruminations and depressive realism represent a preemptive strike strategy, a preparedness to respond to the worst-case scenario? If we have suffered an early loss, social rejection, or abandonment, could ruminations and perseverative thinking be an attempt to think our way out of this predicament? One would need time to sift through the autobiographical memories, looking for the explanation for current woes. Did we do something to create this wretchedness? In normal physiological circumstances it would be a respite, a period of self-reflection, reorientation, and future planning. In these times of change and uncertainty, it may be self-preserving to have a greater sensitivity to threatening environmental cues and negative emotions that signal their presence. The autonomic nervous system, HPA axis, and immune system are all in a state of heightened alert. Given dire circumstances, all these integrated defensive responses may increase our chances of survival.

There may be yet another intriguing aspect of the mind-body interaction in depression. Much as reverberations within the SN–DMN-based ruminative cycle amplify the emotional echo of adversity, thereby instantiating and subsequently perpetuating the defensive repertoire, patterns of mind-body communication in the context of depression may fulfill a similar role. Sympathetic neurotransmitters, parasympathetic signals, cortisol, and inflammatory cytokines all signal back to the brain.[69,269,296] Catecholamines, cortisol, and inflammatory cytokines jointly alter neurotransmission and neurotrophic processes in the brain.[69,72,269,297,298] There is solid evidence that this mind–body–mind cycle also actively shapes the symptoms of depression.[72,236,237,299] As we have previously stated, inflammatory cytokines increase activity in brain areas that form the SN and DMN,[70,268,300] while autonomic changes and cortisol particularly impact SN brain regions.[301] Accumulating evidence suggests that inflammation may be a consequence as well as a precursor of depression.[269,296,302,303] Could the bidirectional mind-body dialogue in depression also act as an amplifier of the "fight-or-flight" distress signals and inflammation amongst them? Is depression a consequence of an adaptive mechanism, evolved in different times and circumstances, which has gone awry? Is depression a price that we are paying for too rapid development of our civilization?

MDD has also been associated with an enduring insufficiency in corticosteroid signaling[301] and alterations of norepinephrine transmission.[304] Both inflammatory cytokines and corticosteroids, in a direct and indirect fashion (via alterations in the glutamate signaling), impact neurotrophic factors and in thus influence neuroplasticity.[72,269,297,299] One can appreciate the adaptive value of our brains creating an enduring record of the life-threatening illnesses and early-life tribulations. It is clearly germane for our survival to either avoid similar circumstances in the future or promptly activate a defensive repertoire, should they be inevitable. Intriguingly, the immune system and neurotrophic signals are intertwined. Inflammatory cytokines, in normal physiological circumstances, support synaptic scaling and memory processes in the brain,[298,305] while brain-derived neurotrophic factor (BDNF), a prototypical neurotrophic factor, has an immune-modulatory influence in the body.[306,307] It appears likely that depression has emerged as a distortion of adaptive mechanisms intended to help us survive infections, early-life adversities, and social hardships. Against this normative backdrop, distributed genetic and epigenetic vulnerabilities interact with the environmental factors to produce the aberrant functional connectivity and eventual structural brain changes that give rise to depression.[72,308–313] Some of the genes implicated in the pathogenesis of depression, such as the 5HTTLPR variant of the serotonin transporter and genes controlling the synthesis of the BDNF, are reported to have a significant influence on the structure, activity level, and connectivity of several key SN, EN, and DMN areas.[309,311,313–315]

Once manifest, depression tends to become self-perpetuating, becoming progressively less dependent on stress and other triggers.[287,310] This pattern points to the possibility that depression might be profitably conceptualized as a consequence of aberrant learning.[316] Even in remission, exaggerated connectedness between the amygdala, hippocampus, ventral ACC, and vmPFC in response to sad stimuli increases the risk of subsequent depressive relapse.[18,209,254] We can safely conclude from these converging lines of evidence that, sadly, once activated, depression never sleeps. When stress, adversity, or illness activates the integrated mind-body defensive repertoire, distributed faulty micro- and macroscopic routines are also triggered and the trap door of depression slams shut. Sometimes it is the case that the regulatory routines are not in sync and proportional with the intensity of the precipitant; at other times they do not properly deactivate—either way adaptive responses are morphed into pathological mechanisms.

In summary, structural and functional studies support an organic basis for the emotional, cognitive,[105,222] somatic, autonomic, immune, and neuroendocrine[27] symptomatology of MDD. While we may still not be able to explain each individual occurrence of depression, it would be spurious, based on the robust cumulative multidisciplinary evidence, to say that we have no understanding of the shared neurobiological underpinnings of depression as a general phenomenon or, more exactly, as the group of depressions that it actually is.

References

1. Wager TD, Davidson ML, Hughes BL, Lindquist MA, Ochsner KN. Prefrontal-subcortical pathways mediating successful emotion regulation. *Neuron.* 2008;59:1037–1050.
2. Menon V. Large-scale brain networks and psychopathology: a unifying triple network model. *Trends Cogn Sci.* 2011;15:483–506.
3. Bressler SL, Menon V. Large-scale brain networks in cognition: emerging methods and principles. *Trends Cogn Sci.* 2010;14:277–290.
4. Seeley WW, Menon V, Schatzberg AF, et al. Dissociable intrinsic connectivity networks for salience processing and executive control. *J Neurosci.* 2007;27:2349–2356.
5. Blackford JU, Buckholtz JW, Avery SN, Zald DH. A unique role for the human amygdala in novelty detection. *Neuroimage.* 2010;50:1188–1193.
6. Balleine BW, Killcross S. Parallel incentive processing: an integrated view of amygdala function. *Trends Neurosci.* 2006;29:272–279.
7. Kensinger EA, Corkin S. Two routes to emotional memory: distinct neural processes for valence and arousal. *Proc Natl Acad Sci U S A.* 2004;101:3310–3315.
8. Kensinger EA, Krendl AC, Corkin S. Memories of an emotional and a nonemotional event: effects of aging and delay interval. *Exp Aging Res.* 2006;32:23–45.
9. Adolphs R. Fear, faces, and the human amygdala. *Curr Opin Neurobiol.* 2008;18:166–172.
10. Sheline YI, Barch DM, Donnelly JM, Ollinger JM, Snyder AZ, Mintun MA. Increased amygdala response to masked emotional faces in depressed subjects resolves with antidepressant treatment: an fMRI study. *Biol Psychiatry.* 2001;50:651–658.
11. Siegle GJ, Thompson W, Carter CS, Steinhauer SR, Thase ME. Increased amygdala and decreased dorsolateral prefrontal BOLD responses in unipolar depression: related and independent features. *Biol Psychiatry.* 2007;61:198–209.
12. Fu CH, Mourao-Miranda J, Costafreda SG, et al. Pattern classification of sad facial processing: toward the development of neurobiological markers in depression. *Biol Psychiatry.* 2008;63:656–662.
13. Dannlowski U, Ohrmann P, Bauer J, et al. Amygdala reactivity predicts automatic negative evaluations for facial emotions. *Psychiatry Res.* 2007;154:13–20.

14. Hariri AR, Drabant EM, Weinberger DR. Imaging genetics: perspectives from studies of genetically driven variation in serotonin function and corticolimbic affective processing. *Biol Psychiatry*. 2006;59:888–897.

15. Lee BT, Seok JH, Lee BC, et al. Neural correlates of affective processing in response to sad and angry facial stimuli in patients with major depressive disorder. *Prog Neuropsychopharmacol Biol Psychiatry*. 2008;32:778–785.

16. Siegle GJ, Steinhauer SR, Thase ME, Stenger VA, Carter CS. Can't shake that feeling: event-related fMRI assessment of sustained amygdala activity in response to emotional information in depressed individuals. *Biol Psychiatry*. 2002;51:693–707.

17. Chan SW, Norbury R, Goodwin GM, Harmer CJ. Risk for depression and neural responses to fearful facial expressions of emotion. *Br J Psychiatry*. 2009;194:139–145.

18. Ramel W, Goldin PR, Eyler LT, Brown GG, Gotlib IH, McQuaid JR. Amygdala reactivity and mood-congruent memory in individuals at risk for depressive relapse. *Biol Psychiatry*. 2007;61:231–239.

19. Frodl T, Meisenzahl E, Zetzsche T, et al. Enlargement of the amygdala in patients with a first episode of major depression. *Biol Psychiatry*. 2002;51:708–714.

20. Frodl T, Meisenzahl EM, Zetzsche T, et al. Larger amygdala volumes in first depressive episode as compared to recurrent major depression and healthy control subjects. *Biol Psychiatry*. 2003;53:338–344.

21. van Eijndhoven P, van Wingen G, van Oijen K, et al. Amygdala volume marks the acute state in the early course of depression. *Biol Psychiatry*. 2009;65:812–818.

22. Hajek T, Kopecek M, Kozeny J, Gunde E, Alda M, Hoschl C. Amygdala volumes in mood disorders—meta-analysis of magnetic resonance volumetry studies. *J Affect Disord*. 2009;115:395–410.

23. Munn MA, Alexopoulos J, Nishino T, et al. Amygdala volume analysis in female twins with major depression. *Biol Psychiatry*. 2007;62:415–422.

24. Sheline YI, Gado MH, Price JL. Amygdala core nuclei volumes are decreased in recurrent major depression. *Neuroreport*. 1998;9:2023–2028.

25. Hamilton JP, Siemer M, Gotlib IH. Amygdala volume in major depressive disorder: a meta-analysis of magnetic resonance imaging studies. *Mol Psychiatry*. 2008;13:993–1000.

26. Frodl TS, Koutsouleris N, Bottlender R, et al. Depression-related variation in brain morphology over 3 years: effects of stress? *Arch Gen Psychiatry*. 2008;65:1156–1165.

27. Drevets WC, Price JL, Bardgett ME, Reich T, Todd RD, Raichle ME. Glucose metabolism in the amygdala in depression: relationship to diagnostic subtype and plasma cortisol levels. *Pharmacol Biochem Behav*. 2002;71:431–447.

28. Sheline Y. 3D MRI studies of neuroanatomic changes in unipolar major depression: the role of stress and medical comorbidity. *Biol Psychiatry*. 2000;48:791–800.

29. Carlezon WA Jr, Thomas MJ. Biological substrates of reward and aversion: a nucleus accumbens activity hypothesis. *Neuropharmacology*. 2009;56(suppl 1):122–132.

30. Levita L, Hare TA, Voss HU, Glover G, Ballon DJ, Casey BJ. The bivalent side of the nucleus accumbens. *Neuroimage*. 2009;44:1178–1187.

31. Lisman JE, Grace AA. The hippocampal-VTA loop: controlling the entry of information into long-term memory. *Neuron*. 2005;46:703–713.

32. Lebrecht S, Badre D. Emotional regulation, or: how I learned to stop worrying and love the nucleus accumbens. *Neuron*. 2008;59:841–843.

33. Pizzagalli DA, Holmes AJ, Dillon DG, et al. Reduced caudate and nucleus accumbens response to rewards in unmedicated individuals with major depressive disorder. *Am J Psychiatry*. 2009;166:702–710.

34. Wacker J, Dillon DG, Pizzagalli DA. The role of the nucleus accumbens and rostral ante-

rior cingulate cortex in anhedonia: integration of resting EEG, fMRI, and volumetric techniques. *Neuroimage.* 2009;46:327–337.

35. Epstein J, Pan H, Kocsis JH, et al. Lack of ventral striatal response to positive stimuli in depressed versus normal subjects. *Am J Psychiatry.* 2006;163:1784–1790.

36. Monk CS, Klein RG, Telzer EH, et al. Amygdala and nucleus accumbens activation to emotional facial expressions in children and adolescents at risk for major depression. *Am J Psychiatry.* 2008;165:90–98.

37. Vythilingam M, Vermetten E, Anderson GM, et al. Hippocampal volume, memory, and cortisol status in major depressive disorder: effects of treatment. *Biol Psychiatry.* 2004; 56:101–112.

38. Strange BA, Fletcher PC, Henson RN, Friston KJ, Dolan RJ. Segregating the functions of human hippocampus. *Proc Natl Acad Sci U S A.* 1999;96:4034–4039.

39. Shohamy D, Wagner AD. Integrating memories in the human brain: hippocampal-midbrain encoding of overlapping events. *Neuron.* 2008;60:378–389.

40. Graham S, Phua E, Soon CS, et al. Role of medial cortical, hippocampal and striatal interactions during cognitive set-shifting. *Neuroimage.* 2009;45:1359–1367.

41. Fanselow MS, Dong HW. Are the dorsal and ventral hippocampus functionally distinct structures? *Neuron.* 2010;65:7–19.

42. Bangasser DA, Shors TJ. The hippocampus is necessary for enhancements and impairments of learning following stress. *Nat Neurosci.* 2007;10:1401–1403.

43. Gianaros PJ, Jennings JR, Sheu LK, Greer PJ, Kuller LH, Matthews KA. Prospective reports of chronic life stress predict decreased grey matter volume in the hippocampus. *Neuroimage.* 2007;35:795–803.

44. MacQueen GM, Campbell S, McEwen BS, et al. Course of illness, hippocampal function, and hippocampal volume in major depression. *Proc Natl Acad Sci U S A.* 2003;100: 1387–1392.

45. Sheline YI, Gado MH, Kraemer HC. Untreated depression and hippocampal volume loss. *Am J Psychiatry.* 2003;160:1516–1518.

46. Colla M, Kronenberg G, Deuschle M, et al. Hippocampal volume reduction and HPA-system activity in major depression. *J Psychiatr Res.* 2007;41:553–560.

47. Chaney A, Carballedo A, Amico F, et al. Effect of childhood maltreatment on brain structure in adult patients with major depressive disorder and healthy participants. *J Psychiatry Neurosci.* 2014;39:50–59.

48. Opel N, Redlich R, Zwanzger P, et al. Hippocampal atrophy in major depression: a function of childhood maltreatment rather than diagnosis? *Neuropsychopharmacology.* 2014;39(12):2723–2731.

49. Block W, Traber F, von Widdern O, et al. Proton MR spectroscopy of the hippocampus at 3 T in patients with unipolar major depressive disorder: correlates and predictors of treatment response. *Int J Neuropsychopharmacol.* 2009;12(3):415–422.

50. Bennett MR. The prefrontal-limbic network in depression: modulation by hypothalamus, basal ganglia and midbrain. *Prog Neurobiol.* 2011;93:468–487.

51. Venkatraman V, Huettel SA, Chuah LY, Payne JW, Chee MW. Sleep deprivation biases the neural mechanisms underlying economic preferences. *J Neurosci.* 2011;31:3712–3718.

52. Bamiou DE, Musiek FE, Luxon LM. The insula (island of Reil) and its role in auditory processing: literature review. *Brain Res Brain Res Rev.* 2003;42:143–154.

53. Craig AD. How do you feel—now? The anterior insula and human awareness. *Nat Rev Neurosci.* 2009;10:59–70.

54. Taylor KS, Seminowicz DA, Davis KD. Two systems of resting state connectivity between the insula and cingulate cortex. *Hum Brain Mapp.* 2009;30:2731–2745.

55. Ortigue S, Grafton ST, Bianchi-Demicheli F. Correlation between insula activation and self-reported quality of orgasm in women. *Neuroimage.* 2007;37:551–560.

56. Morrison I, Bjornsdotter M, Olausson H. Vicarious responses to social touch in posterior insular cortex are tuned to pleasant caressing speeds. *J Neurosci.* 2011;31:9554–9562.

57. Legrain V, Iannetti GD, Plaghki L, Mouraux A. The pain matrix reloaded: a salience detection system for the body. *Prog Neurobiol.* 2011;93:111–124.

58. Graff-Guerrero A, Pellicer F, Mendoza-Espinosa Y, et al. Cerebral blood flow changes associated with experimental pain stimulation in patients with major depression. *J Affect Disord.* 2008;107:161–168.

59. Villemure C, Schweinhardt P. Supraspinal pain processing: distinct roles of emotion and attention. *Neuroscientist.* 2010;16:276–284.

60. Wiech K, Lin CS, Brodersen KH, Bingel U, Ploner M, Tracey I. Anterior insula integrates information about salience into perceptual decisions about pain. *J Neurosci.* 2010;30:16324–16331.

61. Maihofner C, Seifert F, Decol R. Activation of central sympathetic networks during innocuous and noxious somatosensory stimulation. *Neuroimage.* 2011;55:216–224.

62. Peltz E, Seifert F, DeCol R, Dorfler A, Schwab S, Maihofner C. Functional connectivity of the human insular cortex during noxious and innocuous thermal stimulation. *Neuroimage.* 2011;54:1324–1335.

63. Karnath HO, Baier B, Nagele T. Awareness of the functioning of one's own limbs mediated by the insular cortex? *J Neurosci.* 2005;25:7134–7138.

64. Sprengelmeyer R, Steele JD, Mwangi B, et al. The insular cortex and the neuroanatomy of major depression. *J Affect Disord.* 2011;133:120–127.

65. Price CJ. The anatomy of language: contributions from functional neuroimaging. *J Anat.* 2000;197(pt 3):335–359.

66. Ackermann H, Riecker A. The contribution(s) of the insula to speech production: a review of the clinical and functional imaging literature. *Brain Struct Funct.* 2010;214:419–433.

67. Eisenberger NI, Lieberman MD, Williams KD. Does rejection hurt? An FMRI study of social exclusion. *Science.* 2003;302:290–292.

68. Benarroch EE. Autonomic-mediated immunomodulation and potential clinical relevance. *Neurology.* 2009;73:236–242.

69. Taylor AG, Goehler LE, Galper DI, Innes KE, Bourguignon C. Top-down and bottom-up mechanisms in mind-body medicine: development of an integrative framework for psychophysiological research. *Explore (NY).* 2010;6:29–41.

70. Harrison NA, Brydon L, Walker C, et al. Neural origins of human sickness in interoceptive responses to inflammation. *Biol Psychiatry.* 2009;66:415–422.

71. Jabbi M, Bastiaansen J, Keysers C. A common anterior insula representation of disgust observation, experience and imagination shows divergent functional connectivity pathways. *PLoS ONE.* 2008;3:e2939.

72. Maletic V, Raison CL. Neurobiology of depression, fibromyalgia and neuropathic pain. *Front Biosci.* 2009;14:5291–5338.

73. Pacheco-Lopez G, Niemi MB, Kou W, Harting M, Fandrey J, Schedlowski M. Neural substrates for behaviorally conditioned immunosuppression in the rat. *J Neurosci.* 2005;25:2330–2337.

74. Ramirez-Amaya V, Bermudez-Rattoni F. Conditioned enhancement of antibody production is disrupted by insular cortex and amygdala but not hippocampal lesions. *Brain Behav Immun.* 1999;13:46–60.

75. Menon V, Uddin LQ. Saliency, switching, attention and control: a network model of insula function. *Brain Struct Funct.* 2010;214:655–667.

76. Sridharan D, Levitin DJ, Menon V. A critical role for the right fronto-insular cortex in switching between central-executive and default-mode networks. *Proc Natl Acad Sci U S A.* 2008;105:12569–12574.

77. Perico CA, Skaf CR, Yamada A, et al. Relationship between regional cerebral blood flow and separate symptom clusters of major depression: a single photon emission computed tomography study using statistical parametric mapping. *Neurosci Lett.* 2005;384:265–270.

78. Lee BT, Seong Whi C, Hyung Soo K, et al. The neural substrates of affective processing toward positive and negative affective pictures in patients with major depressive disorder. *Prog Neuropsychopharmacol Biol Psychiatry.* 2007;31:1487–1492.

79. Feinstein JS, Stein MB, Paulus MP. Anterior insula reactivity during certain decisions is associated with neuroticism. *Soc Cogn Affect Neurosci.* 2006;1:136–142.

80. Kuhn S, Gallinat J. Resting-state brain activity in schizophrenia and major depression: a quantitative meta-analysis. *Schizophr Bull.* 2013;39(2):358–365.

81. Townsend JD, Eberhart NK, Bookheimer SY, et al. fMRI activation in the amygdala and the orbitofrontal cortex in unmedicated subjects with major depressive disorder. *Psychiatry Res.* 2010;183:209–217.

82. Strigo IA, Matthews SC, Simmons AN. Right anterior insula hypoactivity during anticipation of homeostatic shifts in major depressive disorder. *Psychosom Med.* 2010;72:316–323.

83. Liu Z, Xu C, Xu Y, et al. Decreased regional homogeneity in insula and cerebellum: a resting-state fMRI study in patients with major depression and subjects at high risk for major depression. *Psychiatry Res.* 2010;182:211–215.

84. Fitzgerald PB, Laird AR, Maller J, Daskalakis ZJ. A meta-analytic study of changes in brain activation in depression. *Hum Brain Mapp.* 2008;29:683–695.

85. Wang L, LaBar KS, Smoski M, et al. Prefrontal mechanisms for executive control over emotional distraction are altered in major depression. *Psychiatry Res.* 2008;163:143–155.

86. Biver F, Wikler D, Lotstra F, Damhaut P, Goldman S, Mendlewicz J. Serotonin 5-HT2 receptor imaging in major depression: focal changes in orbito-insular cortex. *Br J Psychiatry.* 1997;171:444–448.

87. Takahashi T, Yucel M, Lorenzetti V, et al. Volumetric MRI study of the insular cortex in individuals with current and past major depression. *J Affect Disord.* 2010;121:231–238.

88. Paus T. Primate anterior cingulate cortex: where motor control, drive and cognition interface. *Nat Rev Neurosci.* 2001;2:417–424.

89. Vogt BA. Pain and emotion interactions in subregions of the cingulate gyrus. *Nat Rev Neurosci.* 2005;6:533–544.

90. Bush G, Luu P, Posner MI. Cognitive and emotional influences in anterior cingulate cortex. *Trends Cogn Sci.* 2000;4:215–222.

91. McCormick LM, Ziebell S, Nopoulos P, Cassell M, Andreasen NC, Brumm M. Anterior cingulate cortex: an MRI-based parcellation method. *Neuroimage.* 2006;32:1167–1175.

92. Nielsen FA, Balslev D, Hansen LK. Mining the posterior cingulate: segregation between memory and pain components. *Neuroimage.* 2005;27:520–532.

93. Thomason ME, Hamilton JP, Gotlib IH. Stress-induced activation of the HPA axis predicts connectivity between subgenual cingulate and salience network during rest in adolescents. *J Child Psychol Psychiatry*. 2011;52:1026–1034.

94. Bissiere S, Plachta N, Hoyer D, et al. The rostral anterior cingulate cortex modulates the efficiency of amygdala-dependent fear learning. *Biol Psychiatry*. 2008;63:821–831.

95. Shackman AJ, Salomons TV, Slagter HA, Fox AS, Winter JJ, Davidson RJ. The integration of negative affect, pain and cognitive control in the cingulate cortex. *Nat Rev Neurosci*. 2011;12:154–167.

96. Grabenhorst F, Rolls ET. Value, pleasure and choice in the ventral prefrontal cortex. *Trends Cogn Sci*. 2011;15:56–67.

97. Pearson JM, Heilbronner SR, Barack DL, Hayden BY, Platt ML. Posterior cingulate cortex: adapting behavior to a changing world. *Trends Cogn Sci*. 2011;15:143–151.

98. Pearson JM, Hayden BY, Raghavachari S, Platt ML. Neurons in posterior cingulate cortex signal exploratory decisions in a dynamic multioption choice task. *Curr Biol*. 2009;19:1532–1537.

99. Hayden BY, Nair AC, McCoy AN, Platt ML. Posterior cingulate cortex mediates outcome-contingent allocation of behavior. *Neuron*. 2008;60:19–25.

100. Hayden BY, Smith DV, Platt ML. Cognitive control signals in posterior cingulate cortex. *Front Hum Neurosci*. 2010;4:223.

101. Vogt BA, Laureys S. Posterior cingulate, precuneal and retrosplenial cortices: cytology and components of the neural network correlates of consciousness. *Prog Brain Res*. 2005;150:205–217.

102. Wiebking C, de Greck M, Duncan NW, Heinzel A, Tempelmann C, Northoff G. Are emotions associated with activity during rest or interoception? An exploratory fMRI study in healthy subjects. *Neurosci Lett*. 2011;491:87–92.

103. Buckner RL, Andrews-Hanna JR, Schacter DL. The brain's default network: anatomy, function, and relevance to disease. *Ann N Y Acad Sci*. 2008;1124:1–38.

104. Pizzagalli DA. Frontocingulate dysfunction in depression: toward biomarkers of treatment response. *Neuropsychopharmacology*. 2011;36:183–206.

105. Drevets WC. Neuroimaging and neuropathological studies of depression: implications for the cognitive-emotional features of mood disorders. *Curr Opin Neurobiol*. 2001;11:240–249.

106. Mayberg HS, Liotti M, Brannan SK, et al. Reciprocal limbic-cortical function and negative mood: converging PET findings in depression and normal sadness. *Am J Psychiatry*. 1999;156:675–682.

107. Hamilton JP, Chen G, Thomason ME, Schwartz ME, Gotlib IH. Investigating neural primacy in major depressive disorder: multivariate Granger causality analysis of resting-state fMRI time-series data. *Mol Psychiatry*. 2011;16:763–772.

108. Matthews SC, Strigo IA, Simmons AN, Yang TT, Paulus MP. Decreased functional coupling of the amygdala and supragenual cingulate is related to increased depression in unmedicated individuals with current major depressive disorder. *J Affect Disord*. 2008;111:13–20.

109. Chen CH, Ridler K, Suckling J, et al. Brain imaging correlates of depressive symptom severity and predictors of symptom improvement after antidepressant treatment. *Biol Psychiatry*. 2007;62:407–414.

110. Lisiecka DM, Carballedo A, Fagan AJ, et al. Altered inhibition of negative emotions in subjects at family risk of major depressive disorder. *J Psychiatr Res*. 2012;46:181–188.

111. Phillips ML, Ladouceur CD, Drevets WC. A neural model of voluntary and automatic

emotion regulation: implications for understanding the pathophysiology and neuro-development of bipolar disorder. *Mol Psychiatry.* 2008;13:829, 833–857.

112. Whittle S, Allen NB, Lubman DI, Yucel M. The neurobiological basis of temperament: towards a better understanding of psychopathology. *Neurosci Biobehav Rev.* 2006;30: 511–525.

113. Mayberg HS. Modulating dysfunctional limbic-cortical circuits in depression: towards development of brain-based algorithms for diagnosis and optimised treatment. *Br Med Bull.* 2003;65:193–207.

114. Sheline YI, Price JL, Yan Z, Mintun MA. Resting-state functional MRI in depression unmasks increased connectivity between networks via the dorsal nexus. *Proc Natl Acad Sci U S A.* 2010;107:11020–11025.

115. Hamilton JP, Furman DJ, Chang C, Thomason ME, Dennis E, Gotlib IH. Default-mode and task-positive network activity in major depressive disorder: implications for adaptive and maladaptive rumination. *Biol Psychiatry.* 2011;70:327–333.

116. Berman MG, Peltier S, Nee DE, Kross E, Deldin PJ, Jonides J. Depression, rumination and the default network. *Soc Cogn Affect Neurosci.* 2011;6:548–555.

117. Berman MG, Nee DE, Casement M, et al. Neural and behavioral effects of interference resolution in depression and rumination. *Cogn Affect Behav Neurosci.* 2011;11:85–96.

118. Zhu X, Wang X, Xiao J, et al. Evidence of a dissociation pattern in resting-state default mode network connectivity in first-episode, treatment-naive major depression patients. *Biol Psychiatry.* 2012;71(7)611–617.

119. Grimm S, Boesiger P, Beck J, et al. Altered negative BOLD responses in the default-mode network during emotion processing in depressed subjects. *Neuropsychopharmacology.* 2009;34:932–843.

120. Stoessel C, Stiller J, Bleich S, et al. Differences and similarities on neuronal activities of people being happily and unhappily in love: a functional magnetic resonance imaging study. *Neuropsychobiology.* 2011;64:52–60.

121. Gusnard DA, Akbudak E, Shulman GL, Raichle ME. Medial prefrontal cortex and self-referential mental activity: relation to a default mode of brain function. *Proc Natl Acad Sci U S A.* 2001;98:4259–4264.

122. Vollm BA, Taylor AN, Richardson P, et al. Neuronal correlates of theory of mind and empathy: a functional magnetic resonance imaging study in a nonverbal task. *Neuroimage.* 2006;29:90–98.

123. Schmitz TW, Johnson SC. Relevance to self: A brief review and framework of neural systems underlying appraisal. *Neurosci Biobehav Rev.* 2007;31:585–596.

124. Johnson MK, Nolen-Hoeksema S, Mitchell KJ, Levin Y. Medial cortex activity, self-reflection and depression. *Social Cogn Affect Neurosci.* 2009;4:313–327.

125. Qin P, Northoff G. How is our self related to midline regions and the default-mode network? *Neuroimage.* 2011;57:1221–1233.

126. Burgess PW, Gilbert SJ, Dumontheil I. Function and localization within rostral prefrontal cortex (area 10). *Philos Trans R Soc Lond B Biol Sci.* 2007;362:887–899.

127. Lemogne C, Delaveau P, Freton M, Guionnet S, Fossati P. Medial prefrontal cortex and the self in major depression. *J Affect Disord.* 2012;136:e1–e11.

128. Lemogne C, Gorwood P, Bergouignan L, Pelissolo A, Lehericy S, Fossati P. Negative affectivity, self-referential processing and the cortical midline structures. *Social Cogn Affect Neurosci.* 2011;6:426–433.

129. Zhou Y, Yu C, Zheng H, et al. Increased neural resources recruitment in the intrinsic organization in major depression. *J Affect Disord.* 2010;121:220–230.

130. Grimm S, Ernst J, Boesiger P, et al. Increased self-focus in major depressive disorder is related to neural abnormalities in subcortical-cortical midline structures. *Hum Brain Mapp.* 2009;30:2617–2627.

131. Barbas H, Saha S, Rempel-Clower N, Ghashghaei T. Serial pathways from primate prefrontal cortex to autonomic areas may influence emotional expression. *BMC Neurosci.* 2003;4:25.

132. Milad MR Wright CI, Orr SP, Pitman RK, Quirk GJ, Rauch SL. Recall of fear extinction in humans activates ventro-medial prefrontal cortex and hippocampus in concert. *Biol Psychiatry.* 2007;62(5):446–454.

133. Maletic V, Robinson M, Oakes T, Iyengar S, Ball SG, Russell J. Neurobiology of depression: an integrated view of key findings. *Int J Clin Pract.* 2007;61:2030–2040.

134. Ongur D, Ferry AT, Price JL. Architectonic subdivision of the human orbital and medial prefrontal cortex. *J Comp Neurol.* 2003;460:425–449.

135. Wong SW, Masse N, Kimmerly DS, Menon RS, Shoemaker JK. Ventral medial prefrontal cortex and cardiovagal control in conscious humans. *Neuroimage.* 2007;35:698–708.

136. Amat J, Baratta MV, Paul E, Bland ST, Watkins LR, Maier SF. Medial prefrontal cortex determines how stressor controllability affects behavior and dorsal raphe nucleus. *Nat Neurosci.* 2005;8:365–371.

137. Vazquez-Borsetti P, Celada P, Cortes R, Artigas F. Simultaneous projections from prefrontal cortex to dopaminergic and serotonergic nuclei. *Int J Neuropsychopharmacol.* 2011;14:289–302.

138. Rempel-Clower NL. Role of orbitofrontal cortex connections in emotion. *Ann N Y Acad Sci.* 2007;1121:72–86.

139. Ongur D, Price JL. The organization of networks within the orbital and medial prefrontal cortex of rats, monkeys and humans. *Cereb Cortex.* 2000;10:206–219.

140. Goel V, Dolan RJ. Reciprocal neural response within lateral and ventral medial prefrontal cortex during hot and cold reasoning. *Neuroimage.* 2003;20:2314–2321.

141. Cox SM, Andrade A, Johnsrude IS. Learning to like: a role for human orbitofrontal cortex in conditioned reward. *J Neurosci.* 2005;25:2733–2740.

142. Milad MR, Wright CI, Orr SP, Pitman RK, Quirk GJ, Rauch SL. Recall of fear extinction in humans activates the ventromedial prefrontal cortex and hippocampus in concert. *Biol Psychiatry.* 2007;62:446–454.

143. Hansel A, von Kanel R. The ventro-medial prefrontal cortex: a major link between the autonomic nervous system, regulation of emotion, and stress reactivity? *Biopsychosoc Med.* 2008;2:21.

144. Banich MT, Mackiewicz KL, Depue BE, Whitmer AJ, Miller GA, Heller W. Cognitive control mechanisms, emotion and memory: a neural perspective with implications for psychopathology. *Neurosci Biobehav Rev.* 2009;33:613–630.

145. Urry HL, van Reekum CM, Johnstone T, et al. Amygdala and ventromedial prefrontal cortex are inversely coupled during regulation of negative affect and predict the diurnal pattern of cortisol secretion among older adults. *J Neurosci.* 2006;26:4415–4425.

146. Johnstone T, van Reekum CM, Urry HL, Kalin NH, Davidson RJ. Failure to regulate: counterproductive recruitment of top-down prefrontal-subcortical circuitry in major depression. *J Neurosci.* 2007;27:8877–8884.

147. Veer IM, Oei NY, Spinhoven P, van Buchem MA, Elzinga BM, Rombouts SA. Endogenous cortisol is associated with functional connectivity between the amygdala and medial prefrontal cortex. *Psychoneuroendocrinology.* 2012;37(7):1039–1047.

148. Oei NY, Veer IM, Wolf OT, Spinhoven P, Rombouts SA, Elzinga BM. Stress shifts brain activation towards ventral "affective" areas during emotional distraction. *Soc Cogn Affect Neurosci.* 2012;7(4):403–412.

149. Veer IM, Oei NY, Spinhoven P, van Buchem MA, Elzinga BM, Rombouts SA. Beyond acute social stress: increased functional connectivity between amygdala and cortical midline structures. *Neuroimage.* 2011;57:1534–1541.

150. Bishop SJ. Trait anxiety and impoverished prefrontal control of attention. *Nat Neurosci.* 2009;12:92–98.

151. Levin RJ, Heller W, Mohanty A, et al. Cognitive deficits in depression and functional specificity of regional brain activity. *Cogn Ther Res.* 2007;31:211–233.

152. Whitmer AJ, Banich MT. Inhibition versus switching deficits in different forms of rumination. *Psychol Sci.* 2007;18:546–553.

153. Philippot P, Brutoux F. Induced rumination dampens executive processes in dysphoric young adults. *J Behav Ther Exp Psychiatry.* 2008;39:219–227.

154. Gray JR, Braver TS, Raichle ME. Integration of emotion and cognition in the lateral prefrontal cortex. *Proc Natl Acad Sci U S A.* 2002;99:4115–4120.

155. Sheline YI, Barch DM, Price JL, et al. The default mode network and self-referential processes in depression. *Proc Natl Acad Sci U S A.* 2009;106:1942–1947.

156. Maroun M. Stress reverses plasticity in the pathway projecting from the ventromedial prefrontal cortex to the basolateral amygdala. *Eur J Neurosci.* 2006;24:2917–2922.

157. Mayberg HS. Positron emission tomography imaging in depression: a neural systems perspective. *Neuroimaging Clin N Am.* 2003;13:805–815.

158. Drevets WC, Ongur D, Price JL. Neuroimaging abnormalities in the subgenual prefrontal cortex: implications for the pathophysiology of familial mood disorders. *Mol Psychiatry.* 1998;3:220–226, 190–191.

159. Zald DH, Mattson DL, Pardo JV. Brain activity in ventromedial prefrontal cortex correlates with individual differences in negative affect. *Proc Natl Acad Sci U S A.* 2002;99:2450–2454.

160. Harvey PO, Pruessner J, Czechowska Y, Lepage M. Individual differences in trait anhedonia: a structural and functional magnetic resonance imaging study in nonclinical subjects. *Mol Psychiatry.* 2007;12:703, 767–775.

161. Killgore WD, Yurgelun-Todd DA. Ventromedial prefrontal activity correlates with depressed mood in adolescent children. *Neuroreport.* 2006;17(2):167–171.

162. Haas BW, Constable RT, Canli T. Stop the sadness: neuroticism is associated with sustained medial prefrontal cortex response to emotional facial expressions. *Neuroimage.* 2008;42:385–392.

163. Smoski MJ, Felder J, Bizzell J, et al. fMRI of alterations in reward selection, anticipation, and feedback in major depressive disorder. *J Affect Disord.* 2009;118:69–78.

164. Dichter GS, Felder JN, Smoski MJ. Affective context interferes with cognitive control in unipolar depression: an fMRI investigation. *J Affect Disord.* 2009;114:131–142.

165. Bremner JD, Vythilingam M, Vermetten E, et al. Reduced volume of orbitofrontal cortex in major depression. *Biol Psychiatry.* 2002;51:273–279.

166. Kempton MJ, Salvador Z, Munafo MR, et al. Structural neuroimaging studies in major depressive disorder. Meta-analysis and comparison with bipolar disorder. *Arch Gen Psychiatry.* 2011;68:675–690.

167. Lacerda AL, Keshavan MS, Hardan AY, et al. Anatomic evaluation of the orbitofrontal cortex in major depressive disorder. *Biol Psychiatry.* 2004;55:353–358.

168. Goldin PR, McRae K, Ramel W, Gross JJ. The neural bases of emotion regulation: reappraisal and suppression of negative emotion. *Biol Psychiatry.* 2008;63:577–586.

169. Forbes CE, Grafman J. The role of the human prefrontal cortex in social cognition and moral judgment. *Annu Rev Neurosci.* 2010;33:299–324.

170. Wendelken C, Nakhabenko D, Donohue SE, Carter CS, Bunge SA. "Brain is to thought as stomach is to ??": investigating the role of rostrolateral prefrontal cortex in relational reasoning. *J Cogn Neurosci.* 2008;20:682–693.

171. Steele JD, Currie J, Lawrie SM, Reid I. Prefrontal cortical functional abnormality in major depressive disorder: a stereotactic meta-analysis. *J Affect Disord.* 2007;101:1–11.

172. Drevets WC. Neuroimaging studies of mood disorders. *Biol Psychiatry.* 2000;48:813–829.

173. Lorenzetti V, Allen NB, Fornito A, Yucel M. Structural brain abnormalities in major depressive disorder: a selective review of recent MRI studies. *J Affect Disord.* 2009;117:1–17.

174. Vasic N, Walter H, Hose A, Wolf RC. Gray matter reduction associated with psychopathology and cognitive dysfunction in unipolar depression: a voxel-based morphometry study. *J Affect Disord.* 2008;109:107–116.

175. Ray RD, Zald DH. Anatomical insights into the interaction of emotion and cognition in the prefrontal cortex. *Neurosci Biobehav Rev.* 2012;36:479–501.

176. MacDonald AW 3rd, Cohen JD, Stenger VA, Carter CS. Dissociating the role of the dorsolateral prefrontal and anterior cingulate cortex in cognitive control. *Science.* 2000;288:1835–1838.

177. Mansouri FA, Tanaka K, Buckley MJ. Conflict-induced behavioural adjustment: a clue to the executive functions of the prefrontal cortex. *Nat Rev Neurosci.* 2009;10:141–152.

178. Badre D. Cognitive control, hierarchy, and the rostro-caudal organization of the frontal lobes. *Trends Cogn Sci.* 2008;12:193–200.

179. Wittfoth M, Schardt DM, Fahle M, Herrmann M. How the brain resolves high conflict situations: double conflict involvement of dorsolateral prefrontal cortex. *Neuroimage.* 2009;44:1201–1209.

180. Haggard P. Human volition: towards a neuroscience of will. *Nat Rev Neurosci.* 2008;9:934–946.

181. Kompus K, Hugdahl K, Ohman A, Marklund P, Nyberg L. Distinct control networks for cognition and emotion in the prefrontal cortex. *Neurosci Lett.* 2009;467:76–80.

182. van den Bos W, Guroglu B, van den Bulk BG, Rombouts SA, Crone EA. Better than expected or as bad as you thought? The neurocognitive development of probabilistic feedback processing. *Front Hum Neurosci.* 2009;3:52.

183. Ohira H, Fukuyama S, Kimura K, et al. Regulation of natural killer cell redistribution by prefrontal cortex during stochastic learning. *Neuroimage.* 2009;47:897–907.

184. Ohira H, Ichikawa N, Nomura M, et al. Brain and autonomic association accompanying stochastic decision-making. *Neuroimage.* 2010;49:1024–1037.

185. Fleming SM, Weil RS, Nagy Z, Dolan RJ, Rees G. Relating introspective accuracy to individual differences in brain structure. *Science.* 2010;329:1541–1543.

186. Fitzgerald PB, Srithiran A, Benitez J, et al. An fMRI study of prefrontal brain activation during multiple tasks in patients with major depressive disorder. *Hum Brain Mapp.* 2008;29:490–501.

187. Werner NS, Meindl T, Materne J, et al. Functional MRI study of memory-related brain regions in patients with depressive disorder. *J Affect Disord.* 2009;119:124–131.

188. Matsuo K, Glahn DC, Peluso MA, et al. Prefrontal hyperactivation during working memory task in untreated individuals with major depressive disorder. *Mol Psychiatry.* 2007;12:158–166.

189. Brody AL, Barsom MW, Bota RG, Saxena S. Prefrontal-subcortical and limbic circuit mediation of major depressive disorder. *Semin Clin Neuropsychiatry.* 2001;6:102–112.

190. Videbech P. PET measurements of brain glucose metabolism and blood flow in major depressive disorder: a critical review. *Acta Psychiatr Scand.* 2000;101:11–20.

191. Wagner G, Sinsel E, Sobanski T, et al. Cortical inefficiency in patients with unipolar depression: an event-related FMRI study with the Stroop task. *Biol Psychiatry.* 2006;59: 958–965.

192. Walter H, Wolf RC, Spitzer M, Vasic N. Increased left prefrontal activation in patients with unipolar depression: an event-related, parametric, performance-controlled fMRI study. *J Affect Disord.* 2007;101:175–185.

193. Fales CL, Barch DM, Rundle MM, et al. Altered emotional interference processing in affective and cognitive-control brain circuitry in major depression. *Biol Psychiatry.* 2008;63:377–384.

194. Grimm S, Beck J, Schuepbach D, et al. Imbalance between left and right dorsolateral prefrontal cortex in major depression is linked to negative emotional judgment: an fMRI study in severe major depressive disorder. *Biol Psychiatry.* 2008;63:369–376.

195. Holmes AJ, Pizzagalli DA. Spatiotemporal dynamics of error processing dysfunctions in major depressive disorder. *Arch Gen Psychiatry.* 2008;65:179–188.

196. Caetano SC, Fonseca M, Olvera RL, et al. Proton spectroscopy study of the left dorsolateral prefrontal cortex in pediatric depressed patients. *Neurosci Lett.* 2005;384:321–326.

197. Bora E, Yucel M, Fornito A, et al. White matter microstructure in opiate addiction. *Addict Biol.* 2012;17:141–148.

198. Peterson BS, Warner V, Bansal R, et al. Cortical thinning in persons at increased familial risk for major depression. *Proc Natl Acad Sci U S A.* 2009;106:6273–6278.

199. Beyer JL, Krishnan KR. Volumetric brain imaging findings in mood disorders. *Bipolar Disord.* 2002;4:89–104.

200. Guillery RW. Anatomical pathways that link perception and action. *Prog Brain Res.* 2005;149:235–256.

201. Price JL, Drevets WC. Neural circuits underlying the pathophysiology of mood disorders. *Trends Cogn Sci.* 2012;16:61–71.

202. Furman DJ, Hamilton JP, Gotlib IH. Frontostriatal functional connectivity in major depressive disorder. *Biol Mood Anxiety Disord.* 2011;1:11.

203. Haber SN, Calzavara R. The cortico-basal ganglia integrative network: the role of the thalamus. *Brain Res Bull.* 2009;78:69–74.

204. Krebs RM, Boehler CN, Roberts KC, Song AW, Woldorff MG. The involvement of the dopaminergic midbrain and cortico-striatal-thalamic circuits in the integration of reward prospect and attentional task demands. *Cereb Cortex.* 2012;22:607–615.

205. Ramnani N, Miall C. Expanding cerebellar horizons. *Trends Cogn Sci.* 2001;5:135–136.

206. Schmahmann JD. Dysmetria of thought: clinical consequences of cerebellar dysfunction on cognition and affect. *Trends Cogn Sci.* 1998;2:362–371.

207. Aggleton JP, O'Mara SM, Vann SD, Wright NF, Tsanov M, Erichsen JT. Hippocampal-anterior thalamic pathways for memory: uncovering a network of direct and indirect actions. *Eur J Neurosci.* 2010;31:2292–2307.

208. Soei E, Koch B, Schwarz M, Daum I. Involvement of the human thalamus in relational and non-relational memory. *Eur J Neurosci.* 2008;28:2533–2541.

209. Hamilton JP, Chen MC, Gotlib IH. Neural systems approaches to understanding major depressive disorder: an intrinsic functional organization perspective. *Neurobiol Dis.* 2013;52:4–11.

210. Hamilton JP, Etkin A, Furman DJ, Lemus MG, Johnson RF, Gotlib IH. Functional neuroimaging of major depressive disorder: a meta-analysis and new integration of base line activation and neural response data. *Am J Psychiatry.* 2012;169:693–703.

211. Greicius MD, Flores BH, Menon V, et al. Resting-state functional connectivity in major depression: abnormally increased contributions from subgenual cingulate cortex and thalamus. *Biol Psychiatry.* 2007;62:429–437.

212. Dichter GS, Kozink RV, McClernon FJ, Smoski MJ. Remitted major depression is characterized by reward network hyperactivation during reward anticipation and hypoactivation during reward outcomes. *J Affect Disord.* 2012;136:1126–1134.

213. Monkul ES, Silva LA, Narayana S, et al. Abnormal resting state corticolimbic blood flow in depressed unmedicated patients with major depression: a ^{15}O-H(2)O PET study. *Hum Brain Mapp.* 2012;33:272–279.

214. Lui S, Wu Q, Qiu L, et al. Resting-state functional connectivity in treatment-resistant depression. *Am J Psychiatry.* 2011;168:642–648.

215. Du MY, Wu QZ, Yue Q, et al. Voxelwise meta-analysis of gray matter reduction in major depressive disorder. *Prog Neuropsychopharmacol Biol Psychiatry.* 2012;36: 11–16.

216. Bielau H, Trubner K, Krell D, et al. Volume deficits of subcortical nuclei in mood disorders A postmortem study. *Eur Arch Psychiatry Clin Neurosci.* 2005;255:401–412.

217. Schmahmann JD, Weilburg JB, Sherman JC. The neuropsychiatry of the cerebellum—insights from the clinic. *Cerebellum.* 2007;6:254–267.

218. Schmahmann JD. Disorders of the cerebellum: ataxia, dysmetria of thought, and the cerebellar cognitive affective syndrome. *J Neuropsychiatry Clin Neurosci.* 2004;16: 367–378.

219. Hoppenbrouwers SS, Schutter DJ, Fitzgerald PB, Chen R, Daskalakis ZJ. The role of the cerebellum in the pathophysiology and treatment of neuropsychiatric disorders: a review. *Brain Res Rev.* 2008;59:185–200.

220. Fields RD. White matter in learning, cognition and psychiatric disorders. *Trends Neurosci.* 2008;31:361–370.

221. Fields RD. Neuroscience. Change in the brain's white matter. *Science.* 2010;330: 768–769.

222. Sheline YI, Price JL, Vaishnavi SN, et al. Regional white matter hyperintensity burden in automated segmentation distinguishes late-life depressed subjects from comparison subjects matched for vascular risk factors. *Am J Psychiatry.* 2008;165:524–532.

223. Zhu X, Wang X, Xiao J, Zhong M, Liao J, Yao S. Altered white matter integrity in first-episode, treatment-naive young adults with major depressive disorder: a tract-based spatial statistics study. *Brain Res.* 2011;1369:223–229.

224. Wang Y, Jia Y, Xu G, Ling X, Liu S, Huang L. Frontal white matter biochemical abnormalities in first-episode, treatment-naive patients with major depressive disorder: a proton magnetic resonance spectroscopy study. *J Affect Disord.* 2012;136:620–626.

225. Cullen KR, Klimes-Dougan B, Muetzel R, et al. Altered white matter microstructure in adolescents with major depression: a preliminary study. *J Am Acad Child Adolesc Psychiatry.* 2010;49:173–183.

226. Anand A, Li Y, Wang Y, et al. Activity and connectivity of brain mood regulating circuit in depression: a functional magnetic resonance study. *Biol Psychiatry.* 2005;57: 1079–1088.

227. Chen CH, Suckling J, Ooi C, et al. Functional coupling of the amygdala in depressed patients treated with antidepressant medication. *Neuropsychopharmacology.* 2008;33: 1909–1918.

228. Papakostas GI, Iosifescu DV, Renshaw PF, et al. Brain MRI white matter hyperintensi-

ties and one-carbon cycle metabolism in non-geriatric outpatients with major depressive disorder (part II). *Psychiatry Res.* 2005;140:301–307.

229. Blood AJ, Iosifescu DV, Makris N, et al. Microstructural abnormalities in subcortical reward circuitry of subjects with major depressive disorder. *PLoS ONE.* 2010;5:e13945.

230. Videbech P, Ravnkilde B, Gammelgaard L, et al. The Danish PET/depression project: performance on Stroop's test linked to white matter lesions in the brain. *Psychiatry Res.* 2004;130:117–130.

231. Tham MW, Woon PS, Sum MY, Lee TS, Sim K. White matter abnormalities in major depression: evidence from post-mortem, neuroimaging and genetic studies. *J Affect Disord.* 2011;132:26–36.

232. Zhang A, Leow A, Ajilore O, et al. Quantitative tract-specific measures of uncinate and cingulum in major depression using diffusion tensor imaging. *Neuropsychopharmacology.* 2012;37:959–967.

233. Brody AL, Saxena S, Mandelkern MA, Fairbanks LA, Ho ML, Baxter LR. Brain metabolic changes associated with symptom factor improvement in major depressive disorder. *Biol Psychiatry.* 2001;50:171–178.

234. Kessler H, Traue H, Wiswede D. Why we still don't understand the depressed brain—not going beyond snapshots. *Psychosoc Med.* 2011;8:Doc06.

235. Etkin A, Schatzberg AF. Common abnormalities and disorder-specific compensation during implicit regulation of emotional processing in generalized anxiety and major depressive disorders. *Am J Psychiatry.* 2011;168:968–978.

236. Raison CL, Capuron L, Miller AH. Cytokines sing the blues: inflammation and the pathogenesis of depression. *Trends Immunol.* 2006;27:24–31.

237. Alesci S, Martinez PE, Kelkar S, et al. Major depression is associated with significant diurnal elevations in plasma interleukin-6 levels, a shift of its circadian rhythm, and loss of physiological complexity in its secretion: clinical implications. *J Clin Endocrinol Metab.* 2005;90:2522–2530.

238. Drevets WC, Price JL, Furey ML. Brain structural and functional abnormalities in mood disorders: implications for neurocircuitry models of depression. *Brain Struct Funct.* 2008;213:93–118.

239. Davidson RJ, Pizzagalli D, Nitschke JB, Putnam K. Depression: perspectives from affective neuroscience. *Annu Rev Psychol.* 2002;53:545–574.

240. Seminowicz DA, Mayberg HS, McIntosh AR, et al. Limbic-frontal circuitry in major depression: a path modeling metanalysis. *Neuroimage.* 2004;22:409–418.

241. Savitz JB, Drevets WC. Imaging phenotypes of major depressive disorder: genetic correlates. *Neuroscience.* 2009;164:300–330.

242. Rajkowska G, Miguel-Hidalgo JJ. Gliogenesis and glial pathology in depression. *CNS Neurol Disord Drug Targets.* 2007;6:219–233.

243. Andrews-Hanna JR, Reidler JS, Huang C, Buckner RL. Evidence for the default network's role in spontaneous cognition. *J Neurophysiol.* 2010;104:322–335.

244. Andrews-Hanna JR, Reidler JS, Sepulcre J, Poulin R, Buckner RL. Functional-anatomic fractionation of the brain's default network. *Neuron.* 2010;65:550–562.

245. Smallwood J, Brown K, Baird B, Schooler JW. Cooperation between the default mode network and the frontal-parietal network in the production of an internal train of thought. *Brain Res.* 2012;1428:60–70.

246. Christoff K. Undirected thought: neural determinants and correlates. *Brain Res.* 2012; 1428:51–59.

247. Gerlach KD, Spreng RN, Gilmore AW, Schacter DL. Solving future problems: default network and executive activity associated with goal-directed mental simulations. *Neuroimage.* 2011;55:1816–1824.

248. Ellamil M, Dobson C, Beeman M, Christoff K. Evaluative and generative modes of thought during the creative process. *Neuroimage.* 2012;59:1783–1794.

249. Lutz A, Slagter HA, Dunne JD, Davidson RJ. Attention regulation and monitoring in meditation. *Trends Cogn Sci.* 2008;12:163–169.

250. Hasenkamp W, Barsalou LW. Effects of meditation experience on functional connectivity of distributed brain networks. *Front Hum Neurosci.* 2012;6:38.

251. Hasenkamp W, Wilson-Mendenhall CD, Duncan E, Barsalou LW. Mind wandering and attention during focused meditation: a fine-grained temporal analysis of fluctuating cognitive states. *Neuroimage.* 2012;59:750–760.

252. Brewer JA, Worhunsky PD, Gray JR, Tang YY, Weber J, Kober H. Meditation experience is associated with differences in default mode network activity and connectivity. *Proc Natl Acad Sci U S A.* 2011;108:20254–20259.

253. Taylor VA, Daneault V, Grant J, et al. Impact of meditation training on the default mode network during a restful state. *Soc Cogn Affect Neurosci.* 2013;8(1):4–14.

254. Farb NA, Anderson AK, Segal ZV. The mindful brain and emotion regulation in mood disorders. *Can J Psychiatry.* 2012;57:70–77.

255. Ives-Deliperi VL, Solms M, Meintjes EM. The neural substrates of mindfulness: an fMRI investigation. *Soc Neurosci.* 2011;6:231–242.

256. Brefczynski Lewis JA, Lutz A, Schaefer HS, Levinson DB, Davidson RJ. Neural correlates of attentional expertise in long-term meditation practitioners. *Proc Natl Acad Sci U S A.* 2007;104:11483–11488.

257. Dickenson J, Berkman ET, Arch J, Lieberman MD. Neural correlates of focused attention during a brief mindfulness induction. *Soc Cogn Affect Neurosci.* 2013;8(1):40–47.

258. Holzel BK, Ott U, Gard T, et al. Investigation of mindfulness meditation practitioners with voxel-based morphometry. *Soc Cogn Affect Neurosci.* 2008;3:55–61.

259. Sharot T, Riccardi AM, Raio CM, Phelps EA. Neural mechanisms mediating optimism bias. *Nature.* 2007;450:102–105.

260. Zoccola PM, Dickerson SS, Lam S. Eliciting and maintaining ruminative thought: the role of social-evaluative threat. *Emotion.* 2012;12(4):673–677.

261. Dawes CT, Loewen PJ, Schreiber D, et al. Neural basis of egalitarian behavior. *Proc Natl Acad Sci U S A.* 2012;109(17):6479–6483.

262. Masten CL, Morelli SA, Eisenberger NI. An fMRI investigation of empathy for "social pain" and subsequent prosocial behavior. *Neuroimage.* 2011;55:381–388.

263. Dewall CN, Macdonald G, Webster GD, et al. Acetaminophen reduces social pain: behavioral and neural evidence. *Psychol Sci.* 2010;21:931–937.

264. Immordino-Yang MH, McColl A, Damasio H, Damasio A. Neural correlates of admiration and compassion. *Proc Natl Acad Sci U S A.* 2009;106:8021–8026.

265. Kersting A, Ohrmann P, Pedersen A, et al. Neural activation underlying acute grief in women after the loss of an unborn child. *Am J Psychiatry.* 2009;166:1402–1410.

266. Gundel H, O'Connor MF, Littrell L, Fort C, Lane RD. Functional neuroanatomy of grief: an fMRI study. *Am J Psychiatry.* 2003;160:1946–1953.

267. O'Connor MF, Gundel H, McRae K, Lane RD. Baseline vagal tone predicts BOLD response during elicitation of grief. *Neuropsychopharmacology.* 2007;32:2184–2189.

268. O'Connor MF, Irwin MR, Wellisch DK. When grief heats up: pro-inflammatory cytokines predict regional brain activation. *Neuroimage.* 2009;47:891–896.

269. Miller AH, Maletic V, Raison CL. Inflammation and its discontents: the role of cytokines in the pathophysiology of major depression. *Biol Psychiatry.* 2009;65:732–741.

270. Freed PJ, Yanagihara TK, Hirsch J, Mann JJ. Neural mechanisms of grief regulation. *Biol Psychiatry.* 2009;66:33–40.

271. Hamilton JP, Gotlib IH. Neural substrates of increased memory sensitivity for negative stimuli in major depression. *Biol Psychiatry*. 2008;63:1155–1162.

272. Zhang J, Wang J, Wu Q, et al. Disrupted brain connectivity networks in drug-naive, first-episode major depressive disorder. *Biol Psychiatry*. 2011;70:334–342.

273. Jin C, Gao C, Chen C, et al. A preliminary study of the dysregulation of the resting networks in first-episode medication-naive adolescent depression. *Neurosci Lett*. 2011; 503:105–109.

274. Bar M. A cognitive neuroscience hypothesis of mood and depression. *Trends Cogn Sci*. 2009;13:456–463.

275. Harrison NA, Brydon L, Walker C, Gray MA, Steptoe A, Critchley HD. Inflammation causes mood changes through alterations in subgenual cingulate activity and meso-limbic connectivity. *Biol Psychiatry*. 2009;66:407–414.

276. Epstein J, Perez DL, Ervin K, et al. Failure to segregate emotional processing from cognitive and sensorimotor processing in major depression. *Psychiatry Res*. 2011;193: 144–150.

277. Marchetti I, Koster EH, Sonuga-Barke EJ, De Raedt R. The default mode network and recurrent depression: a neurobiological model of cognitive risk factors. *Neuropsychol Rev*. 2012;22:229–251.

278. Reppermund S, Ising M, Lucae S, Zihl J. Cognitive impairment in unipolar depression is persistent and non-specific: further evidence for the final common pathway disorder hypothesis. *Psychol Med*. 2009;39(4):603–614.

279. Gorwood P, Corruble E, Falissard B, Goodwin GM. Toxic effects of depression on brain function: impairment of delayed recall and the cumulative length of depressive disorder in a large sample of depressed outpatients. *Am J Psychiatry*. 2008;165:731–739.

280. Nixon NL, Liddle PF, Nixon E, Worwood G, Liotti M, Palaniyappan L. Biological vulnerability to depression: linked structural and functional brain network findings. *Br J Psychiatry*. 2014;204:283–289.

281. Tang YY, Lu Q, Geng X, Stein EA, Yang Y, Posner MI. Short-term meditation induces white matter changes in the anterior cingulate. *Proc Natl Acad Sci U S A*. 2010; 107:15649–15652.

282. Moussavi S, Chatterji S, Verdes E, Tandon A, Patel V, Ustun B. Depression, chronic diseases, and decrements in health: results from the World Health Surveys. *Lancet*. 2007;370:851–858.

283. Pasco JA, Nicholson GC, Williams LJ, et al. Association of high-sensitivity C-reactive protein with de novo major depression. *Br J Psychiatry*. 2010;197:372–377.

284. Gimeno D, Kivimaki M, Brunner EJ, et al. Associations of C-reactive protein and interleukin-6 with cognitive symptoms of depression: 12-year follow-up of the Whitehall II study. *Psychol Med*. 2009;39:413–423.

285. Danese A, Moffitt TE, Harrington H, et al. Adverse childhood experiences and adult risk factors for age-related disease: depression, inflammation, and clustering of metabolic risk markers. *Arch Pediatr Adolesc Med*. 2009;163:1135–1143.

286. Zhang X, Yaseen ZS, Galynker, II, Hirsch J, Winston A. Can depression be diagnosed by response to mother's face? A personalized attachment-based paradigm for diagnostic fMRI. *PLoS ONE*. 2011;6:e27253.

287. Kendler KS, Thornton LM, Gardner CO. Stressful life events and previous episodes in the etiology of major depression in women: an evaluation of the "kindling" hypothesis. *Am J Psychiatry*. 2000;157:1243–1251.

288. Johnson L, Andersson-Lundman G, Aberg-Wistedt A, Mathe AA. Age of onset in affective disorder: its correlation with hereditary and psychosocial factors. *J Affect Disord*. 2000;59:139–148.

289. Maletic V. Pathophysiology of pain and depression: the role of dual-acting antidepressants. *CNS Spectr.* 2005;10:7–9.

290. Johansson L, Skoog I, Gustafson DR, et al. Midlife psychological distress associated with late-life brain atrophy and white matter lesions: a 32-year population study of women. *Psychosom Med.* 2012;74:120–125.

291. Brosschot JF, Gerin W, Thayer JF. The perseverative cognition hypothesis: a review of worry, prolonged stress-related physiological activation, and health. *J Psychosom Res.* 2006;60:113–124.

292. Wisco BE, Nolen-Hoeksema S. Valence of autobiographical memories: the role of mood, cognitive reappraisal, and suppression. *Behav Res Ther.* 2010;48:335–340.

293. Brosschot JF. Markers of chronic stress: prolonged physiological activation and (un)conscious perseverative cognition. *Neurosci Biobehav Rev.* 2010;35:46–50.

294. Brosschot JF, Verkuil B, Thayer JF. Conscious and unconscious perseverative cognition: is a large part of prolonged physiological activity due to unconscious stress? *J Psychosom Res.* 2010;69:407–416.

295. Seidel EM, Satterthwaite TD, Eickhoff SB, et al. Neural correlates of depressive realism—an fMRI study on causal attribution in depression. *J Affect Disord.* 2012;138:268–276.

296. Irwin MR, Cole SW. Reciprocal regulation of the neural and innate immune systems. *Nat Rev Immunol.* 2011;11:625–632.

297. McNally L, Bhagwagar Z, Hannestad J. Inflammation, glutamate, and glia in depression: a literature review. *CNS Spectr.* 2008;13:501–510.

298. Besedovsky HO, del Rey A. Central and peripheral cytokines mediate immune-brain connectivity. *Neurochem Res.* 2011;36:1–6.

299. Maes M, Mihaylova I, Kubera M, Ringel K. Activation of cell-mediated immunity in depression: association with inflammation, melancholia, clinical staging and the fatigue and somatic symptom cluster of depression. *Prog Neuropsychopharmacol Biol Psychiatry.* 2012;36:169–175.

300. Harrison PJ, Tunbridge EM. Catechol-*O*-methyltransferase (COMT): a gene contributing to sex differences in brain function, and to sexual dimorphism in the predisposition to psychiatric disorders. *Neuropsychopharmacology.* 2008;33:3037–3045.

301. Raison CL, Miller AH. When not enough is too much: the role of insufficient glucocorticoid signaling in the pathophysiology of stress-related disorders. *Am J Psychiatry.* 2003;160:1554–1565.

302. Liu Y, Ho RC, Mak A. Interleukin (IL)-6, tumour necrosis factor alpha (TNF-alpha) and soluble interleukin-2 receptors (sIL-2R) are elevated in patients with major depressive disorder: a meta-analysis and meta-regression. *J Affect Disord.* 2012;139(3):230–239.

303. Maier SF. Bi-directional immune-brain communication: implications for understanding stress, pain, and cognition. *Brain Behav Immun.* 2003;17:69–85.

304. Barton DA, Dawood T, Lambert EA, et al. Sympathetic activity in major depressive disorder: identifying those at increased cardiac risk? *J Hypertens.* 2007;25:2117–2124.

305. McAfoose J, Baune BT. Evidence for a cytokine model of cognitive function. *Neurosci Biobehav Rev.* 2009;33:355–366.

306. Asami T, Ito T, Fukumitsu H, Nomoto H, Furukawa Y, Furukawa S. Autocrine activation of cultured macrophages by brain-derived neurotrophic factor. *Biochem Biophys Res Commun.* 2006;344:941–947.

307. Cao L, Liu X, Lin EJ, et al. Environmental and genetic activation of a brain-adipocyte BDNF/leptin axis causes cancer remission and inhibition. *Cell.* 2010;142:52–64.

308. Hasler G, Northoff G. Discovering imaging endophenotypes for major depression. *Mol Psychiatry.* 2011;16:604–619.

309. Meyer-Lindenberg A. Neural connectivity as an intermediate phenotype: brain networks under genetic control. *Hum Brain Mapp.* 2009;30:1938–1946.

310. Post RM. Mechanisms of illness progression in the recurrent affective disorders. *Neurotox Res.* 2010;18:256–271.

311. Glahn DC, Winkler AM, Kochunov P, et al. Genetic control over the resting brain. *Proc Natl Acad Sci U S A.* 2010;107:1223–1228.

312. Post RM. Kindling and sensitization as models for affective episode recurrence, cyclicity, and tolerance phenomena. *Neurosci Biobehav Rev.* 2007;31:858–873.

313. Thomason ME, Yoo DJ, Glover GH, Gotlib IH. BDNF genotype modulates resting functional connectivity in children. *Front Hum Neurosci.* 2009;3:55.

314. Ohira H, Matsunaga M, Isowa T, et al. Polymorphism of the serotonin transporter gene modulates brain and physiological responses to acute stress in Japanese men. *Stress.* 2009;12:533–543.

315. Murakami H, Matsunaga M, Ohira H. Association of serotonin transporter gene polymorphism and emotion regulation. *Neuroreport.* 2009;20:414–418.

316. Nissen C, Holz J, Blechert J, et al. Learning as a model for neural plasticity in major depression. *Biol Psychiatry.* 2010;68:544–552.

CHAPTER 9

Changes in Neurotransmission and Subcellular Function in Depression

Or, The Secret of the Shogun's Box

When Joseph Schildkraut published his seminal review of evidence supporting the monoamine hypothesis of depression in 1965,[1] little was known about extraneuronal monoamine transport, glia monoamine receptors, or the role of monoamines in regulating glutamate, gamma-aminobutyric acid (GABA), inflammatory, and neurotrophic signaling. Unfortunately, the last two papers published by Schildkraut and his coauthors received much less attention.[2,3] In these two papers, published in 2004 and 2008 (posthumously), Schildkraut and John Mooney brought to our attention a very important discovery: they proposed several steps in the mechanism of action of desipramine (DMI). Before this, the initial rise in the synaptic levels of norepinephrine (NE) had been attributed to DMI antagonism of the NE transporter (NET, a.k.a. Uptake-1); consequent accumulation of synaptic NE interacted with the presynaptic inhibitory alpha-2 adrenergic autoreceptor, temporarily diminishing further NE release; and eventual desensitization of inhibitory presynaptic alpha-2 receptors resulted in an increase in synaptic NE content. In contrast, Schildkraut and Mooney introduced an entirely new idea about the mechanism of DMI action. They postulated that delay in antidepressant action, presumably linked to NE accumulation, may also be related to an uninterrupted activity of extraneuronal uptake mechanisms, including glial Uptake-2 conducted by organic cation transporter-3, which is regulated by the SLC22A3 gene, and the plasma membrane monoamine transporter. Although DMI effectively blocks the activity of NET, it has virtually no impact on its glial NET counterpart, Uptake-2. The initial increase in glial NE metabolism and the ensuing production of normetanephrine (NMN) were necessary for the subsequent antidepressant effect. Namely, while DMI has little capacity to block the glial equivalent of NET, NMN possesses robust glial transporter antagonistic properties. Therefore, delay in action of DMI was in part explained by the time necessary for NMN accumulation to occur, followed by glial transporter blockade, which in turn produces a greater accumulation of extra-neuronal NE, which putatively coincides with the clinical onset of antidepressant action.[2,3] Subsequent preclinical research supported and extended these findings by demonstrating that the combination of NMN and venlafaxine effects a greater release of cortical NE than the antidepressant alone.[4]

Although some of the later research on the impact of antidepressants on monoamine turnover in part contradicted Schildkraut and Mooney's work, they pioneered several intriguing ideas. Exclusive focus on neuronal transporters and receptors may not be sufficient to provide us with an accurate understanding of the mechanism of antidepressant action. Glial cells (which represent 90 percent of the cellular population of the brain) and their uptake sites may play an important role in the pathophysiology of major depressive disorder (MDD) and its treatment. The majority of monoamine release (>80 percent) is extrasynaptic and therefore out of reach of mostly presynaptically located neuronal transporters.

While monoamine theory has generated an abundance of fruitful research and advances in the understanding and treatment of MDD, it has also left great gaps in our understanding of the pathophysiology of this condition. Or, should we more properly define MDD as a syndrome? Despite six decades of development of monoamine-modulating antidepressant medications, remission rates have not exceeded those seen with tricyclic antidepressants and monoamine oxidase (MAO) inhibitors in the 1960s. Although safety and tolerability of antidepressants have indeed improved, improvement in efficacy continues to elude our research efforts.

Medieval Japanese lore describes an interesting tradition taking place when local visiting dignitaries paid respects to the shogun. Their servants would bring a large gift box into the reception hall. The shogun would lift the lid, revealing a tray filled with edible delicacies featuring the shogun's favorite dishes. Below the tray, concealed from the public eye, was a deeper compartment filled with gold coins. Can we get beyond the delicacy of monoamine signaling and uncover the hidden gold underneath?

The yin and yang of glutamate and GABA opposition extends beyond neural excitation and inhibition. Glutamate propagates inflammatory signaling in the brain, whereas GABA opposes it. Neurotransmission, glial transmission, and immune signaling represent a mutually integrated processing system providing a bidirectional flow of information. In other words, not only is inflammation capable of enhancing glutamate efflux from neural cells, but the opposite is also true. Glia-released GABA counters not only excitatory but also proinflammatory effects of glutamate. Monoamines act as slow modulators of rapidly signaling glutamate and GABA neurons. Glutamate, GABA, and monoamines all jointly regulate intracellular signaling cascades, which ultimately regulate gene transcription of neurotrophic factors.

Glutamate and GABA in MDD

Multiple lines of evidence implicate aberrant glutamate and GABA transmission in the etiopathogenesis of MDD.

GLUTAMATERGIC DYSFUNCTION IN MDD

As the principal excitatory neurotransmitter in the circuitry linking limbic and cortical areas, glutamate is virtually ubiquitous in the brain. Cortical glutamatergic projections have a principal role in modulating activity in the brainstem mono-amine nuclei, giving origin to NE in the locus ceruleus (LC), serotonin (5-hydroxytryptamine, 5HT) in the raphe nuclei (RN), and dopamine (DA) in the sub-stantia nigra and ventral tegmental area (VTA).

Several classes of receptors are involved in mediating glutamatergic neuro-transmission. Ionotropic receptors, as the name suggests, are coupled to ion channels and include receptors for N-methyl-D-aspartate (NMDAR), alpha-amino-3-hydroxyl-5 methyl-4-isoxazolepropionate (AMPAR), and kainite. For NMDARs to be activated, neural membranes must also express AMPARs. NMDARs uncoupled from AMPARs are often referred to as "silent" NMDARs.[5] Increased glutamatergic activity leads to repeated activation of the synaptic NMDARs, promoting the synthesis of brain-derived neurotrophic factor (BDNF). Binding of BDNF to cognate tyrosine receptor kinase B (TrkB) receptors facilitates synaptic delivery of AMPAR, thereby mediating neural plasticity and long-term potentiation, key mechanisms for translating experience into enduring modi-fication of synaptic transmission.[5,6] Additionally, BDNF modulates dendritic arborization and synaptic spine density and morphology, contributing to a micro-feed-forward circuit that allows the brain to rewire in response to increased neu-ral activity.[6] Furthermore, indirect evidence suggests that glutamate signaling via NMDARs on the precursor cells may support neurogenesis.[7,8] Moreover, engage-ment of synaptic NMDARs promotes resistance to oxidative stress.[9]

In contradistinction to activation of the *synaptic* NMDAR, glutamate binding to *extrasynaptic* NMDARs has the opposite effect: it shuts off the intracellular cyclical adenosine monophosphate (cAMP) response element binding protein (CREB) signaling pathway and thus suppresses BDNF synthesis.[10,11] Additionally, extrasynaptic NMDAR activation causes loss of mitochondrial membrane poten-tial, an early harbinger of apoptosis.[10] Excessive glutamate signaling and engage-ment of NMDARs (especially the extrasynaptic receptors) induce toxic cell destruction, termed *excitotoxicity*. Excitotoxicity is characterized by mitochon-drial dysfunction, leading to its collapse, and morphological changes of neurons, including focal swelling of dendrites, as well as loss of synaptic spines.[12]

NMDAR-mediated glutamate transmission is further modulated by several potentiators. Astrocytes are active partners with neurons in transmission. D-serine released by astrocytes binds to the glycine site associated with NMDAR and facilitates its activation.[13] Because astrocyte processes "coat" neurons, the degree of coverage defines the accessibility of glycine sites and therefore NMDAR-mediated neuroplasticity.[13] Furthermore, inflammatory cytokines, released primarily by microglia (although some are of astrocytic origin), significantly modulate glutamatergic transmission. Tumor necrosis factor-alpha (TNF) causes rapid translocation of AMPARs to the cell membrane, enabling NMDAR-mediated signaling.[14] Moreover, TNF also triggers endocytosis of GABA-A receptors, thus actively shaping the GABA/glutamate balance and neuroplasticity.[14] TNF critically regulates glutamate release from astrocytes. Glutamate released by astrocytes engages neuronal presynaptic NMDARs, which in a feed-forward fashion facilitate glutamate release.[15] Additionally, preclinical studies have substantiated that interleukin-6 (IL-6) administration upregulated NMDAR-mediated functions, potentially contributing to neurotoxicity.[16] Thus, glia cells and immune molecules collaborate in potentiating glutamate transmission.

Furthermore, glutamate also binds to three different classes of presynaptic and postsynaptic metabotropic glutamate receptors (mGluRs), which are G-protein-coupled receptors with a role in modulating neurotransmitter release and postsynaptic activation of AMPARs and NMDARs.[17] The group I mGluRs include mGlu-1 and -5; group II, mGlu-2 and -3; and group III, mGlu-4, -6, -7, and -8.[18] Group I mGluRs are coupled to the phosphatidylinositol hydrolysis/Ca^{2+} signal transduction pathway. Group II and III mGluRs are both coupled in an inhibitory fashion to the adenylyl cyclase (AC) signaling cascade.[17]

Mostly preclinical evidence suggests that mGluRs may have a role in the pathophysiology of MDD and its treatment. Glutamate interacts with astrocytic group I mGluRs in the basal forebrain, precipitating BDNF release from astrocytes, which supports the function of the local cholinergic neurons.[19] Activation of basal forebrain mGluRs may also be important for the memory processes. On the other hand, evidence suggests that both chronic imipramine treatment and electroconvulsive therapy (ECT) suppress responsiveness of group I mGluRs, an effect associated with antidepressant behavioral effects in preclinical studies.[17,20] Group II and III mGluRs are most often located on presynaptic glutamatergic terminals, where they act to diminish excessive glutamate release.[21] Aversive stimuli upregulate group II mGluRs in the key limbic areas implicated in depression: the amygdala and insula. Not surprisingly, behavioral sensitization induced by aversive stimuli is suppressed by group II mGluR agonists.[21] Group II mGluR antagonists have demonstrated antidepressant behavioral effects in preclinical models, presumably by modulating glutamate release in the serotonergic dorsal raphe nucleus (DRN).[22] Preclinical evidence has implicated group III mGluR-7 in the regulation of amygdala plasticity and fear extinction. Activation of mGluR-7 blocked fear learning and acquisition of aversive memories.[23] Group III mGluR agonists have been shown to have antidepressant and anxiolytic-like effects in animal studies.[24]

There are five types of glutamate transporters on the neural and glia cellular membranes, also known as excitatory amino acid transporters (EAAT) 1 through 5.[25,26] Glutamate transporters play a key role in regulating glutamate transmission and keeping the neurotransmitter concentration within its narrow physiological boundaries, between 1 and 3 µM.[25,27] Dysfunction of EAATs may lead to excitotoxicity and neurodegeneration; glial EAATs may play a particularly important role in this respect.[28] Proinflammatory cytokines, such as IL-1, IL-6, and TNF, may in part produce their neuropsychiatric effects, including fatigue, by interfering with the function of EAATs.[27] Nuclear factor kappa-beta, one of the principal targets of the intracellular cascade activated by inflammatory cytokines, is also a potent regulator of EAAT expression.[28] A postmortem study of MDD patients found diminished hippocampal expression of SLCA2 and -3 and increased expression of SLCA7 (genes coding respectively for glial EAAT-2, glial EAAT-1, and neuronal vesicular glutamate transporter, respectively), compared with controls.[26] These findings support the proposed glutamate uptake dysfunction in MDD.

Stress, glucocorticoids, and monoamines may in a reciprocal way interact with glutamatergic transmission, altering neuroplasticity and neurogenesis. Adrenal steroids and stress have been shown to cause excessive NMDA activation and increase intracellular Ca^{2+}, suppress neurogenesis through NMDA-dependent process, and enhance glutamate release via presynaptic NMDA-related mechanisms.[29–31] Stress-precipitated alterations in glutamate signaling may have an enduring impact on adaptive neuroplasticity, especially if stressful events occurred earlier in life.[32] Evidence suggests that stress and glucocorticoid amplification of glutamate signaling may be responsible for dendritic remodeling, and changes in emotional responses, memory, and cognition characteristic of mood and anxiety disorders.[33] Furthermore, chronic treatment with conventional antidepressants reduces NMDA- and AMPA-mediated glutamate transmission and presynaptic glutamate release, while NMDA antagonists, such as ketamine, exert rapid and robust antidepressant effect.[33]

Glutamate and DA mutually regulate each other's signaling in limbic areas, including the nucleus accumbens (NAcc). Glutamate release in the shell of the NAcc stimulates AMPARs and upregulates DA transmission. Elevation of DA transmission, in the same location, precipitates an increase in the extracellular glutamate levels.[34] Glutamate signaling via mGluRs modulates release of not only DA but also 5HT and NE.[22] Moreover, dopaminergic stimulation of astrocytes attenuates the endogenous release of kynurenic acid, which acts as a functional NMDA antagonist, therefore indirectly enhancing glutamatergic transmission.[35] Furthermore, DA, NE, and 5HT neurons may be equipped for "double duty": they have been shown to possess vesicles filled with glutamate and vesicular glutamate transporters.[36]

5HT is involved in complex bimodal regulation of glutamate transmission. Activation of 5HT1A receptors on pyramidal neurons has an inhibitory effect and suppresses NMDA function. Conversely, 5HT2A stimulation enhances presynaptic glutamate release.[37] Preclinical studies have demonstrated that endogenous 5HT, acting via 5HT1B receptors, potentiates glutamatergic transmission in the rodent hippocampus. This serotonergic potentiation of excitatory transmission is altered in animal models of depression and restored by chronic antidepressant administration.[38] Interaction between 5HT and glutamate tends to have a regionally specific character. Magnetic resonance spectroscopic (MRS) studies have discovered that serotonergic stimulation of the hypothalamus results in depletion of the local glutamate/glutamine stores (Glx signal), which temporally coincides with the release of adrenocorticotropic hormone and cortisol in healthy volunteers.[39]

Cross talk between NE and glutamate systems is extremely complex and regionally specific. Exhaustive review of the topic is beyond the scope of this text, so we limit our discussion to a few examples. Emotional stress and subsequent activation of beta adrenergic receptors (ARs) increases the synaptic strength by facilitating the insertion of AMPARs into the neuronal membrane. NE-mediated activation of alpha-2 ARs on glutamatergic neurons closes hyperpolarization-activated cyclic-nucleotide-gated channels (HCNs), decreasing the action potential threshold and facilitating sustained firing.[40] Some researchers have postulated that alpha-2 AR–mediated closure of HCNs and subsequent sustained firing of cortical pyramidal neurons form the physiological underpinning of working memory.[41] HCNs and alpha-2 ARs are colocalized on pyramidal dendritic spines,[41] demonstrating the "location is everything" principle.

Here are a few more examples of the "location is everything" principle. Temporal cortical NE activation of alpha-1 ARs results in diminished glutamate neuron firing, while beta-AR stimulation increases excitatory responses. In the prefrontal cortex (PFC), the roles are completely reversed: alpha-1 AR activation has an excitatory effect, while beta AR stimulation leads to inhibition of glutamatergic transmission.[40] The bed nucleus of stria terminalis (BNST) is one of the main recipients of central NE innervation; it is also a main "effector" organ of stress response, coordinating input from the amygdala and orchestrating hypothalamic-pituitary-adrenal (HPA) axis and sympathetic response to stress and threat.[42] NE influx and activation of alpha-2 ARs in the ventral BNST produce inhibition, while stimulation of beta-2 ARs in the dorsal BNST increases glutamate signaling in this region.[43] If we were to further incorporate NE regulation of astroglia and microglia (discussed later in this chapter) and their influence on glutamate synapses, we would be confronted with daunting complexity.

Although little direct clinical evidence supports glutamatergic involvement in MDD, convergent results of the imaging, biochemical, preclinical, and treatment studies all point in the same direction. Early studies evaluating serum and plasma glutamate levels in MDD generated equivocal findings.[11] Very few researchers examined cerebrospinal fluid (CSF) glutamate levels in depressed patients. One of these studies discovered significantly higher CSF glutamine concentrations in depressed patients than in the control group. The authors speculated that glutamine elevation in the patient group may be attributable either to glial dysfunction or to neuronal inability to convert glia-produced glutamine into glutamate.[44] Further extending these findings, a postmortem study observed increased glutamate levels in the frontal cortex of MDD and bipolar disorder patients. Additionally, a positive correlation was noted between D-serine and glutamate levels.[45] Because D-serine is a coactivator of the NMDARs, one would assume an increase in NMDA-mediated glutamatergic transmission in this group of mood-disordered patients. Other postmortem studies have described reduced expression of glutamate transporters in frontal cortical areas of depressed patients.[46] Moreover, a study compared CSF levels of glutamate and corticotropin-releasing factor (CRF) in a group of depressed patients and healthy controls. In the depressed group higher suicidal ratings at baseline correlated with higher glutamate levels. Although there were no overall significant differences in the CSF measures of glutamate and CRF between the control and patient group, either at baseline or after treatment, there was a significant posttreatment reduction in glutamine.[47] A contrasting report indicated a significant reduction in CSF glutamate and glycine concentrations in a group of refractory affective disorder patients (bipolar I and II and MDD) versus controls.[48]

MRS studies have noted decreased Glx (a measure combining glutamate, homocarnosine, GABA, and glutamine spectroscopic signatures) in the anterior cingulate cortex (ACC) and amygdala of depressed adults, children, and elderly patients.[11] Furthermore, both ACC Glx and glutamate were significantly decreased in the subgroup of severely depressed patients.[49] In one of these studies, aberrant Glx measures normalized with successful ECT treatment (see ref[11] and ref[50] for a review). Moreover, duration of illness and remission status likely have a bearing on glutamatergic transmission. A group of authors utilized MRS to evaluate glutamate in the ventromedial PFC (vmPFC) of 45 depressed patients (10 first-episode MDD, 16 remitted-recurrent MDD, and 19 chronic MDD) and 15 healthy controls. Levels of glutamate were significantly reduced in both remitted-recurrent and chronic-MDD patients relative to first-episode MDD patients and controls. The decrease of glutamate in the remitted-recurrent and chronic-MDD groups was substantial (up to 28 percent mean reduction) and was negatively correlated with illness duration.[51] The same group later reported significant Glx and N-acetylaspartate (a measure of neuronal integrity) reductions in patients with treatment-resistant/chronic and remitted-recurrent MDD compared with controls, which was especially pronounced in the right hippocampal region. The decrease in the hippocampal Glx levels was again proportional to illness duration.[52] Reduced cortical glutamate and N-acetylaspartate in MDD patients, relative to controls, has been described by other authors.[53]

Contrasting these findings, another research group discovered a significantly higher glutamine:GABA ratio in the occipital cortex of depressed individuals than in matched healthy controls. Additional reports indicate changes in the NMDAR glycine binding site in depressed suicide victims and in NMDAR subunits in LC of depressed subjects.[11] Furthermore, dysregulation of cortical pyramidal neuron signaling may have a bearing on the function of the remote brain areas to which they project. Abnormal function of glutamatergic fibers originating from the vmPFC and projecting to sympathetic and parasympathetic brainstem centers has also been discovered in MDD patients.[54] This finding may provide a link between emotional dysregulation and the excessive stress reactivity, which has been repeatedly noted in depressed individuals.[54] Unfortunately, this cycle of glutamatergic dysfunction may be self-perpetuating, as stress and glucocorticoids excessively enhance glutamate transmission in limbic and cortical areas involved with mood regulation, interfering with neuroplasticity and precipitating substantial pathological changes in these formations.[55] The rapid effect of glucocorticoids on glutamatergic transmission in the PFC is mediated by glucocorticoid and mineralocorticoid receptors, respectively.[55] While acute stress increases the membrane expression of AMPARs, chronic stress downregulates both AMPAR- and NMDAR-mediated signaling. Chronic stress may also interfere with glutamate clearance, thereby compounding on the synaptic dysfunction.[55,56]

Preclinical studies of different classes of antidepressants and electroconvulsive seizures in a variety of animal models of depression also provide indirect evidence implicating glutamatergic disturbance in MDD.[56] Chronic administration of conventional monoamine-modulating antidepressants is associated with a reduction in membrane expression of the NMDAR subunits.[55,56] Furthermore, chronic, but not acute, administration of antidepressants reduced glutamate release, most likely by interfering with synaptic protein function.[56] Chronic antidepressant administration in the preclinical models blocked glutamate release, induced by stressful stimuli, in the key limbic areas, including the amygdala and hippocampus.[56] Additionally, several classes of antidepressant medications normalized stress-induced expression of NMDARs and AMPARs on the cell surface and prevented ensuing reduction in dendritic arborization.[56] A novel class of positive AMPA-modulating agents have shown ability to mitigate the negative impact of stress on AMPA expression and restore stress-impaired long-term potentiation. Preliminary evidence stemming from preclinical studies suggests that AMPA-modulating compounds show promise as potential antidepressant, procognitive agents.[57–59] Open label studies of lamotrigine and rizulole (both inhibitors of glutamate release), as well as controlled randomized trials of ketamine (an NMDA antagonist), in treatment-resistant depressed (TRD) patients provide preliminary evidence of efficacy of glutamatergic modulators in the treatment of MDD.[60] Burgeoning clinical evidence supporting ketamine benefits in MDD has been extensively reviewed in literature.[56,59,61,62] Both ketamine and a newer NMDAR antagonist, traxoprodil, have established antidepressants effects in randomized controlled trials.[59,60] The antidepressant effect following intravenous infusion of ketamine was rapid (within a matter of hours), robust, sustained over at least 72 hours and was replicated in studies of depressed suicidal patients, TRD patients, and bipolar depressed patients.[46,59]

Interestingly, reviews suggest that ketamine response in depressed patients may be based on an "all-or-nothing" principle. In a study utilizing three doses of ketamine over a 12-day period to treat TRD, the response rate (>50 percent reduction in the score on a standardized scale) was 71 percent. The initial response was maintained with multiple doses; however, the patients who failed to respond to the initial response continued to be nonresponders with subsequent administrations.[63] The antidepressant effect of ketamine may in part be mediated by its ability to increase the presynaptic glutamate release and then "reroute" it by blocking NMDARs and directing glutamate transmission toward AMPARs.[55] Preclinical studies have additionally evidenced that ketamine administration results in elevation of BDNF and its downstream target, mTOR (mammalian target of rapamycin), a known regulator of activity-dependent synaptogenesis.[64–66] Furthermore, initial clinical evidence supports the ameliorating effect of ketamine on neurotrophic signaling. A group of patients suffering from TRD who experienced a response to ketamine infusion showed a significant increase in plasma BDNF compared with nonresponders. The degree of plasma BDNF elevation correlated with decreases in Montgomery-Åsberg Depression Rating Scale (MADRS) scores, indicating clinical improvement.[67] Moreover, ketamine suppresses proapoptotic glycogen synthase 3-beta (GSK-3b), decreases GABA transmission (most likely via antagonism of facilitatory presynaptic NMDARs), and reduces proinflammatory IL-1 and IL-6 in rodent PFC and hippocampus. Further extending these findings, ketamine reduces depressive-like behaviors in the animal models of depression.[64,66,68] Indirect enhancement of glutamate release, mediated by suppression of inhibitory GABA transmission, may be an important aspect of ketamine-related antidepressant activity. Lamotrigine, a glutamate release modulator, successfully mitigated perceptual disturbances related to excessive glutamatergic transmission following ketamine administration, suggesting that these agents in some instances may have opposing actions.[69]

Neural correlates of ketamine response are still open to debate due to lack of consistency in the results of imaging studies evaluating its effect on cerebral function. Earlier studies reported reduction in the activity of the vmPFC, subgenual ACC, and orbitofrontal cortex, which strongly predicted its dissociative effects. Pretreatment with lamotrigine (see above) abrogated most of the functional brain changes and largely prevented psychotic-like symptoms. Intriguingly, risperidone (an atypical antipsychotic) also blocked ketamine-induced reduction in subgenual ACC activity.[70] These findings may be relevant for understanding the mode of ketamine action in MDD, given that subgenual ACC hyperactivity is one of the most consistent imaging findings in this disease state. Other imaging evidence suggests that ketamine may be a modulator of medial and orbital prefrontal network activity in MDD.[71] Chapter 8, focusing on the functional and structural brain changes in MDD, discusses the dysfunction of resting networks and their clinical correlates. It appears that ketamine administration produces a significant reduction in the aberrant connectivity between the "dorso-medial nexus," subgenual ACC (a hub of the salience network), and the default mode network (DMN). Ketamine also reduced dysfunctional connectivity between the two principal components of the DMN: the posterior cingulate cortex and the medial PFC (mPFC).[72] Abnormal connectivity between the components of the DMN and the salience network was strongly associated with rumination, cognitive dysfunction, and the intensity of depression.

Initial clinical evidence suggests that zinc and magnesium, both functional NMDAR antagonists, may have a role as adjuncts in the treatment of MDD. Zinc (25 mg/daily) effectively augmented imipramine in addressing TRD.[59] Preclinical and preliminary clinical investigations have provided proof of antidepressant-like properties of mGlu-2/3 agonists and antagonists, mGlu-5 antagonists, and mGlu-7 positive modulators.[55,56,59] Antagonists of mGlu-2/3 may increase synaptic levels of glutamate, potentiate AMPAR signaling, and elevate 5HT and DA transmission.[56] Acamprosate, a functional NMDA and mGlu-5 antagonist currently used in the treatment of alcoholism, has demonstrated some antidepressant-like activity.[59] Tianeptine, approved for treatment of MDD in several countries, but not in the United States, has been shown to suppress glutamate surge following stress in preclinical models of depression.[59]

We have discussed the role of glutamate in MDD in some detail. Multiple layers of evidence indicate its central role in the pathophysiology of this disease. Here we briefly summarize the key findings. Known precipitants of depression, such as stress and inflammation, have a significant impact on glutamatergic transmission in the key limbic and cortical areas involved in mood regulation. Elevation of inflammatory cytokines and glucocorticoids is associated with increase in glutamate signaling. Additionally, dysregulated glutamatergic transmission can precipitate inflammatory cytokine release from glia cells. Furthermore, glia cells express ionotropic glutamate receptors and mGluRs and actively participate in regulating synaptic transmission. One of the main pathohistological findings in MDD is decreased density of astrocytes in several limbic and cortical areas implicated in the pathophysiology of depression by imaging studies. Decline in glial numbers and function is likely to profoundly impact glutamate transmission in the affected areas. Postmortem studies evaluating glutamate levels and transporter density in the brain tissue, CSF analyses of glutamate in MDD patients, and MRI have all detected glutamatergic abnormalities in depressed populations. Pharmacological manipulation of NMDAR has produced dramatic relief of depressive symptomatology, within a matter of minutes to hours. Even conventional antidepressant agents have been shown to influence glutamate transmission. By contrast, monoamine-modulating antidepressants require weeks to provide symptomatic relief, and even then in only about half of the depressed patients. Thus, convergent evidence points to the primacy of glutamatergic disturbance in the pathophysiology of MDD.

ALTERATIONS IN GABA-MEDIATED TRANSMISSION IN MDD

We now turn our attention to the role of GABA in MDD. GABA neurons are widely distributed in virtually all brain areas. They account for up to 20–40 percent of all neurons, depending on the brain region.[73] GABA concentrations in the central nervous system (CNS) are approximately a thousand times greater than concentrations of monoamine transmitters.[74] The amygdala, hippocampus, hypothalamus, and PFC are all endowed with dense GABA neuronal projections.[74] Although GABAergic neurons are perhaps best known for their short local projections and their role as interneurons, there are also longer GABAergic tracts. GABA cells sometimes have specialized names, such as Purkinje cells in the cerebellum; basket cells are cortical GABA neurons that receive signals from the thalamus and form axosomatic synapses; cortical GABA chandelier cells participate in axoaxonal synapses with local pyramidal neurons; double bouquet cells compose axodendritic synapses in cortical minicolumns; and spiny neurons reside in the striatum.[74,75] Aside from the shorter inhibitory GABAergic projections linking basal ganglia substructures and the thalamus, there are also longer bidirectional GABA pathways connecting the hippocampus and entorhinal cortex, as well as neocortical long-range GABA projections.[74,75] Basalocortical GABA projection neurons target other GABA cells in the PFC and cingulate cortex.[75] The consequences of GABA neuron activation can be dramatically different, depending on their targets: if GABA neurons synapse with an excitatory pyramidal neuron. they will produce a "true" inhibitory effect, as opposed to GABA neurons projecting to another GABA neuron, which may ultimately generate a disinhibiting effect. Cortical GABA interneurons have a unique property: they are capable of adult neurogenesis (albeit limited).[76] The functional impact of new neocortical GABA interneurons is still uncertain.

Not all GABA cells in the brain are neurons. Astrocytes are endowed with GABA receptors, synthetic and catabolic enzymes, transporters, and release mechanisms.[77] Furthermore, GABA of astrocyte origin may play an "unorthodox" role: it exercises an anti-inflammatory influence by stabilizing microglial cells. Much more information on this subject can be found in the Chapter 7, Astrocyte transmitters.

GABA is synthesized by two different forms of glutamate decarboxylase (GAD), 67- and 65-kDa forms. Its levels are regulated by the catabolic enzyme GABA-α-ketoglutaric acid aminotransferase.[77] Pyridoxine (vitamin B6) is a cofactor in the synthesis of GABA.[74] Two distinct classes of GABA receptors mediate GABA transmission. GABA-A receptors are ligand-gated ionotropic chloride channel-linked receptors, while GABA-B receptors belong to a class of metabotropic G-protein-coupled inhibitory receptors.[74]

Monoamine-secreting neurons and GABA neurons are engaged in a rich cross talk. Activation of GABA-B receptors exerts an inhibitory influence on 5HT and NE release.[74] 5HT in turn, via 5HT1A and 5HT1C receptors, inhibits GABA and glutamate transmission, respectively,[78] while activation of 5HT2A/2C receptors on GABA neurons has an excitatory impact.[79] 5HT may indirectly influence NE, acetylcholine, and its own release by binding to 5HT3 receptors on the inhibitory GABA neurons.[80]

The relationship between NE and GABA transmission is complex. Presynaptic beta ARs and somatodendritic alpha-1 ARs both facilitate GABA transmission, contrary to activation of axon-terminal alpha-2 ARs, which inhibit GABA signaling.[81,82] Furthermore, research has revealed that stress-related noradrenergic signaling via beta ARs located on excitatory neurons may in turn initiate glutamatergic signaling to mGlu-1 receptors on GABA neurons, converting them into an excitatory status.[83] These neuroplastic changes may contribute to stress-related neuroendocrine sensitization.[83] Moreover, NE may have a capacity to decrease GABA synthesis in the limbic stress circuits.[84]

Additional preclinical studies have offered evidence of the importance of GABA transmission in neuroendocrine regulation. In one study genetically lesioned mice were rendered incapable of synthesizing fully functional GABA-A receptors. Baseline corticosterone concentrations in GABA-deficient mice were elevated regardless whether the genetic lesion was induced during embryogenesis or delayed until adolescence. However, the manifestation of anxious-depressive behavioral phenotype correlated only with early postnatal onset of HPA axis hyperactivity. Chronic, but not acute, DMI and fluoxetine treatment of genetically altered mice normalized anxiety-like behavior. In addition, DMI normalized both depression-like behavior and HPA axis function. By contrast, fluoxetine was ineffective as an antidepressant and failed to normalize HPA axis function.[85] This study provides preliminary evidence that effective HPA regulation requires proper GABA function. Furthermore, antidepressants that modulate NE and 5HT may have differential effects on anxious and depressive phenotypes, as well as on normalization of the HPA activity. In aggregate, preclinical evidence supports involvement of complex, reciprocal, and iterative communication among monoamine/GABA/glutamate signaling and endocrine systems in modulation of stress- and mood-regulating corticolimbic networks.

Several studies have reported reduction of plasma GABA levels in MDD (see ref[86] for a review). One of these studies compared plasma GABA levels in a group of MDD patients before and after treatment with those of healthy volunteers. At baseline GABA levels were lower in patient samples, whereas glutamate and glutamine levels were higher. An increase in plasma GABA levels and a decrease in glutamate and glutamine levels were observed following a 10-day course of two different selective serotonin reuptake inhibitor (SSRI) agents. No difference was detected between the drug treatments. This is a preliminary indication that plasma GABA levels may be considered as a marker of treatment response in MDD.[87] Additionally, researchers have established that GABA CSF levels were significantly more reduced in the groups of depressed patients relative to control subjects.[74,88] Further extending these findings, postmortem studies detected decreased GABA neurons in the lateral orbital PFC and dorsolateral PFC (dlPFC) of depressed individuals, relative to controls.[88,89] A postmortem study found strong molecular evidence of a combined GABA and BDNF dysfunction in the amygdala of female subjects who suffered from MDD. Compared with the control group, depressed subjects had diminished amygdala gene transcripts of peptides related to GABA interneurons and a parallel reduction in BDNF RNA and protein levels.[90] Possibly contradicting these findings, Bielau et al.,[91] using the GABA synthetic enzyme GAD-65/67 as a marker, reported higher GABA neuronal densities in MDD patients compared with controls in the dlPFC, superior temporal cortex, orbitofrontal cortex, and hippocampus. Interestingly, in depressed patients, dose equivalents of antidepressant agents given prior to death correlated positively with neuronal density in the superior temporal cortex and hippocampus.[91]

In aggregate, data point to dysregulation of the GABAergic system in corticolimbic regions in MDD patients. It is possible that antidepressant treatment may ameliorate or even overcompensate for deficits of GABAergic neurotransmission. Further supporting the compensating effect of antidepressant treatment on GABA transmission, another group of researchers noted a substantial reduction of GAD-67 (34 percent drop) in the dlPFC (Brodmann area 9) of depressed subjects compared with matched controls, which was absent in depressed individuals treated with antidepressants.[92] These are particularly intriguing findings, given the previously described role of dlPFC and lateral orbital PFC in cognition, voluntary regulation of emotion, and suppression of maladaptive affect.

Imaging studies provided further proof of GABA involvement in MDD. Early MRS studies suggested that altered cortical GABA and glutamate concentrations may not only differentiate MDD patients from controls but also differentiate melancholy and atypical depressive subtypes from each other.[93] Depressed patients had significantly lower occipital cortex GABA and increased glutamate concentrations than did healthy controls. Alterations in GABA and glutamate concentrations were more pronounced in patients with melancholy than in patients with atypical MDD. This study demonstrated that an altered ratio of excitatory to inhibitory neurotransmitter levels in the cortex of depressed subjects may be a correlate of abnormal brain function in this condition. Furthermore, MRS GABA measures may serve as a biological marker for a subtype of MDD.[93]

Other evidence points to anomalies of GABA transmission early in MDD and their association with particular symptomatic manifestations of the disorder. A group of investigators using MRS imaging discovered a significant decrease in

ACC GABA signal in adolescents with MDD, relative to control subjects. More-over, ACC GABA levels were negatively correlated with anhedonia scores for the whole MDD group.[94] Another study comparing GABA levels in unmedicated depressed patients and healthy controls showed reduced GABA levels in the dor-sal and pregenual ACC, dlPFC, and frontopolar cortex (Brodmann area 10) of affected individuals.[95] These are the same brain areas in which pathohistological studies established alterations in glial density in MDD patients, compared with healthy controls.[95]

Furthermore, the age of onset and duration of illness may influence cortical GABA concentrations. While researchers found no difference in the GABA con-centrations between remitted MDD subjects and healthy controls in the vmPFC and dlPFC, additional analyses provided evidence of a negative relationship between the Glx:GABA ratio in the vmPFC and the age of onset of MDD.[96] Other studies have also provided evidence that treatment response status may have some bearing on brain GABA levels. A study comparing a depressed cohort with TRD patients and healthy controls noted a decrease in occipital cortex GABA levels in the TRD group compared with both healthy volunteers (20.2 percent mean reduction) and non-TRD depressed subjects (16.4 percent mean reduction). The same study detected a similar effect of diagnosis on ACC GABA levels.[97] Sev-eral preclinical and clinical studies have noted that antidepressants and ECT may improve GABA deficits.[84,88]

In conclusion, convergent evidence from preclinical, postmortem, clinical, and imaging studies has implicated GABA dysfunction in the pathophysiology of MDD. There is some indication that deficits in CNS GABA signaling and even reductions in GABA neuron density may be more state markers rather than trait markers, because these alterations tend to normalize with successful antidepres-sant treatments.

Monoamine Neurotransmitters in MDD

Our brief review of the brain monoamine signaling is not intended to be compre-hensive or exhaustive. Instead, we provide a cogent background for a discussion of altered monoamine transmission in MDD and the mechanism of action of antide-pressant medications.

SEROTONIN TRANSMISSION

More than one label can be appropriately assigned to designate the role of 5HT. Although it is most often considered to be a neurotransmitter, achieving its physi-ological role by binding to pre- and postsynaptic receptors, 5HT can also act as a neuromodulator and a neurohormone, via "volume transmission" and enduring action.[98] Much like other monoamines, 80 percent of 5HT is released into extracellular space in a paracrine manner, not into the synapse.[99] Despite this "sprinkler" type release, functional concentrations of 5HT are maintained over the span of several micrometers.[100] In other words, 5HT does not appear to have been designed to deliver messages with a pinpoint accuracy; instead, it influences assemblies of neurons and glial cells.

5HT is an ancient molecule. Estimates suggest that its receptors appeared some 800 million years ago in single-cell organisms such as paramecia and amoebas.[101] Through evolution it has developed into an extensive neurosignaling system, aside from glutamatergic transmission.[102] Multiple roles of 5HT include endocrine regulation; modulation of affect and stress response; sensory gating; regulation of sleep and appetite; synapse formation; pain modulation; gastrointestinal, sexual, and vascular function; and platelet aggregation.[100,101,103]

There are only approximately 250,000 5HT neurons in the human brain, which is a relatively humble number given that the brain numbers one hundred *billion* nerve cells. Most 5HT neurons originate from the DRN, median RN, and mesencephalic/pontine nuclei, from which they project to virtually all cortical and limbic areas, as well as basal ganglia, hypothalamus, and thalamus (see figure 9.1).[102,104,105] Other serotonergic fibers innervating the cerebellum originate

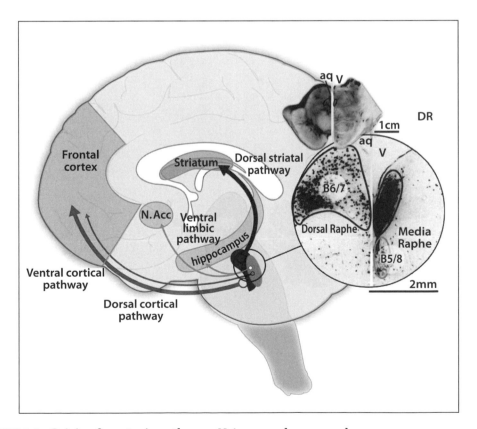

FIGURE 9.1. Origin of serotonin pathways. N.Acc = nucleus accumbens.

from the lower brainstem nuclei.[103] Although there are relatively few 5HT neurons, they have a disproportionately robust impact due to the high density of 5HT-releasing axonal varicosities, up to 100,000 per cubic millimeter of neocortical tissue.[102]

Both in the CNS, and in peripheral tissues, 5HT is synthesized first from l-tryptophan to 5-hydroxytryptophan, mediated by tryptophan hydroxylase, and then to 5HT, with assistance from l-amino acid decarboxylase.[98] In the pineal gland 5HT serves as a substrate for the synthesis of melatonin.[106] Surplus 5HT may either be removed from the synapse by a 5HT transporter (5HTT) or undergo endocellular degradation to 5-hydroxyindoleacetic acid (5HIAA), primarily by MAOA, although MAOB may also be involved.[98] In the CNS, 5HT breakdown takes place either in neurons or in astrocytes.

5HT achieves its physiological actions by signaling via seven different receptor classes, which are composed of 14 distinct receptors.[102,103] Our review focuses on the 5HT receptors with established relevance in pathophysiology of MDD or its treatment. All of the 5HT receptors are G-protein-coupled receptors aside from 5HT3, which is a ionotropic receptor, coupled to cation channels, much like nicotinic receptors and several of the glutamate and some glycine and GABA receptors.

There are three subtypes of 5HT1 receptors, labeled A through C. All three are linked to inhibition of adenylate cyclase and are localized as pre- and postsynaptic auto- and heteroreceptors. 5HT1A autoreceptors have a somatodendritic distribution and mediate regulation of 5HT release predominantly in the RN. Activation of 5HT1A presynaptic autoreceptors produces hyperpolarization, reduced firing rate and subsequently diminished 5HT synthesis and release.[101–103,105,107] 5HT-induced activation of the postsynaptic 5HT1A receptors located on GABA, glutamate, and cholinergic neurons results in hyperpolarization of corresponding neurons and inhibited transmission.[101–103,105,107] 5HT1A-mediated inhibition of GABA interneurons can also indirectly disinhibit the release of acetylcholine, glutamate, and DA.[101–103,105,107]

5HT1B receptors can also have a presynaptic and postsynaptic location. 5HT binding to terminal/axonal presynaptic 5HT1B/D autoreceptors inhibits 5HT release. 5HT1B heteroreceptors have been found on GABA interneurons, glutamatergic pyramidal neurons, and cholinergic neurons. Direct effects of 5HT1B activation produce inhibition of the cognate transmitter release, while activation of 5HT1B heteroreceptors on GABA neurons can inhibit their activity and therefore indirectly disinhibit the release of glutamate, acetylcholine, and other neurotransmitters. Signaling via 5HT1B and 5HT4 receptors is regulated by a p11 protein that colocalizes with these 5HT receptors and increases their function.[101–103,105,107]

Significant concentrations of 5HT2A receptors are found in cerebral cortices, brainstem nuclei, limbic areas, and basal ganglia. 5HT2A receptors are coupled to a stimulatory Gq/11 protein, initiating an increase in inositol phosphates and cytosolic Ca^{2+}. Hallucinogens, including LSD, have agonistic properties at the 5HT2A receptors. Activation of 5HT2A postsynaptic heteroreceptors stimulates glutamate, GABA, and DA release. 5HT2A-mediated activation of GABA interneurons can ultimately produce an inhibitory effect on glutamatergic, dopaminergic, noradrenergic, serotonergic, and cholinergic transmission, while 5HT2A-mediated activation of glutamatergic projections to monoaminergic brainstem nuclei would have an opposite effect.[101–103,105,107,108] Serotonergic stimulation of 5HT2C receptors located on GABA interneurons supports tonic inhibition of NE, DA, and 5HT. Therefore, 5HT2C antagonism may produce an enduring increase in monoamine release.[79,101,102,105,107]

Postsynaptic 5HT3 receptors gate the function of cation channels. They are located predominantly on dendrites of GABA interneurons. 5HT3 activation leads to a rapid depolarization associated with release of GABA and downstream inhibition of excitatory glutamatergic neurons, mediated by GABA-A and GABA-B receptors. Thus, direct 5HT3-driven inhibitory GABA effects, and indirect effects via GABA-mediated glutamatergic modulation (whereby GABA dampens glutamate-driven transmitter release), regulate DA, 5HT, and acetylcholine transmission.[101–103,105,107]

5HT4, 5HT6, and 5HT7 receptors are preferentially coupled to G_s proteins and activate various adenylate cyclases. Primary locations of the 5HT4 neurons are in the basal ganglia, especially the caudate and putamen, ventral striatum (including the NAcc), and substantia nigra. Lesser concentrations of 5HT4 have been described in the neocortex, amygdala, and hippocampus. Like 5HT1B, 5HT4 also requires the presence of p11 protein for optimal function. Activation of 5HT4 receptors on the cortical pyramidal neurons may be involved in feedback control of midbrain serotonergic neurons and also DA transmission. Early preclinical evidence supports the role of 5HT4 receptors in the early antidepressant response, memory, and neuroplasticity.[101–103,105,107]

5HT6 receptors are also postsynaptic receptors expressed with high density in the striatum, NAcc, and cortex and with lesser density in the hippocampus, amygdala, thalamus, hypothalamus, and cerebellum. Activation of the 5HT6 receptors mediates processes related to circadian regulation, feeding behavior, learning, memory, neuroplasticity (BDNF synthesis), and mood regulation. Preclinical evidence suggests that 5HT6 receptors modulate GABA, glutamate, DA, NE, and acetylcholine release. Application of 5HT6 antagonists in the preclinical models produces increases in acetylcholine release, which may contribute to precognitive effects of these agents. Preliminary evidence also supports antidepressant effect of 5HT6 antagonist in the animal models. Antidepressant effects may be mediated by indirect increases in release of DA and NE.[101,102,105,107]

Like 5HT6, 5HT7 receptors are also positively coupled to adenylate cyclase. They are highly expressed in the cortex, thalamus, hypothalamus, hippocampus, and suprachiasmatic nucleus. Postsynaptic somatodendritic 5HT7 heterore-ceptors have been identified on both GABA and pyramidal glutamate neurons. Axonally located 5HT7 receptors were identified on corticoraphe neurons. They presumably participate in glutamatergic modulation of 5HT transmission. Although their activation, based on the location of the receptor, has a potential t o be either excitatory (via glutamate) or inhibitory (via GABA); the net effect in healthy rodents appears to be mostly excitatory. Additionally, preclinical research has found evidence of 5HT7 participation in the regulation of the sleep–wakefulness cycle, sensory processing, temperature regulation, cognition, and mood (see figure 9.2).[101,102,105,107,109,110]

5HT transmission, originating from the RN, is to a significant degree regu-lated through complex feedback loops, reciprocally connecting it with the mPFC. Activation of the densely distributed postsynaptic 5HT1A receptors may inhibit cortical GABA interneurons, thus disinhibiting mPFC pyramidal glutamate neu-rons. Furthermore, mPFC glutamatergic neurons may be directly stimulated by an RN–mPFC serotonergic pathway via excitatory 5HT2A receptors. Excitatory glutamatergic feedback projections from the mPFC may directly stimulate 5HT neurons in the RN or inhibit them after interfacing with the local GABA neurons. Therefore, the yin-and-yang principle is represented in both afferent 5HT fibers and the efferent glutamatergic neurons feeding back to the RN. In this manner, 5HT neurons are simultaneously regulated by the local, immediate feedback loops involving 5HT1A autoreceptors and 5HT2A and -2C heteroreceptors on the local RN GABA neurons, but also in a delayed fashion, by either a facilitatory or inhibitory feedback from the remote mPFC pyramidal neurons.[105] Additionally, activation of the cortical 5HT4 receptors appears to elicit a rapid excitatory feed-back to the midbrain serotonergic neurons.

A "sensitivity hierarchy," prioritizing 5HT affinity for the 5HT1A receptors over 5HT2A and 5HT2C receptors, may provide an additional opportunity for fine-tuning in these regulatory loops. Moreover, 5HT2A receptors are not active during tonic 5HT neuron firing, they seem to be more responsive to the bursts of diffuse 5HT release (volume transmission) in the mPFC.[105] mPFC areas, espe-cially the vmPFC, are crucial for adaptive emotional regulation and stress response. As we noted in earlier chapters, the vmPFC is at the crossroads between more lateral and dorsal cognitive circuits and more ventral limbic and paralim-bic structures. Therefore, a sum of diverse signals converging on the mPFC indi-rectly influences the cortical glutamatergic feedback fibers projecting back to midbrain serotonergic nuclei, which in turn orchestrate the stress response. In this respect, evidence of compromised cortical 5HT1A postsynaptic function may help us to understand elevated emotional reactivity in the context of MDD.[105]

Convergent lines of evidence point to serotonergic dysfunction in MDD. Chap-ter 4 reviewed at length the genetic evidence implicating alleles regulating the synthesis of 5HTT, tryptophan hydroxylase (a synthesizing enzyme), and several

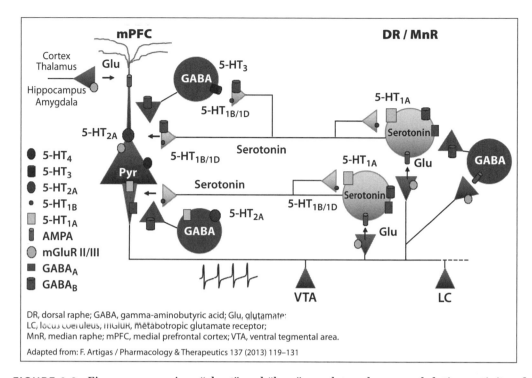

DR, dorsal raphe; GABA, gamma-aminobutyric acid; Glu, glutamate;
LC, locus coeruleus, mGluR, metabotropic glutamate receptor;
MnR, median raphe; mPFC, medial prefrontal cortex; VTA, ventral tegmental area.

Adapted from: F. Artigas / Pharmacology & Therapeutics 137 (2013) 119–131

FIGURE 9.2. Figure summarizes "short" and "long" regulatory loops modulating activity of brainstem monoamine nuclei. Serotonin nuclei in the midbrain, dorsal and median raphe nuclei (DR and MnR) provide a "short" collateral feedback loop ending in proximity of somato-dendritic 5HT1A autoreceptors. Excessive accumulation of 5HT in the synaptic cleft engages 5HT1A inhibitory autoreceptors, resulting in a reduced 5HT synthesis and diminished neuronal firing rate. Some of the longer serotonin projections innervate medial prefrontal cortex (mPFC). Terminal 5HT1B/1D autoreceptors respond to elevated 5HT concentration in mPFC synapses by suppressing further serotonin release. In addition to activation of postsynaptic 5HT receptors on glutamatergic neurons, serotonin projections also interface with GABAergic interneurons. Activation of 5HT3 and 5HT7 postsynaptic receptors on GABAergic interneurons leads to increased GABA release and consequently to inhibition of mPFC pyramidal glutamatergic neurons. Thus, through direct activation of postsynaptic 5HT2A receptors on mPFC glutamate neurons and inhibitory input mediated by 5HT3/7 stimulation of GABAergic interneurons, serotonin projections can fine-tune mPFC pyramidal neuron activity. The "long" feedback loop originates from pyramidal neurons in the mPFC which innervate the DR and MnR via excitatory synapses with 5-HT neurons. and. Activation of the mPFC results may increase 5-HT neuronal firing rate via excitation mediated by NMDA and AMPA glutamate receptors on 5HT neurons or lead to suppression of DR and MnR serotonin neurons due to activation of 5HT7 receptors on inhibitory GABAergic neurons. Therefore, brainstem 5HT neurons can modulate their own activity via the "short" auto-regulatory loop or via "long" regulatory loop which also involves serotoninergic modulation of mPFC pyramidal glutamatergic neuronal activity. AMPA = alpha-amino-3-hydroxy-5-methyl-4 isoxazolepropionic acid glutamatergic receptor; NMDA = N-methyl-D-aspartate glutamatergic receptor

different 5HT receptors in propagating the vulnerability toward MDD.[111-113] Early studies have reported lower levels of 5HT precursor tryptophan and diminished platelet 5HT uptake and 5HT2A receptor binding in depressed patients relative to healthy controls.[111] 5HT facilitates the release of prolactin by the pituitary gland; therefore, serotonergic agents, such as SSRIs and *d*-fenfluramine, can be utilized as chemical probes to indirectly assess the efficiency of serotonergic transmission. While some of the studies noted a compromised prolactin response to serotonergic agents among depressed patients, others have identified 5HT dysfunction only in a subgroup of depressed individuals (~40 percent), compared with healthy controls.[111,114] Studies of 5HT metabolites in the CSF of depressed patients have yielded highly contradictory results (discussed in some detail later in this chapter).

Imaging studies have provided more consistent evidence of reduced postsynaptic 5HT1A binding in the brains of depressed patients relative to controls; furthermore, this was even true in recovered patients.[109,111,113] Decreased density of 5HT1A receptors was associated with severe depression.[109] Persistently diminished 5HT1A binding in depressed individuals is therefore more likely a trait rather than a state marker. Findings of the postmortem studies generally echo the positron emission tomography (PET) imaging data, also revealing reduced 5HT1A density.[109]

PET imaging studies have found increased density of presynaptic 5HT1A in the RN, in contradistinction to postsynaptic receptors.[112] Increased expression of presynaptic 5HT1A receptors has been correlated with both depressed mood and increased amygdala reactivity in response to threatening stimuli. Similar to the pattern with the postsynaptic 5HT1A receptors, presynaptic receptors retained increased density even in remitted patients.[109,112] Although a hasty review of these findings might suggest a discrepancy, reports regarding density of pre- and postsynaptic 5HT1A receptors are actually consistent. Both increased inhibitory presynaptic 5HT1A autoreceptors and decreased postsynaptic 5HT1A heteroreceptors reflect insufficient 5HT signaling.

Imaging data on 5HT2A and 5HTT binding, comparing depressed patients with healthy controls, are fairly contradictory and may be regionally specific.[109,111,113] Most of the reports from postmortem and imaging studies indicate increased expression of the cortical postsynaptic 5HT2A receptors.[109,111,113,115] Increased cortical 5HT2A heteroreceptor binding was described in depressed suicide victims, depressed individuals, and recovered patients, compared with healthy subjects.[109,111,113] Other researchers have reported the opposite findings: lower cortical 5HT2A levels in the brain tissue of depressed patients and depressed individuals who committed suicide, relative to matched controls.[116] Unlike cortical 5HT2A receptors, hippocampal 5HT2A receptors appear to have decreased density in the depressed patients compared with the control group.[109] Divergent findings may be due to differences in methodology but may also reflect a substantial biological diversity inherent in MDD.[109,111]

Imaging studies comparing 5HTT densities between depressed patients and healthy subjects have had inconsistent findings. While some have found diminished 5HTT binding in MDD, which normalized with treatment, others have had contrary findings.[113,115,117] 5HT depletion studies and CSF metabolite assays are discussed later in the chapter.

NOREPINEPHRINE TRANSMISSION

Central noradrenergic fibers originate from seven brainstem nuclei, labeled A1 to A7 (see figure 9.3).[118,119] Noradrenergic nuclei can be further subdivided into three groups: caudal (medullary; A1 and A2), rostral (pontine; A6), and central (medullo-pontine group; A5 and A7). Caudal and central nuclei give rise to both ascending and descending fibers. Ascending fibers form the ventral noradrenergic bundle that projects to the midbrain reticular formation, hypothalamus (including the periventricular nucleus [PVN]), and parts of the limbic system. Descending fibers innervate the spinal cord.[118]

The most relevant noradrenergic nucleus, from the perspective of MDD pathophysiology, is A6, also known as the locus ceruleus (LC). Named after its bluish-

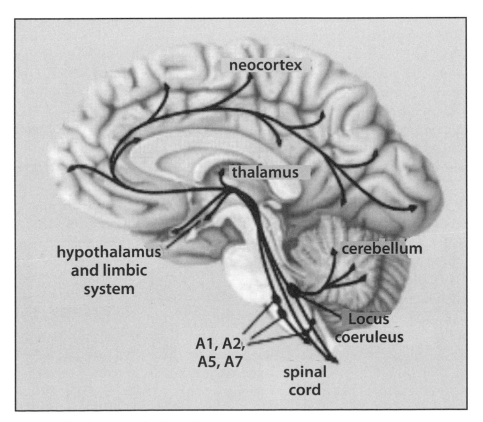

FIGURE 9.3. **Noradrenergic brain pathways.**

grayish color, the LC is the largest noradrenergic nucleus, giving rise to 50 percent of NE neurons.[118] The LC is approximately 14.5 mm long and 2.5 mm thick.[120] It contains as many as 60,000 neurons in younger and 40,000 in older individuals, or as few as 15,000 neurons, according to differing sources.[120,121] There are substantial gender differences in the number of NE neurons in the LC: women may have as many as 20 percent more NE neurons than do men in the LC.[122] It is not certain if and how this gender-related anatomical difference influences the risk of acquiring stress-related disorders, such as MDD.

The NE fibers from the LC project to the cortex, cingulate, amygdala, hippocampus, basal ganglia, thalamus, and hypothalamus.[120,121] The LC has bidirectional connections with CRF-producing neurons in the hypothalamic PVN. Both CRF and glutamate facilitate NE release from the LC in stressful situations, while, in turn, NE release in PVN stimulates CRF signaling.[118,119] Furthermore, the LC inhibits the hypothalamic sleep-promoting ventrolateral preoptic area, while GABA neurons in the ventrolateral preoptic area provide inhibitory feedback to the LC. Moreover, both lateral hypothalamic (LH) orexinergic and tuberomammilary histaminergic neurons provide excitatory input to LC NE neurons.[118] These complex LC–hypothalamic feedback loops have a principal role in regulation of the stress response, as well as sleep and wakefulness. Brain noradrenergic projections subserve multiple neural functions, including regulation of arousal, sleep and wakefulness, stress response, emotional regulation, attention, executive function, decision making, learning and memory, sensory processing, reward, regulation of motor activity, endocrine function, autonomic modulation, and neuroplasticity, respiratory, gastrointestinal, and immune activity.[104,118–121,123,124]

NE is synthesized from tyrosine, which is a common precursor for all three catecholamines, DA, NE, and epinephrine. Tyrosine hydroxylase (TH) converts tyrosine to 3,4-dihydroxyphenylalanine (DOPA), which is subsequently converted to DA and then, with enzymatic mediation of dopamine-beta-hydroxylase, to NE. Once synthesized, NE is stored in vesicles, also known as vesicular monoamine transporters (VMATs). While VMAT-1 stores monoamines in the periphery of the body, central catecholamines are stored in VMAT-2. Increase of intracellular calcium assists the merger of VMATs with cellular membranes.[125] The process of exocytosis, or neurotransmitter release, is further assisted by several synaptic proteins.

Much like other monoamines, NE is mostly released from extrasynaptic varicosities. NE passively diffuses in the extracellular space, reaching its cogent receptors.[99,118] Only about 20 percent of the NE in the brain is released in a typical neurotransmitter-like "neurocrine" manner, from the presynaptic nerve terminal into the synaptic cleft.[99,118] The described pattern of release would suggest that NE in the brain acts more like a neurohormone while participating in paracrine "volume transmission." Noradrenergic neurons may also release the cotransmitters neuropeptide Y (NPY) and galanin.[118] These cotransmitters may modulate NE signaling at both the presynaptic and postsynaptic end (more detailed discussion of neuropeptides appears later in this chapter). Galanin release accompanying excessive NE signaling, for example, under chronically stressful circumstances, may suppress DA release.[121] Anhedonia, fatigue, and compromised cognitive function in chronic stress may be partially attributable to galanin-mediated suppression of DA signaling.

Central noradrenergic neurons additionally have a rich "conversation" with astrocytes, microglia, and oligodendroglia. Glial cells express a multitude of noradrenergic receptors, which have an important role in regulation of their function. Noradrenergic receptors on astrocytes influence their energy utilization and immune and neurotrophic signaling.[126] Microglial NE receptors regulate synthesis and release of inflammatory cytokines,[127] while noradrenergic innervation of oligodendrocytes plays an important role in myelination.[118] Furthermore, astrocytes also express NE uptake sites.[128]

Once their mission is accomplished, monoamines, including NE, are taken up from the synaptic cleft by their respective uptake pumps or transporters. NETs are expressed on the presynaptic terminals of NE neurons and on the membranes of glial cells. Transporter function is significantly influenced by the level of polarization of the neural membrane. Hyperpolarization of the cellular membrane enhances the velocity of the transporter, while depolarization decreases it.[125] In addition to the high-affinity NET, low-affinity, high-capacity biogenic amine transporters, such as organic cation transporters and plasma membrane monoamine transporters, assist in NE clearance. Their role may be especially important in removing extrasynaptic transmitter molecules that participate in volume transmission, or in the circumstances of compromised function of the primary high-affinity transporters.[129] Additionally, catechol O-methyltransferase, a catabolic enzyme, may inactivate any extracellular NE that has not been promptly removed by the uptake pump.

Furthermore, endocellular NE not stored in the vesicles can be broken down by MAO, which is readily available in the mitochondria of nerve terminals.[130] Two isoforms of MAO, MAOA and MAOB, have different affinities for monoamine compounds. While MAOA preferentially catabolizes 5HT and NE, MAOB prefers benzylamine and beta-phenylethylamine. Both MAOA and MAOB metabolize DA and tryptamine.[125] In contrast to MAOA, which is mostly located in the catecholaminergic nerve terminals, MAOB is predominantly found in glia cells.[121] NE is initially metabolized to NMN, and subsequently into several transitional metabolites, including its principal brain metabolite, 3-methoxy-4-hydroxyphenylglycol (MHPG).[130]

Physiological activity of NE is mediated by the three families of G-protein-coupled receptors: alpha-1, alpha-2, and beta ARs. The alpha-1 AR has three subclasses: alpha-1A, alpha-1B, and alpha-1D.[118] There are also three subtypes of alpha-2 receptors: alpha-2A, -2B, and -2C, located either as somatodendritic and axonal autoreceptors or as postsynaptic and extrasynaptic (outside the synapse) heteroreceptors.[131,132] Beta ARs also manifest in three subtypes: beta-1, -2, and -3.[118] In addition to alpha-2 ARs, beta-2 ARs can also have presynaptic locations.[133] Alpha-2 and beta ARs have opposite effects on the intracellular activation of the adenylate cyclase. While beta ARs elevate intracellular levels of cAMP and have a predominantly stimulatory effect on neural transmission, alpha-2 ARs suppress intracellular cAMP and have mostly an inhibitory influence on neural function.[133] Alpha-1 ARs initiate a sequence that leads to increased availability of intracellular phospholipase-C (PLC) and consequently the release of intracellular Ca^{2+}. Activation of alpha-1 ARs generally produces a stimulatory effect.[133]

The alpha-2 autoreceptor provides feedback inhibition if there is excessive NE release, as in circumstances of NET inhibition. There is a controversy regarding alpha-2 autoreceptor desensitization: some of the evidence suggests that, while terminal alpha-2 ARs lose their sensitivity in the face of extended NET blockade and ensuing accumulation of NE in the synapse, somatodendritic alpha-2 autoreceptors do not appear to desensitize as readily.[132] Furthermore, postsynaptic alpha-1 and alpha-2 ARs do not generally desensitize even in the presence of substantial synaptic NE accumulation, as can be encountered following NE reuptake inhibitor (NRI) usage. In contrast, beta ARs tend to desensitize following prolonged NRI or dual-acting antidepressant use.[132]

ARE ALPHA-ADRENERGIC RECEPTOR SUBTYPES CLINICALLY RELEVANT?

Alpha AR subtypes often have opposing physiological functions. While alpha-1A stimulation may mediate learning, memory, neurogenesis, and antidepressant action of medications and ECT, alpha-1B activation may interfere with learning, produce apoptosis, lead to anhedonia, and mediate CRF response to chronic stress. In a similar fashion, alpha-2A ARs may be involved in the analgesic effects of noradrenergic antidepressants, via activation of descending pain pathways, as well as enhanced attention and working memory, while alpha-2C activation may interfere with cognition and mediate stress-induced depression and anxiety.[134–140]

THE IMPACT OF ADRENERGIC RECEPTOR BINDING
ON OTHER NEUROTRANSMITTERS

Stimulation of alpha-1 ARs on VTA DA and RN 5HT neurons results in tonic activation of these monoaminergic nuclei.[141–143] In contradistinction to alpha-1 ARs, alpha-2 postsynaptic heteroreceptors have an inhibitory influence on 5HT, DA, and acetylcholine neurons.[121,132,141,144] Furthermore, NE may inhibit DA signaling by binding directly to inhibitory presynaptic D2 receptors on DA fibers.[121] Additionally, stimulation of alpha-1 and beta-1 ARs activates wakefulness-promoting cholinergic neurons in the brainstem.[118] Furthermore, noradrenergic stimulation of orexigenic neurons via alpha-1 ARs activates them, thereby promoting wakefulness, while alpha-2 stimulation suppresses their activity.[118]

CHANGES IN NORADRENERGIC SIGNALING IN MDD

One of the studies of patients suffering from melancholy depression reported elevated CSF levels of NE, and plasma levels of cortisol in MDD patients relative to healthy control subjects.[145] Samples obtained around the clock demonstrated that NE and cortisol levels were strongly correlated to each other.[145] Another study by the same group replicated the previous findings and noted that CSF NE, plasma NE, and cortisol all rose in parallel during the night and peaked in the morning hours. All NE and cortisol levels were normalized after ECT treatment.[146]

Postmortem studies have detected increased NE levels in the brains of unipolar and bipolar depressed patients[147] and diminished NET binding in the LC.[148] One group utilized internal jugular vein catheterization to indirectly evaluate the release of brain monoamines and concentration of their metabolites in a group of treatment refractory depressed patients.[149] Compared with a group of healthy volunteers, depressed patients had lower levels of venoarterial NE and MHPG, its principal metabolite.[149]

Other postmortem studies demonstrated that both the affinity and density of the presynaptic alpha-2 ARs were increased in the brains of depressed suicide victims relative to controls.[150] Several of the earlier histopathological studies focusing on the noradrenergic LC have reported increased numbers of alpha-2 ARs, elevated levels of TH (a synthesizing enzyme), and reduced density of NETs, but no change in the number of noradrenergic neurons, in MDD subjects compared with controls.[151–153] One of these studies found no difference in alpha-2 AR density in the serotonergic RN of depressed individuals compared with control subjects.[151] A subsequent study by the same group evaluated alpha-2 binding in the amygdala and orbitofrontal cortex (Brodmann area 47) of deceased depressed patients. Relative to the control group, depressed patients had decreased density of alpha-2 ARs in the orbitofrontal cortex, which did not reach a statistical significance, and no difference in amygdala alpha-2 binding.[154]

Furthermore, studies evaluating growth hormone response to alpha-2 agonists have had equivocal findings. In physiological circumstances, NE via alpha-2 ARs augments growth hormone release. Several groups have noted a blunted growth hormone response to alpha-2 agonists in depressed populations compared with healthy controls;[155,153] other researchers found a blunted growth hormone response only in about 40 percent of depressed subjects.[114] Other studies have described diminished cAMP levels in the brains of depressed suicide victims relative to control groups.[109] Because activation of alpha-2 ARs reduces cAMP quantities, lower cAMP levels could also be a consequence of greater alpha-2–mediated signaling. In aggregate, it is not easy to interpret changes in the presynaptic inhibitory alpha-2 ARs, because either they could reflect increased inhibition of NE efflux, and therefore reduced transmitter levels, or it could be a homeostatic response to compensate for the excessive NE release (higher activity of TH might support this hypothesis). It is also possible that divergent findings reflect regional differences in alpha-2 activity, possibly due to diverse regulation of local NE signaling. We have previously mentioned that the brainstem monoamine signaling is regulated by the short, "local" feedback loops, as well as by the distant prefrontal excitatory and inhibitory inputs. It is also not inconceivable that changes in receptor density may be a reflection of inadequate intracellular signaling (cAMP levels in depressed patients are altered).

Much as is the case with alpha-2 ARs, studies have not found consistent evidence of beta AR abnormalities in MDD. Reduction of beta-AR-coupled Gs protein function in the mononuclear leukocytes of depressed patients relative to controls may reflect diminished beta AR density or a primary deficit in depressed patients.[156] Interestingly, symptoms of depression and fatigue, lower socioeconomic status, and elevation of C-reactive protein, an inflammatory marker, all correlated with decreased responsiveness of beta ARs in a sample of healthy participants.[157–159] Depressive symptoms, fatigue, and elevated inflammation are all also associated with chronic stress and MDD.[160] A postmortem study detected significantly reduced adenylate cyclase (the enzyme facilitating synthesis of cAMP) response to beta-1 ARs in deceased subject suffering from MDD relative to controls.[161] Other studies have found no difference in the binding of beta-1 and -2 ARs in the hippocampus[162] and pineal glands[163] of depressed subjects compared with controls.

In aggregate, available research does not point to a simple relationship between derangement in noradrenergic signaling and symptoms of depression. Research has also noted, in addition to significant regional differences, evidence of both elevated and suppressed activity of NE in MDD. It may prove more fruitful to consider alterations in NE transmission as disturbances in signal-to-noise tuning of GABA and glutamate signaling[148] affecting mood-regulating corticolimbic circuits. Inconsistent findings could also reflect biologically different subtypes of MDD, generating similar enough phenotypes to be subsumed under the same diagnostic umbrella.

THE ROLE OF DOPAMINE IN MDD

Synthesis of DA was described in the preceding section, as it is also a transitional step in the process of NE anabolism from the amino acids phenylalanine and tyrosine. Decarboxylation of DOPA generates DA.[130] Although there are 10 groups of dopaminergic neurons in the mammalian brain (A8 through A17), mesencephalic nuclei have by far the greatest importance in the study of pathophysiology of MDD.[164] The mesencephalon contains two major dopaminergic nuclei, nigral neurons (A9) projecting to the striatum along the nigrostriatal tract and VTA DA neurons (A10) projecting to limbic (including NAcc) and cortical areas via mesolimbic and mesocortical pathways, respectively.[165,166] Mesolimbic fibers, as the name suggests, project from the mesencephalic VTA to limbic regions such as the NAcc in the ventral striatum, amygdala, and hippocampus.[165] The mesocortical pathway connects the VTA with the ACC and frontal and temporal cortices and has an important role in attention and working memory.[165] Studies have provided evidence that substantia nigra DA neurons have a more complex network of projections than was initially appreciated. Some of the substantia nigra neurons project to limbic and cortical areas. Moreover, the A8 group of neurons, adjacent to and extending the substantia nigra grouping, has extensive projections to the striatum, limbic, and cortical areas. Beyond its well-known role in motor planning and regulation of movement, the nigrostriatal system also plays a part in cognitive function.[165]

The mesencephalon contains the largest population of DA neurons; in humans there are more than 200,000 dopaminergic nerve cells, on each side of the brain. Over 70 percent of these neurons are located in the substantia nigra.[166] The third major group of DA neurons is located in the hypothalamic arcuate nucleus (A12) and PVN (A14).[167] Projections from these neurons, in addition to some originating from the A8 group, form the tuberoinfundibular tract.[168,169] The principal role of tuberoinfundibular neurons is neuroendocrine regulation.[169] In addition to regulation of prolactin release, this pathway (figure 9.4) is also involved in control of growth hormone secretion.[165] Furthermore, A13 DA neurons from the subthalamic zona incerta modulate the release of gonadotropins and have a major role in initiation of puberty and sexual function.[165,170] Dopaminergic neurons originating from the posterior hypothalamus (A11) project to the spinal column and are believed to play a role in restless leg syndrome.[170] Some of the dopaminergic axons originating from the mesencephalon can be up to 1.5 meters (almost 5 feet) long, making them very vulnerable in the context of head trauma.[164]

Inactivation of DA for the most part parallels the process previously described for NE. There are some notable differences, however. In addition to involvement of the DA transporter (DAT), in the areas lacking of cognate transporter, such as the PFC and hippocampus, DA is taken up by NET.[129,165] Much like NE, DA is also metabolized by MAO and catechol *O*-methyltransferase. In DA nerve terminals, DA is metabolized into 3,4-dihydroxyphenylacetaldehyde and subsequently to 3,4-dihydroxyphenylacetic acid (DOPAC). Excessive accumulation of DOPAC in the nerve endings, as might be the case in methamphetamine users, is concerning, given that DOPAC is a neurotoxic compound.[121] In physiological circumstances, the final end product of DA catabolism is homovanillic acid (HVA), which is excreted in urine.[171]

Dopaminergic projections have a key role in regulation of affect, motivation, motor activity, sleep and wakefulness, neuroendocrine and immune activity,

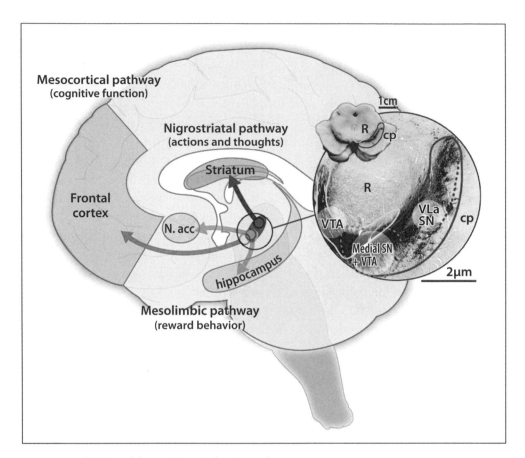

FIGURE 9.4. Origin of dopaminergic brain pathways.

attention, memory, pain, feeding, and sexual behavior.[166,168,169,172,173] Functions of CNS dopaminergic tracts are mediated by five distinct G-protein coupled receptors, divided into two families: D1-like and D2-like. Members of the D1 family (D1 and D5) stimulate cAMP production, while D2-like receptors (D2, D3, and D4) inhibit it.[165] Unlike the D1 family, D2 and D3 are expressed both pre- and postsynaptically. There are two genetic variants of D2 receptors, short and long. While the short form has mostly presynaptic locations, long forms are predominantly postsynaptic.[168]

D1 receptors are expressed in high concentrations in the mesocortical (including PFC structures), mesolimbic, and nigrostriatal areas. Lower densities of D1 can be found in the hippocampus, thalamus, hypothalamus, and cerebellum. D5 receptors, in general, have substantially lower density than D1 receptors and have been detected in cortical areas, including the premotor cortex and cingulate, but also in the hippocampus, hypothalamus, and basal ganglia.[168] While D1 receptors have mostly dendritic localization, D5 receptors are localized on the soma of pyramidal neurons.[124] Many of the cortical D1/D5 receptors are also localized on GABA neurons.[124]

D2-like receptors are densely represented in the striatum (especially NAcc), substantia nigra, VTA (many of the D2 receptors in VTA have presynaptic location), hypothalamus and pituitary (regulating prolactin release), hippocampus, and amygdala. D3 receptors have a more limited distribution. They are represented in limbic areas, the striatum, and hippocampus. D4 receptors have the least dense pattern of distribution and can be found in the cortex, mesotemporal structures (amygdala and hippocampus), basal ganglia, thalamus, and hypothalamus.[168] Most D4 receptors are located on GABA interneurons and have high affinity for NE, leading some authors to suggest that they be classified as catecholamine, rather than DA, receptors.[124]

THE IMPACT OF DOPAMINERGIC SIGNALING ON OTHER NEUROTRANSMITTER SYSTEMS

Most likely, the principal effects of DA are achieved by slow modulation of rapid glutamate and GABA transmission.[168] Both D1 and D2 receptors are expressed on GABA and glutamate neurons, where D1 receptors perform an excitatory role while D2 receptors inhibit neural function.[129] Moderate levels of NE, acting via alpha-2 ARs, and DA interacting with D1 receptors optimize the function of cortical pyramidal glutamatergic neurons. Stressful situations can elevate catecholamines to the point where excessive D1, alpha-1, and beta-1 signaling interferes with PFC executive function, including working memory.[124,142] Our discussion here focuses predominantly on dopaminergic modulation of other monoamine systems, because the role of DA receptors on GABA neurons, glutamate neurons, and glial cells is discussed extensively earlier in this chapter.

NE may also interact with presynaptic D2 autoreceptors, promoting tonic inhibition of midbrain DA neurons.[121] Moreover, DA may inhibit NE release by directly interacting with presynaptic alpha-2 receptors on NE fibers.[147] Preclinical studies have also identified D2-like receptors on LC NE neurons, which most likely mediate an inhibitory influence of VTA DA neurons on LC firing rate, although this effect has not been fully elucidated.[174] Furthermore, D2-like receptors have also been identified on 5HT neurons. Dopaminergic input exerts a direct excitatory effect on DRN 5HT neurons, most likely mediated by postsynaptic D2 heteroreceptors. This effect is not fully understood, because D2 receptors typically mediate inhibitory signals.[175]

Dopaminergic activation of GABA/dynorphin NAcc neurons via D1 receptors produces an increased release of dynorphin from the feedback pathways projecting back to the VTA. Dynorphin binds to kappa-opioid receptors on VTA DA neurons, inhibiting their activity.[176] This feedback circuit connecting the VTA with the NAcc has an important role in the pathophysiology of substance abuse and depression.[176]

DA is also involved in the regulation of wakefulness by providing an input to the histaminergic tuberomammilary nucleus. Dopaminergic activation of D1 receptors has a predictable excitatory impact on histamine neurons. Binding to D2 has an unorthodox consequence: its activation leads to intracellular PLC signaling, generating increased firing frequency of the histamine neurons (typically D2 receptors mediate an inhibitory response).[177]

A study using light microscopy has identified D2 receptors on the cholinergic neurons in the dorsal striatum and NAcc. D2 activation is associated with the inhibition of acetylcholine release.[178] Moreover, an in vitro study has provided additional insight into the mechanism of dopaminergic modulation of striatal cholinergic interneurons. Activation of D1 receptors is associated with excitation of cholinergic neurons, while D2 binding produces their inhibition.[179]

DOPAMINERGIC ALTERATIONS IN MDD

Considerable research has focused on elucidating the links among psychomotor retardation (PMR), anhedonia, decreased motivation, and alteration in dopaminergic reward circuitry in MDD. Preclinical studies have provided direct evidence tying dopaminergic VTA neuron firing to the anticipation and receipt of an award. The NAcc is a key reward-related area of the brain. Its neurons precisely encode phasic VTA dopaminergic firing. Conversely, inhibitory GABA neuron activity in the VTA was linked with aversion and anhedonia. Chronic mild stress, an experimental paradigm known for inducing a depression-like phenotype in rodents, was associated with a reduction of VTA dopaminergic signaling. Moreover, inhibition of VTA DA neurons in rodents was associated with multiple depressive-like behavioral changes, which were subsequently reversed by resumption of VTA dopaminergic activity.[180] Furthermore, VTA DA neurons exercise an inhibitory influence on NE firing via projections to the LC, which appears to be mediated by alpha-2 receptors, and perhaps D2 receptors.[181] This VTA–LC pathway, utilizing alpha-2 receptors, may have a role in antidepressant action. A two-day administration of the putative dopaminergic antidepressant bupropion resulted in a suppression of firing of NE LC neurons. An alpha-2 adrenergic antagonist completely reversed this LC suppression.[181] Hypothetically, dysfunction of the clock genes in the dopaminergic VTA–NAcc circuit may contribute to depressive symptomatology. Furthermore, depression may be linked with an excessive accumulation of CREB, a transcription factor, in the NAcc. This overabundance of CREB in NAcc neurons in depression has been tied to elevated dynorphin (a kappa-opioid agonist) transmission, resulting in suppression of VTA dopaminergic neurons.[182]

An interesting hypothesis has linked anhedonia in MDD to diminished sensitivity of postsynaptic D2/D3 receptors in limbic areas involved in reward processing. Moreover, chronic antidepressant use may produce an increase in the sensitivity of D2/D3 receptors.[168] DA binding to high-affinity D2 receptors in NAcc inhibits it, while activation of low-affinity D1 receptors stimulates this reward area in the ventral striatum. Presence of rewarding or pleasurable stimuli would likely elicit burst firing of mesolimbic VTA neurons and engage D1 receptors.[115] Therefore, deficits in dopaminergic signaling would result in diminished DA elevation during phasic signaling and inadequate NAcc D1 stimulation, producing anhedonia, while even low levels of DA would be still be sufficient to activate low-affinity D2 receptors, thereby suppressing the NAcc.[115]

Indeed, preliminary research has offered an indication that D1 receptor binding may be altered in depressed individuals compared with controls. A PET imaging study compared D1 binding potential (BP) in MDD patients relative to healthy subjects and found significantly reduced NAcc and putamen D1 BP in the depressed group. Reduction in D1 BP was negatively correlated with the illness duration and anhedonia ratings.[183] Somewhat contradicting these suppositions, receptor binding studies have noted greater D2/D3 density in the basal ganglia of depressed patients relative to healthy controls.[168,184] Attempts were made to assess the function of the reward circuitry in MDD by using a dopaminergic probe in the form of 30 mg dextroamphetamine. In support of putative DA receptor hypersensitivity in the reward circuits, administration of amphetamine was associated with a twofold elevation in ventrolateral PFC, vmPFC, caudate, and putamen activity, as assessed by functional MRI, in MDD patients relative to healthy controls.[185] Another study described positive correlation between anhedonia and vmPFC activity and negative correlation with amygdala and ventral striatal activity in response to happy stimuli.[186]

An alternative explanation postulates that cortisol elevation, a common occurrence in MDD, especially among subjects who experienced poor maternal care in early life, may alter dopaminergic transmission in the ventral striatum, negatively influencing subsequent reward response.[165] Moreover, prominent anhedonia, associated with diminished connectivity in the VTA–ventral striatum–ventrolateral PFC reward circuit, established by functional MRI, was associated with nonresponse to repeated transcranial magnetic stimulation of the dorsomedial PFC in MDD patients.[187] Interestingly, both ECT and repeated transcranial magnetic stimulation result in augmented DA release. Deep brain stimulation of areas adjacent to the NAcc has also been associated with a rapid antidepressant effect in TRD patients.[186] Cumulatively, these data point to possible dopaminergic dysfunction in the reward circuitry of a subset of depressed patients. This maladaptive function of the reward circuit in MDD may be linked with symptoms of anhedonia, pessimism, and loss of interest.[187] This intriguing hypothesis awaits additional empirical support.[168]

Emergent evidence has linked dopaminergic dysfunction with the severity of depression and response to antidepressant strategies. A single-photon emission computed tomography study found increased D2/D3 binding in the temporal cortex of the depressed group compared with healthy controls, which correlated with the severity of depression as measured by Hamilton Depression Rating Scale

21-item version (HAMD$_{21}$).[188] Elevated D2/D3 binding may be a consequence of diminished transmitter availability or increased affinity for the ligand.[165] Interestingly, one research group reported that D2/D3 binding in the ACC of depressed patients decreased after ECT.[115] Perhaps paradoxically, studies have also reported upregulation of D2 receptors associated with a treatment response to SSRIs.[169] Several other studies have not detected any difference in D1 and D2 binding between depressed patients and healthy controls.[168,184] Studies evaluating DAT binding in MDD have also been inconclusive, although the most comprehensive PET study noted a reduction in DAT binding in depression.[165] One of the studies reported a reduction in DAT binding in the caudate but not putamen of MDD patients, suggesting that there may be some regional specificity in dopaminergic alterations.[115]

Psychomotor retardation (PMR), especially in the context of melancholy depression, has also been associated with dopaminergic dysfunction. Hypothetically, PMR and even fatigue are related to the dysfunction of the circuitry connecting the PFC (especially dlPFC) with the putamen and caudate.[186,189,190] PET studies have reported that DOPA uptake, possibly reflecting presynaptic DA function, was significantly reduced in depressed patients with significant PMR compared with anxiously depressed patients with high impulsivity, and with healthy controls.[165,189,191] Additionally research has also identified increased D2/D3 binding in the caudate and putamen of depressed patients relative to controls, most likely indicating compensatory hypersensitivity due to diminished dopaminergic tone in these areas.[189] Furthermore, a negative correlation was noted between dlPFC blood flow and clinically rated PMR in depressed patients.[189] Because of negative and divergent findings, one can conclude that the interrelationship between D2/D3 binding in the striatum and the PMR in depression is still equivocal.[189,190] Other studies have established a positive correlation between clinically diagnosed depression with PMR and urinary MHPG (an NE metabolite), additionally implicating dysfunctional noradrenergic transmission as a possible causal factor of PMR in depression.[190]

Neuroendocrine studies attempting to evaluate DA receptor function by assessing prolactin and growth hormone response to various dopaminergic agonists have yielded equivocal results.[165,184] These findings are further confounded by the diversity of methodology and the influence of stress on prolactin secretion.[184] Postmortem studies have provided equivocal evidence about brain DA and concentrations of its principal metabolite, HVA, in suicide victims compared with controls. In suicide attempters, compared with controls, some studies found lower CSF HVA concentrations, whereas others reported elevation in CSF HVA correlated to higher CSF concentrations of proinflammatory IL-6 and TNF.[165,192] Higher cytokine levels were associated with increased suicidality.[192] Another study described reduced DAT density and increased D2/D3 binding in the amygdala of depressed subjects relative to controls.[193]

Treatment studies mostly support the benefits of adjunct DA agonists such as pramipexole and bromocriptine in the treatment of major depressive episodes.[165] Genetic alterations affecting DA signaling in MDD have been discussed in the Genetics chapter while neurochemical studies of monoamine perturbations in MDD will be the focus of the next section.

All in all, the cumulative preclinical, clinical, imaging, biochemical, and postmortem evidence, although equivocal, does support a role of dopaminergic dysfunction in the pathophysiology of at least a segment of depressed patients, more likely the ones presenting with prominent anhedonia, fatigue, and PMR.

REVISITING THE MONOAMINE HYPOTHESIS OF MDD

Despite decades of elaboration, the "monoamine hypothesis" of depression remains beset with controversies. Prompted by the evident treatment efficacy of antidepressant medications, which modulate 5HT, DA, and NE, insufficient monoamine signaling has long been held to have a cardinal role in the etiopathogenesis of MDD.[1,194] In support of this hypothesis, researches have noted alterations of NE and 5HT receptor density in cortical and limbic formations of depressed patients.[194] Chapter 4 on genetics reviews the evidence implicating genes that code for 5HTT, NAT, catechol O-methyltransferase, MAO, and monoamine receptors in perpetuating vulnerability toward depression, especially when interacting with environmental adversity. Meyer et al.[195] have noted elevated levels of MAOA in the brains of depressed patients. Because MAOA is a primary intercellular enzyme involved in the monoamine breakdown, its excessive activity may impede monoamine signaling in MDD.[195]

Additionally, changes in platelet 5HT and NE receptor density have also been noted in depressed and suicidal patients, possibly reflecting a body-wide alteration or adaptation.[194] Pathohistological studies have reported decreased numbers of NE neurons in the LC of depressed patients whose death was unrelated to suicide, compared with healthy controls.[196] The same authors also noted a decrease in the number of 5HT neurons in the DRN of depressed patients compared with healthy controls.[196] Neuromelanin-sensitive MRI imaging has revealed an attenuated signal in the LC of depressed patients.[104]

Research assessing NE and 5HT metabolites in the CSF and plasma has yielded inconsistent results. Levels of 5HIAA have been reported to be lower in depressed and suicidal patients[197] and especially low in victims of violent suicide.[194] However, because MDD is a biologically heterogeneous syndrome, it is not surprising that there are differing reports on the levels of monoamine biomarkers. For example, MHPG, a major NE metabolite, was found to be elevated in the CSF of agitated and anxious depressed patients, while depressed individuals with PMR were found to have lower levels of MHPG and HVA (a primary DA metabolite), compared with healthy controls.[198] Moreover, elevation of CSF MHPG levels was not correlated with the severity of depression.[198] Furthermore, there may be a gender difference in CSF concentrations of monoamine metabolites in depressed populations. One study noted an elevation of CSF MHPG in both genders; women had higher 5HIAA levels, while men had reduced HVA levels, relative to healthy controls.[199] Another study, using catheters placed in the internal jugular vein, noted reduced NE and DA release in the brains of patients suffering from refractory depression compared with healthy volunteers.[149] In contrast to NE and DA findings, the same group, using a similar technique, found elevated brain 5HT turnover in depressed patients compared with healthy subjects.[200]

Several reports noted a reduction of CSF 5HIAA (a 5HT metabolite) and MHPG (the main NE metabolite) following effective antidepressant activity.[201–205] Findings regarding "normalization" of elevated CSF MHPG after antidepressant treatment are surprisingly consistent. It appears that antidepressant-related lowering of CSF MHPG and 5HIAA, most likely reflecting reestablished NE and 5HT turnover homeostasis, tends to be enduring. A reduction in CSF MHPG and 5HIAA, compared with pretreatment levels, has been noted to persist up to 15 weeks after the initiation of antidepressant therapy.[206] Additionally, there appears to be a relationship between elevated pretreatment plasma MHPG and subsequent response to an SSRI.[207] In concert with these findings, a study that evaluated the impact of a MAO-inhibiting antidepressant on the urinary MHPG secretion noted its reduction after four weeks of phenelzine, associated with improvement in depressive symptomatology.[208] Furthermore, a study of TRD patients reported a reduction of plasma HVA levels following five weeks of ECT treatment.[209] Opposing results, whereby ECT was associated with an increase of CSF HVA and 5HIAA in depressed patients, have also been published.[210] Monoamine transporters also seem to be influenced by the disease process. For example, DAT has a 15 percent lower BP in depressed patients compared with controls,[211] and 5HTT BP (which can be considered as a marker of 5HTT density) tends to be elevated during a depressive episode, especially a more severe one.[195]

Pharmacological strategies designed to deplete monoamines suggest that the therapeutic effect of antidepressants may be selectively reversed by depleting the monoamine affected by a particular antidepressant.[212] Namely, acute tryptophan depletion precipitates recurrence of depression in more than half the patients who have been successfully treated with SSRIs, but not in patients who have benefited from NRIs or in healthy controls.[213] Tryptophan is an amino acid precursor of 5HT, and its dietary depletion results in rapid and robust reduction of plasma 5HT: plasma 5HT levels are reduced by as much as 70 percent within a matter of hours.[213,214] Conversely, oral administration of alpha-methylparatyrosine triggered a temporary recurrence of depression in depressed patients who had responded to DMI, a catecholamine-elevating antidepressant, but not in healthy controls or SSRI-treated patients.[213] Alpha-methylparatyrosine is a competitive inhibitor of TH, a rate-limiting enzyme regulating synthesis of DA, NE, and epinephrine. Its administration results in a precipitous reduction of plasma cate-cholamines and transient recurrence of depressive symptoms in as many as 70 percent of NRI-treated patients.[213] Remarkably, both 5HT depletion and catechol-amine depletion produced reduced metabolism, assessed by PET imaging, in the thalamus, orbitofrontal PFC, and dlPFC of patients, coinciding with return of depressive symptomatology.[213]

Subsequent preclinical research has raised some important methodological issues. While acute tryptophan depletion predictably reduces plasma 5HT levels, there is only scant evidence that there is a direct impact on the release of neu-rotransmitter from the brain 5HT neurons. The first study, which evaluated in vivo 5HT efflux from neurons innervating the mPFC, found no effect of acute tryptophan depletion on the brain 5HT release.[215] Tryptophan depletion and DA/NE depletion appear to induce transient depressive feelings primarily in healthy individuals who have a family history of depression, in remitted patients who used SSRIs or NRIs, and in medication-free remitted depressed patients, but not in healthy individuals.[215] Both family members of depressed patients and remit-ted depressed patients who have not been taking their medication experienced a much milder monoamine-depletion-induced depressive relapse than individuals who are currently taking their antidepressants.[215] It is also important to remem-ber that SSRIs may diminish 5HT synthesis and therefore render the individuals taking these medications particularly sensitive to tryptophan depletion.[215] In conclusion, depletion of 5HT and catecholamine does not directly cause depressed mood. More likely it unmasks a monoamine "vulnerability" in depressed indi-viduals, or it interferes with the compensatory change in monoamine transmis-sion, either of endogenous origin or related to antidepressant use.[215]

Studies using pharmacological probes to evaluate the 5HT and NE signaling have provided further evidence of the limited monoamine role in MDD causa-tion.[114] Using the prolactin response to *d*-fenfluramine, a robust serotonergic agent, as an indirect measure of 5HT function, and using growth hormone release precipitated by clonidine, an alpha-2 noradrenergic receptor agonist, as a reflec-tion of an intact NE transmission, allows direct assessment of monoamine func-tion in the context of MDD.[114] Using this methodology, one study found that approximately 11 percent of depressed patients had only 5HT abnormalities (blunted prolactin response to *d*-fenfluramine), 32 percent had insufficient NE signaling (blunted growth hormone response to clonidine), 18 percent had both NE and 5HT abnormalities, and 39 percent had no deficiency of either 5HT or NE transmission.[114]

Therefore, a converging body of evidence brings into question simplistic interpretations of the "monoamine theory." If monoamines are the primary abnor-mality in MDD, it is hard to understand why in the Sequenced Treatment Alter-natives to Relieve Depression (STAR*D) trial 50 percent of the patients failed to respond to first-line SSRI treatment, 65 percent did not achieve remission, and more than a half of those who did still had two or more residual symptoms.[108] While in vivo preclinical evidence describes prompt LC activation following SSRI application,[216] clinical studies have shown that it may take as long as five to eight weeks to attain optimal antidepressant response.[217] Mayberg[218] evaluated SSRI responses utilizing PET imaging. These investigators found no difference between responders and nonresponders following a week of antidepressant treatment. Rather, the pattern of activity associated with depression was reversed only after six weeks of treatment, suggesting an adaptation to chronic antidepressant administration as the basis of therapeutic effect.[218] Furthermore, a variety of antidepressant medications and ECT have been reported to suppress the activity of TH, a key enzyme regulating NE synthesis.[219]

There is also evidence that antidepressant interventions may affect a change by reducing monoamine turnover and brainstem nucleus firing rates. A preclinical study demonstrated a significant reduction in LC electrophysiological activity following 14 days of treatment with a diverse group of antidepressants, including DMI (a predominantly noradrenergic tricyclic antidepressant), paroxetine and citalopram (SSRIs), and mirtazepine (an alpha-2 antagonist).[204] Moreover, Barton et al.[200] reported elevated 5HT turnover in unmedicated MDD patients. Twelve weeks of SSRI treatment resulted in a marked reduction in brain 5HT turnover, accompanied by significant clinical improvement.

Imaging studies have described insufficient activity and reduced volume of the vmPFC in many depressed individuals.[54,218,220–222] Because the vmPFC plays a key role in regulating amygdala activity and sympathetic/parasympathetic balance, it is not surprising that depressed patients tend to exhibit excessive sympathetic activation in response to stressful stimuli.[54,223,224] Furthermore, glutamatergic fibers projecting from vmPFC have a key role in regulating monoamine release from the brainstem nuclei. In a direct fashion, glutamatergic fibers from the vmPFC can stimulate monoamine release, while indirectly, by interfacing with the local GABA neurons, they can also impede monoamine transmission.[79,105,129] Therefore, accumulating evidence suggests that in some instances dysregulation in monoamine signaling may be a consequence of GABA/glutamate imbalance, or an unsuccessful attempt to compensate for it.

Multiple studies have shown that monoamines also regulate one another through complex interactions. For example, dopaminergic input tends to upregulate serotonergic and downregulate noradrenergic activity. Elevated serotonergic activity has a mostly inhibitory effect on NE and DA, while increases in NE tend to suppress DA but can modulate 5HT transmission in either direction.[141,175] Complex cross talk between dopaminergic and noradrenergic systems appears to take place in the VTA, LC, and dorsal hippocampus.[174] Furthermore, more than one monoamine transmitter can be released from the same nerve ending, such that extracellular DA in the PFC originates not only from DA terminals but also from NE terminals.[225] Moreover, not only do monoamines influence one another via complex interactions, but GABA and glutamate tend to have a bidirectional regulatory influence on monoamines.[36,37,78,84,226] In summary, evidence supports the view of a complex dysregulation of interrelated neurotransmitter systems and distributed brain networks involved in regulation of mood, cognition, and the stress response, rather than a simple deficit of monoamine signaling.[227,228]

Endogenous Opioids and Other Peptide Neurotransmitters in MDD

The roles of the peptide neurotransmitters galanin, neuropeptide S (NPS), NPY, orexin/hypocretin, endocannabinoids (ECs), and endogenous opiates in the pathophysiology of MDD have been the focus of vigorous research.[229–234]

GALANIN

Galanin is coexpressed in serotonergic DRN neurons, noradrenergic LC neurons, and cholinergic neurons in the nucleus basalis.[235] Its biological activity is mediated by three types of G-protein-coupled receptors, GalR-1, -2, and -3. These receptors are localized in the PFC, cingulate cortex, insula, amygdala, hippocampus, hypothalamus and the brainstem nuclei LC and DRN.[231,236] Elevation of galanin levels in DRN is associated with diminished 5HT output, most likely due to its interaction with GalR1/R3 and modulation of 5HT1A receptors. Activation of GalR2 probably facilitates 5HT release in DRN.[237] In a similar fashion, galanin may slow LC NE neuron firing by modulating alpha-2 AR signaling.[236] Moreover, galanin may also exercise a complex modulatory, primarily inhibitory influence on dopaminergic VTA and mesolimbic projections.[238] Stress-related activation of LC neurons may cause suppression of DA signaling, mediated by NE projections to the VTA.[232] While mild tonic LC NE activity has facilitatory influence on VTA DA transmission, excessive phasic NE release, accompanied by elevation of VTA galanin, has an inhibitory effect on DA transmission, which is reversed by galanin antagonists.[231]

Through modulation of dopaminergic transmission, galanin may have a role in modulating instrumental behaviors and thus an influence in mood and substance use disorders.[238] Furthermore, a combined influence of elevated galanin/reduced DA transmission may be related to hypersomnolence, cognitive difficulties, decreased motor activity, and anhedonia often associated with depressive episodes.[231] Activation of hippocampal GalR2 may be associated with neurogenesis and neuroprotective processes, while GalR1 may mediate inhibition of cholinergic firing in the same location.[235] Furthermore, galanin may play an important role in regulation of mood, anxiety, sleep, alcohol intake, pain threshold, memory, and cognition.[237–239] That modulation of GalR2 may be important in galanin's antidepressant activity is supported by studies showing elevated galanin mRNA and GalR2 binding in the DRN following SSRI use.[235] There is also an intriguing possibility that antidepressants cause a shift from predominantly inhibitory GalR1 and -R3 signaling to predominantly excitatory GalR2 signaling.[237] Moreover, in the preclinical models of depression, an injection of a nonselective galanin receptor agonist resulted in an antidepressant-like response, possibly due to suppression of LC NE activity.[231]

The regulatory/inhibitory influence of galanin modulating agents may be of interest in the context of MDD treatment, given that a considerable number of depressed patients may have excessive LC NE transmission.[231] GalR3 is expressed in the hypothalamus and amygdala; its antagonists have shown efficacy in the preclinical models of depression and may have a role in the regulation of alcohol intake.[235] Antidepressant-like efficacy of GalR3 antagonists in preclinical models of depression may be based on the reversal of the inhibitory impact of galanin on DRN 5HT neurons.[231] Galanin receptor modulators are showing early promise in preclinical and clinical studies as antidepressant, anxiolytic, and neurogenesis-promoting agents.[231] The antidepressant effect of galanin-modulating compounds is probably exerted through modulation of 5HT, DA, and NE transmission.[231,237] There is very limited evidence from genome-wide association studies linking galanin genes to depression, and a healthy volunteer study demonstrating an "antidepressant-like" effect of the galanin intravenous infusion, supporting its relevance in clinical medicine.[233,237]

NEUROPEPTIDE S

A review emphasizes the pivotal role of NPS in communicating peripheral stress-related inflammatory signals to the brain. The point of emphasis is a central position of NPS in bidirectional signaling involving brain and body, which is important for regulation of mood, stress, and the immune response.[229] Moreover, NPS fibers, and the main neurokinin-1 (NK-1) receptor, are well represented in the PFC and limbic areas, such as the amygdala, hippocampus, and the PVN of the hypothalamus, involved in the regulation of mood, anxiety, and the stress response.[233,240] Studies have demonstrated that emotional stress results in NPS efflux in the amygdala and septal areas.[240] Furthermore, preclinical research has demonstrated that stress induces NPS signaling in the LC, facilitating NE transmission from projection terminals in the mPFC, thus modulating prefrontal stress responses.[240,380] Additionally, NPS modulates the firing rate of serotonergic DRN neurons and dopaminergic VTA neurons.[241]

Preclinical studies utilizing systemic administration of NK-1 receptor antagonists have demonstrated increased firing rates in VTA DA, LC NE, and DRN 5HT neurons, indicating the primarily inhibitory influence of NPS transmission in these structures.[241] Furthermore, chronic administration of NK-1 receptor antagonists produced an increase in the firing rate of DRN serotonergic neurons, most likely by desensitizing inhibitory 5HT1A autoreceptors.[232,241] NPS can also indirectly inhibit 5HT secretion by binding to NK-1 receptors on GABA neurons, which exercise a tonic inhibitory influence on DRN.[232] Moreover, NPS has an important role in the regulation of peripheral inflammation and thus is ideally positioned to be an important mediator in the bidirectional mind-body communication so relevant in the etiopathogenesis of MDD.[229]

In animal models of depression injection of NPS has a less pronounced antidepressant-like effect compared with SSRI treatment.[233] Furthermore, functional MRI studies have demonstrated an increased amygdala response to aversive stimuli in a group of healthy volunteers endowed with the less functional T-allele of the gene coding the NPS receptor.[233] Clinical studies have found elevated peripheral levels of NPS in depressed patients compared with controls, which normalized with successful antidepressant treatment.[242] Although the study measured plasma NPS levels, it may be a relevant indicator of brain NPS activity, because there appears to be a stable correlation between peripheral and central NPS levels.[242] Moreover, a postmortem study reported decreased NK1 binding in the rostral orbitofrontal cortex of deceased depressed individuals compared with controls.[242] These results possibly reflect NK1 downregulation in this PFC area, due to elevated NPS transmission. Initial controlled clinical trials of NK-1 antagonists in MDD have been discontinued, because compounds failed to consistently separate from placebo.[241,242] More conclusive evidence supporting clinical use of NPS modulators is still lacking.

NEUROPEPTIDE Y

NPY is involved in regulation of feeding, energy homeostasis, circadian rhythms, neuronal excitability, cognition, addictive behaviors, and stress response.[233,243,244] NPY is expressed in the brainstem noradrenergic and adrenergic nuclei, amygdala, hippocampus, and BNST.[233,243,244] NPY neurons from the arcuate nucleus project to the hypothalamic PVN, where they are involved in the regulation of CRF release.[233] Additionally, NPY is released into plasma from sympathetic terminals.[244] NPY exerts its action via five G-protein-coupled receptors: Y1, Y2, Y4, Y5, and Y6. Y3 has not yet been cloned, and Y6 has no known relevant function in humans because it mutated in evolution and appears only its truncated form in primates.[233] Y1 mRNA expression is most significant in the frontal cortex, hippocampus, amygdala, and lateral septum. Peptide binding to Y1 produces an anxiolytic effect, while antagonists have been reported to induce anxiety.[233] It appears that Y2 has an opposite function of Y1; injection of Y2 agonists into animal amygdala produces anxiety.[233] Its cerebral distribution parallels that of Y1, with moderate expression in the amygdala, BNST, hypothalamus, and brainstem.[233] NPY binding to brainstem Y1 and Y2 receptors is involved in modulation of NE and 5HT nuclei, and consequently their limbic and cortical projections.[243] NPY projections and receptor localization suggests its primary role in regulation of the stress response. Furthermore,

NPY has an established role in promoting cell proliferation in the hippocampus, a brain structure with a preeminent role in stress response regulation.[245]

Genetic imaging studies have noted an increased rostral ACC response to negative emotional stimuli in a group of depressed patients with a low-NPY-expressing genotype, compared with patients with the high-expressing genotype.[246] The low-NPY-expressing genotype was overrepresented in the MDD group relative to healthy controls. Results of human studies of NPY function in depression are not consistent. Studies have reported decreased plasma and CSF concentrations of NPY during spontaneous depressive episodes.[244] However, NPY levels in remitted depressed patients were indistinguishable from healthy controls.[244] An older study reported an elevation of plasma NPY levels in depressed patients compared with the control group.[247] There are several potential explanations for these discrepant findings. MDD is highly biologically diverse, and different subtypes may have different NPY levels. Furthermore, it is possible that peripheral NPY levels may differ from central levels and that they may represent a state rather than trait marker.

OREXIN/HYPOCRETIN

Orexins, also known as hypocretins, are produced by groups of neurons located in the lateral hypothalamus (LH), dorsomedial hypothalamus, and prefornical hypothalamic area. Orexin-A (OX-A) and OX-B are excitatory peptides secreted broadly in the CNS by their projections in the PFC, hippocampus, thalamus, hypothalamus, and monoaminergic nuclei such as RN (5HT), LC (NE), VTA (DA), and tuberomammilary nucleus (histamine).[232,245,248] Additionally, orexinergic fibers project to pediculopontine tegmental nuclei, which include cholinergic cells involved in regulation of arousal and rapid-eye-movement sleep, and CRF-synthesizing neurons in the hypothalamic PVN.[232] OX-A and OX-B exert their actions by binding to G-protein-coupled receptors, orexin receptor-1 and -2 (OXR-1 and OXR-2). While OX-A preferentially binds to OXR-1, OX-B has a higher affinity for OXR-2.

Orexins play an array of roles important for survival: stabilization of sleep/wakefulness cycle, arousal, feeding behavior, stress response, pleasurable and sexual behavior, motivation and reward, motor activity, and autonomic regulation, via projections to the nucleus of solitary tract and BNST.[245,248] While some of the activity of the orexin signaling system is regulated by the suprachiasmatic nucleus, the main circadian pacemaker, other activity changes are determined by extemporaneous demands.[248] The network of orexinergic projections and their physiological responses indicate that they may have a crucial role in adjusting the level of arousal and coordinating complex endocrine, autonomic, emotional, behavioral, and cognitive responses to both appetitive and aversive conditions.[245,248]

Several clinical studies point to aberrations of orexin signaling in MDD. A rare 24-hour intrathecal collection of CSF has demonstrated that the amplitude of diurnal OX-A variations was significantly reduced in depressed patients compared with healthy controls.[245] There was a tendency for orexin levels to be elevated in depressed subjects compared with controls. This difference was reduced by a five-week course of SSRI.[245] Orexin levels positively correlated with the CSF level of CRF.[245] Preliminary genetic studies have also substantiated a potential role of orexins in the etiology of depression. Individuals carrying the A-allele of the gene coding OXR1 (HCRTR1) had 2.5 times greater risk of developing depressive disorders. Overall, studies evaluating central and peripheral levels of orexin and its mRNA expression have yielded inconsistent results. While some studies reported elevation of orexins, other found reductions, and yet others found no difference in orexin levels compared with control group.

Observed inconsistencies can be potentially explained by a complex relationship between the orexin signaling system and symptoms of depression, as well as by the biological diversity of MDD. Namely, certain preclinical models of depression, such as unpredictable chronic mild stress (UCMS), generate higher activation in one group of orexin neurons, in the dorsomedial hypothalamus–prefornical hypothalamic area, compared with LH neurons. On the other hand, LH orexin neurons seem to be preferentially activated in the context of appetitive/reward-seeking behavior.[248] Therefore, elevated stress/adversity-related orexin signaling in the dorsomedial hypothalamus–prefornical hypothalamic area could account for sleep disturbance and related memory deficits, while low activity in LH orexin neurons may be associated with anhedonia and loss of interest.[245] Furthermore, orexin receptor regulation is also important: while OXR-1 antagonism in preclinical models has an antidepressant-like effect, OXR-2 antagonism is depressogenic.[245] Rather than measuring cross-sectional orexin levels, it may be more useful to evaluate circadian orexin rhythmicity and orexin level changes in response to emotional stimuli.

In the forced-swim-test animal model of depression, intracerebroventricular injection of OX-A produced a reduction in despair behavior, which was pharmacologically reversed by administration of an OXR1 antagonist.[245] Conversely, results from the UCSM paradigm, which is believed to be biologically more akin to human depression, support the hypothesis of orexin elevation as a contributing factor in depression. Chronic administration of dual orexin receptor antagonists ameliorated depressive-like behaviors and HPA disturbance precipitated by the UCMS protocol.[245] Further clinical studies of orexin-modulating agents will be necessary before we can determine their usefulness in the treatment of MDD.

ENDOCANNABINOIDS

The Encocannabinoid (EC) signaling system is composed of several lipid ligands. Best known are anandamide (ANA) and 2-arachydonylglycerol; it also includes two cannabinoid receptors (CB1 and CB2), synthetic and catabolic enzymes (of which fatty acid amide hydrolase is the most significant), and an uptake pump that has not been well characterized.[234,249–251] Biological consequences of EC signaling are sometimes obscured due to ANA binding to transient receptor potential vanilloid-1 receptor (TRPV1), which has signaling properties completely distinct from those of CB1 and CB2.[234,249,250] The EC system is widespread across the neuraxis, the including amygdala, hippocampus, PFC, striatum, and cerebellum.[234,249,250] ECs regulate an array of processes, such as cognition, memory, feeding, motor behavior, sensory signaling, autonomic regulation, neuroendocrine and immune responses, and neuroplasticity. For the most part ECs act as retrograde inhibitors of synaptic signaling. After repeated, at times excessive, glutamate or GABA activity, postsynaptic neurons release ANA or 2-arachydonylglycerol, which in a feedback fashion binds to presynaptic terminal CB1 receptors and diminishes further glutamate or GABA release.[234,249,250] The EC signaling system can also act in an autocrine manner, binding to a postsynaptic CB1 receptor and thereby producing prolonged self-inhibition.[250] In this manner the EC system plays an important role in response extinction and habituation. Activation of CB1 receptors has been associated with 5HT, NE, DA, acetylcholine, and HPA (CRF) modulation.[234,249,250]

EC receptors are coupled with inhibitory G-proteins. Their activity suppresses cAMP activity and influences the operation of ion channels. CB1-precipitated changes in the function of Ca^{2+} channels are believed to be the primary mechanism involved in regulation of neurotransmitter release.[234] While CB1 receptors are predominantly located in the brain, CB2 receptors are mostly distributed in peripheral tissues, primarily in the immune system.[234,249,250] Aside from nerve cells, brain cannabinoid receptors are also found on astrocytes, oligodendroglia, and microglia.[234,249,250] Based on cannabinoid receptor locations, it is understandable how the EC system functions as a metasignaling system, regulating stress response; feedback regulation of monoamine, GABA, and glutamate transmission; reward signaling via modulation of DA transmission in the NAcc; feeding behavior; and inflammation and pain signaling.[234,249,250] An interesting paradox is associated with EC signaling: low doses of CB1 agonists are associated with an anxiolytic effect, but high doses are anxiogenic.[234] The anxiogenic effect induced by higher doses of CB1 agonists is most likely due to activation of TRPV1 receptors.[234,250]

Four single nucleotide polymorphisms of CNR1, the gene regulating CB1 receptor synthesis, have a significant effect on the human emotional response. Individuals who are A-allele homozygous are hyperresponsive to emotional and social stimuli. Interestingly, depressed individuals who are G-allele homozygous, and therefore less responsive to emotional stimuli, showed less response to antidepressant therapy.[250] Moreover, a postmortem study comparing CB1 expression in subjects who suffered from schizophrenia, bipolar disorder, or MDD and in a control group reported a significant reduction in CB1 expression only in the ACC glial cells of depressed subjects, compared with the controls.[252] Furthermore, CB1 antagonists, initially developed for the treatment of obesity, are associated with elevated discontinuation rates due to treatment-emergent anxiety and depression.[234,250] Because of undesirable side effects, direct CB1 modulators may not be suitable for treatment of mood disorders. Multitargeted agents that block ANA degradation by blocking fatty acid amide hydrolase, combined with TRPV1 antagonism, are the most promising therapeutic agents for mood disorders, based on available preclinical data.[234,250]

OPIOIDS

Endogenous opioid signaling is conducted by a complex neuromodulatory network composed of three peptide families and three cognate receptor families.[253,254] Endogenous opioids are products of enzymatic cleavage of large precursor molecules. Proopiomelanocortin is a precursor of beta-endorphin, preproenkephalin gives rise to leucine- and methionine-enkephalins, and preprodynorphin acts as a parent compound for dynorphins (including dynorphins A and B and neoendorphins).[253] While proopiomelanocortin synthesizing neurons generating beta-endorphin are confined to two locations, the hypothalamic arcuate nucleus and nucleus tractus solitarius in the dorsal medulla, preproenkephalin and preprodynorphin neurons are widely distributed in the CNS. Projections of endogenous opioid neurons innervate the neocortex, limbic areas (including the amygdala and NAcc), hippocampus, hypothalamus, thalamus, basal ganglia, periaqueductal gray, and brainstem monoaminergic nuclei.[253] Therefore, virtually all PFC, limbic, and paralimbic areas involved in the stress response and emotional regulation receive rich input from the endogenous opioid system. Different classes of endogenous opioids have their own receptor preferences: beta-endorphins have primary affinity for mu-opioid receptors (MORs) and delta-opioid receptors (DORs), enkephalins show high affinity for DORs, and dynorphins act primarily on kappa-opioid receptors (KORs).[253]

Endogenous opioids have a complex relationship with monoamine systems. At the brainstem level, endogenous opioids exercise an inhibitory effect via MORs on GABA interneurons regulating VTA DA and RN 5HT neurons, thereby disinhibiting monoamine release. Conversely, opioids exercise a direct inhibitory effect via MORs on NE neurons in the LC. DA and NE terminals in the NAcc are additionally modulated via KOR heteroreceptors, whose activation inhibits DA and NE release in this reward-related region.[254] At least in part, anhedonia induced by chronic stress is believed to be caused by KOR-mediated reduction of NE and DA signaling in the NAcc.[254]

Multiple preclinical studies offer indirect evidence of antidepressant-like effects of endorphins and enkephalins in animal models of depression. Antidepressant-like effects are best documented in association with the acute DOR agonist administration, accompanied by increased BDNF and TrkB expression in the rodent frontal cortex, hippocampus, and basolateral amygdala.[255]

Interestingly, unlike chronic antidepressants administration, chronic administration of a DOR agonist failed to elevate BDNF mRNA levels.[256] Furthermore, consistently with our prediction based on the inhibitory role of dynorphin KOR on monoamine signaling, KOR antagonists have demonstrated antidepressant-like benefits and increased hippocampal BDNF mRNA in preclinical models.[254]

The bidirectional relationship between opioid addiction and depression also points to potentially common underlying pathophysiology. Moreover, Kennedy et al., utilizing PET imaging in female MDD patients, found evidence of anomalous endogenous opioid transmission.[230] They also discovered a reduction in MOR binding in the ACC, ventral basal ganglia, hypothalamus, and amygdala of MDD patients compared with healthy subjects.[230] Furthermore, their data demonstrate disturbance of opioid transmission in depressed patients, involving brain areas critical for emotional homeostasis and stress response.

Intracellular Signaling Cascades in MDD

Current antidepressants have repeatedly demonstrated their limitations. Remission rates upon initiation of traditional antidepressant agents have hovered between 30 percent and 40 percent. Even with repeated efforts and advanced augmentation and cotherapy strategies, ultimate remission rates have seldom surpassed 70 percent. Furthermore, even the fortunate individuals who attain remission often have to wait weeks for the clinical benefits to become apparent. Commonly, antidepressants will exact a price. One has to be ready to tolerate sometimes quite bothersome adverse reactions. In fact, sustained well-being is by no means guaranteed. Late loss of efficacy and relapse are often lurking around the corner. So why have we not made greater advances in the last five decades? One of the answers has been repeatedly articulated in the previous chapters: depression is not a biologically homogeneous disease. A one-size-fits-all cure will most likely never be found, as has been the case with other medical conditions with complex etiopathogenesis, such as metabolic syndrome. Another, much simpler reason may be that we have not been looking in all the right places. Could it be that we have been under the spell of monoamine-modulating antidepressants too long? What are the alternatives? It is becoming increasingly evident that current antidepressants confer their benefits not solely through interaction by neuronal membrane surface receptors but, rather, by initiating intracellular signaling cascades that may eventually lead to enduring changes in gene expression and consequent changes in neurotransmission and neuroplasticity. A better understanding of intracellular signaling cascades may therefore be a path to underlying causes of depression and eventually to more successful treatment strategies.

Arguably the most relevant and the best-studied cascade in the MDD context involves the activation of monoamine G-protein receptors, such as D1, beta-1 and beta-2 ARs, and 5HT4, -6, and -7 receptors, which precipitates activation of adenylyl cyclase (AC) via the intracellular Gs domain. AC-mediated conversion of adenosine triphosphate to cAMP leads to activation of protein kinase-A (PKA). CREB, the main target of PKA, is a major transcription factor regulating synthesis of neurotrophic factors, most notably BDNF. The cAMP-initiated cascade is subject to negative regulation by phosphodiesterases (PDEs), of which PDE4 is the most relevant for our story.[257–262] Alternatively, PKA may activate a parallel cascade involving extracellular-regulated kinase (ERK)/mitogen-activated protein kinase (MAPK), discussed in detail further below. Human evidence suggests that depressed patients have lower AC activity, attenuated stimulated cAMP production, and lower PKA levels than do healthy controls.[262] Preclinical studies have demonstrated a change in AC activity influenced by antidepressants and electroconvulsive seizures, an animal equivalent of ECT.[257,258] Furthermore, a global reduction of PDE4 levels (by about 20 percent) was found in the brains of MDD patients, relative to healthy controls.[257]

One of the more MDD-relevant parallel pathways to CREB activation leads from neurotrophic factor binding to their cognate receptors. BDNF binds to TrkB, leading to activation of several parallel cascades. The first one involves TrkB autoactivation and subsequent recruitment of several adaptor proteins, including Sos, a guanine nucleotide exchange protein. Sos participates in conversion from guanosine triphosphate to guanosine diphosphate, which in turn facilitates Ras and Raf activation, ultimately leading to ERK/MAPK initiation and nuclear translocation of transcription factors, including CREB. The second path involves the BDNF/TrkB-initiated PLC-γ/inositol phosphate-3 cascade, while the third one leads to phosphatidylinositol-3 kinase (PI3K)/Akt activation.[257,258]

Postmortem studies have reported reduced Raf/ERK1/2 signaling in the PFC and hippocampus, and MAPK kinase (MEK)/ERK hippocampal activity in MDD patients who committed suicide, relative to control subjects.[258] In contradistinction to hippocampal and PFC findings, elevation of MEK/ERK signaling in the amygdala was associated with depressive and anxious behaviors.[258] Additionally, research has provided evidence that MAPK phosphatase-1 (MKP-1), which targets MAPKs, is overexpressed in the hippocampal region of individuals diagnosed with depression compared with the control group.[263] MAPK substrates include ERK1/2, the c-Jun N-terminal kinases, and p38 MAPKs. These are principal components of intracellular pathways involved in growth factor and cytokine signaling.[263] Therefore, elevated levels of MKP-1 in the brain may precipitate a decline of phosphorylation-activated ERK1/2 and MAPKs and consequently CREB-dependent transcription of BDNF, vascular endothelial growth factor, NPY, CRF, glutamate receptor subunits, and other molecules important in stress response and mood regulation.[259,263] Moreover, antidepressants such as the prototypical SSRI fluoxetine attenuate the upregulation of hippocampal MKP-1 induced by stress. One study found a relationship between MAPK1 polymorphism and remission following antidepressant treatment.[264] The PI3K/Akt pathway is a general signal transduction pathway regulating growth factors, including BDNF, and the neuroprotective compound Bcl-2.[258,265] Postmortem studies have also established lower PI3K/Akt signaling in the ventral PFC of depressed individuals who committed suicide, which can be reversed by antidepressant treatment.[258,266]

Another pathway that also converges on CREB regulation involves glutamate signaling via NMDARs. Activation of glutamate NMDARs is one of the key regulators of long-term potentiation and neuroplasticity, which constitute the neurobiological basis for learning and experience-driven rewiring of the brain. Glutamate binding to NMDAR initiates influx of Ca^{2+} into the cell. Calcium signal is initially propagated by calmodulin and then by one of the isoforms of calmodulin-dependent kinase (CaMK), which subsequently regulates CREB activity.[257–259] The two CaMK isoforms may have opposing actions. CaMK-II phosphorylates CREB, thus interrupting gene transcription, while CaMK-IV promotes CREB-based transcription.[259] Acute stress and stress-related glucocorticoid signaling are also coupled to downstream CaMK, ERK, PLC-γ, Akt, CREB, BDNF, and TrkB activation, and subsequent long-term memory formation.[267] On the other hand, chronic stress and repeated corticosteroid administration, much like preclinical learned helplessness models, have an opposite effect by lowering PKA and subsequently CREB and BDNF signaling.[258]

Human postmortem studies have reported that CREB is reduced in the PFC and hippocampus of depressed individuals who committed suicide.[258,259,262] Behavioral chronic stress models have also been associated with a reduction of CREB activity. Duplicating the scenario with MEK/ERK, increased CREB activity in the amygdala and NAcc was associated with anxious and depressive behaviors.[258,259] Sustained NAcc elevation of CREB in animal models was additionally linked with anhedonia and behavioral despair.[259] Several preclinical studies have reported increases in CREB following chronic antidepressant and ketamine administration. Furthermore, an antidepressant response in a group of MDD patients was accompanied by a significant increase in T-lymphocyte CREB phosphorylation.[258,261]

Recent decades have brought forth a body of information about the role of the Wnt (wingless)/frizzled/disheveled/GSK-3 cascade in the etiology and treatment of MDD. (The exotic-sounding names of the cascade components reflect the early stages of research on these molecules involving fruit flies.) The GSK-3 signaling pathway modulates apoptosis, neurotransmission, cytoskeletal reorganization, and synaptic plasticity.[257,268–272] While increased activity in the GSK pathway supports apoptosis, attenuation of GSK-3 activity leads to upregulation of Bcl-2 and beta-catenin, with consequent enhancement of neuroplasticity and cellular resilience.[268,271–273] Wnt signaling is an important modulator of adult hippocampal neurogenesis.[274] This pathway is also involved in circadian regulation.[271] A postmortem study has reported elevation of GSK-3 in the ventral PFC of depressed suicide victims but not in nondepressed suicide victims.[275]

As a point of interest, inhibition of the GSK-3 pathway results in both anti-manic and antidepressant effect. A diverse group of antidepressants and mood-stabilizing agents, including lithium, valproate, and atypical antipsychotics, directly and indirectly interact with the GSK-3 pathway.[257,268,269,271–273,276] Serotonergic antidepressants are believed to inhibit GSK-3 via its action 5HT1A receptors.[276] Benefit from adjunct mood-stabilizing medications in MDD patients has been linked to polymorphisms of the genes regulating GSK-3 function.[277] The rapid antidepressant action of ketamine is supposedly mediated by stimulation of BDNF release and subsequent activation of the Akt pathway, leading to phosphorylation and inhibition of GSK-3.[276]

Conclusion

The voluminous evidence reviewed in this chapter offers no smoking guns. No specific neurotransmitters or neuromodulators are affected in a similar fashion in all depressed patients—most likely we are dealing with distributed vulnerabilities. Because of the interconnectedness of the neural signaling systems, it is virtually impossible to detect individual "faults." Monoamines, peptides, GABA, and glutamate mutually regulate one another in complex, intricate ways. Rather then viewing individual transmitter systems as separate entities, it may be more helpful to consider them as components of a highly integrated system underpinning immensely complex neural functions. We have come to understand that neural structures receive homeostatic inputs from local neural circuits, as well as from the remote brain areas. For example, if we were to detect an elevated level of glutamatergic transmission in a certain brain area, is it because local GABA interneurons or their receptors are not functioning well? Could it be that astrocyte glutamate transporters are not doing their job? Perhaps remote monoamine neurons are not providing proper modulation? Or have local peptides failed in their mission? As you can see, this quandary may not have a plausible resolution. To make things even more impenetrable, we are dealing with a structure with multiple levels.

At the level of transcending neurotransmission and cellular communication are the higher neural processes such as cognition, sensation, and emotion. Although these psychological phenomena are ostensibly underpinned by the function of neural networks and communication among their cellular components, they cannot be reasonably reduced to the function of these elements. This form of reductionism would be akin to attempting to explain the structure of Dostoevski's novels by the distribution of ink on the paper or the sensibility of Fellini's films by the flickering of pixels. Psychological phenomena have their own laws, which may both arise from and descend to the cellular signaling level, but they are not ultimately translatable to the lower levels of processing.

At the subcellular level, inadequate neurotransmission may be a consequence of improper translation of chemical signals from cell-surface receptors to intracellular signaling cascades, the result of maladaptive gene expression and protein synthesis. Biological heterogeneity of MDD and individual differences in its expression, shaped by unique life experiences, further compound our predicament. So why bother? If the puzzle of depression cannot be solved, why should we continue with this exercise in futility? Because solution of this problem is not hopeless—as a matter of fact, it is becoming much more hopeful. Understanding these intricate connections in the biological underpinnings of MDD provides more opportunities to detect and intervene. In other words, complicated problems require complex and integrated solutions.

References

1. Schildkraut JJ. The catecholamine hypothesis of affective disorders: a review of supporting evidence. *Am J Psychiatry*. 1965;122:509–522.
2. Schildkraut JJ, Mooney JJ. Toward a rapidly acting antidepressant: the normetanephrine and extraneuronal monoamine transporter (uptake 2) hypothesis. *Am J Psychiatry*. 2004;161:909–911.
3. Mooney JJ, Samson JA, Hennen J, et al. Enhanced norepinephrine output during long-term desipramine treatment: a possible role for the extraneuronal monoamine transporter (SLC22A3). *J Psychiatr Res*. 2008;42:605–611.
4. Rahman Z, Ring RH, Young K, et al. Inhibition of uptake 2 (or extraneuronal monoamine transporter) by normetanephrine potentiates the neurochemical effects of venlafaxine. *Brain Res*. 2008;1203:68–78.
5. Citri A, Malenka RC. Synaptic plasticity: multiple forms, functions, and mechanisms. *Neuropsychopharmacology*. 2008;33:18–41.
6. Carvalho AL, Caldeira MV, Santos SD, Duarte CB. Role of the brain-derived neurotrophic factor at glutamatergic synapses. *Br J Pharmacol*. 2008;153(suppl 1):S310–S324.
7. Nacher J, McEwen BS. The role of N-methyl-D-aspartate receptors in neurogenesis. *Hippocampus*. 2006;16:267–270.
8. Nacher J, Varea E, Miguel Blasco-Ibanez J, et al. N-methyl-D-aspartate receptor expression during adult neurogenesis in the rat dentate gyrus. *Neuroscience*. 2007;144:855–864.
9. Papadia S, Soriano FX, Leveille F, et al. Synaptic NMDA receptor activity boosts intrinsic antioxidant defenses. *Nat Neurosci*. 2008;11:476–487.
10. Hardingham GE, Fukunaga Y, Bading H. Extrasynaptic NMDARs oppose synaptic NMDARs by triggering CREB shut-off and cell death pathways. *Nat Neurosci*. 2002;5:405–414.
11. Kugaya A, Sanacora G. Beyond monoamines: glutamatergic function in mood disorders. *CNS Spectr*. 2005;10:808–819.
12. Greenwood SM, Connolly CN. Dendritic and mitochondrial changes during glutamate excitotoxicity. *Neuropharmacology*. 2007;53:891–898.
13. Panatier A, Theodosis DT, Mothet JP, et al. Glia-derived D-serine controls NMDA receptor activity and synaptic memory. *Cell*. 2006;125:775–784.
14. Stellwagen D, Beattie EC, Seo JY, Malenka RC. Differential regulation of AMPA receptor and GABA receptor trafficking by tumor necrosis factor-alpha. *J Neurosci*. 2005;25:3219–3228.
15. Santello M, Bezzi P, Volterra A. TNFalpha controls glutamatergic gliotransmission in the hippocampal dentate gyrus. *Neuron*. 2011;69:988–1001.

16. Qiu Z, Sweeney DD, Netzeband JG, Gruol DL. Chronic interleukin-6 alters NMDA receptor-mediated membrane responses and enhances neurotoxicity in developing CNS neurons. *J Neurosci.* 1998;18:10445–10456.

17. Palucha A, Pilc A. On the role of metabotropic glutamate receptors in the mechanisms of action of antidepressants. *Pol J Pharmacol.* 2002;54:581–586.

18. Nicoletti F, Bockaert J, Collingridge GL, et al. Metabotropic glutamate receptors: from the workbench to the bedside. *Neuropharmacology.* 2011;60:1017–1041.

19. Jean YY, Lercher LD, Dreyfus CF. Glutamate elicits release of BDNF from basal forebrain astrocytes in a process dependent on metabotropic receptors and the PLC pathway. *Neuron Glia Biol.* 2008;4:35–42.

20. Smialowska M, Szewczyk B, Branski P, et al. Effect of chronic imipramine or electroconvulsive shock on the expression of mGluR1a and mGluR5a immunoreactivity in rat brain hippocampus. *Neuropharmacology.* 2002;42:1016–1023.

21. Stam R, de Lange RP, Graveland H, Verhave PS, Wiegant VM. Involvement of group II metabotropic glutamate receptors in stress-induced behavioural sensitization. *Psychopharmacology (Berl).* 2007;191:365–375.

22. McEwen BS, Chattarji S, Diamond DM, et al. The neurobiological properties of tianeptine (Stablon): from monoamine hypothesis to glutamatergic modulation. *Mol Psychiatry.* 2010;15:237–249.

23. Fendt M, Schmid S, Thakker DR, et al. mGluR7 facilitates extinction of aversive memories and controls amygdala plasticity. *Mol Psychiatry.* 2008;13:970–979.

24. Tatarczynska E, Palucha A, Szewczyk B, Chojnacka-Wojcik E, Wieronska J, Pilc A. Anxiolytic- and antidepressant-like effects of group III metabotropic glutamate agonist (1S,3R,4S)-1-aminocyclopentane-1,3,4-tricarboxylic acid (ACPT-I) in rats. *Pol J Pharmacol.* 2002;54:707–710.

25. Tzingounis AV, Wadiche JI. Glutamate transporters: confining runaway excitation by shaping synaptic transmission. *Nat Rev Neurosci.* 2007;8:935–947.

26. Medina A, Burke S, Thompson RC, et al. Glutamate transporters: a key piece in the glutamate puzzle of major depressive disorder. *J Psychiatr Res.* 2013;47:1150–1156.

27. Ronnback L, Hansson E. On the potential role of glutamate transport in mental fatigue. *J Neuroinflamm.* 2004;1:22.

28. Kim K, Lee SG, Kegelman TP, et al. Role of excitatory amino acid transporter-2 (EAAT2) and glutamate in neurodegeneration: opportunities for developing novel therapeutics. *J Cell Physiol.* 2011;226:2484–2493.

29. Cameron HA, Tanapat P, Gould E. Adrenal steroids and N-methyl-D-aspartate receptor activation regulate neurogenesis in the dentate gyrus of adult rats through a common pathway. *Neuroscience.* 1998;82:349–354.

30. Takahashi T, Kimoto T, Tanabe N, Hattori TA, Yasumatsu N, Kawato S. Corticosterone acutely prolonged N-methyl-D-aspartate receptor-mediated Ca2+ elevation in cultured rat hippocampal neurons. *J Neurochem.* 2002;83:1441–1451.

31. Kuzmiski JB, Marty V, Baimoukhametova DV, Bains JS. Stress-induced priming of glutamate synapses unmasks associative short-term plasticity. *Nat Neurosci.* 2010;13:1257–1264.

32. Timmermans W, Xiong H, Hoogenraad CC, Krugers HJ. Stress and excitatory synapses: from health to disease. *Neuroscience.* 2013;248:626–636.

33. Musazzi L, Racagni G, Popoli M. Stress, glucocorticoids and glutamate release: effects of antidepressant drugs. *Neurochem Int.* 2011;59:138–149.

34. Ikeda H, Akiyama G, Fujii Y, Minowa R, Koshikawa N, Cools AR. Role of AMPA and

NMDA receptors in the nucleus accumbens shell in turning behaviour of rats: interaction with dopamine receptors. *Neuropharmacology*. 2003;44:81–87.

35. Poeggeler B, Rassoulpour A, Wu HQ, Guidetti P, Roberts RC, Schwarcz R. Dopamine receptor activation reveals a novel, kynurenate-sensitive component of striatal N-methyl-D-aspartate neurotoxicity. *Neuroscience*. 2007;148:188–197.

36. Trudeau LE. Glutamate co-transmission as an emerging concept in monoamine neuron function. *J Psychiatry Neurosci*. 2004;29:296–310.

37. Yuen EY, Jiang Q, Chen P, Feng J, Yan Z. Activation of 5-HT2A/C receptors counteracts 5-HT1A regulation of n-methyl-D-aspartate receptor channels in pyramidal neurons of prefrontal cortex. *J Biol Chem*. 2008;283:17194–17204.

38. Cai X, Kallarackal AJ, Kvarta MD, et al. Local potentiation of excitatory synapses by serotonin and its alteration in rodent models of depression. *Nat Neurosci*. 2013;16: 464–472.

39. Jacobs GE, der Grond J, Teeuwisse WM, et al. Hypothalamic glutamate levels following serotonergic stimulation: a pilot study using 7-Tesla magnetic resonance spectroscopy in healthy volunteers. *Prog Neuropsychopharmacol Biol Psychiatry*. 2010;34:486–491.

40. O'Donnell J, Zeppenfeld D, McConnell E, Pena S, Nedergaard M. Norepinephrine: a neuromodulator that boosts the function of multiple cell types to optimize CNS performance. *Neurochem Res*. 2012;37:2496–2512.

41. Wang M, Ramos BP, Paspalas CD, et al. Alpha2A-adrenoceptors strengthen working memory networks by inhibiting cAMP-HCN channel signaling in prefrontal cortex. *Cell*. 2007;129:397–410.

42. Forray MI, Gysling K. Role of noradrenergic projections to the bed nucleus of the stria terminalis in the regulation of the hypothalamic-pituitary-adrenal axis. *Brain Res Brain Res Rev*. 2004;47:145–160.

43. Egli RE, Kash TL, Choo K, et al. Norepinephrine modulates glutamatergic transmission in the bed nucleus of the stria terminalis. *Neuropsychopharmacology*. 2005;30:657–668.

44. Levine J, Panchalingam K, Rapoport A, Gershon S, McClure RJ, Pettegrew JW. Increased cerebrospinal fluid glutamine levels in depressed patients. *Biol Psychiatry*. 2000; 47:586–593.

45. Hashimoto K, Sawa A, Iyo M. Increased levels of glutamate in brains from patients with mood disorders. *Biol Psychiatry*. 2007;62:1310–1316.

46. Catena-Dell'osso M, Fagiolini A, Rotella F, Baroni S, Marazziti D. Glutamate system as target for development of novel antidepressants. *CNS Spectr*. 2013;18:188–198.

47. Garakani A, Martinez JM, Yehuda R, Gorman JM. Cerebrospinal fluid levels of glutamate and corticotropin releasing hormone in major depression before and after treatment. *J Affect Disord*. 2013;146:262–265.

48. Frye MA, Tsai GE, Huggins T, Coyle JT, Post RM. Low cerebrospinal fluid glutamate and glycine in refractory affective disorder. *Biol Psychiatry*. 2007;61:162–166.

49. Auer DP, Putz B, Kraft E, Lipinski B, Schill J, Holsboer F. Reduced glutamate in the anterior cingulate cortex in depression: an in vivo proton magnetic resonance spectroscopy study. *Biol Psychiatry*. 2000;47:305–313.

50. Sanacora G, Rothman DL, Mason G, Krystal JH. Clinical studies implementing glutamate neurotransmission in mood disorders. *Ann N Y Acad Sci*. 2003;1003:292–308.

51. Portella MJ, de Diego-Adelino J, Gomez-Anson B, et al. Ventromedial prefrontal spectroscopic abnormalities over the course of depression: a comparison among first episode, remitted recurrent and chronic patients. *J Psychiatr Res*. 2011;45:427–434.

52. de Diego-Adelino J, Portella MJ, Gomez-Anson B, et al. Hippocampal abnormalities of

glutamate/glutamine, N-acetylaspartate and choline in patients with depression are related to past illness burden. *J Psychiatry Neurosci.* 2013;38:107–116.

53. Jarnum H, Eskildsen SF, Steffensen EG, et al. Longitudinal MRI study of cortical thickness, perfusion, and metabolite levels in major depressive disorder. *Acta Psychiatr Scand.* 2011;124:435–446.

54. Hansel A, von Kanel R. The ventro-medial prefrontal cortex: a major link between the autonomic nervous system, regulation of emotion, and stress reactivity? *Biopsychosoc Med.* 2008;2:21.

55. Sanacora G, Treccani G, Popoli M. Towards a glutamate hypothesis of depression: an emerging frontier of neuropsychopharmacology for mood disorders. *Neuropharmacology.* 2012;62:63–77.

56. Musazzi L, Treccani G, Mallei A, Popoli M. The action of antidepressants on the glutamate system: regulation of glutamate release and glutamate receptors. *Biol Psychiatry.* 2013;73:1180–1188.

57. Black MD. Therapeutic potential of positive AMPA modulators and their relationship to AMPA receptor subunits: a review of preclinical data. *Psychopharmacology (Berl).* 2005;179:154–163.

58. Zhang H, Etherington LA, Hafner AS, et al. Regulation of AMPA receptor surface trafficking and synaptic plasticity by a cognitive enhancer and antidepressant molecule. *Mol Psychiatry.* 2013;18:471–484.

59. Pilc A, Wieronska JM, Skolnick P. Glutamate-based antidepressants: preclinical psychopharmacology. *Biol Psychiatry.* 2013;73:1125–1132.

60. Zarate CA Jr, Singh JB, Carlson PJ, et al. A randomized trial of an N-methyl-D-aspartate antagonist in treatment-resistant major depression. *Arch Gen Psychiatry.* 2006;63:856–864.

61. Zarate C Jr, Machado-Vieira R, Henter I, Ibrahim L, Diazgranados N, Salvadore G. Glutamatergic modulators: the future of treating mood disorders? *Harv Rev Psychiatry.* 2010;18:293–303.

62. Krystal JH, Sanacora G, Duman RS. Rapid-acting glutamatergic antidepressants: the path to ketamine and beyond. *Biol Psychiatry.* 2013;73:1133–1141.

63. Salvadore G, Singh JB. Ketamine as a fast acting antidepressant: current knowledge and open questions. *CNS Neurosci Ther.* 2013;19:428–436.

64. Duman RS, Aghajanian GK. Synaptic dysfunction in depression: potential therapeutic targets. *Science.* 2012;338:68–72.

65. Li N, Lee B, Liu RJ, et al. mTOR-dependent synapse formation underlies the rapid antidepressant effects of NMDA antagonists. *Science.* 2010;329:959–964.

66. Yang C, Hu YM, Zhou ZQ, Zhang GF, Yang JJ. Acute administration of ketamine in rats increases hippocampal BDNF and mTOR levels during forced swimming test. *Upsala J Med Sci.* 2013;118:3–8.

67. Haile CN, Murrough JW, Iosifescu DV, et al. Plasma brain derived neurotrophic factor (BDNF) and response to ketamine in treatment-resistant depression. *Int J Neuropsychopharmacol.* 2014;17(2):331–336.

68. Yang C, Hong T, Shen J, et al. Ketamine exerts antidepressant effects and reduces IL-1beta and IL-6 levels in rat prefrontal cortex and hippocampus. *Exp Ther Med.* 2013; 5:1093–1096.

69. Anand A, Charney DS, Oren DA, et al. Attenuation of the neuropsychiatric effects of ketamine with lamotrigine: support for hyperglutamatergic effects of N-methyl-D-aspartate receptor antagonists. *Arch Gen Psychiatry.* 2000;57:270–276.

70. Doyle OM, De Simoni S, Schwarz AJ, et al. Quantifying the attenuation of the ketamine

pharmacological magnetic resonance imaging response in humans: a validation using antipsychotic and glutamatergic agents. *J Pharmacol Exp Ther.* 2013;345:151–160.

71. Carlson PJ, Diazgranados N, Nugent AC, et al. Neural correlates of rapid antidepressant response to ketamine in treatment-resistant unipolar depression: a preliminary positron emission tomography study. *Biol Psychiatry.* 2013;73:1213–1221.

72. Scheidegger M, Walter M, Lehmann M, et al. Ketamine decreases resting state functional network connectivity in healthy subjects: implications for antidepressant drug action. *PLoS One.* 2012;7:e44799.

73. Luscher B, Shen Q, Sahir N. The GABAergic deficit hypothesis of major depressive disorder. *Mol Psychiatry.* 2011;16:383–406.

74. Croarkin PE, Levinson AJ, Daskalakis ZJ. Evidence for GABAergic inhibitory deficits in major depressive disorder. *Neurosci Biobehav Rev.* 2011;35:818–825.

75. Caputi A, Melzer S, Michael M, Monyer H. The long and short of GABAergic neurons. *Curr Opin Neurobiol.* 2013;23:179–186.

76. Cameron HA, Dayer AG. New interneurons in the adult neocortex: small, sparse, but significant? *Biol Psychiatry.* 2008;63:650–655.

77. Yoon BE, Woo J, Lee CJ. Astrocytes as GABA-ergic and GABA-ceptive cells. *Neurochem Res.* 2012;37:2474–2479.

78. Lee JJ, Hahm ET, Lee CH, Cho YW. Serotonergic modulation of GABAergic and glutamatergic synaptic transmission in mechanically isolated rat medial preoptic area neurons. *Neuropsychopharmacology.* 2008;33:340–352.

79. Millan MJ. Multi-target strategies for the improved treatment of depressive states: conceptual foundations and neuronal substrates, drug discovery and therapeutic application. *Pharmacol Ther.* 2006;110:135–370.

80. Bang-Andersen B, Ruhland T, Jorgensen M, et al. Discovery of 1-[2-(2,4-dimethylphenyl sulfanyl)phenyl]piperazine (Lu AA21004): a novel multimodal compound for the treatment of major depressive disorder. *J Med Chem.* 2011;54:3206–3221.

81. Han SK, Chong W, Li LH, Lee IS, Murase K, Ryu PD. Noradrenaline excites and inhibits GABAergic transmission in parvocellular neurons of rat hypothalamic paraventricular nucleus. *J Neurophysiol.* 2002;87:2287–2296.

82. Saitow F, Satake S, Yamada J, Konishi S. beta-Adrenergic receptor-mediated presynaptic facilitation of inhibitory GABAergic transmission at cerebellar interneuron-Purkinje cell synapses. *J Neurophysiol.* 2000;84:2016–2025.

83. Inoue W, Baimoukhametova DV, Fuzesi T, et al. Noradrenaline is a stress-associated metaplastic signal at GABA synapses. *Nat Neurosci.* 2013;16:605–612.

84. Herman JP, Renda A, Bodie B. Norepinephrine-gamma-aminobutyric acid (GABA) interaction in limbic stress circuits: effects of reboxetine on GABAergic neurons. *Biol Psychiatry.* 2003;53:166–174.

85. Shen Q, Lal R, Luellen BA, Earnheart JC, Andrews AM, Luscher B. gamma-Aminobutyric acid-type A receptor deficits cause hypothalamic-pituitary-adrenal axis hyperactivity and antidepressant drug sensitivity reminiscent of melancholic forms of depression. *Biol Psychiatry.* 2010;68:512–520.

86. Kalueff AV, Nutt DJ. Role of GABA in anxiety and depression. *Depress Anxiety.* 2007; 24:495–517.

87. Kucukibrahimoglu E, Saygin MZ, Caliskan M, Kaplan OK, Unsal C, Goren MZ. The change in plasma GABA, glutamine and glutamate levels in fluoxetine- or S-citalopram-treated female patients with major depression. *Eur J Clin Pharmacol.* 2009;65:571–577.

88. Krystal JH, Sanacora G, Blumberg H, et al. Glutamate and GABA systems as targets for

novel antidepressant and mood-stabilizing treatments. *Mol Psychiatry.* 2002;7(suppl 1):S71–S80.

89. Rajkowska G, O'Dwyer G, Teleki Z, Stockmeier CA, Miguel-Hidalgo JJ. GABAergic neurons immunoreactive for calcium binding proteins are reduced in the prefrontal cortex in major depression. *Neuropsychopharmacology.* 2007;32:471–482.

90. Guilloux JP, Douillard-Guilloux G, Kota R, et al. Molecular evidence for BDNF- and GABA-related dysfunctions in the amygdala of female subjects with major depression. *Mol Psychiatry.* 2012;17:1130–1142.

91. Bielau H, Steiner J, Mawrin C, et al. Dysregulation of GABAergic neurotransmission in mood disorders: a postmortem study. *Ann N Y Acad Sci.* 2007;1096:157–169.

92. Karolewicz B, Maciag D, O'Dwyer G, Stockmeier CA, Feyissa AM, Rajkowska G. Reduced level of glutamic acid decarboxylase-67 kDa in the prefrontal cortex in major depression. *Int J Neuropsychopharmacol.* 2010;13:411–420.

93. Sanacora G, Gueorguieva R, Epperson CN, et al. Subtype-specific alterations of gamma-aminobutyric acid and glutamate in patients with major depression. *Arch Gen Psychiatry.* 2004;61:705–713.

94. Gabbay V, Mao X, Klein RG, et al. Anterior cingulate cortex gamma-aminobutyric acid in depressed adolescents: relationship to anhedonia. *Arch Gen Psychiatry.* 2012;69:139–149.

95. Hasler G, van der Veen JW, Tumonis T, Meyers N, Shen J, Drovcts WC. Reduced prefrontal glutamate/glutamine and gamma-aminobutyric acid levels in major depression determined using proton magnetic resonance spectroscopy. *Arch Gen Psychiatry.* 2007;64:193–200.

96. Hasler G, Neumeister A, van der Veen JW, et al. Normal prefrontal gamma-aminobutyric acid levels in remitted depressed subjects determined by proton magnetic resonance spectroscopy. *Biol Psychiatry.* 2005;58:969–973.

97. Price RB, Shungu DC, Mao X, et al. Amino acid neurotransmitters assessed by proton magnetic resonance spectroscopy: relationship to treatment resistance in major depressive disorder. *Biol Psychiatry.* 2009;65:792–800.

98. Murphy DL, Andrews AM, Wichems CH, Li Q, Tohda M, Greenberg B. Brain serotonin neurotransmission: an overview and update with an emphasis on serotonin subsystem heterogeneity, multiple receptors, interactions with other neurotransmitter systems, and consequent implications for understanding the actions of serotonergic drugs. *J Clin Psychiatry.* 1998;59(suppl 15):4–12.

99. Kiss JP. Theory of active antidepressants: a nonsynaptic approach to the treatment of depression. *Neurochem Int.* 2008;52:34–39.

100. Daubert EA, Condron BG. Serotonin: a regulator of neuronal morphology and circuitry. *Trends Neurosci.* 2010;33:424–434.

101. Hannon J, Hoyer D. Molecular biology of 5-HT receptors. *Behav Brain Res.* 2008;195:198–213.

102. Artigas F. Serotonin receptors involved in antidepressant effects. *Pharmacol Ther.* 2013;137:119–131.

103. Fink KB, Gothert M. 5-HT receptor regulation of neurotransmitter release. *Pharmacol Rev.* 2007;59:360–417.

104. Sasaki M, Shibata E, Tohyama K, et al. Monoamine neurons in the human brain stem: anatomy, magnetic resonance imaging findings, and clinical implications. *Neuroreport.* 2008;19:1649–1654.

105. Sharp T, Boothman L, Raley J, Queree P. Important messages in the "post": recent discoveries in 5-HT neurone feedback control. *Trends Pharmacol Sci.* 2007;28:629–636.

106. Oxenkrug GF. Genetic and hormonal regulation of tryptophan kynurenine metabolism: implications for vascular cognitive impairment, major depressive disorder, and aging. *Ann N Y Acad Sci.* 2007;1122:35–49.

107. Carr GV, Lucki I. The role of serotonin receptor subtypes in treating depression: a review of animal studies. *Psychopharmacology (Berl).* 2011;213:265–287.

108. Trivedi MH, Hollander E, Nutt D, Blier P. Clinical evidence and potential neurobiological underpinnings of unresolved symptoms of depression. *J Clin Psychiatry.* 2008;69:246–258.

109. Hamon M, Blier P. Monoamine neurocircuitry in depression and strategies for new treatments. *Prog Neuropsychopharmacol Biol Psychiatry.* 2013;45:54–63.

110. Pehrson AL, Sanchez C. Serotonergic modulation of glutamate neurotransmission as a strategy for treating depression and cognitive dysfunction. *CNS Spectr.* 2014;19(2): 121–133.

111. Cowen PJ. Serotonin and depression: pathophysiological mechanism or marketing myth? *Trends Pharmacol Sci.* 2008;29:433–436.

112. Albert PR, Benkelfat C. The neurobiology of depression—revisiting the serotonin hypothesis. II. Genetic, epigenetic and clinical studies. *Philos Trans R Soc Lond B Biol Sci.* 2013;368:20120535.

113. Sharp T, Cowen PJ. 5-HT and depression: is the glass half-full? *Curr Opin Pharmacol.* 2011;11:45–51.

114. Duval F, Mokrani MC, Bailey P, et al. Serotonergic and noradrenergic function in depression: clinical correlates. *Dialogues Clin Neurosci.* 2000;2:299–308.

115. Savitz JB, Drevets WC. Neuroreceptor imaging in depression. *Neurobiol Dis.* 2013;52: 49–65.

116. Dean B, Tawadros N, Seo MS, et al. Lower cortical serotonin 2A receptors in major depressive disorder, suicide and in rats after administration of imipramine. *Int J Neuropsychopharmacol.* 2014;17(6):895–906.

117. Joensuu M, Tolmunen T, Saarinen PI, et al. Reduced midbrain serotonin transporter availability in drug-naive patients with depression measured by SERT-specific [(123)I] nor-beta-CIT SPECT imaging. *Psychiatry Res.* 2007;154:125–131.

118. Szabadi E. Functional neuroanatomy of the central noradrenergic system. *J Psychopharmacol.* 2013;27:659–693.

119. Itoi K, Sugimoto N. The brainstem noradrenergic systems in stress, anxiety and depression. *J Neuroendocrinol.* 2010;22:355–361.

120. Chamberlain SR, Robbins TW. Noradrenergic modulation of cognition: therapeutic implications. *J Psychopharmacol.* 2013;27:694–718.

121. Ferrucci M, Giorgi FS, Bartalucci A, Busceti CL, Fornai F. The effects of locus coeruleus and norepinephrine in methamphetamine toxicity. *Curr Neuropharmacol.* 2013; 11:80–94.

122. Bangasser DA, Wiersielis KR, Khantsis S. Sex differences in the locus coeruleus-norepinephrine system and its regulation by stress. *Brain Res.* 2016;1641:177–188.

123. Stone EA, Lin Y, Sarfraz Y, Quartermain D. The role of the central noradrenergic system in behavioral inhibition. *Brain Res Rev.* 2011;67:193–208.

124. Arnsten AF. Catecholamine influences on dorsolateral prefrontal cortical networks. *Biol Psychiatry.* 2011;69:e89–e99.

125. Elhwuegi AS. Central monoamines and their role in major depression. *Prog Neuropsychopharmacol Biol Psychiatry.* 2004;28:435–451.

126. Quesseveur G, Gardier AM, Guiard BP. The monoaminergic tripartite synapse: a puta-

tive target for currently available antidepressant drugs. *Curr Drug Targets*. 2013;14: 1277–1294.

127. Kato TA, Yamauchi Y, Horikawa H, et al. Neurotransmitters, psychotropic drugs and microglia: clinical implications for psychiatry. *Curr Med Chem*. 2013;20:331–344.

128. Pav M, Kovaru H, Fiserova A, Havrdova E, Lisa V. Neurobiological aspects of depressive disorder and antidepressant treatment: role of glia. *Physiol Res*. 2008;57:151–164.

129. Hensler JG, Artigas F, Bortolozzi A, et al. Catecholamine/serotonin interactions: systems thinking for brain function and disease. *Adv Pharmacol*. 2013;68:167–197.

130. Glowinski J, Baldessarini RJ. Metabolism of norepinephrine in the central nervous system. *Pharmacol Rev*. 1966;18:1201–1238.

131. Arnsten AF, Pliszka SR. Catecholamine influences on prefrontal cortical function: relevance to treatment of attention deficit/hyperactivity disorder and related disorders. *Pharmacol Biochem Behav*. 2011;99:211–216.

132. Tremblay P, Blier P. Catecholaminergic strategies for the treatment of major depression. *Curr Drug Targets*. 2006;7:149–158.

133. Drago A, Crisafulli C, Sidoti A, Serretti A. The molecular interaction between the glutamatergic, noradrenergic, dopaminergic and serotoninergic systems informs a detailed genetic perspective on depressive phenotypes. *Prog Neurobiol*. 2011;94:418–460.

134. Doze VA, Papay RS, Goldenstein BL, et al. Long-term alpha1A-adrenergic receptor stimulation improves synaptic plasticity, cognitive function, mood, and longevity. *Mol Pharmacol*. 2011;80:747–758.

135. Gyires K, Zadori ZS, Shujaa N, et al. Pharmacological analysis of alpha(2)-adrenoceptor subtypes mediating analgesic, anti-inflammatory and gastroprotective actions. *Inflammopharmacology*. 2009;17:171–179.

136. Gyires K, Zadori ZS, Torok T, Matyus P. alpha(2)-Adrenoceptor subtypes-mediated physiological, pharmacological actions. *Neurochem Int*. 2009;55:447–453.

137. Kalkman HO, Subramanian N, Hoyer D. Extended radioligand binding profile of iloperidone: a broad spectrum dopamine/serotonin/norepinephrine receptor antagonist for the management of psychotic disorders. *Neuropsychopharmacology*. 2001;25:904–914.

138. Nalepa I, Kreiner G, Bielawski A, Rafa-Zablocka K, Roman A. alpha1-Adrenergic receptor subtypes in the central nervous system: insights from genetically engineered mouse models. *Pharmacol Rep*. 2013;65:1489–1497.

139. Perez DM, Doze VA. Cardiac and neuroprotection regulated by alpha(1)-adrenergic receptor subtypes. *J Recept Signal Transduct Res*. 2011;31:98–110.

140. Pertovaara A. The noradrenergic pain regulation system: a potential target for pain therapy. *Eur J Pharmacol*. 2013;716:2–7.

141. Hopwood SE, Stamford JA. Noradrenergic modulation of serotonin release in rat dorsal and median raphe nuclei via alpha(1) and alpha(2A) adrenoceptors. *Neuropharmacology*. 2001;41:433–442.

142. El Mansari M, Guiard BP, Chernoloz O, Ghanbari R, Katz N, Blier P. Relevance of norepinephrine-dopamine interactions in the treatment of major depressive disorder. *CNS Neurosci Ther*. 2010;16:e1–e17.

143. Vazquez-Borsetti P, Celada P, Cortes R, Artigas F. Simultaneous projections from prefrontal cortex to dopaminergic and serotonergic nuclei. *Int J Neuropsychopharmacol*. 2011;14:289–302.

144. Millan MJ. Dual- and triple-acting agents for treating core and co-morbid symptoms of major depression: novel concepts, new drugs. *Neurotherapeutics*. 2009;6:53–77.

145. Wong ML, Kling MA, Munson PJ, et al. Pronounced and sustained central hypernor-adrenergic function in major depression with melancholic features: relation to hyper-cortisolism and corticotropin-releasing hormone. *Proc Natl Acad Sci U S A.* 2000; 97:325–330.

146. Gold PW, Wong ML, Goldstein DS, et al. Cardiac implications of increased arterial entry and reversible 24-h central and peripheral norepinephrine levels in melancho-lia. *Proc Natl Acad Sci U S A.* 2005;102:8303–8308.

147. Dremencov E, el Mansari M, Blier P. Brain norepinephrine system as a target for anti-depressant and mood stabilizing medications. *Curr Drug Targets.* 2009;10:1061–1068.

148. Goddard AW, Ball SG, Martinez J, et al. Current perspectives of the roles of the central norepinephrine system in anxiety and depression. *Depress Anxiety.* 2010;27:339–350.

149. Lambert G, Johansson M, Agren H, Friberg P. Reduced brain norepinephrine and dopamine release in treatment-refractory depressive illness: evidence in support of the catecholamine hypothesis of mood disorders. *Arch Gen Psychiatry.* 2000;57: 787–793.

150. Brunello N, Mendlewicz J, Kasper S, et al. The role of noradrenaline and selective noradrenaline reuptake inhibition in depression. *Eur Neuropsychopharmacol.* 2002; 12:461–475.

151. Ordway GA, Schenk J, Stockmeier CA, May W, Klimek V. Elevated agonist binding to alpha2-adrenoceptors in the locus coeruleus in major depression. *Biol Psychiatry.* 2003;53:315–323.

152. Rajkowska G. Histopathology of the prefrontal cortex in major depression: what does it tell us about dysfunctional monoaminergic circuits? *Prog Brain Res.* 2000;126: 397–412.

153. Ressler KJ, Nemeroff CB. Role of serotonergic and noradrenergic systems in the patho-physiology of depression and anxiety disorders. *Depress Anxiety.* 2000;12(suppl 1):2–19.

154. Piletz JE, Ordway GA, Rajkowska G, et al. Differential expression of alpha2-adrenoceptor vs. imidazoline binding sites in postmortem orbitofrontal cortex and amygdala of depressed subjects. *J Psychiatr Res.* 2003;37:399–409.

155. Correa H, Duval F, Claude MM, et al. Noradrenergic dysfunction and antidepressant treatment response. *Eur Neuropsychopharmacol.* 2001;11:163–168.

156. Avissar S, Barki-Harrington L, Nechamkin Y, Roitman G, Schreiber G. Reduced beta-adrenergic receptor-coupled Gs protein function and Gs alpha immunoreactivity in mononuclear leukocytes of patients with depression. *Biol Psychiatry.* 1996;39:755–760.

157. Euteneuer F, Mills PJ, Rief W, Ziegler MG, Dimsdale JE. Association of in vivo beta-adrenergic receptor sensitivity with inflammatory markers in healthy subjects. *Psy-chosom Med.* 2012;74:271–277.

158. Euteneuer F, Mills PJ, Rief W, Ziegler MG, Dimsdale JE. Subjective social status pre-dicts in vivo responsiveness of beta-adrenergic receptors. *Health Psychol.* 2012;31: 525–529.

159. Euteneuer F, Ziegler MG, Mills PJ, Rief W, Dimsdale JE. In vivo beta-adrenergic recep-tor responsiveness: ethnic differences in the relationship with symptoms of depres-sion and fatigue. *Int J Behav Med.* 2014;21(5):843–850.

160. Miller AH, Maletic V, Raison CL. Inflammation and its discontents: the role of cyto-kines in the pathophysiology of major depression. *Biol Psychiatry.* 2009;65:732–741.

161. Valdizan EM, Gutierrez O, Pazos A. Adenylate cyclase activity in postmortem brain of

suicide subjects: reduced response to beta-adrenergic stimulation. *Biol Psychiatry.* 2003;54:1457–1464.

162. Klimek V, Rajkowska G, Luker SN, et al. Brain noradrenergic receptors in major depression and schizophrenia. *Neuropsychopharmacology.* 1999;21:69–81.

163. Little KY, Ranc J, Gilmore J, Patel A, Clark TB. Lack of pineal beta-adrenergic receptor alterations in suicide victims with major depression. *Psychoneuroendocrinology.* 1997;22:53–62.

164. Tritsch NX, Sabatini BL. Dopaminergic modulation of synaptic transmission in cortex and striatum. *Neuron.* 2012;76:33–50.

165. Dunlop BW, Nemeroff CB. The role of dopamine in the pathophysiology of depression. *Arch Gen Psychiatry.* 2007;64:327–337.

166. Bjorklund A, Dunnett SB. Dopamine neuron systems in the brain: an update. *Trends Neurosci.* 2007;30:194–202.

167. Ben-Jonathan N, Hnasko R. Dopamine as a prolactin (PRL) inhibitor. *Endocrine Rev.* 2001;22:724–763.

168. Beaulieu JM, Gainetdinov RR. The physiology, signaling, and pharmacology of dopamine receptors. *Pharmacol Rev.* 2011;63:182–217.

169. Kienast T, Heinz A. Dopamine and the diseased brain. *CNS Neurol Disord Drug Targets.* 2006;5:109–131.

170. Paulus W, Schomburg ED. Dopamine and the spinal cord in restless legs syndrome: does spinal cord physiology reveal a basis for augmentation? *Sleep Med Rev.* 2006;10:185–196.

171. Eisenhofer G, Kopin IJ, Goldstein DS. Catecholamine metabolism: a contemporary view with implications for physiology and medicine. *Pharmacol Rev.* 2004;56:331–349.

172. Sarkar C, Basu B, Chakroborty D, Dasgupta PS, Basu S. The immunoregulatory role of dopamine: an update. *Brain Behav Immun.* 2010;24:525–528.

173. Wood PB, Schweinhardt P, Jaeger E, et al. Fibromyalgia patients show an abnormal dopamine response to pain. *Eur J Neurosci.* 2007;25:3576–3582.

174. Guiard BP, El Mansari M, Blier P. Cross-talk between dopaminergic and noradrenergic systems in the rat ventral tegmental area, locus ceruleus, and dorsal hippocampus. *Mol Pharmacol.* 2008;74:1463–1475.

175. Guiard BP, El Mansari M, Merali Z, Blier P. Functional interactions between dopamine, serotonin and norepinephrine neurons: an in-vivo electrophysiological study in rats with monoaminergic lesions. *Int J Neuropsychopharmacol.* 2008;11:625–639.

176. Berton O, Nestler EJ. New approaches to antidepressant drug discovery: beyond monoamines. *Nat Rev Neurosci.* 2006;7:137–151.

177. Yanovsky Y, Li S, Klyuch BP, et al. L-Dopa activates histaminergic neurons. *J Physiol.* 2011;589:1349–1366.

178. Alcantara AA, Chen V, Herring BE, Mendenhall JM, Berlanga ML. Localization of dopamine D2 receptors on cholinergic interneurons of the dorsal striatum and nucleus accumbens of the rat. *Brain Res.* 2003;986:22–29.

179. Szalisznyo K, Muller L. Dopamine induced switch in the subthreshold dynamics of the striatal cholinergic interneurons: a numerical study. *J Theor Biol.* 2009;256:547–560.

180. Tye KM, Mirzabekov JJ, Warden MR, et al. Dopamine neurons modulate neural encoding and expression of depression-related behaviour. *Nature.* 2013;493:537–541.

181. Guiard BP, El Mansari M, Blier P. Prospect of a dopamine contribution in the next

generation of antidepressant drugs: the triple reuptake inhibitors. *Curr Drug Targets.* 2009;10:1069–1084.

182. Nestler EJ, Carlezon WA Jr. The mesolimbic dopamine reward circuit in depression. *Biol Psychiatry.* 2006;59:1151–1159.

183. Cannon DM, Klaver JM, Peck SA, Rallis-Voak D, Erickson K, Drevets WC. Dopamine type-1 receptor binding in major depressive disorder assessed using positron emission tomography and [(11)C]NNC-112. *Neuropsychopharmacology.* 2009;34(5):1277–1287.

184. Galani VJ, Rana DJ. Depression and antidepressants with dopamine hypothesis—a review. *IJPFR.* 2011;1:45–60.

185. Tremblay LK, Naranjo CA, Graham SJ, et al. Functional neuroanatomical substrates of altered reward processing in major depressive disorder revealed by a dopaminergic probe. *Arch Gen Psychiatry.* 2005;62:1228–1236.

186. Stein DJ. Depression, anhedonia, and psychomotor symptoms: the role of dopaminergic neurocircuitry. *CNS Spectr.* 2008;13:561–565.

187. Downar J, Geraci J, Salomons TV, et al. Anhedonia and reward-circuit connectivity distinguish nonresponders from responders to dorsomedial prefrontal repetitive transcranial magnetic stimulation in major depression. *Biol Psychiatry.* 2014;76(3):176–185.

188. Lehto SM, Kuikka J, Tolmunen T, et al. Temporal cortex dopamine D2/3 receptor binding in major depression. *Psychiatry Clin Neurosci.* 2008;62:345–348.

189. Bennabi D, Vandel P, Papaxanthis C, Pozzo T, Haffen E. Psychomotor retardation in depression: a systematic review of diagnostic, pathophysiologic, and therapeutic implications. *Biomed Res Int.* 2013;2013:158746.

190. Buyukdura JS, McClintock SM, Croarkin PE. Psychomotor retardation in depression: biological underpinnings, measurement, and treatment. *Prog Neuropsychopharmacol Biol Psychiatry.* 2011;35:395–409.

191. Martinot M, Bragulat V, Artiges E, et al. Decreased presynaptic dopamine function in the left caudate of depressed patients with affective flattening and psychomotor retardation. *Am J Psychiatry.* 2001;158:314–316.

192. Lindqvist D, Janelidze S, Hagell P, et al. Interleukin-6 is elevated in the cerebrospinal fluid of suicide attempters and related to symptom severity. *Biol Psychiatry.* 2009;66: 287–292.

193. Klimek V, Schenck JE, Han H, Stockmeier CA, Ordway GA. Dopaminergic abnormalities in amygdaloid nuclei in major depression: a postmortem study. *Biol Psychiatry.* 2002;52:740–748.

194. Delgado PL. Depression: the case for a monoamine deficiency. *J Clin Psychiatry.* 2000; 61(suppl 6):7–11.

195. Meyer JH, Ginovart N, Boovariwala A, et al. Elevated monoamine oxidase a levels in the brain: an explanation for the monoamine imbalance of major depression. *Arch Gen Psychiatry.* 2006;63:1209–1216.

196. Baumann B, Bogerts B. Neuroanatomical studies on bipolar disorder. *Br J Psychiatry Suppl.* 2001;41:s142–s147.

197. Jokinen J, Nordstrom AL, Nordstrom P. CSF 5-HIAA and DST non-suppression—orthogonal biologic risk factors for suicide in male mood disorder inpatients. *Psychiatry Res.* 2009;165:96–102.

198. Redmond DE Jr, Katz MM, Maas JW, Swann A, Casper R, Davis JM. Cerebrospinal fluid amine metabolites: relationships with behavioral measurements in depressed, manic, and healthy control subjects. *Arch Gen Psychiatry.* 1986;43:938–947.

199. Koslow SH, Maas JW, Bowden CL, Davis JM, Hanin I, Javaid J. CSF and urinary bio-

genic amines and metabolites in depression and mania: a controlled, univariate analysis. *Arch Gen Psychiatry.* 1983;40:999–1010.

200. Barton DA, Esler MD, Dawood T, et al. Elevated brain serotonin turnover in patients with depression: effect of genotype and therapy. *Arch Gen Psychiatry.* 2008;65:38–46.

201. Martensson B, Wagner A, Beck O, Brodin K, Montero D, Asberg M. Effects of clomipramine treatment on cerebrospinal fluid monoamine metabolites and platelet 3H-imipramine binding and serotonin uptake and concentration in major depressive disorder. *Acta Psychiatr Scand.* 1991;83:125–133.

202. Sheline Y, Bardgett ME, Csernansky JG. Correlated reductions in cerebrospinal fluid 5-HIAA and MHPG concentrations after treatment with selective serotonin reuptake inhibitors. *J Clin Psychopharmacol.* 1997;17:11–14.

203. Nikisch G, Mathe AA, Czernik A, et al. Stereoselective metabolism of citalopram in plasma and cerebrospinal fluid of depressive patients: relationship with 5-HIAA in CSF and clinical response. *J Clin Psychopharmacol.* 2004;24:283–290.

204. West CH, Ritchie JC, Boss-Williams KA, Weiss JM. Antidepressant drugs with differing pharmacological actions decrease activity of locus coeruleus neurons. *Int J Neuropsychopharmacol.* 2009;12(5):627–641.

205. Sharma RP, Javaid JI, Faull K, Davis JM, Janicak PG. CSF and plasma MHPG, and CSF MHPG index: pretreatment levels in diagnostic groups and response to somatic treatments. *Psychiatry Res.* 1994;51:51–60.

206. Backman J, Alling C, Alsen M, Regnell G, Traskman-Bendz L. Changes of cerebrospinal fluid monoamine metabolites during long-term antidepressant treatment. *Eur Neuropsychopharmacol.* 2000;10:341–349.

207. Ko HC, Lu RB, Shiah IS, Hwang CC. Plasma free 3-methoxy-4-hydroxyphenylglycol predicts response to fluoxetine. *Biol Psychiatry.* 1997;41:774–781.

208. Sharma RP, Janicak PG, Javaid JI, Pandey GN, Gierl B, Davis JM. Platelet MAO inhibition, urinary MHPG, and leukocyte beta-adrenergic receptors in depressed patients treated with phenelzine. *Am J Psychiatry.* 1990;147:1318–1321.

209. Okamoto T, Yoshimura R, Ikenouchi-Sugita A, et al. Efficacy of electroconvulsive therapy is associated with changing blood levels of homovanillic acid and brain-derived neurotrophic factor (BDNF) in refractory depressed patients: a pilot study. *Prog Neuropsychopharmacol Biol Psychiatry.* 2008;32:1185–1190.

210. Nikisch G, Mathe AA. CSF monoamine metabolites and neuropeptides in depressed patients before and after electroconvulsive therapy. *Eur Psychiatry.* 2008;23:356–359.

211. Meyer JH, Goulding VS, Wilson AA, Hussey D, Christensen BK, Houle S. Bupropion occupancy of the dopamine transporter is low during clinical treatment. *Psychopharmacology (Berl).* 2002;163:102–105.

212. Delgado PL. How antidepressants help depression: mechanisms of action and clinical response. *J Clin Psychiatry.* 2004;65(suppl 4):25–30.

213. Bremner JD, Vythilingam M, Ng CK, et al. Regional brain metabolic correlates of alpha-methylparatyrosine-induced depressive symptoms: implications for the neural circuitry of depression. *JAMA.* 2003;289:3125–3134.

214. van der Plasse G, Meerkerk DT, Lieben CK, Blokland A, Feenstra MG. Lack of evidence for reduced prefrontal cortical serotonin and dopamine efflux after acute tryptophan depletion. *Psychopharmacology (Berl).* 2007;195:377–385.

215. Ruhe HG, Mason NS, Schene AH. Mood is indirectly related to serotonin, norepinephrine and dopamine levels in humans: a meta-analysis of monoamine depletion studies. *Mol Psychiatry.* 2007;12:331–359.

216. Schwarz AJ, Gozzi A, Reese T, Bifone A. In vivo mapping of functional connectivity in

neurotransmitter systems using pharmacological MRI. *Neuroimage*. 2007;34:1627–1636.

217. Paez-Pereda M. New drug targets in the signaling pathways activated by antidepressants. *Prog Neuropsychopharmacol Biol Psychiatry*. 2005;29:1010–1016.

218. Mayberg HS. Modulating dysfunctional limbic-cortical circuits in depression: towards development of brain-based algorithms for diagnosis and optimised treatment. *Br Med Bull*. 2003;65:193–207.

219. Nestler EJ, McMahon A, Sabban EL, Tallman JF, Duman RS. Chronic antidepressant administration decreases the expression of tyrosine hydroxylase in the rat locus coeruleus. *Proc Natl Acad Sci U S A*. 1990;87:7522–7526.

220. Fitzgerald PB, Laird AR, Maller J, Daskalakis ZJ. A meta-analytic study of changes in brain activation in depression. *Hum Brain Mapp*. 2008;29:683–695.

221. Mayberg HS. Positron emission tomography imaging in depression: a neural systems perspective. *Neuroimaging Clin N Am*. 2003;13:805–815.

222. Bremner JD, Vythilingam M, Vermetten E, et al. Reduced volume of orbitofrontal cortex in major depression. *Biol Psychiatry*. 2002;51:273–279.

223. Heim C, Ehlert U, Hellhammer DH. The potential role of hypocortisolism in the pathophysiology of stress-related bodily disorders. *Psychoneuroendocrinology*. 2000;25:1–35.

224. Barton DA, Dawood T, Lambert EA, et al. Sympathetic activity in major depressive disorder: identifying those at increased cardiac risk? *J Hypertens*. 2007;25:2117–2124.

225. Devoto P, Flore G. On the origin of cortical dopamine: is it a co-transmitter in noradrenergic neurons? *Curr Neuropharmacol*. 2006;4:115–125.

226. Tao R, Auerbach SB. Regulation of serotonin release by GABA and excitatory amino acids. *J Psychopharmacol*. 2000;14:100–113.

227. Wager TD, Davidson ML, Hughes BL, Lindquist MA, Ochsner KN. Prefrontal-subcortical pathways mediating successful emotion regulation. *Neuron*. 2008;59:1037–1050.

228. Stone EA, Lin Y, Quartermain D. A final common pathway for depression? Progress toward a general conceptual framework. *Neurosci Biobehav Rev*. 2008;32:508–524.

229. Rosenkranz MA. Substance P at the nexus of mind and body in chronic inflammation and affective disorders. *Psychol Bull*. 2007;133:1007–1037.

230. Kennedy SE, Koeppe RA, Young EA, Zubieta JK. Dysregulation of endogenous opioid emotion regulation circuitry in major depression in women. *Arch Gen Psychiatry*. 2006;63:1199–1208.

231. Lu X, Sharkey L, Bartfai T. The brain galanin receptors: targets for novel antidepressant drugs. *CNS Neurol Disord Drug Targets*. 2007;6:183–192.

232. Belzung C, Yalcin I, Griebel G, Surget A, Leman S. Neuropeptides in psychiatric diseases: an overview with a particular focus on depression and anxiety disorders. *CNS Neurol Disord Drug Targets*. 2006;5:135–145.

233. Kormos V, Gaszner B. Role of neuropeptides in anxiety, stress, and depression: from animals to humans. *Neuropeptides*. 2013;47:401–419.

234. Micale V, Di Marzo V, Sulcova A, Wotjak CT, Drago F. Endocannabinoid system and mood disorders: priming a target for new therapies. *Pharmacol Ther*. 2013;138:18–37.

235. Mitsukawa K, Lu X, Bartfai T. Galanin, galanin receptors and drug targets. *Cell Mol Life Sci*. 2008;65:1796–1805.

236. Kuteeva E, Wardi T, Lundstrom L, et al. Differential role of galanin receptors in the regulation of depression-like behavior and monoamine/stress-related genes at the cell body level. *Neuropsychopharmacology*. 2008;33:2573–2585.

237. Kuteeva E, Hokfelt T, Wardi T, Ogren SO. Galanin, galanin receptor subtypes and depression-like behaviour. *Cell Mol Life Sci.* 2008;65:1854–1863.

238. Robinson JK, Brewer A. Galanin: a potential role in mesolimbic dopamine-mediated instrumental behavior. *Neurosci Biobehav Rev.* 2008;32:1485–1493.

239. Karlsson RM, Holmes A. Galanin as a modulator of anxiety and depression and a therapeutic target for affective disease. *Amino Acids.* 2006;31:231–239.

240. Ebner K, Singewald N. The role of substance P in stress and anxiety responses. *Amino Acids.* 2006;31:251–272.

241. Adell A. Antidepressant properties of substance P antagonists: relationship to mono-aminergic mechanisms? *Curr Drug Targets CNS Neurol Disord.* 2004;3:113–121.

242. McLean S. Do substance P and the NK1 receptor have a role in depression and anxiety? *Curr Pharm Des.* 2005;11:1529–1547.

243. Cohen H, Liu T, Kozlovsky N, Kaplan Z, Zohar J, Mathe AA. The neuropeptide Y (NPY)-ergic system is associated with behavioral resilience to stress exposure in an animal model of post-traumatic stress disorder. *Neuropsychopharmacology.* 2012;37:350–363.

244. Czermak C, Hauger R, Drevets WC, et al. Plasma NPY concentrations during trypto-phan and sham depletion in medication-free patients with remitted depression. *J Affect Disord.* 2008;110:277–281.

245. Nollet M, Leman S. Role of orexin in the pathophysiology of depression: potential for pharmacological intervention. *CNS Drugs.* 2013;27:411–422.

246. Mickey BJ, Zhou Z, Heitzeg MM, et al. Emotion processing, major depression, and functional genetic variation of neuropeptide Y. *Arch Gen Psychiatry.* 2011;68:158–166.

247. Irwin M, Brown M, Patterson T, Hauger R, Mascovich A, Grant I. Neuropeptide Y and natural killer cell activity: findings in depression and Alzheimer caregiver stress. *FASEB J.* 1991;5:3100–3107.

248. Berridge CW, Espana RA, Vittoz NM. Hypocretin/orexin in arousal and stress. *Brain Res.* 2010;1314:91–102.

249. Svizenska I, Dubovy P, Sulcova A. Cannabinoid receptors 1 and 2 (CB1 and CB2), their distribution, ligands and functional involvement in nervous system structures—a short review. *Pharmacol Biochem Behav.* 2008;90:501–511.

250. Lutz B. Endocannabinoid signals in the control of emotion. *Curr Opin Pharmacol.* 2009;9:46–52.

251. Ganon-Elazar E, Akirav I. Cannabinoids prevent the development of behavioral and endocrine alterations in a rat model of intense stress. *Neuropsychopharmacology.* 2012;37:456–466.

252. Koethe D, Llenos IC, Dulay JR, et al. Expression of CB1 cannabinoid receptor in the anterior cingulate cortex in schizophrenia, bipolar disorder, and major depression. *J Neural Transm.* 2007;114:1055–1063.

253. Benarroch EE. Endogenous opioid systems: current concepts and clinical correlations. *Neurology.* 2012;79:807–814.

254. Lutz PE, Kieffer BL. Opioid receptors: distinct roles in mood disorders. *Trends Neuro-sci.* 2013;36:195–206.

255. Torregrossa MM, Isgor C, Folk JE, Rice KC, Watson SJ, Woods JH. The delta-opioid receptor agonist (+)BW373U86 regulates BDNF mRNA expression in rats. *Neuropsy-chopharmacology.* 2004;29:649–659.

256. Torregrossa MM, Folk JE, Rice KC, Watson SJ, Woods JH. Chronic administration of the delta opioid receptor agonist (+)BW373U86 and antidepressants on behavior in the

forced swim test and BDNF mRNA expression in rats. *Psychopharmacology (Berl).* 2005;183:31–40.

257. Niciu MJ, Ionescu DF, Mathews DC, Richards EM, Zarate CA. Second messenger/signal transduction pathways in major mood disorders: moving from membrane to mechanism of action, part I: major depressive disorder. *CNS Spectr.* 2013;18(5):231–241.

258. Marsden WN. Synaptic plasticity in depression: molecular, cellular and functional correlates. *Prog Neuropsychopharmacol Biol Psychiatry.* 2013;43:168–184.

259. Carlezon WA Jr, Duman RS, Nestler EJ. The many faces of CREB. *Trends Neurosci.* 2005;28:436–445.

260. Fukuchi M, Tabuchi A, Tsuda M. Transcriptional regulation of neuronal genes and its effect on neural functions: cumulative mRNA expression of PACAP and BDNF genes controlled by calcium and cAMP signals in neurons. *J Pharmacol Sci.* 2005;98:212–218.

261. Koch JM, Kell S, Hinze-Selch D, Aldenhoff JB. Changes in CREB-phosphorylation during recovery from major depression. *J Psychiatr Res.* 2002;36:369–375.

262. Young LT. Postreceptor pathways for signal transduction in depression and bipolar disorder. *J Psychiatry Neurosci.* 2001;26(suppl):S17–S22.

263. Duric V, Banasr M, Licznerski P, et al. A negative regulator of MAP kinase causes depressive behavior. *Nat Med.* 2010;16:1328–1332.

264. Calati R, Crisafulli C, Balestri M, et al. Evaluation of the role of MAPK1 and CREB1 polymorphisms on treatment resistance, response and remission in mood disorder patients. *Prog Neuropsychopharmacol Biol Psychiatry.* 2013;44:271–278.

265. Einat H, Yuan P, Gould TD, et al. The role of the extracellular signal-regulated kinase signaling pathway in mood modulation. *J Neurosci.* 2003;23:7311–7316.

266. Duman CH, Schlesinger L, Kodama M, Russell DS, Duman RS. A role for MAP kinase signaling in behavioral models of depression and antidepressant treatment. *Biol Psychiatry.* 2007;61:661–670.

267. Chen DY, Bambah-Mukku D, Pollonini G, Alberini CM. Glucocorticoid receptors recruit the CaMKIIalpha-BDNF-CREB pathways to mediate memory consolidation. *Nat Neurosci.* 2012;15:1707–1714.

268. Carlson PJ, Singh JB, Zarate CA Jr, Drevets WC, Manji HK. Neural circuitry and neuroplasticity in mood disorders: insights for novel therapeutic targets. *NeuroRx.* 2006;3:22–41.

269. Charney DS, Manji HK. Life stress, genes, and depression: multiple pathways lead to increased risk and new opportunities for intervention. *Sci STKE.* 2004;2004:re5.

270. Manji HK DW, Charney DS. The cellular neurobiology of depression. *Nat Med.* 2001;7:541–547.

271. Carter CJ. Multiple genes and factors associated with bipolar disorder converge on growth factor and stress activated kinase pathways controlling translation initiation: implications for oligodendrocyte viability. *Neurochem Int.* 2007;50:461–490.

272. Bachmann RF, Schloesser RJ, Gould TD, Manji HK. Mood stabilizers target cellular plasticity and resilience cascades: implications for the development of novel therapeutics. *Mol Neurobiol.* 2005;32:173–202.

273. Manji HK, Quiroz JA, Payne JL, et al. The underlying neurobiology of bipolar disorder. *World Psychiatry.* 2003;2:136–146.

274. Lie DC, Colamarino SA, Song HJ, et al. Wnt signalling regulates adult hippocampal neurogenesis. *Nature.* 2005;437:1370–1375.

275. Karege F, Perroud N, Burkhardt S, et al. Alteration in kinase activity but not in protein

levels of protein kinase B and glycogen synthase kinase-3beta in ventral prefrontal cortex of depressed suicide victims. *Biol Psychiatry*. 2007;61:240–245.

276. Duman RS, Voleti B. Signaling pathways underlying the pathophysiology and treatment of depression: novel mechanisms for rapid-acting agents. *Trends Neurosci*. 2012;35:47–56.

277. Adli M, Hollinde DL, Stamm T, et al. Response to lithium augmentation in depression is associated with the glycogen synthase kinase 3-beta-50T/C single nucleotide polymorphism. *Biol Psychiatry*. 2007;62:1295–1302.

CHAPTER 10

Pathogen-Host Defense in the Evolution of Depression and Its Risk Genes

In Chapter 3, we argued that the environmental factors most likely to cause depression share in common the fact that they reliably reduced survival and/or reproduction (which together constitute overall evolutionary fitness) across human evolution. Further, we noted that these factors could be broadly grouped into those associated with infection and those involving psychosocial stressors, especially stressors related to conflict, isolation, diminished status/influence, and the perception of being trapped in these types of negative circumstances without the ability to escape. The idea that we become depressed today in response to circumstances that recall ancestral conditions that really were life-and-death issues we have formalized as the "threat to overall evolutionary fitness" model of depressive pathogenesis.

But identifying that threats to overall evolutionary fitness promote depression does not in and of itself answer the deeper question of why these threats should produce depression. If a first response is that these conditions (sickness and social threats) cause depression because they are so depressing, we would have to agree, noting that this response gets at something important—these conditions are so depressing that it seems natural that they should cause depression. But, of course, this type of circular reasoning doesn't take us where we want to go. In fact, when one thinks about it for a while it is rather remarkable that depression so often results from these types of adversities. One might imagine that genes promoting optimistic, proactive, and problem-solving approaches to these environmental conditions would have undergone enough positive selection over time that depression would now be rare instead of extremely common. The logic of natural selection forces us to ask, therefore, whether depressive responses to infectious and psychosocial adversities (and the genes that promote these responses) might have been retained because they conferred some type of advantage in these situations.

The cogency of this possibility is heightened by the fact that not all threats to survival and reproduction in ancestral environments so reliably produce depression. For example, humans were not infrequently hunted by predatory animals across much of our evolution,[1] and yet exposure to these animals, although frightening, does not induce depression on any regular basis (if it did, zoos would be out of business). Rather, in all indigenous cultures predatory animals were venerated and often considered exemplars and teachers. Thus, the fact that only certain ancient threats to overall fitness induce depression provides additional support for the possibility that depressive responses to these particular threats may be so common because depression conferred survival advantages not readily apparent in the modern world.

Before turning to the details, let us here state in the broadest terms how we have come to think about possible evolutionary explanations for the persistence of depression risk genes in human populations. As we discuss below, the vast majority of studies done to date have attempted to identify social benefits of depression that might outweigh its obvious social cost. Although different in detail, these ideas are united by the hypothesis that developing some level of depressive symptoms in response to ancient psychosocial threats to overall evolutionary fitness is a strategy with a high enough adaptive payoff (whatever its costs) that genes promoting this response have been retained in the human gene pool. While we don't disagree with this possibility, we devote the rest of this chapter to laying out a complementary but alternative vision.

This vision, which grows out of our work on the association between depression and inflammation, suggests that depression may have evolved primarily as an adaptive response to infection and the risk of infection, rather than as a winning strategy for navigating social threats. Any situations in which depression benefited both infectious and stress-related dangers would have increased the positive selection pressure on genetic variants that promote the disorder. But an important implication of the ideas we discuss in this chapter is that depression did not have to confer any social benefits at all across human evolution if its value in protecting against pathogens was high enough to outweigh its associated social costs. These ideas were summed up succinctly by our colleague Steve Maier many years ago when he observed that depression makes more sense in the context of sickness than it does in the context of stress. That is the essence of the argument we make in this chapter.

Strengths and Weaknesses of Adaptive and Nonadaptive Explanations for the Persistence of Depression Risk Alleles

Like many people of genius, Charles Darwin struggled with mental illness, and were he to be resurrected today and tell the inner story of his life, he would certainly earn a diagnosis of recurrent Major Depression. But of the people essential to the discovery of evolution, he didn't have the worst of it. That distinction would undoubtedly go to Robert FitzRoy, captain of the *Beagle*, the ship that launched evolution by taking Darwin to the Galapagos Islands and other places where the evidence for natural selection was especially striking. Darwin ended up on the *Beagle* because FitzRoy, who came from a family haunted by suicide, wanted intellectual company as a bulwark against the risk of depression on his long ocean voyage. By all accounts Darwin served admirably in this regard, although depression descended upon FitzRoy in the years following the voyage of the *Beagle*. In the end he embraced the destiny he so greatly feared and committed suicide.

So perhaps any discussion of the evolutionary benefits of depression should start by recognizing that the theory of evolution by natural selection itself evolved, in part, out of a nineteenth-century attempt to ward off depression's horrors. Had FitzRoy not feared depression, Darwin would have stayed home. It does not appear that Darwin recognized this association himself, but in his later years he more than once contemplated the possibility that depression might confer evolutionary advantages. In this he was the first of a long line of theorists who have wrestled with the question of why depression, which clearly runs in families and appears to have a strong genetic component, has not been extinguished by natural selection.

The crux of the issue is this. Major depressive disorder (MDD) is a highly prevalent condition associated with significant decrements in survival and reproduction, at least in the modern world. Indeed, depression reduces fertility, impairs fitness-enhancing social behaviors, and increases the risk for morbidity and mortality from other disease states.[2] And yet, many genes implicated in the disorder are present at high rates in the human genome, suggesting that they serve some adaptive purpose. Consider, for example, the most famous of depression-associated genes, the gene that codes for the serotonin transporter protein and its short versus long alleles. If it is indeed true that having short versions of the serotonin transporter protein gene increases the risk of depression in the context of environmental adversity, why do rates of this allelic variant approach 100 percent in some Asian cultures?[3] Why wouldn't natural selection have culled this variant of the gene from the human genome? Why, in fact, does it appear that this variant has actually been increasing in prevalence across human evolution?[4] The only consistent explanation is that it is conferring some type of survival and/or reproductive advantage either by increasing depression risk or because it has other effects that offset its cost in terms of depression. (This type of balance of plusses and minuses is called pleiotropy.)

Multiple theories have been expounded over the years to address this conundrum. These theories fall into two broad categories based on whether they view depressogenic alleles as being adaptive and therefore promoting survival and/or reproduction in ways that balance their costs, or as being maladaptive but for one reason or another are being beyond the power of natural selection to them cull from the human genome.[5–19] Most adaptive theories elaborated to date attempt to demonstrate that, appearances to the contrary, depressive symptoms themselves actually benefit survival and/or reproduction by positively affecting the depressed person's relations with fellow humans. Nonadaptive theories have invoked various genetic mechanisms, including polygenic mutation balance and genomic imprinting, to account for how MDD could be nonadaptive and yet remain beyond the reach of natural selection.[18,19]

Of most relevance to our discussion is the fact that each of these theoretical positions has limitations, which we briefly enumerate here. Most theories that ascribe adaptive functions to depressive symptoms emphasize the potential value of normal negative emotions for a variety of social negotiations, such as abandoning unattainable goals, yielding in dominance struggles, and so forth, and relegate clinical depression to the realm of nonadaptive pathology.[5–7,10–14,16,18,20] Plenty of examples exist for this type of pattern. As we discuss further below, fever protects animals during infection, so the ability to mount a fever is clearly adaptive from an evolutionary perspective. However, like all good things, there is such a thing as too much fever. When too high, febrile temperatures can damage the brain and lead to death. Perhaps depression, like fever, is adaptive at low levels and becomes maladaptive only when extreme.

However, while attractive at first glance, this type of explanation does not work nearly as well for depression as it does for fever. Most damning is the fact that even minor levels of depression impair social functioning in ways likely to reduce fitness, whereas mild to moderate increases in body temperature are exactly the changes most likely to enhance protection against pathogens.[21–23] Moreover, unlike the ability to mount mild fevers, which poses no significant risk for developing catastrophic fevers, mild depressive symptoms powerfully promote the development of pathological depression.[23,24] Thus, even if they conferred some advantages, these would have to outweigh the hugely increased risk for developing levels of depression that powerfully reduce fitness. Finally, to complicate things further, studies have been unable to demonstrate any discrete point at which the severity or number of depressive symptoms transitions from adaptive or neutral to impairing.[22,23,25]

One of the few theoretical approaches to claim an explicit adaptive function for clinical depression itself suggests that MDD may prove adaptive by focusing cognitive resources in a ruminative fashion on the specific survival/reproduction-relevant challenges facing an individual.[16] Variously known as the social navigation or analytical rumination hypothesis, the theory suggests that, by inhibiting potentially distracting activities, other depressive symptoms are understood as aiding this process. Some studies provide support for this idea. However, while provocative, this theory leaves many important questions unanswered. For example, how would other core depressive symptoms, such as fatigue, sleep disturbance, and appetite changes, fit into this paradigm, given that these abnormalities might be expected to impair one's ability to maintain the type of sustained focused attention that is depression's raison d'être in this model. Similarly, this theory has yet to provide tractable ways of examining whether any purported benefits of increased rumination outweigh the well-established survival costs associated with other important aspects of depression, including attendant social deficits expected to reduce individual and inclusive fitness (e.g., by being less able to aid relatives) in prime reproductive years,[26] reduced fertility rates, and markedly increased risk of developing a number of other life-threatening health conditions.[27–39] Nonetheless, it may well be that the value of depression-induced "analytic rumination" combines with other adaptive aspects of depression to increase the prevalence of its risk alleles.

Nonadaptive theories, such as polygenic mutation balance, face their own challenges. For example, because polygenic mutation balance theory is consistent with the possibility that all levels of depressive symptoms are purely maladaptive, it has the strength of requiring no historical or adaptive context whatsoever to justify the disorder's existence. However, the theory does require that risk alleles, while extremely numerous, be individually rare, because a higher prevalence of any of these alleles would be more consistent with one form or other of balanced selection and hence some type of adaptive advantage.[18] In this regard, it is difficult to reconcile polygenic mutation balance with the fact that most of the putative vulnerability alleles for depression identified to date exist at far higher rates in the human genome than would be predicted if they were purely maladaptive.[40]

While most of the remainder of this chapter is devoted to expounding a novel adaptive theory for commonly occurring depressive risk alleles, we would be remiss not to emphasize two important points that support nonadaptive explanations. First, a number of important studies over the last few years have made it increasingly plausible that major mental illnesses may serve no appreciable adaptive functions and may have arisen from simple genetic mistakes. Thus, it is becoming increasingly clear that many cases of schizophrenia and autism may arise from mutations that either are very recent in the family of the patient or are entirely new with the afflicted person.[41] Individually, each of these specific genetic changes is very rare, but when one occurs it typically confers a huge risk for disease development. A corollary to this is that there are likely thousands of different genetic mutations that cause disease states we now label as schizophrenia, bipolar disorder, or major depression. Because people with serious mental disorders generally reproduce less successfully than others in the population, one would predict that any one of these innumerable high-impact genetic "mistakes" would be removed from the gene pool relatively quickly, but because so many new mutations pop up that can produce any given psychiatric disease, the disease persists even while the individual genetic variations causing it die.[18] A second important point to bear in mind is that, in fact, no genes that conclusively cause depression have been identified. This lack of certainty makes any discussion of the genetics of depression somewhat speculative.

Overview of a Pathogen-Host Defense (PATHOS-D) Theory of Depression

Let's start with an assumption that may be wrong. Despite the failure of gold-standard genome-wide association studies (GWAS) to unambiguously identify any clear-cut risk genes for depression that replicate either across studies or between different ethnic/racial groups, let's assume that there is at least some truth behind the many candidate gene studies that have identified a small army of commonly occurring genetic variants as risks for depression. Moreover, let's assume that common genetic variants repeatedly found to be almost associated with depression by GWAS may in fact really increase the risk for the disorder. If we make these two assumptions, then we are back where we started in this chapter: why do genes that increase the risk for developing depression seem to be so common and so prevalent in the human genome despite their apparent costs to survival and reproduction?

To address this question one of us (C. Raison), in collaboration with Andrew H. Miller at Emory University, proposed a set of ideas we called the pathogen-host defense (PATHOS-D) theory of depression. The PATHOS-D theory proposes that depressogenic risk alleles originated and have been largely retained in the human genome not because depression is adaptive for social functioning but because *these alleles enhance host defense against pathogens* (i.e., viruses, bacteria, protozoa, and worms) via both their direct physiological effects and their effects on behavior. Many processes contribute to host defense, including many biological processes abnormal in depression that are not typically conceptualized as being parts of the immune system. However, at the core of the PATHOS-D idea is that the enhanced pathogen defense associated with depression is accomplished primarily via the types of heightened innate immune activation discussed in Chapter 6. This innate immune activation leads to more robust sickness behavior, which results in reduced death from infectious causes,[42–45] especially in infancy when selection pressure from infection is strongest,[46] the adaptive immune system is not fully operational,[46–49] and long-term immunocompetence has yet to be established.[50–55] Because infection has been a primary cause of early mortality and hence reproductive failure across human evolution,[49,56–60] one would expect that if depressogenic alleles conferred even minor benefits in this regard, they would have undergone strong positive selection pressure and would thus be both numerous and prevalent, as indeed they appear to be based on the candidate gene literature.

However, any potential survival benefits of inflammatory processes come at a cost to reproductive fitness. Inflammation induces septic shock in response to severe infection, which is a significant cause of mortality.[61,62] Innate immune inflammatory processes can be manipulated by pathogens for their own benefits and usually at a cost to us.[60,63] Especially when chronic, inflammation leads to the types of long-term tissue damage that are at the heart of most modern maladies, including cardiovascular disease, stroke, cancer, and dementia. For all these reasons, prevalence of depressogenic risk alleles would be predicted to be not 100 percent but an intermediate prevalence reflecting the benefit of enhanced host defense in any given environment minus attendant costs. Again, this is consistent with current findings in the genetics of depression.

Before examining data that might support the PATHOS-D theory, let us step back and recognize the larger context in which these ideas are situated. In this regard, Paul Ewald and colleagues have succinctly articulated the overarching rationale for PATHOS-D theorizing:

> When diseases have been common in human populations for many generations and still have a substantial negative impact on fitness, they are likely to have infectious causes. These considerations suggest that the most important of the human diseases that are not now thought to be caused by infection will eventually be shown to have infectious causes. These infectious causes may be causes in the proximate sense (e.g., *Mycobacterium tuberculosis* causes tuberculosis) or in an evolutionary sense (*Plasmodium falciparum* is an evolutionary cause of sickle cell anemia). . . . The only such compensating fitness benefit that has been documented for major human genetic diseases is *resistance to infection.* (italics added)[64]

Consistent with Ewald's observations, the central tenants of PATHOS-D theory might suggest that depression is analogous to a condition like sickle cell anemia, a devastating and lethal illness for those who carry two copies of the risk allele but one that, by happy coincidence, protects against another devastating and lethal disease (malaria) in individuals with a single copy of that allele. However, from a PATHOS-D perspective, comparing depression with a condition like sickle cell anemia falsifies as much as it reveals. For while it is true that the PATHOS-D theory conceptualizes depression as a devastating condition caused (at least in part) by genes retained in the genome because they enhance host defense, we are not suggesting that depression is a purely maladaptive condition like sickle cell anemia. We are saying something more radical: that the genes that promote depression have been retained not in spite of but because they promote depressive symptoms, which themselves promote host defense.

A Brief Detour: Might Associations Between Inflammation, Genes, and Depression Be Explained by Depression Being an Infectious Disease?

Before exploring evidence that depression may have evolved as an adaptive response to avoid and/or combat infection, let us take a moment to consider the other possible way that depression and pathogens might be related. What if, rather than being a defense against infection, depression was caused by infection? Ten years ago we would have dismissed this idea without further comment. But there is much wisdom in Ewald's observation that as time has passed more and more diseases have been linked to infectious agents.

The primary argument against an infectious etiology for depression is that no one has ever found one, if by this we mean that active infection accounts for any significant portion of the depressed population. (This is different from the question of whether an acute infection might change functioning in the brain and body that promote chronic depression—data are better for that.) Moreover, it seems increasingly clear that many environmental factors can cause depression, making it highly unlikely that a single (or even multiple) infectious agent(s) would be responsible for the bulk of depressive illness in the world.

Arguments in support of infection are more circumstantial in nature and in toto not very convincing, but they are intriguing nonetheless. Some studies have found increased rates of chronic infection with pathogens in people with depression. The most examined infectious agent in this regard is the bornavirus; however, the most rigorously conducted study finds no association of this pathogen with depression.[65] *Toxoplasma gondii* is a neurotropic protozoan parasite that chronically infects approximately a third of the world's population. Although people with depression do not seem to have higher rates of *T. gondii* infection than others,[66] people infected with *T. gondii* have been shown in several studies to have markedly increased rates of suicide,[67] which at the least suggests that chronic CNS infection with *T. gondii* might increase the risk of impulsive behavior in the context of depression. Other data suggest that pathogens may be capable of manipulating human behavior in ways relevant to emotional well-being and hence, at least theoretically, to depression. For example, people show a significant spike in sociability three days following receipt of the flu vaccine at exactly the time when they would be most contagious had they contracted the actual virus.[68] Although we argue in the rest of this chapter that depression evolved to fight pathogens, it is not beyond the realm of possibility that in some instances a pathogen might depress us for reasons of its own.

Putting the PATHOS-D Theory to the Test: Examining the Evidence

We turn now to demonstrating that the PATHOS-D theory parsimoniously accounts for multiple aspects of MDD not adequately addressed by other theoretical orientations. To accomplish this, we propose a series of propositions that follow directly from the hypothesis that MDD is common because risk alleles for the condition have undergone positive selection as a result of enhancing survival during infection in ancestral environments.

PROPOSITION 1: INFLAMMATORY ACTIVATION SHOULD INDUCE DEPRESSION, AND DEPRESSION SHOULD BE ASSOCIATED WITH INCREASED INFLAMMATION

In Chapter 6 we discuss associations between depression and inflammation in some detail. Here we review the key points of this association, both as a reminder and to set the stage for other aspects of PATHOS-D theory. If you have all this firmly in hand, skip to proposition 2. If not, read on.

Microbial activation of the mammalian inflammatory response reliably produces a highly regulated suite of symptoms and behaviors known as sickness behavior that bears a striking resemblance to behavioral changes induced by stress in laboratory animals, as well as to the symptoms of MDD in humans.[2,69–79] Many of these symptoms and behaviors can be blocked or attenuated in animal models via antidepressant administration,[80–84] further suggesting that cytokine-induced behavioral changes are either closely aligned with or identical to MDD in humans.

Significant data suggest that cytokine exposure predisposes to the development of depression in humans, too. For example, studies report that 20–70 percent of patients undergoing chronic cytokine activation as a result of treatment with interferon-alpha (IFN-α) meet symptom criteria for MDD.[70,85] Moreover, IFN-α–induced depression shares symptom homology with idiopathic MDD[86] and responds to treatment with standard antidepressants.[70,87–90] In addition to a remarkable symptom overlap, sickness and depression during cytokine exposure also appear to be causally linked, given the strong association between sickness in the first week of treatment with IFN-α and the development of cognitive/emotional symptoms of depression over the ensuing six months of therapy.[91] Finally, peripheral inflammatory activation induces many, if not all, of the most replicated central nervous system (CNS) and neuroendocrine abnormalities observed in MDD.[92–99]

A huge literature reports cross-sectional associations between depressive symptoms and/or MDD and increases in various markers of peripheral inflammatory activation,[2] with meta-analyses reporting the most consistent findings for plasma concentrations of interleukin-6 (IL-6), C-reactive protein (CRP), and haptoglobin, and some evidence for tumor necrosis factor-alpha (TNF).[100–103] Longitudinal studies extend these cross-sectional observations by reporting that increased inflammatory markers in nondepressed individuals predict the later development of depression.[104–107]

Most studies conducted to date have examined proinflammatory cytokines and CRP, which explains in part why these inflammatory mediators are overrepresented in the meta-analytic literature. But, consistent with PATHOS-D theory, emerging data suggest that a far wider array of host immune response elements are linked to MDD, with an overall pattern of increased inflammatory/host defense activation and reduced immune tolerogenic pathway activity.[108–117] A clear prediction of PATHOS-D theory is that as novel innate immune antipathogen mechanisms are identified they will be found to be enhanced in depressed individuals. For example, studies indicate that antimicrobial peptides upregulated by inflammatory cytokines (e.g., ribonuclease 7, psoriasin, human beta-defensin-2 and -3)[118] are increased in the skin of patients with inflammatory skin conditions, such as atopic dermatitis and psoriasis,[119,120] that are comorbid with MDD.[121,122] One would predict a similar increase in these peptides, although perhaps to a lesser degree, in medically healthy individuals with MDD.

As we note in Chapter 6, inflammatory biomarkers are not elevated in all individuals with MDD, and typically more variance in these biomarkers is observed in depressed populations than in normal comparison groups.[123] Whether patients with increased inflammation represent a biologically and evolutionary distinct subset of MDD is an area of active research. If this turns out to be the case, it may be that selection for enhanced pathogen-host defense is relevant primarily to these individuals and is thus only one adaptive factor driving the persistence of depressogenic alleles. On the other hand, findings from patients undergoing treatment with the cytokine IFN-α suggest a more inclusive scenario for the role of pathogen defense in the evolution/persistence of depressogenic alleles. Although standardized dosages of IFN-α are employed, a wide range of behavioral responses are observed during treatment, from mild neurovegetative/sickness symptoms, such as fatigue, to completed suicide in response to catastrophic Major Depression. Individuals who develop significant depressive symptoms evince changes in CNS and neuroendocrine functioning that are also observed in idiopathic MDD[94–99] but that are not observed to a significant degree in patients on IFN-α who do not develop depression.

These findings raise an intriguing possibility. In addition to being a frank inflammatory condition in some people, depression may have been driven across human evolution even in situations when the condition is not characterized by heightened immune system activity per se, given that other biological abnormalities seen in depression may have antipathogen effects. If so, depressogenic risk alleles that do not promote a direct increase in inflammatory biomarkers may nonetheless have undergone positive selection because they enhanced pathogen-host defense via sensitization of downstream CNS/neuroendocrine pathways that themselves promote survival during infection. To date, few data support this possibility, although it is intriguing to note that glucocorticoid resistance, which is common in MDD[124] and is associated with the development of depressive symptoms during IFN-α treatment,[125] has been associated with improved T cell function in infection with human immunodeficiency virus[126] and that enrichment paradigms known to enhance glucocorticoid sensitivity in animal models increase mortality in response to *Escherichia coli* infection.[127] Moreover, a large study found that stress-related reductions in glucocorticoid receptor resistance were associated with increased cold symptoms in response to experimental rhinovirus exposure. While most of us think of catching a cold as a travail rather than a benefit, the types of increased inflammatory responses that promote the common cold may well have helped clear viruses from the body across human evolution.[128]

Seen in this way, any genes (or epigenetic changes) that promote glucocorticoid resistance might both promote depression and enhance the immune system's ability to fight invading pathogens. Although these types of concrete examples are not available for other bodily systems implicated in depression, multiple studies have shown that depression-relevant systems such as monoamine neurotransmitters have profound and complex effects on immune function,[129] consistent with the possibility that depression-related alterations in these systems might have been selected across human evolution, at least in part, for their impact on protection from pathogens.

PROPOSITION 2: ON THE WHOLE, PATTERNS OF INCREASED IMMUNE ACTIVITY ASSOCIATED WITH MDD SHOULD RESULT IN DECREASED MORTALITY FROM INFECTION IN ANCESTRAL ENVIRONMENTS

This proposition faces a pretty stiff challenge from data indicating that depression worsens the outcome of a number of infections[130–137] and is associated with impairments in adaptive immune mechanisms important for protection against both viruses and bacteria.[102,138,139] So, on the face of things, it would seem unlikely that biological and/or behavioral changes associated with depression might actually help more than hurt host defense against pathogens. But as is always the case with evolved systems, immune protection involves trade-offs and imperfections, given that limited energy is available to organisms and the demands upon them are almost endless. Thus, the immune changes associated with depression might come with real costs in terms of immune protection and still, over long evolutionary time, have provided more benefit than risk.

To begin our examination of whether the types of immune activation reported in depression might enhance host defense, let's first ask whether these types of immune activation might produce the patterns of infectious vulnerability and adaptive immune impairment that are apparent in depression. Surprisingly, the answer is yes.[140,141] Although essential for activating adaptive immunity in response to pathogen invasion, chronic inflammation can actually suppress T and B cell function through various mechanisms.[140–147] Consistent with this, rates of infection are often increased, not decreased, in autoimmune conditions characterized by chronic inflammation.[148] However, as noted above, PATHOS-D theory requires only that across evolutionary time the survival benefits of enhanced inflammatory activity characteristic of depression outweigh any costs imposed by associated reductions in other aspects of immune functioning. Several lines of evidence support this possibility.

One line of evidence comes from Ghana, a country in which some regions rely on contaminated rivers for drinking water and others have access to far purer water from wells. As would be expected, death rates from infection are far higher in regions with polluted drinking water than in areas with clean well water. Consistent with the prediction that increased inflammatory signaling is protective in the type of high-infection environments that were common during human evolution (and especially common since the origin of agriculture and the rise of cities),[149] a form (haplotype) of the gene for the anti-inflammatory cytokine IL-10 associated with increased inflammation was found to be significantly more prevalent in populations that rely on river water than in populations that drink from wells, suggesting positive selection driven by enhanced pathogen protection.[42] Consistent with this possibility, during a five-year follow-up period, the high-inflammation IL-10 haplotype was associated with increased survival in populations that drank from rivers but reduced survival in individuals who drank from wells.[42] As in industrialized societies, the negative impact of increased inflammation on survival was seen only toward the end of life, whereas the protective effect of increased inflammation was evident across the entire adult life-span. This point is significant, because it suggests that indeed the protective effects of increased inflammation in high-pathogen environments occur at exactly the ages when it would contribute maximally to survival and reproduction.

PROPOSITION 3: ENVIRONMENTAL RISK FACTORS FOR MDD SHOULD BE ASSOCIATED WITH INCREASED RISK OF INFECTION AND ATTENDANT INFLAMMATORY ACTIVATION

If the genes that promote depression also contribute to protection against infectious morbidity and mortality, then circumstances in which infection was likely or had already happened should be especially potent activators of these genes and hence especially likely to induce depression. Moreover, because these alleles may heighten host defense in part by increasing inflammation, inflammatory mediators released in response to environments rife with pathogen danger would be expected to induce depressive symptoms. These predictions are confirmed by many studies demonstrating the depressogenic effects of inflammatory mediators,[2,69–79,150] as well as the diverse array of conditions that activate inflammatory processes and also increase the risk for depression, including obesity, sedentary lifestyle, chronic poor sleep, psychosocial stress, a diet replete with processed foods, and, of course, medical illness (see Table 3.1 in Chapter 3).[151–198]

Because inflammation is central to infectious disease and most other medical conditions,[2] it is no surprise, from a PATHOS-D perspective, that medical illness has been reported by the World Health Organization to be the most potent risk factor for the development of MDD worldwide.[199] However, while quite consistent with a PATHOS-D perspective, this observation is not readily explained by theories that privilege psychosocial explanations for the persistence of depressogenic alleles. If depression evolved primarily as an adaptive strategy for managing complex social problems, why should immune stimuli be at least as powerful as social ones for inducing the disorder? At the very least this observation suggests that there might be two evolved pathways into depression, one that results from psychosocial factors and a second that arises from immune challenges. But as we describe below, much evidence suggests that this type of dichotomous thinking belies a deeper truth that psychosocial and infectious adversity may be best conceptualized as two sides of the same coin.

Psychosocial stress is a second universal and powerful risk for the development of depression.[199–202] This squares nicely with social theories of depression and at first glance appears to challenge the perspective that host-defense requirements might have been the primary driver of depression across human evolution. But if we consider that the vast majority of "psychological stressors" in mammals over evolutionary time boiled down to risks inherent in hunting, being hunted, or fighting other members of the same species in dominance hierarchies for reproductive access/status, it is not surprising that these states are also circumstances in which the risk of pathogen invasion, and subsequent death from infection, was greatly increased as a result of wounding and a resultant traumatic opening of the protective skin barrier.[203] Such wounding is common in social species and was a significant source of morbidity and mortality among humans in the ancestral environment.[204,205]

Given this, it is not surprising that, as noted by Firdaus Dhabhar, "stress perception by the brain may serve as an 'early warning signal' to activate the immune system in preparation for a markedly increased likelihood of subsequent infection."[206] And while chronic stress can suppress certain measures of immune function,[207] the types of acute and/or psychosocial stressors most likely to be associated with immediate risk of wounding and hence infection activate both innate and adaptive immunity.[208–218] From a PATHOS-D perspective, then, illness and psychosocial stress increase the risk for depression because they activate host-defense mechanisms that reliably induce depressive symptoms, and do so, as we show below, because these symptoms promoted survival in the context of infection across hominin evolution.

In addition to providing an explanation for why illness and stress are primary risk factors for the development of depression, PATHOS-D theory offers a unifying perspective on why many other facets of modern life are also depressogenic, a perspective not readily provided by theories focused more exclusively on the social realm. Indeed, if the adaptive value of depression is to be found primarily in its effects on social functioning, it is hard to understand why so many risks for depression, including obesity, sedentary lifestyle, dietary factors, diminished sleep, air pollution, and smoking, are nonsocial in nature. On the other hand, these conditions are all associated with increased inflammation,[151–198] suggesting that they may be depressogenic because they tap into pathways that initially evolved to fight infection.

To sum up, a PATHOS-D perspective accounts for why depression has the risk factors it does and, moreover, makes the testable prediction that any environmental factor that is proinflammatory and activates host defenses will on balance be depressogenic, whereas any factor (or intervention) that is anti-inflammatory will, in general, have antidepressant properties, especially in individuals suffering from chronic inflammation, as is the case with many of us in the modern world.

PROPOSITION 4: FORMS OF GENES THAT INCREASE THE RISK FOR DEPRESSION SHOULD ENHANCE HOST-DEFENSE MECHANISMS IN GENERAL AND INNATE IMMUNE INFLAMMATORY RESPONSES IN PARTICULAR

Several years ago we were presenting the ideas in this chapter at an academic meeting. Following our talk one of the world's leading researchers into genetic and environmental risk factors for MDD approached us. "Very good talk," she said. "Only problem is that no one has ever discovered a gene for depression." Studies increasingly point to an additional complication. If there are genes for depression, they are almost certainly not risk genes for the disorder per se but, rather, likely increase the risk for psychopathology more generally. For example, allelic variants in the CACNA1C gene, which we discuss at some length below, have been shown to increase the risk for other major psychiatric disorders in addition to MDD.[219]

With these caveats in mind, let us proceed as if many of the genetic variants implicated (although imperfectly) in MDD actually contribute in incremental ways to risk of developing the disorder. If we start with this assumption, it is clear that to be fully consistent with PATHOS-D theory, allelic risk variants should meet three criteria:

1. Be located in genes with known immune effects
2. Increase signaling in inflammatory/host-defense pathways
3. Increase survival in the context of infection

Although a number of candidate gene studies have identified depression risk alleles that are associated with inflammatory processes,[220–224] to evaluate in the most conservative manner whether putative risk alleles meet the three criteria above, we limit our examination here to candidate genes confirmed either by GWAS or by meta-analysis of candidate gene studies.

Depression Risk Genes Supported by GWAS

Currently, GWAS has confirmed only four candidate single-nucleotide polymorphisms (SNPs) for MDD, rs12520799 in DCNP1 (dendritic cell nuclear protein-1), rs16139 in NPY (neuropeptide Y), rs12415800 in SIRT1 (sirtuin 1), and rs35936514 in LHPP (phospholysine phosphohistadine inorganic pyrophosphate phosphatase); and one candidate gene for MDD, TNF—although the two GWAS publications providing these findings do not replicate each other's findings.[225,226] It is striking that, with the exception of LHPP, each of these genes is known to play important roles in processes central to host defense, including proinflammatory cytokine signaling (TNF), antigen presentation (DCNP1), T helper 1 (Th1) cell differentiation, and function (NPY) and limiting the extent and duration of acute inflammation (SIRT1). Of these SNPs, functionality has been established only for rs16139 in NPY. Although NPY has numerous and contrasting effects on innate and adaptive immune functioning, its primary actions appear to be anti-inflammatory in both the brain and periphery.[227–229] Given this, PATHOS-D theory predicts that MDD should be characterized by reduced NPY activity and that the depression risk T allele at rs16139 should be associated with reduced NPY production. Significant data support both predictions.[230–234]

Unlike for rs16139 in NPY, the functionality of rs76917 in *TNF* is currently unknown. A clear prediction of PATHOS-D theory is that this SNP should be associated with increased TNF production, given that TNF is increased in MDD and appears to be especially relevant to enhanced survival from infection in the types of pathogen-dense environments that were normative during human evolution. A separate SNP (–308G/A) in the promoter region for TNF is worthy of comment in this regard. Although not found to be significant by GWAS,[225] several studies have associated the high-production A allele at position –308[235] with depression and related states such as anger.[223,224,236] As predicted by PATHOS-D theory, the –308A allele has also been associated with reduced risk for infection with a number of pathogens, including *Mycobacterium tuberculosis*, parvovirus B19, and hepatitis B virus (HBV),[237–239] and with an increased likelihood of survival in critically ill hospitalized patients.[240] On a population level, Canadian First Peoples, who are highly susceptible to tuberculosis, have a markedly reduced prevalence of the A allele compared with Caucasians.[241]

DCNP1 was initially considered to be unique to dendritic cells,[242] although it has subsequently been identified in neurons.[243] The rs12520799 T-allele, which is associated with MDD, codes for a truncated version of the protein. No data are available regarding the effect of this allele on either inflammatory signaling or infection outcomes, but given strong patterns of comorbidity between asthma/atopy and MDD, it is intriguing that the allele has been associated with increased levels of immunoglobulin E for common specific antigens in individuals with asthma.[244]

SIRT1 codes for sirtuin 1, a class III histone deacetylase enzyme that serves as an important sensor of cellular energy and redox states.[245] Via epigenetic mechanisms, sirtuin 1 plays important roles in limiting the extent and duration of acute inflammation by promoting a shift from inflammation-driven glycolytic activity to adaptation-phase fatty-acid metabolism. Sirtuin 1 suppresses nuclear factor kappa-beta activity, represses cyclooxygenase 2 gene expression,[246] and silences at the promoters of proinflammatory genes, including TNF and IL-1β, as well as the promoter for hypoxia-inducible factor-1-alpha, a signaling factor important for maintenance of proinflammatory glycolytic activity.[247] In addition, sirtuin 1 increases the production of peroxisome proliferator-activated receptor gamma coactivator 1-alpha and -beta, which promotes the fatty acid metabolism essential for resolution of the inflammatory response.[248] The end result of these activities is that sirtuin 1 inhibits the transformation of monocytes to macrophages and promotes anti-inflammatory M2 macrophages and regulatory T cells at the expense of proinflammatory M1-type macrophages and effector T cells.[249,250]

However, conflicting data suggest that in at least some contexts sirtuin 1 may have inflammatory and adaptive immune-stimulating effects. For example, sirtuin 1 inhibition has been reported to stimulate Foxp3 expression in regulatory T cells.[251] Despite these complexities, evidence of diminished sirtuin 1 activity in medical conditions characterized by chronic inflammation suggests that its function might also be reduced in MDD, especially in patients with elevated peripheral inflammatory biomarkers. But to our knowledge, no data are available to support or disprove this idea. Similarly, given the association of MDD with chronic inflammation, one would predict that the depression risk allele near the SIRT1 gene should reduce sirtuin 1 activity, if it is found to have a functional effect, which is currently unknown.

But these predictions should be balanced by findings suggesting a complex and contradictory role for sirtuin 1 in protection against pathogens. In certain situations, such as the hypoinflammatory phase of sepsis, sirtuin 1 blockade has been reported to reduce bacterial load and enhance survival. Sirtuin 1 blockade also inhibits HRV replication in hepatocytes.[252] Similarly, sirtuin-deficient mice demonstrate improved intestinal antibacterial defense mechanisms.[253] On the other hand, the use of the cyclooxygenase-2 inhibitor celecoxib to stimulate sirtuin 1 within macrophages resulted in an enhanced ability of ampicillin to clear *Staphylococcus aureus* from these cells,[254] consistent with the observation that low levels of sirtuin 1 within macrophages associates with bacterial infection in these cells.[246,255] Sirtuin 1 also appears to be essential for optimal immune clearance of respiratory syncytial virus and has been shown to suppress human T-cell leukemia virus type 1 transcription.[256,257]

Candidate Genes Confirmed by Meta-analysis

Although findings of candidate genes for depression have proven remarkably difficult to replicate,[225] a meta-analysis provides at least some additional support for several allelic variants being risk factors for MDD, including GNB3 825T, MTHFR (methylenetetrahydrofolate reductase) 677T, APOE (apolipoprotein E) ε2 allele, SLC6A3 (solute carrier family 6 member 3) 40-bp variable number tandem repeat (VNTR) 9/10 genotype, and SLC6A4 44-bp ins/del short allele.[258]Although not traditionally considered primarily immune-related, each of these genes has well-documented immunological effects and hence meets the first of the three criteria for consistency with PATHOS-D theory. In addition, each to a varying degree has some evidence consistent with either the second or third criterion.

GNB3 825T produces a shortened splice variant of the guanine nucleotide-binding protein beta-3 subunit that has enhanced signal transduction properties.[259] It has been reported to enhance in vitro cellular immune responses to recall antigens and IL-2 stimulation, to increase neutrophil chemotaxis in response to IL-8, and to increase both lymphocyte chemotaxis and the number of circulating CD4+ T cells.[259,260] These immune-enhancing effects come at the price of increased rates of microalbuminuria, hypertension, and cardiovascular disease in T-allele carriers.[261,262] However, as predicted by PATHOS-D theory, these effects also appear to translate into improved host defense, given associations between the T-allele and reduced death from infection in infancy and evidence of positive selection for the T-allele in geographical areas with high rates of infectious pathology.[263,264] Also consistent with enhanced host-defense responses, the T-allele is associated with improved antiviral responses following IFN-α treatment for hepatitis C virus (HCV) and highly active retroviral treatment for human immunodeficiency virus.[265–267] In addition, following HBV booster vaccination, the T-allele increases in vitro lymphocyte proliferative responses to HBV surface antigen.[268]

The MTHFR 677T allele produces a version of the methylenetetrahydrofolate reductase enzyme with reduced activity,[269] leading to elevations in plasma concentrations of homocysteine and other markers of inflammation.[270–276] Animal and human data suggest that this reduced MTHFR activity and concomitant increase in inflammatory tone may enhance host defense in at least some situations. For example, in a mouse model, MTHFR deficiency protects against cytomegalovirus infection,[269] and in pregnant females increased methylenetetrahydrofolate is associated with the presence of a sexually transmitted disease and bacterial vaginosis.[277] Directly supporting a protective role for the T-allele are data demonstrating that the allele protects against HBV infection in African populations.[276] Moreover, the hyperhomocysteinemia associated with reduced MTHFR activity has been posited as protective against malaria and has been suggested as selection factor for the T-allele in sub-Saharan Africa.[278] Interestingly, however, the prevalence of the T-allele is actually far lower in sub-Saharan populations than in other ethnic/geographical groups despite these potential benefits, likely because homozygosity for the allele is lethal in situations of low folate availability such as pertain throughout much of the region.[276] On the other hand, given the array of disease states that has been associated with MTHFR 677T,[279–284] as well as reduced fertility,[285] its increased prevalence in environments of ready folate availability may reflect more substantial benefits for host defense than are currently recognized.

APOE, a glycoprotein central to lipid transport and metabolism, has been implicated as a risk and/or protective factor in a wide range of illnesses. The APOE gene has three primary alleles; termed ε2, ε3, and ε4, with ε3 being the most common worldwide, but with significant data suggesting that ε4 is the ancestral human allele.[286–289] APOE impacts immune functioning in complex and apparently contradictory ways, with both immune-enhancing and immune-suppressing effects reported. The depression-protective ε2 allele does not appear to be associated with reduced inflammation per se, as PATHOS-D theory would predict, but may meet the third criterion required by PATHOS-D theory by being a risk factor for diseases known to have exerted significant selection pressure on humans, including tuberculosis and malaria.[290] Conversely, the ε4 allele, which increases the risk for MDD compared with ε2, is associated with increases in many measures of inflammation and related processes such as oxidative stress[286–289] and has been reported to protect against the development of childhood diarrhea in high-pathogen environments.

Dopamine and serotonin are pivotal neurotransmitters in mood regulation, and yet like other factors linked to depression, these monoamines both affect and are affected by the immune system. The bulk of available evidence suggests that MDD is best characterized as a condition of low dopamine availability, at least in CNS regions linked to motivation and reward.[291–294] The possibility that reduced dopamine availability in MDD may serve host-defense purposes is suggested by animal studies showing that hyperdopaminemia is associated with reductions in both innate and adaptive Th1-type cellular immunity, with resultant increased susceptibility to infection.[295,296] That dopamine transporter activity in particular may be important for host defense in humans is suggested by findings from two genome-wide linkage analyses of risk factors for tuberculosis in geographic areas in which the disease is endemic. Both studies localized a genetic protective factor to a locus of chromosome 15.[297,298] Fine mapping of this locus identified an SNP (rs250682) within the dopamine transporter gene (SLC6A3) as conferring the strongest protective effect.[297] The G-allele of rs250682 was associated with reduced skin reactions to the tuberculin test, which predicts reduced risk of later active disease in endemic areas.[297] However, no data indicated that rs250682 is in linkage disequilibrium with the SLC6A3 40-bp VNTR, which has been associated with MDD. Nor do any data address whether the 9-repeat allele of the VNTR has immunological effects that would enhance host defense. Indeed, even the question of whether this putative depression risk allele is a gain- or loss-of-function variant for the dopamine transporter remains to be definitively clarified.[299,300]

The SLC6A4 44-bp ins/del polymorphism (often referred to as 5HTTLPR) is by far the most extensively studied and debated genetic risk factor for MDD. Significant data suggest that the "short" allele of this serotonin transporter polymorphism (which is less efficient in the reuptake of serotonin) increases the risk for developing depression in response to psychosocial adversity, both during development and in adulthood. Less well known, but consistent with PATHOS-D predictions, the short allele has also been shown to protect against sudden infant death syndrome, a condition often associated with unrecognized infectious morbidity.[301–304] Given the PATHOS-D prediction that stress should activate inflammation as a prepotent protection against risk of wounding (see below), it is intriguing that the SLC6A4 short allele is associated with an increase in the ratio of circulating proinflammatory (e.g., IL-6) to anti-inflammatory (e.g., IL-10) cytokines following a psychosocial stressor.[305] Further supporting a role for SLC6A4 in host defense is the finding that the gene might account for 10 percent of the correlation between depressive symptoms and circulating levels of IL-6 in a group of medically healthy adults.[306] Finally, the prevalence of the short allele in cultures around the world is strongly correlated with historical burden of disease-causing pathogens in these cultures,[307] consistent with the possibility that the short allele has undergone positive selection as a result of enhancing host defense.[3]

Alleles Identified by Meta-analyses of GWAS Data

Far less is known about the general functionality of alleles identified in GWAS, let alone which physiological effects may be relevant to MDD. It should not be surprising, therefore, that limited data are available regarding whether these potentially depressogenic SNPs impact immunity to enhance host defense. On the other hand, it is intriguing that associations with immune/inflammatory function or other aspects of host defense against pathogens have been demonstrated for 8 of the top 10 genes (or their very close homologs) identified in the largest GWAS meta-analysis of MDD conducted to date.[308–343] Many other depression-relevant genes identified in earlier large GWAS studies (as well as meta-analyses of these studies), including PBRM1, GNL3, ATP6V1B2, SP4, AK294384, LY86, KSP37, SMG7, NFKB1, LOC654346, LAMC2, ATG7, CUGBP1, NFE2L3, LOC647167, VCAN, NLGN1, BBOX1, ATF3, RORA, EIF3F, CDH13, ITGB1, and GRM8, have also been linked to immune system and/or host-defense functions.

An exception to the general lack of knowledge regarding GWAS-identified depression risk alleles is provided by the rs1006737 SNP in the CACNA1C gene, which codes for the alpha-1 subunit of the L-type voltage-gated calcium channel (Cav1.2).[344] CACNA1C has been identified as a potential depression risk gene in several GWAS studies,[308,345,346] and convergent validity for its role in depression is provided by data demonstrating that carriers of the risk A-allele have changes in brain function and morphology relevant to MDD.[347–349]

As with other genes, SIRT1 in particular, an examination of the immune effects of CACNA1C highlights both the promise and complexities of a PATHOS-D perspective. Calcium signaling pathways play central and essential roles in multiple aspects of immune function, and the Cav1.2 channel in particular contributes to the function of a variety of immune cell types, including dendritic cells, CD4+ and CD8+ T cells, mast cells, and macrophages.[350–358] Consistent with an overall proinflammatory effect for Cav1.2, agents that block this calcium channel have been repeatedly observed to have anti-inflammatory properties.[359] Given these findings, PATHOS-D theory predicts that the depressogenic A-allele at rs1006737 should be a gain-of-function variant with an overall proinflammatory effect. In support of this, the A-allele has been associated with reduced activation of the anti-inflammatory intracellular messenger Akt,[360] which is known from in vitro studies to downregulate TNF and inducible nitric oxide synthase production in response to challenge with bacterial endotoxin.[361] Moreover, if Cav1.2 activation promotes host defense via activation of inflammatory processes, one would predict that the A-allele should be associated with increased CACNA1C protein production. Although this has yet to be confirmed, data from postmortem brain tissue indicate that carriers of the A-allele have increased CACNA1C mRNA production in the CNS.[348]

These data suggest that the A-allele of CACNA1C meets the first two criteria for consistency with a PATHOS-D perspective: it is located in a gene with known immune effects and is associated with increased signaling in inflammatory/host-defense pathways. The finding that Cav1.2 activation is necessary for T-cell defense against *Leishmania major* infection is consistent with the third criterion,[352] given that the A-allele appears to be a gain-of-function variant. However, other lines of circumstantial evidence undermine any straightforward association between allelic variants that increase Cav1.2 function and enhanced host defense. In fact, the opposite appears to be the case, given that Timothy syndrome, caused by a rare gain-of-function variant in CACNA1C,[362] is associated with a strikingly increased risk of infection.[358] Similarly, activation of Cav1.2 channels appears to actually impede host defense against *M. tuberculosis* by reducing the bactericidal activity of dendritic-cell-activated T cells.[353] These results appear paradoxical given that calcium influx into immune cells is essential for eradication of *M. tuberculosis*, and significant data indicate that L-type voltage-gated channels play an important role in this regard.[354] However, conflicting data suggest that L-type calcium channels may actually downregulate overall calcium influx, given that blocking these channels increased calcium signaling and bactericidal activity in *M. tuberculosis*–infected macrophages.[353] These findings are consistent with the observation that bacterial endotoxin acutely downregulates L-type calcium channel mRNA, as would be expected if Cav1.2 has an anti-inflammatory function.[363]

These considerations introduce a critically important complication into our discussion of the immune effects of depressogenic gene variants. Up to this point we have proceeded as though pathogen-host defense is a monolithic process, which is a simplification exposed by the bivalent effects of L-type intracellular calcium signaling on infectious outcomes. Because calcium signaling activates multiple facets of the immune system, it is not surprising that this signaling has been shown to contribute to the antipathogen capacities of a variety of cell types. For example, macrophages rely on L-type calcium channel activation in response to *Chlamydia pneumoniae* lipopolysaccharide to kill the microorganism.[364] However, other microbes have evolved to manipulate this host-defense system to their own benefit, such as *Legionella pneumophila*, which requires L-type calcium signaling to replicate within infected host cells.[365] These examples demonstrate that the same physiological process can enhance host defense to one pathogen while increasing vulnerability to another.

PROPOSITION 5: DEPRESSIVE SYMPTOMS SHOULD OVERLAP WITH
THE SYMPTOMS OF SICKNESS AND SHOULD THEREFORE ENHANCE SURVIVAL
IN THE CONTEXT OF ACUTE INFECTION AND IN SITUATIONS IN WHICH
RISK OF INFECTION FROM WOUNDING IS HIGH

PATHOS-D theory asserts that depressogenic alleles are common not because depression may or may not be adaptive in managing social negotiations but because these alleles promote symptoms and behaviors that decreased mortality from infectious causes across mammalian evolution. However, from an evolutionary perspective there is no a priori reason why these antipathogen effects should overlap with the depressogenic effects of these risk alleles. That they do so is powerful evidence, we suggest, for the primacy of immune defense in the pathogenesis of depression, regardless of the environmental adversity that initiates the disorder in individual cases. In keeping with this perspective, let's examine the possibility that depression has the symptoms it does because these symptoms promote survival in response to infection.

Fever and Hypoferremia

Although once viewed as a maladaptive consequence of immune activation,[366] several decades of research have produced a consensus that sickness behavior is an adaptive central motivational state evolved to promote survival and necessitated to a large degree by the metabolic costs of mounting a fever.[69,75,366–369] Fever, in turn, has been shown to enhance resistance to both viral and bacterial pathogens, over and above other antipathogen effects of the inflammatory mechanisms by which fever is induced. In addition to retarding pathogen replication/spread,[370–373] febrile range temperatures have multiple stimulatory effects on the immune system that enhance host defense.[374–380] Because these effects are augmented in conditions of low iron availability, it should not be surprising that, in addition to causing fever, inflammatory cytokines deplete bodily iron stores,[381] or that sickness is associated with reduced iron (hypoferremia),[382,383] which, after fever, is probably the feature of sickness that has been best established as of adaptive value.[384–386] For example, low bodily iron stores protect against infection in children in the developing world,[387] and multiple studies suggest that iron supplementation worsens an array of infection-related health outcomes and increases infectious mortality.[388–392] From this perspective hypoferremia can be understood as an evolved adaptive sickness response that prevents iron from being readily available to invading pathogens that need it to survive and multiply within the infected host.

If depressive symptoms aid in pathogen defense and if fever and hypoferremia are important in this regard, one would expect that MDD should be associated with elevated body temperature and reduced bodily iron stores, even in individuals with no evidence of an infectious process. Similarly, PATHOS-D theory predicts that because psychosocial stressors promote depressive symptoms, at least in part, because they signal danger of wounding, these stressors should also increase body temperature and lower iron stores to preemptively prepare for infection. Consistent with these predictions, acute and chronic stressors increase body temperature and reduce gastrointestinal iron absorption and peripheral iron levels in laboratory animals.[393–400] Similarly, the phenomenon of "psychogenic fever" has been repeatedly demonstrated in humans exposed to stress,[401,402] and at least one study reports reduced bodily iron stores following an intense five-day psychosocial stressor in young males in the military.[403] Given the centrality of fever to the adaptive function of sickness behavior,[75,370,404] it is surprising that so little attention has been paid to the fact that MDD appears to be reliably characterized by an elevation in body temperature into the range known to be maximally protective in the context of infection.[405–412] As with elevated body temperature, a number of studies have reported that depressive symptoms are associated with reductions in various measures of bodily iron stores.[413–417]

Because fever and hypoferremia are central to the adaptive purposes of sickness, their presence in depression is mandated from a PATHOS-D perspective, and their absence would strongly argue against the validity of this approach. On the other hand, their presence in depression is not parsimoniously explained by theories that focus on potential social benefits of depression. Similarly, if depression is simply a nonadaptive phenomenon, why would such an ancient, highly conserved, and highly complex physiological response be a hallmark of the disorder?

Evolutionary Trade-offs: Conservation-Withdrawal Versus Behavioral Activation and Hypervigilance

Proinflammatory cytokines induce a behavioral/emotional state characterized by depressed mood, anhedonia, psychomotor retardation, fatigue, social avoidance, and anorexia.[69,418,419] Immune activation can also promote sleepiness, with increased slow-wave sleep and suppression of rapid-eye-movement sleep.[420–424] Together these symptoms can be understood as comprising a behavioral state of conservation-withdrawal.[425] This state is an integral component of depressive disorders and has been widely considered to develop in the context of infection and/or tissue injury as a means of marshaling limited metabolic resources for the expensive tasks of immune activation, fever generation, and tissue repair.[366]

In addition to energy allocation, conservation-withdrawal symptoms may have also proved adaptive by reducing interpersonal contact and thereby limiting infectious exposure. Because ancestral humans typically lived in small groups of genetically related individuals, the logic of inclusive fitness suggests that social withdrawal might have been adaptive for an individual's genes by reducing the risk of infection in kin, even if such withdrawal limited the provision of much needed care from others and thus reduced individual survival. However, significant data demonstrate that viral infections promote aggressive immune responses to bacterial superinfections that can greatly increase mortality;[426–432] therefore, any decrement in survival from loss of social aid might have been more than offset by reduced risk of exposure to other pathogens while in a vulnerable immune state. Moreover, social withdrawal and reduced environmental exploration might also have promoted individual survival by limiting a sick person's contact with immunologically dissimilar out-group members who potentially harbored pathogens against which the sick person would have had reduced immunity compared with pathogens endemic in the home group.[433]

While withdrawal-conservation behavior is prominent in MDD (and especially in younger people), depressed individuals also often manifest metabolically expensive symptoms more consistent with behavioral activation, including anxiety/agitation, insomnia, and anger/irritability.[434] By siphoning energy away from immune activity, these symptoms would be expected to impair host defense and hence to argue against a PATHOS-D perspective. However, sickness behavior, while of benefit for surviving infection, would have carried its own its own survival and reproduction costs across human evolution, as a result of increased risk for predation and reduced ability to care for one's young, as well as potential loss of status in a social species and/or loss of breeding territory.[435] Therefore, evolutionary logic dictates that inflammatory processes, especially when chronic, might promote hypervigilant behavior, which, while shunting energy away from fighting infection, would nonetheless serve adaptive purposes by protecting against environmental dangers engendered by sickness.

In fact, significant data demonstrate that chronic cytokine activation reliably produces just these types of hypervigilant behaviors/symptoms, including anxiety/agitation, anger/irritability, and insomnia.[436,437] And although acute immune activation has been associated with hypersomnia and increased slow-wave sleep, we have shown in a polysomnographic study that patients receiving chronic IFN-α demonstrate reduced sleep continuity and slow-wave sleep, as well as decreased ability to nap during the day, despite poor nighttime sleep—all of which are consistent with cytokine-induced increases in vigilance.[94] Neurobiological substrates for the mixture of withdrawal-conservation and behavioral activation/hypervigilance symptoms that are common to chronic inflammation/medical illness and MDD have also been identified. In multiple studies, immune activation (typhoid vaccine, lipopolysaccharide, IFN-α)[92,438–443] has reliably altered activity in the cingulate cortex, often considered the brain's error detection region (hence vigilance), as well as in the basal ganglia, which play important roles in fatigue and psychomotor retardation.

Anorexia, Depression, and Host Defense

Loss of appetite/interest in food can be understood as potentially enhancing survival during infection by redirecting energy away from food procurement to the metabolic demands of immune activation/fever. But these very metabolic demands make the anorexic response to infection a paradox in need of a more robust adaptive explanation. Why would metabolically expensive inflammatory processes[444] have as an integral component the behavioral effect of depriving an organism of the very metabolic resources needed by the immune system to fight infection? And yet if cytokine-induced anorexia is not adaptive, why is it ubiquitous across phyla as divergent as mammals and insects?[445] Anorexia is also more common in MDD than is hyperphagia,[446] again pointing to its primacy as the feeding abnormality that links sickness with depression.

Although it remains unclear whether food restriction protects against the development of infection,[447] animal data indicate that force-feeding rodents once they are infected increases mortality.[448] Similarly, the provision of total parenteral nutrition (TPN) in animal models and to critically ill patients has been associated with increased risk for infection and subsequent mortality.[449–451] Interestingly, rats injected with lipopolysaccharide consume proportionately more carbohydrates, even though more energy is available from ingesting lipids.[452] This suggests that lipid consumption may be counterproductive during an infection. Consistent with this possibility, preclinical data demonstrate that lipid consumption increases infectious mortality,[445] and a meta-analysis of TPN use in hospitals found that infected patients provided lipids in their feedings had higher complication rates than those receiving TPN without lipids.[453] Moreover, critically ill patients provided TPN were more likely to develop serious infections in hospital. Omega-3 fatty acids, which were highly represented in ancestral human diets and have been widely touted for their potential anti-inflammatory and antidepressant properties, have immune properties that may have compromised host defense against pathogens during human evolution. Given the tremendous selection pressure placed on the human genome by tuberculosis, it is intriguing that omega-3 fatty acids have been shown to activate peroxisome proliferator-activated receptor-gamma signaling in dendritic cells, with a resultant downregulation of CD1a receptor expression.[332] CD1a expression in dendritic cells is crucial for the presentation of *M. tuberculosis* antigens to cells of the adaptive immune system.[454] CD1a receptors also play an essential role in activating T-cell responses to other pathogens, as demonstrated by the ability of *Leishmania donovani* to survive in host cells by downregulating these receptors.[455]

PROPOSITION 6: AGE AND SEX DIFFERENCES IN DEPRESSIVE SYMPTOM PROFILES SHOULD BE UNDERSTANDABLE IN TERMS OF TRADE-OFFS BETWEEN THE BENEFITS AND RISKS OF SICKNESS IN THE ANCESTRAL ENVIRONMENT

Why So Young?

With the exception of asthma and allergies, inflammatory conditions typically strike after the age of reproduction, and thus alleles that promote them are subject to minimal selective pressure, even in modern environments.[456] If depression is also often a condition of chronic low-grade inflammation, why does it follow such a different time course, with an incident peak in the twenties and thirties,[457–459] an age of primary reproductive/childrearing responsibilities? PATHOS-D theory provides a startling answer to this question that is diametrically opposed to other evolutionary theories linking inflammation to depression.[17] From a PATHOS-D perspective, depression is common early in life for the same reason that sickness is also prevalent, and that is because these years were associated with a high infectious burden, and subsequent morbidity/mortality, in ancestral environments.[46,57] Indeed, across most of human history, 50 percent of those born were dead from infectious causes by completion of adolescence. In the context of pathogen-host defense, depressive symptoms are no less adaptive than are sickness symptoms. They do not represent an aberrant phenomenon resulting from an evolutionary mismatch between current conditions and ancestral environments. They are an evolved behavioral phenotype induced by immune activation to aid in both preventing and battling infection. In this regard they are quite different from late-life, inflammatory "wear-and-tear" conditions, such as cardiovascular disease and dementia that comprise part of the price humans pay for robust host-defense mechanisms earlier in life.[460,461]

This perspective provides a parsimonious explanation for evidence that, when compared with depression that occurs during reproductive years, depression with onset late in life follows a different clinical course and is associated with different patterns of CNS vascular and morphological change. Whereas conditions of chronic depression that commence early in life are characterized primarily by loss of glial elements and sparing of neurons in the CNS, late-life depression is more reliably associated with neuronal death. PATHOS-D theory suggests that the glial changes characteristic of early-life depression (i.e., astrocytic and oligodendroglial cell loss and increased microglial density/numbers) would be well worth studying for their potential pathogen defense characteristics. From a PATHOS-D perspective, early-life depression is an evolved biological/behavioral phenotype that serves host-defense functions. Depression with a late-life onset would be expected to be a more heterogeneous amalgam of adaptive immunological states and conditions that reflect nothing more than the consequences of a lifetime's worth of wear and tear on CNS tissue.

Why Is the Depressive Phenotype Affected by Sex and Age?

Most people with depression experience impaired sleep and reduced appetite,[446] but a significant minority manifest hypersomnia and hyperphagia instead.[462] These symptoms are most frequent in females between adolescence and middle age.[463–465] How might PATHOS-D theory account for the existence of these reversed neurovegetative symptoms, as well as their age and sex distribution? A first step is to establish that cytokine pathways known to be activated by infection are capable of producing both hypersomnia and hyperphagia. Hypersomnia has been recognized for years as a primary behavioral manifestation of proinflammatory cytokine activation,[420–424] and studies in healthy adolescents and adults indicate that chronically increased sleep is associated with increased saliva and blood concentrations of IL-6 and CRP.[466,467] In terms of feeding behavior, we have already presented evidence from animal models that inflammation promotes carbohydrate preference,[452] such as is typical in depressive hyperphagia. Less well known are data that high-fat diets induce leptin and insulin resistance, as well as obesity, in response to activation of inflammatory mediators in the hypothalamus.[468,469] Conversely, blocking hypothalamic inflammation prevents obesity and other stigmata of metabolic syndrome in rodents, even in the context of high fat consumption.[469–471] In rodents, exposure to either TNF or IL-6 in utero results in adulthood obesity,[472] again suggesting that cytokines can induce hyperphagia/weight gain under certain circumstances. Although we know of no data showing that females are more likely than males to respond to inflammatory signaling with hyperphagia, female rodents have less anorexia than do males in response to influenza infection.[473]

Because the presence of widespread obesity is recent, the question arises as to whether more ancient signals for inflammatory activation (and hence depression) might also promote hyperphagia instead of anorexia. We know of no data that directly address this issue in terms of infection, but certain adenoviruses have been associated with weight gain.[474,475] In terms of depressogenic psychosocial factors, preclinical studies suggest that stressors associated with a high degree of wounding, such as chronic social defeat, induce hypothalamic resistance to leptin,[468,476] consistent with their known ability to activate inflammatory pathways.[208,210,214,477] As in depression, where hyperphagia and weight gain are associated with disease chronicity,[464] chronic social defeat leads initially to weight loss but to weight gain over time.[476] Given the role of leptin resistance in hyperphagia, it is intriguing that increased peripheral leptin levels (consistent with leptin resistance) have been observed more consistently in women than in men with MDD[478–482] and are more common in atypical than in nonatypical depression.[483]

Why might younger individuals in general, and females in particular, be more likely to develop depressive conditions characterized by hypersomnia and hyperphagia? From a PATHOS-D perspective the simplest answer may be because, in ancestral environments, they could. In primate species youth and females are frequently more protected from predation and have food supplied to them by others, raising the possibility that in ancestral environments these individuals enjoyed sufficient security to partake of the recuperative effects of sleep and to eat without having to expend energy searching for food.

Given data presented earlier about potential antipathogen effects of anorexia, might similar benefits accrue to hyperphagia, especially in youth and females, under at least some evolutionarily relevant situations? While admittedly speculative, several lines of evidence suggest that by promoting hypothalamic resistance to leptin, genes associated with increased inflammatory signaling might enhance host defense by driving ongoing leptin production despite malnutrition in conditions of food scarcity. This increased leptin production would both augment the drive to seek and consume food and lower the set point at which food consumption initiated the types of inflammatory responses that are all too common in the obese, but that appear to be lifesaving in the face of an infection such as tuberculosis, which is most lethal for females of reproductive age and for which low body weight and reduced leptin are deadly.[484–489]

Summary

In this chapter we have marshaled evidence from multiple disciplines to support the theory that depressogenic risk alleles evolved and have been retained in the human genome at least in part because they enhance host defense against pathogens, primarily via promotion of innate immune system activity, which is especially relevant to survival in infancy, when infectious mortality is traditionally highest and the adaptive immune system is not fully functional. Moreover, we have provided data demonstrating that many depressive symptoms may themselves be adaptive as a result of enhancing pathogen defense over and above direct antipathogen activities of the immune, neuroendocrine, and CNS processes from which these symptoms arise.

It is increasingly recognized that, rather than producing depression directly, many vulnerability alleles are better classified as modifiers of sensitivity to environmental conditions, and especially conditions characterized by social interactions (or their lack). In this sense depression can be understood not as inhering within the afflicted individual only but, rather, as being, at least to some degree, a product of the larger social system in which the individual is a ensconced. Depression is inherently a relational disorder. PATHOS-D theory can be seen as radically expanding this idea by suggesting that depression is also a social disorder vis-à-vis our relationships with the microbial and parasitic world. This perspective suggests that depression more is the result of a long-standing conversation (or battle!) with a huge array of life forms than the result of any fixed, maladaptive physiological pattern that inheres within individuals. By expanding the depth and breadth of beings that are relevant to depressogenesis, PATHOS-D theory does not require that depression be adaptive primarily within the very narrow range of our relationships with conspecifics; thus, the theory avoids many of the conceptual gyrations required to make a disorder so damaging to the human world appear to be of benefit in the same arena. Moreover, by recognizing that depression evolved in a complex and ongoing dialogue with the microbial and parasitic world, PATHOS-D theory offers a welcome antidote to the widespread tendency in both psychiatry and psychoimmunology to view the immune alterations characteristic of depression as mere pathophysiological "lesions."

Finally, PATHOS-D theory adds an important dimension to theorizing regard-

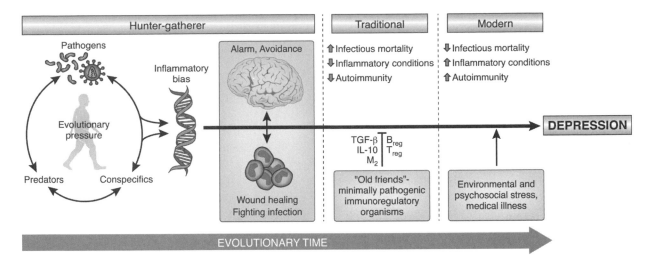

FIGURE 10.1. Antidepressant effects of whole-body hyperthermia (WBH) compared with sham treatment. Error bars represent standard deviations of the mean score at each assessment point; numbers in parentheses indicate the number of participants in each group at that assessment. Abbreviations: 17-item HDRS, 17-item Hamilton Depression Rating Scale; WBH, whole body hyperthermia.

ing the etiological role of excessive hygiene in the pathogenesis of psychiatric disorders, including MDD. Building upon many years' data regarding associations between enhanced hygiene and the explosive increase of autoimmune/ allergic/asthmatic conditions in the modern world, researchers have proposed that loss of contact with immunotolerogenic microorganisms that were widespread during human evolution may be contributing to the increased inflammation, and consequent increased MDD, observed in First-World societies.[490] Thus, as shown in Figure 10.1, modern humans have inherited an inflammatory bias that has been exacerbated by modern living conditions. Combining hygiene theorizing with PATHOS-D theory points to an important truth for health care of the future. If future modalities treat depression by reducing inflammatory signaling, these strategies will require that we maintain sanitation practices/modern medicine as a type of extended phenotype that, by doing much of the work that was traditionally the sole province of the immune system, will continue to make it safe to reduce our evolved defense mechanisms against pathogens in the name of enhanced emotional well-being. A primary challenge of the twenty-first century will revolve around how to create environments that protect against infection while avoiding the types of widespread sterility that drive enhanced inflammation precisely when we need it least. However we resolve this dilemma, PATHOS-D theory suggests that mental health and public health will be forever inextricably linked.

References

1. Hart D, Sussman RW. *Man the hunted: primates, predators, and human evolution.* Boulder, CO: Westview Press; 2009.

2. Miller AH, Maletic V, Raison CL. Inflammation and its discontents: the role of cytokines in the pathophysiology of major depression. *Biol Psychiatry.* 2009;65(9):732–741.

3. Chiao JY, Blizinsky KD. Culture-gene coevolution of individualism-collectivism and the serotonin transporter gene. *Proc Biol Sci.* 2010;277(1681):529–537.

4. Crespi B, Summers K, Dorus S. Adaptive evolution of genes underlying schizophrenia. *Proc Biol Sci.* 2007;274(1627):2801–2810.

5. Price J, Sloman L, Gardner R, Gilbert P, Rohde P. The social competition hypothesis of depression. *Br J Psychiatry.* 1994;164(3):309–315.

6. Price J. Darwinian dynamics of depression. *Aust N Z J Psychiatry.* 2009;43(11):1029–1037.

7. Nesse RM. Is depression an adaptation? *Arch Gen Psychiatry.* 2000;57(1):14–20.

8. Klinger E. Consequences of commitment to and disengagement from incentives. *Psychol Rev.* 1975;82(1–25).

9. Leahy RL. Depression and resistance: an investment model of decision-making. *Behav Ther.* 1997;20:3–6.

10. Keller MC, Nesse RM. The evolutionary significance of depressive symptoms: different adverse situations lead to different depressive symptom patterns. *J Pers Soc Psychol.* 2006;91(2):316–330.

11. Allen NB, Badcock PB. The social risk hypothesis of depressed mood: evolutionary, psychosocial, and neurobiological perspectives. *Psychol Bull.* 2003;129(6):887–913.

12. Allen NB, Badcock PB. Darwinian models of depression: a review of evolutionary accounts of mood and mood disorders. *Prog Neuropsychopharmacol Biol Psychiatry.* 2006;30(5):815–826.

13. Sloman L, Gilbert P, Hasey G. Evolved mechanisms in depression: the role and interaction of attachment and social rank in depression. *J Affect Disord.* 2003;74(2):107–121.

14. Sloman L. A new comprehensive evolutionary model of depression and anxiety. *J Affect Disord.* 2008;106(3):219–228.

15. Watson PJ, Andrews PW. Toward a revised evolutionary adaptationist analysis of depression: the social navigation hypothesis. *J Affect Disord.* 2002;72(1):1–14.

16. Andrews PW, Thomson JA Jr. The bright side of being blue: depression as an adaptation for analyzing complex problems. *Psychol Rev.* 2009;116(3):620–654.

17. Kinney DK, Tanaka M. An evolutionary hypothesis of depression and its symptoms, adaptive value, and risk factors. *J Nerv Ment Dis.* 2009;197(8):561–567.

18. Keller MC, Miller G. Resolving the paradox of common, harmful, heritable mental disorders: which evolutionary genetic models work best? *Behav Brain Sci.* 2006;29(4):385–452.

19. Wilkins JF. Antagonistic coevolution of two imprinted loci with pleiotropic effects. *Evolution.* 2010;64(1):142–151.

20. Nesse RM. The smoke detector principle: natural selection and the regulation of defensive responses. *Ann N Y Acad Sci.* 2001;935:75–85.

21. Rapaport MH, Judd LL. Minor depressive disorder and subsyndromal depressive symptoms: functional impairment and response to treatment. *J Affect Disord.* 1998;48(2–3):227–232.

22. Ayuso-Mateos JL, Nuevo R, Verdes E, Naidoo N, Chatterji S. From depressive symptoms

to depressive disorders: the relevance of thresholds. *Br J Psychiatry.* 2010;196(5):365–371.

23. Fergusson DM, Horwood LJ, Ridder EM, Beautrais AL. Subthreshold depression in adolescence and mental health outcomes in adulthood. *Arch Gen Psychiatry.* 2005;62(1):66–72.

24. Horwath E, Johnson J, Klerman GL, Weissman MM. Depressive symptoms as relative and attributable risk factors for first-onset major depression. *Arch Gen Psychiatry.* 1992;49(10):817–823.

25. Kendler KS, Gardner CO, Jr. Boundaries of major depression: an evaluation of *DSM-IV* criteria. *Am J Psychiatry.* 1998;155(2):172–177.

26. Hamilton BA, Naismith SL, Scott EM, Purcell S, Hickie IB. Disability is already pronounced in young people with early stages of affective disorders: data from an early intervention service. *J Affect Disord.* 2011;131(1–3):84–91.

27. Williams KE, Marsh WK, Rasgon NL. Mood disorders and fertility in women: a critical review of the literature and implications for future research. *Hum Reprod Update.* 2007;13(6):607–616.

28. Gurhan N, Akyuz A, Atici D, Kisa S. Association of depression and anxiety with oocyte and sperm numbers and pregnancy outcomes during in vitro fertilization treatment. *Psychol Rep.* 2009;104(3):796–806.

29. Meller W, Burns LH, Crow S, Grambsch P. Major depression in unexplained infertility. *J Psychosom Obstet Gynaecol.* 2002;23(1):27–30.

30. Drosdzol A, Skrzypulec V. Depression and anxiety among Polish infertile couples—an evaluative prevalence study. *J Psychosom Obstet Gynaecol.* 2009;30(1):11–20.

31. Vaccarino V, Johnson BD, Sheps DS, et al. Depression, inflammation, and incident cardiovascular disease in women with suspected coronary ischemia: the National Heart, Lung, and Blood Institute-sponsored WISE study. *J Am Coll Cardiol.* 2007;50(21):2044–2050.

32. Janszky I, Ahnve S, Lundberg I, Hemmingsson T. Early-onset depression, anxiety, and risk of subsequent coronary heart disease: 37-year follow-up of 49,321 young Swedish men. *J Am Coll Cardiol.* 2010;56(1):31–37.

33. Frasure-Smith N, Lesperance F, Talajic M. Depression following myocardial infarction: impact on 6-month survival [erratum appears in *JAMA* 1994;271(14):1082]. *JAMA.* 1993;270(15):1819–1825.

34. Steptoe A, Strike PC, Perkins-Porras L, McEwan JR, Whitehead DL. Acute depressed mood as a trigger of acute coronary syndromes. *Biol Psychiatry.* 2006;60(8):837–842.

35. Pan A, Lucas M, Sun Q, et al. Bidirectional association between depression and type 2 diabetes mellitus in women. *Arch Intern Med.* 2010;170(21):1884–1891.

36. Engum A. The role of depression and anxiety in onset of diabetes in a large population-based study. *J Psychosom Res.* 2007;62(1):31–38.

37. Penninx BW, Guralnik JM, Pahor M, et al. Chronically depressed mood and cancer risk in older persons. *J Natl Cancer Inst.* 1998;90(24):1888–1893.

38. Ritchie K, Carriere I, Ritchie CW, Berr C, Artero S, Ancelin ML. Designing prevention programmes to reduce incidence of dementia: prospective cohort study of modifiable risk factors. *BMJ.* 2010;341:c3885.

39. Gatz JL, Tyas SL, St John P, Montgomery P. Do depressive symptoms predict Alzheimer's disease and dementia? *J Gerontol A Biol Sci Med Sci.* 2005;60(6):744–747.

40. Gelernter J, Kranzler H, Cubells JF. Serotonin transporter protein (SLC6A4) allele and haplotype frequencies and linkage disequilibria in African- and European-American

and Japanese populations and in alcohol-dependent subjects. *Hum Genet.* 1997;101(2): 243–246.

41. Takata A, Ionita-Laza I, Gogos JA, Xu B, Karayiorgou M. De novo synonymous mutations in regulatory elements contribute to the genetic etiology of autism and schizophrenia. *Neuron.* 2016;89(5):940–947.

42. Kuningas M, May L, Tamm R, et al. Selection for genetic variation inducing pro-inflammatory responses under adverse environmental conditions in a Ghanaian population. *PLoS ONE.* 2009;4(11):e7795.

43. van Dissel JT, van Langevelde P, Westendorp RG, Kwappenberg K, Frolich M. Anti-inflammatory cytokine profile and mortality in febrile patients. *Lancet.* 1998;351(9107): 950–953.

44. Bermejo-Martin JF, Martin-Loeches I, Rello J, et al. Host adaptive immunity deficiency in severe pandemic influenza. *Crit Care.* 2010;14(5):R167.

45. Westendorp RG, Langermans JA, Huizinga TW, et al. Genetic influence on cytokine production and fatal meningococcal disease. *Lancet.* 1997;349(9046):170–173.

46. McDade TW. Life history theory and the immune system: steps toward a human ecological immunology. *Am J Phys Anthropol.* 2003;suppl 37:100–125.

47. Pedron B, Guerin V, Cordeiro DJ, Masmoudi S, Dalle JH, Sterkers G. Development of cytomegalovirus and adenovirus-specific memory CD4 T-cell functions from birth to adulthood. *Pediatr Res.* 2011;69(2):106–111.

48. Nwachuku N, Gerba CP. Health risks of enteric viral infections in children. *Rev Environ Contam Toxicol.* 2006;186:1–56.

49. Chen LC, Rahman M, Sarder AM. Epidemiology and causes of death among children in a rural area of Bangladesh. *Int J Epidemiol.* 1980;9(1):25–33.

50. Collinson AC, Ngom PT, Moore SE, Morgan G, Prentice AM. Birth season and environmental influences on blood leucocyte and lymphocyte subpopulations in rural Gambian infants. *BMC Immunol.* 2008;9:18.

51. Moore SE, Collinson AC, Tamba N'Gom P, Aspinall R, Prentice AM. Early immunological development and mortality from infectious disease in later life. *Proc Nutr Soc.* 2006;65(3):311–318.

52. Moore SE, Cole TJ, Collinson AC, Poskitt EM, McGregor IA, Prentice AM. Prenatal or early postnatal events predict infectious deaths in young adulthood in rural Africa. *Int J Epidemiol.* 1999;28(6):1088–1095.

53. Avitsur R, Sheridan JF. Neonatal stress modulates sickness behavior. *Brain Behav Immun.* 2009;23(7):977–985.

54. McDade TW. Life history, maintenance, and the early origins of immune function. *Am J Hum Biol.* 2005;17(1):81–94.

55. Kiecolt-Glaser JK, Gouin JP, Weng NP, Malarkey WB, Beversdorf DQ, Glaser R. Childhood adversity heightens the impact of later-life caregiving stress on telomere length and inflammation. *Psychosom Med.* 2011;73(1):16–22.

56. Finch CE. Evolution in health and medicine Sackler colloquium: evolution of the human lifespan and diseases of aging: roles of infection, inflammation, and nutrition. *Proc Natl Acad Sci U S A.* 2010;107(suppl 1):1718–1724.

57. Dobson AP, Carper ER. Infectious diseases and human population history. *Bioscience.* 1996;46(2):115–126.

58. Wolfe ND, Dunavan CP, Diamond J. Origins of major human infectious diseases. *Nature.* 2007;447(7142):279–283.

59. Lovel H. Targeted interventions and infant mortality. *Trans R Soc Trop Med Hyg.* 1989; 83(1):10–18.

60. Kavaliers M, Colwell DD, Choleris E. Parasites and behavior: an ethopharmacological analysis and biomedical implications. *Neurosci Biobehav Rev.* 1999;23(7):1037–1045.

61. Goncalves GM, Zamboni DS, Camara NO. The role of innate immunity in septic acute kidney injuries. *Shock.* 2010;34(suppl 1):22–26.

62. Oberholzer A, Oberholzer C, Moldawer LL. Sepsis syndromes: understanding the role of innate and acquired immunity. *Shock.* 2001;16(2):83–96.

63. Klein SL. Parasite manipulation of the proximate mechanisms that mediate social behavior in vertebrates. *Physiol Behav.* 2003;79(3):441–449.

64. Cochran GM, Ewald PW, Cochran KD. Infectious causation of disease: an evolutionary perspective. *Perspect Biol Med.* 2000;43(3):406–448.

65. Hornig M, Briese T, Licinio J, et al. Absence of evidence for bornavirus infection in schizophrenia, bipolar disorder and major depressive disorder. *Mol Psychiatry.* 2012; 17(5):486–493.

66. Pearce BD, Kruszon-Moran D, Jones JL. The relationship between *Toxoplasma gondii* infection and mood disorders in the third National Health and Nutrition Survey. *Biol Psychiatry.* 2012;72(4):290–295.

67. Pedersen MG, Mortensen PB, Norgaard-Pedersen B, Postolache TT. *Toxoplasma gondii* infection and self-directed violence in mothers. *Arch Gen Psychiatry.* 2012;69(11): 1123–1130.

68. Reiber C, Shattuck EC, Fiore S, Alperin P, Davis V, Moore J. Change in human social behavior in response to a common vaccine. *Ann Epidemiol.* 2010;20(10):729–733.

69. Dantzer R, O'Connor JC, Freund GG, Johnson RW, Kelley KW. From inflammation to sickness and depression: when the immune system subjugates the brain. *Nat Rev Neurosci.* 2008;9(1):46–56.

70. Musselman DL, Lawson DH, Gumnick JF, et al. Paroxetine for the prevention of depression induced by high-dose interferon alfa. *N Engl J Med.* 2001;344(13):961–966.

71. Raison CL, Borisov AS, Broadwell SD, et al. Depression during pegylated interferon-alpha plus ribavirin therapy: prevalence and prediction. *J Clin Psychiatry.* 2005;66(1): 41–48.

72. Kraus MR, Schafer A, Csef H, Scheurlen M. Psychiatric side effects of pegylated interferon alfa-2b as compared to conventional interferon alfa-2b in patients with chronic hepatitis C. *World J Gastroenterol.* 2005;11(12):1769–1774.

73. Reichenberg A, Gorman JM, Dieterich DT. Interferon-induced depression and cognitive impairment in hepatitis C virus patients: a 72 week prospective study. *AIDS.* 2005; 19(suppl 3):S174–S178.

74. Andreasson A, Arborelius L, Erlanson-Albertsson C, Lekander M. A putative role for cytokines in the impaired appetite in depression. *Brain Behav Immun.* 2007;21(2): 147–152.

75. Maier SF, Watkins LR. Cytokines for psychologists: implications of bidirectional immune-to-brain communication for understanding behavior, mood, and cognition. *Psychol Rev.* 1998;105(1):83–107.

76. Yirmiya R, Weidenfeld J, Pollak Y, et al. Cytokines, "depression due to a general medical condition," and antidepressant drugs. *Adv Exp Med Biol.* 1999;461:283–316.

77. Hayley S, Merali Z, Anisman H. Stress and cytokine-elicited neuroendocrine and neurotransmitter sensitization: implications for depressive illness. *Stress.* 2003;6(1):19–32.

78. Gibb J, Audet MC, Hayley S, Anisman H. Neurochemical and behavioral responses to inflammatory immune stressors. *Front Biosci (Schol Ed).* 2009;1:275–295.

79. Maes M, Yirmyia R, Noraberg J, et al. The inflammatory and neurodegenerative (I&ND)

hypothesis of depression: leads for future research and new drug developments in depression. *Metab Brain Dis.* 2009;24(1):27–53.

80. Yirmiya R, Pollak Y, Barak O, et al. Effects of antidepressant drugs on the behavioral and physiological responses to lipopolysaccharide (LPS) in rodents. *Neuropsychopharmacology.* 2001;24(5):531–544.

81. Merali Z, Brennan K, Brau P, Anisman H. Dissociating anorexia and anhedonia elicited by interleukin-1beta: antidepressant and gender effects on responding for "free chow" and "earned" sucrose intake. *Psychopharmacology (Berl).* 2003;165(4):413–418.

82. Dunn AJ, Swiergiel AH. The reductions in sweetened milk intake induced by interleukin-1 and endotoxin are not prevented by chronic antidepressant treatment. *Neuroimmunomodulation.* 2001;9(3):163–169.

83. Castanon N, Bluthe RM, Dantzer R. Chronic treatment with the atypical antidepressant tianeptine attenuates sickness behavior induced by peripheral but not central lipopolysaccharide and interleukin-1beta in the rat. *Psychopharmacology.* 2001;154(1):50–60.

84. Shen Y, Connor TJ, Nolan Y, Kelly JP, Leonard BE. Differential effect of chronic antidepressant treatments on lipopolysaccharide-induced depressive-like behavioural symptoms in the rat. *Life Sci.* 1999;65(17):1773–1786.

85. Raison CL, Demetrashvili M, Capuron L, Miller AH. Neuropsychiatric adverse effects of interferon-alpha: recognition and management. *CNS Drugs.* 2005;19(2):105–123.

86. Capuron L, Fornwalt FB, Knight BT, Harvey PD, Ninan PT, Miller AH. Does cytokine-induced depression differ from idiopathic major depression in medically healthy individuals? *J Affect Disord.* 2009;119(1–3):181–185.

87. Raison CL, Woolwine BJ, Demetrashvili MF, et al. Paroxetine for prevention of depressive symptoms induced by interferon-alpha and ribavirin for hepatitis C. *Aliment Pharm Ther.* 2007;25(10):1163–1174.

88. Kraus MR, Schafer A, Al-Taie O, Scheurlen M. Prophylactic SSRI during interferon alpha re-therapy in patients with chronic hepatitis C and a history of interferon-induced depression. *J Viral Hepat.* 2005;12(1):96–100.

89. Kraus MR, Schafer A, Faller H, Csef H, Scheurlen M. Paroxetine for the treatment of interferon-alpha-induced depression in chronic hepatitis C. *Aliment Pharm Ther.* 2002;16(6):1091–1099.

90. Hauser P, Khosla J, Aurora H, et al. A prospective study of the incidence and open-label treatment of interferon-induced major depressive disorder in patients with hepatitis C. *Mol Psychiatry.* 2002;7(9):942–947.

91. Wichers MC, Koek GH, Robaeys G, Praamstra AJ, Maes M. Early increase in vegetative symptoms predicts IFN-alpha-induced cognitive-depressive changes. *Psychol Med.* 2005;35(3):433–441.

92. Eisenberger NI, Berkman ET, Inagaki TK, Rameson LT, Mashal NM, Irwin MR. Inflammation-induced anhedonia: endotoxin reduces ventral striatum responses to reward. *Biol Psychiatry.* 2010;68(8):748–754.

93. Harrison NA, Brydon L, Walker C, Gray MA, Steptoe A, Critchley HD. Inflammation causes mood changes through alterations in subgenual cingulate activity and mesolimbic connectivity. *Biol Psychiatry.* 2009;66(5):407–414.

94. Raison CL, Rye DB, Woolwine BJ, et al. Chronic interferon-alpha administration disrupts sleep continuity and depth in patients with hepatitis C: association with fatigue, motor slowing, and increased evening cortisol. *Biol Psychiatry.* 2010;68(10):942–949.

95. Raison CL, Dantzer R, Kelley KW, et al. CSF concentrations of brain tryptophan and kynurenines during immune stimulation with IFN-alpha: relationship to CNS immune responses and depression. *Mol Psychiatry.* 2010;15(4):393–403.

96. Raison CL, Borisov AS, Woolwine BJ, Massung B, Vogt G, Miller AH. Interferon-alpha effects on diurnal hypothalamic-pituitary-adrenal axis activity: relationship with proinflammatory cytokines and behavior. *Mol Psychiatry.* 2010;15(5):535–547.

97. Raison CL, Borisov AS, Majer M, et al. Activation of central nervous system inflammatory pathways by interferon-alpha: relationship to monoamines and depression. *Biol Psychiatry.* 2009;65(4):296–303.

98. Capuron L, Pagnoni G, Demetrashvili MF, et al. Basal ganglia hypermetabolism and symptoms of fatigue during interferon-alpha therapy. *Neuropsychopharmacology.* 2007;32(11):2384–2392.

99. Capuron L, Pagnoni G, Demetrashvili M, et al. Anterior cingulate activation and error processing during interferon-alpha treatment. *Biol Psychiatry.* 2005;58(3):190–196.

100. Howren MB, Lamkin DM, Suls J. Associations of depression with C-reactive protein, IL-1, and IL-6: a meta-analysis. *Psychosom Med.* 2009;71(2):171–186.

101. Dowlati Y, Herrmann N, Swardfager W, et al. A meta-analysis of cytokines in major depression. *Biol Psychiatry.* 2010;67(5):446–457.

102. Zorrilla EP, Luborsky L, McKay JR, et al. The relationship of depression and stressors to immunological assays: a meta-analytic review. *Brain Behav Immun.* 2001;15(3): 199–226.

103. Haapakoski R, Mathieu J, Ebmeier KP, Alenius H, Kivimaki M. Cumulative meta-analysis of interleukins 6 and 1beta, tumour necrosis factor alpha and C-reactive protein in patients with major depressive disorder. *Brain Behav Immun.* 2015;49:206–215.

104. Gimeno D, Kivimaki M, Brunner EJ, et al. Associations of C-reactive protein and interleukin-6 with cognitive symptoms of depression: 12-year follow-up of the Whitehall II study. *Psychol Med.* 2009;39(3):413–423.

105. van den Biggelaar AH, Gussekloo J, de Craen AJ, et al. Inflammation and interleukin-1 signaling network contribute to depressive symptoms but not cognitive decline in old age. *Exp Gerontol.* 2007;42(7):693–701.

106. Pasco JA, Nicholson GC, Williams LJ, et al. Association of high-sensitivity C-reactive protein with de novo major depression. *Br J Psychiatry.* 2010;197:372–377.

107. Valkanova V, Ebmeier KP, Allan CL. CRP, IL-6 and depression: a systematic review and meta-analysis of longitudinal studies. *J Affect Disord.* 2013;150(3):736–744.

108. Noponen M, Sanfilipo M, Samanich K, et al. Elevated PLA2 activity in schizophrenics and other psychiatric patients. *Biol Psychiatry.* 1993;34(9):641–649.

109. Piletz JE, Halaris A, Iqbal O, et al. Pro-inflammatory biomarkers in depression: treatment with venlafaxine. *World J Biol Psychiatry.* 2009;10(4):313–323.

110. Sutcigil L, Oktenli C, Musabak U, et al. Pro- and anti-inflammatory cytokine balance in major depression: effect of sertraline therapy. *Clin Dev Immunol.* 2007;2007:76396.

111. Suarez EC, Krishnan RR, Lewis JG. The relation of severity of depressive symptoms to monocyte-associated proinflammatory cytokines and chemokines in apparently healthy men. *Psychosom Med.* 2003;65(3):362–368.

112. Dhabhar FS, Burke HM, Epel ES, et al. Low serum IL-10 concentrations and loss of regulatory association between IL-6 and IL-10 in adults with major depression. *J Psychiatr Res.* 2009;43(11):962–969.

113. Hashioka S, Klegeris A, Monji A, et al. Antidepressants inhibit interferon-gamma-induced microglial production of IL-6 and nitric oxide. *Exp Neurol.* 2007;206(1):33–42.

114. Gabbay V, Klein RG, Alonso CM, et al. Immune system dysregulation in adolescent major depressive disorder. *J Affect Disord.* 2009;115(1–2):177–182.

115. Shelton RC, Claiborne J, Sidoryk-Wegrzynowicz M, et al. Altered expression of genes

involved in inflammation and apoptosis in frontal cortex in major depression. *Mol Psychiatry.* 2011;16(7):751–762.

116. Myint AM, Leonard BE, Steinbusch HW, Kim YK. Th1, Th2, and Th3 cytokine alterations in major depression. *J Affect Disord.* 2005;88(2):167–173.

117. Maes M. Depression is an inflammatory disease, but cell-mediated immune activation is the key component of depression. *Prog Neuropsychopharmacol Biol Psychiatry.* 2011;35(3):664–675.

118. Harder J, Glaser R, Schroder JM. The role and potential therapeutical applications of antimicrobial proteins in infectious and inflammatory diseases. *Endocr Metab Immune Disord Drug Targets.* 2007;7(2):75–82.

119. Harder J, Dressel S, Wittersheim M, et al. Enhanced expression and secretion of antimicrobial peptides in atopic dermatitis and after superficial skin injury. *J Invest Dermatol.* 2010;130(5):1355–1364.

120. Harder J, Schroder JM. Psoriatic scales: a promising source for the isolation of human skin-derived antimicrobial proteins. *J Leukoc Biol.* 2005;77(4):476–486.

121. Yang YW, Tseng KC, Chen YH, Yang JY. Associations among eczema, asthma, serum immunoglobulin E and depression in adults: a population-based study. *Allergy.* 2010; 65(6):801–802.

122. Gili M, Garcia-Toro M, Vives M, et al. Medical comorbidity in recurrent versus first-episode depressive patients. *Acta Psychiatr Scand.* 2011;123(3):220–227.

123. Kling MA, Alesci S, Csako G, et al. Sustained low-grade pro-inflammatory state in unmedicated, remitted women with major depressive disorder as evidenced by elevated serum levels of the ascute phase proteins C-reactive protein and serum amyloid A. *Biol Psychiat.* 2007;62(4):309–313.

124. Raison CL, Miller AH. When not enough is too much: the role of insufficient glucocorticoid signaling in the pathophysiology of stress-related disorders. *Am J Psychiatry.* 2003;160(9):1554–1565.

125. Felger JC, Haroon E, Woolwine BJ, Raison CL, Miller AH. Interferon-alpha-induced inflammation is associated with reduced glucocorticoid negative feedback sensitivity and depression in patients with hepatitis C virus. *Physiol Behav.* 2015.

126. Norbiato G, Bevilacqua M, Vago T, Taddei A, Clerici. Glucocorticoids and the immune function in the human immunodeficiency virus infection: a study in hypercortisolemic and cortisol-resistant patients. *J Clin Endocrinol Metabol.* 1997;82(10):3260–3263.

127. Huff GR, Huff WE, Balog JM, Rath NC. The effects of behavior and environmental enrichment on disease resistance of turkeys. *Brain Behav Immun.* 2003;17(5):339–349.

128. Cohen S, Janicki-Deverts D, Doyle WJ, et al. Chronic stress, glucocorticoid receptor resistance, inflammation, and disease risk. *Proc Natl Acad Sci U S A.* 2012;109(16):5995–5999.

129. Raison CL, Miller AH. The evolutionary significance of depression in pathogen host defense (PATHOS-D). *Mol Psychiatry.* 2013;18(1):15–37.

130. Leutscher PD, Lagging M, Buhl MR, et al. Evaluation of depression as a risk factor for treatment failure in chronic hepatitis C. *Hepatology.* 2010;52(2):430–435.

131. Raison CL, Broadwell SD, Borisov AS, et al. Depressive symptoms and viral clearance in patients receiving interferon-alpha and ribavirin for hepatitis C. *Brain Behav Immun.* 2005;19(1):23–27.

132. Doering LV, Martinez-Maza O, Vredevoe DL, Cowan MJ. Relation of depression, natural killer cell function, and infections after coronary artery bypass in women. *Eur J Cardiovasc Nurs.* 2008;7(1):52–58.

133. Faulkner S, Smith A. A longitudinal study of the relationship between psychological distress and recurrence of upper respiratory tract infections in chronic fatigue syndrome. *Br J Health Psychol.* 2008;13(pt 1):177–186.

134. Cruess DG, Petitto JM, Leserman J, et al. Depression and HIV infection: impact on immune function and disease progression. *CNS Spectr.* 2003;8(1):52–58.

135. Leserman J. Role of depression, stress, and trauma in HIV disease progression. *Psychosom Med.* 2008;70(5):539–545.

136. Evans DL, Ten Have TR, Douglas SD, et al. Association of depression with viral load, CD8 T lymphocytes, and natural killer cells in women with HIV infection. *Am J Psychiatry.* 2002;159(10):1752–1759.

137. Zorrilla EP, McKay JR, Luborsky L, Schmidt K. Relation of stressors and depressive symptoms to clinical progression of viral illness. *Am J Psychiatry.* 1996;153(5):626–635.

138. Herbert TB, Cohen S. Depression and immunity: a meta-analytic review. *Psychol Bull.* 1993;113(3):472–486.

139. Castilla-Cortazar I, Castilla A, Gurpegui M. Opioid peptides and immunodysfunction in patients with major depression and anxiety disorders. *J Physiol Biochem.* 1998;54(4):203–215.

140. Blume J, Douglas SD, Evans DL. Immune suppression and immune activation in depression. *Brain Behav Immun.* 2011;25(2):221–229.

141. Vaknin I, Blinder L, Wang L, et al. A common pathway mediated through Toll-like receptors leads to T- and natural killer-cell immunosuppression. *Blood.* 2008;111(3):1437–1447.

142. Moraska A, Campisi J, Nguyen KT, Maier SF, Watkins LR, Fleshner M. Elevated IL-1beta contributes to antibody suppression produced by stress. *J Apple Physiol.* 2002;93(1):207–215.

143. Cope AP, Liblau RS, Yang XD, et al. Chronic tumor necrosis factor alters T cell responses by attenuating T cell receptor signaling. *J Exp Med.* 1997;185(9):1573–1584.

144. Cope AP. Exploring the reciprocal relationship between immunity and inflammation in chronic inflammatory arthritis. *Rheumatology (Oxf).* 2003;42(6):716–731.

145. Eleftheriadis T, Kartsios C, Yiannaki E, et al. Decreased CD3+CD16+ natural killer-like T-cell percentage and zeta-chain expression accompany chronic inflammation in haemodialysis patients. *Nephrology (Carlton).* 2009;14(5):471–475.

146. Muller AJ, Sharma MD, Chandler PR, et al. Chronic inflammation that facilitates tumor progression creates local immune suppression by inducing indoleamine 2,3 dioxygenase. *Proc Natl Acad Sci U S A.* 2008;105(44):17073–17078.

147. Clark J, Vagenas P, Panesar M, Cope AP. What does tumour necrosis factor excess do to the immune system long term? *Ann Rheum Dis.* 2005;64(suppl 4):iv70–iv76.

148. Doran MF, Crowson CS, Pond GR, O'Fallon WM, Gabriel SE. Frequency of infection in patients with rheumatoid arthritis compared with controls: a population-based study. *Arthritis Rheum.* 2002;46(9):2287–2293.

149. Armelagos GJ, Brown PJ, Turner B. Evolutionary, historical and political economic perspectives on health and disease. *Soc Sci Med.* 2005;61(4):755–765.

150. Reichenberg A, Yirmiya R, Schuld A, et al. Cytokine-associated emotional and cognitive disturbances in humans. *Arch Gen Psychiatry.* 2001;58(5):445–452.

151. Simon GE, Ludman EJ, Linde JA, et al. Association between obesity and depression in middle-aged women. *Gen Hosp Psychiatry.* 2008;30(1):32–39.

152. Simon GE, Von Korff M, Saunders K, et al. Association between obesity and psychiatric disorders in the US adult population. *Arch Gen Psychiatry.* 2006;63(7):824–830.

153. Miller GE, Freedland KE, Carney RM, Stetler CA, Banks WA. Pathways linking depression, adiposity, and inflammatory markers in healthy young adults. *Brain Behav Immun.* 2003;17(4):276–285.

154. Lampert R, Bremner JD, Su S, et al. Decreased heart rate variability is associated with higher levels of inflammation in middle-aged men. *Am Heart J.* 2008;156(4):759.

155. Ranjit N, Diez-Roux AV, Shea S, et al. Psychosocial factors and inflammation in the multi-ethnic study of atherosclerosis. *Arch Int Med.* 2007;167(2):174–181.

156. Kloiber S, Ising M, Reppermund S, et al. Overweight and obesity affect treatment response in major depression. *Biol Psychiatry.* 2007;62(4):321–326.

157. Himmerich H, Fulda S, Linseisen J, et al. TNF-alpha, soluble TNF receptor and interleukin-6 plasma levels in the general population. *Eur Cytokine Netw.* 2006;17(3):196–201.

158. Suarez EC. C-reactive protein is associated with psychological risk factors of cardiovascular disease in apparently healthy adults. *Psychosom Med.* 2004;66(5):684–691.

159. Douglas KM, Taylor AJ, O'Malley PG. Relationship between depression and C-reactive protein in a screening population. *Psychosom Med.* 2004;66(5):679–683.

160. Roberts RE, Deleger S, Strawbridge WJ, Kaplan GA. Prospective association between obesity and depression: evidence from the Alameda County Study. *Int J Obes Relat Metab Disord.* 2003;27(4):514–521.

161. Pine DS, Goldstein RB, Wolk S, Weissman MM. The association between childhood depression and adulthood body mass index. *Pediatrics.* 2001;107(5):1049–1056.

162. Kern PA, Ranganathan S, Li C, Wood L, Ranganathan G. Adipose tissue tumor necrosis factor and interleukin-6 expression in human obesity and insulin resistance. *Am J Physiology Endocrinol Metabol.* 2001;280(5):E745–E751.

163. Katz JR, Taylor NF, Goodrick S, Perry L, Yudkin JS, Coppack SW. Central obesity, depression and the hypothalamo-pituitary-adrenal axis in men and postmenopausal women. *Int J Obes Relat Metab Disord.* 2000;24(2):246–251.

164. Haack M, Hinze-Selch D, Fenzel T, et al. Plasma levels of cytokines and soluble cytokine receptors in psychiatric patients upon hospital admission: effects of confounding factors and diagnosis. *J Psychiatr Res.* 1999;33(5):407–418.

165. Vieira VJ, Valentine RJ, McAuley E, Evans E, Woods JA. Independent relationship between heart rate recovery and C-reactive protein in older adults. *J Am Geriatr Soc.* 2007;55(5):747–751.

166. Moyna NM, Bodnar JD, Goldberg HR, Shurin MS, Robertson RJ, Rabin BS. Relation between aerobic fitness level and stress induced alterations in neuroendocrine and immune function. *Int J Sports Med.* 1999;20(2):136–141.

167. Kohut ML, McCann DA, Russell DW, et al. Aerobic exercise, but not flexibility/resistance exercise, reduces serum IL-18, CRP, and IL-6 independent of beta-blockers, BMI, and psychosocial factors in older adults. *Brain Behav Immun.* 2006;20(3):201–209.

168. Balducci S, Zanuso S, Nicolucci A, et al. Anti-inflammatory effect of exercise training in subjects with type 2 diabetes and the metabolic syndrome is dependent on exercise modalities and independent of weight loss. *Nutr Metab Cardiovasc Dis.* 2010;20(8):608–617.

169. Ghosh S, Khazaei M, Moien-Afshari F, et al. Moderate exercise attenuates caspase-3 activity, oxidative stress, and inhibits progression of diabetic renal disease in db/db mice. *Am J Physiol Renal Physiol.* 2009;296(4):F700–F708.

170. Anton SD, Newton RL Jr, Sothern M, Martin CK, Stewart TM, Williamson DA. Association of depression with body mass index, sedentary behavior, and maladaptive eating attitudes and behaviors in 11 to 13-year old children. *Eat Weight Disord.* 2006;11(3):e102–e108.

171. Colditz GA. Economic costs of obesity and inactivity. *Med Sci Sports Exerc.* 1999;31(11 suppl):S663–S667.

172. Rajala U, Uusimaki A, Keinanen-Kiukaanniemi S, Kivela SL. Prevalence of depression in a 55-year-old Finnish population. *Soc Psychiatry Psychiatr Epidemiol.* 1994;29(3): 126–130.

173. Tanskanen A, Hibbeln JR, Tuomilehto J, et al. Fish consumption and depressive symptoms in the general population in Finland. *Psychiatr Serv.* 2001;52(4):529–531.

174. Maes M, Christophe A, Delanghe J, Altamura C, Neels H, Meltzer HY. Lowered omega3 polyunsaturated fatty acids in serum phospholipids and cholesteryl esters of depressed patients. *Psychiatry Res.* 1999;85(3):275–291.

175. Maes M, Smith R, Christophe A, Cosyns P, Desnyder R, Meltzer H. Fatty acid composition in major depression: decreased omega 3 fractions in cholesteryl esters and increased C20: 4 omega 6/C20:5 omega 3 ratio in cholesteryl esters and phospholipids. *J Affect Disord.* 1996;38(1):35–46.

176. Williams LL, Kiecolt-Glaser JK, Horrocks LA, Hillhouse JT, Glaser R. Quantitative association between altered plasma esterified omega-6 fatty acid proportions and psychological stress. *Prostaglandins Leukotr Essent Fatty Acids.* 1992;47(2):165–170.

177. Dai J, Miller AH, Bremner JD, et al. Adherence to the Mediterranean diet is inversely associated with circulating interleukin-6 among middle-aged men: a twin study. *Circulation.* 2008;117(2):169–175.

178. Zampelas A, Panagiotakos DB, Pitsavos C, et al. Fish consumption among healthy adults is associated with decreased levels of inflammatory markers related to cardiovascular disease: the ATTICA study. *J Am Coll Cardiol.* 2005;46(1):120–124.

179. Chrysohoou C, Panagiotakos DB, Pitsavos C, Das UN, Stefanadis C. Adherence to the Mediterranean diet attenuates inflammation and coagulation process in healthy adults: the ATTICA Study. *J Am Coll Cardiol.* 2004;44(1):152–158.

180. Westover AN, Marangell LB. A cross-national relationship between sugar consumption and major depression? *Depress Anxiety.* 2002;16(3):118–120.

181. O'Keefe JH, Gheewala NM, O'Keefe JO. Dietary strategies for improving post-prandial glucose, lipids, inflammation, and cardiovascular health. *J Am Coll Cardiol.* 2008;51(3): 249–255.

182. Schulze MB, Hoffmann K, Manson JE, et al. Dietary pattern, inflammation, and incidence of type 2 diabetes in women. *Am J Clin Nutr.* 2005;82(3):675–684.

183. Lee O, Bruce WR, Dong Q, Bruce J, Mehta R, O'Brien PJ. Fructose and carbonyl metabolites as endogenous toxins. *Chem Biol Interact.* 2009;178(1–3):332–339.

184. O'Connor MF, Bower JE, Cho HJ, et al. To assess, to control, to exclude: effects of biobehavioral factors on circulating inflammatory markers. *Brain Behav Immun.* 2009;23(7): 887–897.

185. Ford DE, Kamerow DB. Epidemiologic study of sleep disturbances and psychiatric disorders: an opportunity for prevention? *JAMA.* 1989;262(11):1479–1484.

186. Livingston G, Blizard B, Mann A. Does sleep disturbance predict depression in elderly people? A study in inner London. *Br J Gen Pract.* 1993;43(376):445–448.

187. Breslau N, Roth T, Rosenthal L, Andreski P. Sleep disturbance and psychiatric disorders: a longitudinal epidemiological study of young adults. *Biol Psychiat.* 1996;39(6): 411–418.

188. Gillin JC. Are sleep disturbances risk factors for anxiety, depressive and addictive disorders? *Acta Psychiatr Scand Suppl.* 1998;393:39–43.

189. Irwin MR, Wang M, Ribeiro D, et al. Sleep loss activates cellular inflammatory signaling. *Biol Psychiatry.* 2008;64(6):538–540.

190. McDade TW, Hawkley LC, Cacioppo JT. Psychosocial and behavioral predictors of

inflammation in middle-aged and older adults: the Chicago Health, Aging, and Social Relations Study. *Psychosom Med.* 2006;68(3):376–381.

191. Irwin MR, Wang M, Campomayor CO, Collado-Hidalgo A, Cole S. Sleep deprivation and activation of morning levels of cellular and genomic markers of inflammation. *Arch Int Med.* 2006;166(16):1756–1762.

192. Meier-Ewert HK, Ridker PM, Rifai N, et al. Effect of sleep loss on C-reactive protein, an inflammatory marker of cardiovascular risk. *J Am Coll Cardiol.* 2004;43(4):678–683.

193. Friedman EM, Hayney MS, Love GD, et al. Social relationships, sleep quality, and interleukin-6 in aging women. *Proc Natl Acad Sci U S A.* 2005;102(51):18757–18762.

194. Irwin M, Rinetti G, Redwine L, Motivala S, Dang J, Ehlers C. Nocturnal proinflammatory cytokine-associated sleep disturbances in abstinent African American alcoholics. *Brain Behav Immun.* 2004;18(4):349–360.

195. Vgontzas AN, Zoumakis M, Papanicolaou DA, et al. Chronic insomnia is associated with a shift of interleukin-6 and tumor necrosis factor secretion from nighttime to daytime. *Metabolism.* 2002;51(7):887–892.

196. Redwine L, Hauger RL, Gillin JC, Irwin M. Effects of sleep and sleep deprivation on interleukin-6, growth hormone, cortisol, and melatonin levels in humans. *J Clin Endocrinol Metabol.* 2000;85(10):3597–3603.

197. Saules KK, Pomerleau CS, Snedecor SM, et al. Relationship of onset of cigarette smoking during college to alcohol use, dieting concerns, and depressed mood: results from the Young Women's Health Survey. *Addict Behav.* 2004;29(5):893–899.

198. Lenz BK. Tobacco, depression, and lifestyle choices in the pivotal early college years. *J Am Coll Health.* 2004;52(5):213–219.

199. Moussavi S, Chatterji S, Verdes E, Tandon A, Patel V, Ustun B. Depression, chronic diseases, and decrements in health: results from the World Health Surveys. *Lancet.* 2007;370(9590):851–858.

200. Handwerker WP. Cultural diversity, stress, and depression: working women in the Americas. *J Womens Health Gend Based Med.* 1999;8(10):1303–1311.

201. Brown GW, Harris TO, Hepworth C. Life events and endogenous depression: a puzzle reexamined. *Arch Gen Psychiat.* 1994;51(7):525–534.

202. Kendler KS, Thornton LM, Gardner CO. Stressful life events and previous episodes in the etiology of major depression in women: an evaluation of the "kindling" hypothesis. *Am J Psychiatry.* 2000;157(8):1243–1251.

203. DiPietro LA. Wound healing: the role of the macrophage and other immune cells. *Shock.* 1995;4(4):233–240.

204. Ross SR, Bloomsmith MA, Bettinger TL, Wagner KE. The influence of captive adolescent male chimpanzees on wounding: management and welfare implications. *Zoo Biol.* 2009;28(6):623–634.

205. Eshed V, Gopher A, Pinhasi R, Hershkovitz I. Paleopathology and the origin of agriculture in the Levant. *Am J Phys Anthropol.* 2010;143(1):121–133.

206. Dhabhar FS. Enhancing versus suppressive effects of stress on immune function: implications for immunoprotection and immunopathology. *Neuroimmunomodulation.* 2009;16(5):300–317.

207. Herbert TB, Cohen S. Stress and immunity in humans: a meta-analytic review. *Psychosom Med.* 1993;55(4):364–379.

208. Bailey MT, Kinsey SG, Padgett DA, Sheridan JF, Leblebicioglu B. Social stress enhances IL-1beta and TNF-alpha production by *Porphyromonas gingivalis* lipopolysaccharide-stimulated CD11b+ cells. *Physiol Behav.* 2009;98(3):351–358.

209. Pace TW, Mletzko TC, Alagbe O, et al. Increased stress-induced inflammatory responses in male patients with major depression and increased early life stress. *Am J Psychiatry.* 2006;163(9):1630–1633.

210. Powell ND, Mays JW, Bailey MT, Hanke ML, Sheridan JF. Immunogenic dendritic cells primed by social defeat enhance adaptive immunity to influenza A virus. *Brain Behav Immun.* 2011;25(1):46–52.

211. Mays JW, Bailey MT, Hunzeker JT, et al. Influenza virus-specific immunological memory is enhanced by repeated social defeat. *J Immunol.* 2010;184(4):2014–2025.

212. Steptoe A, Hamer M, Chida Y. The effect of acute psychological stress on circulating inflammatory factors in humans: a review and meta-analysis. *Brain Behav Immun.* 2007;7:901–912.

213. Bierhaus A, Wolf J, Andrassy M, et al. A mechanism converting psychosocial stress into mononuclear cell activation. *Proc Natl Acad Sci U S A.* 2003;100(4):1920–1925.

214. Avitsur R, Kavelaars A, Heijnen C, Sheridan JF. Social stress and the regulation of tumor necrosis factor-alpha secretion. *Brain Behav Immun.* 2005;19(4):311–317.

215. Quan N, Avitsur R, Stark JL, et al. Social stress increases the susceptibility to endotoxic shock. *J Neuroimmunol.* 2001;115(1–2):36–45.

216. Rosenberger PH, Ickovics JR, Epel E, et al. Surgical stress-induced immune cell redistribution profiles predict short-term and long-term postsurgical recovery: a prospective study. *J Bone Joint Surg Am.* 2009;91(12):2783–2794.

217. Joachim RA, Handjiski B, Blois SM, Hagen E, Paus R, Arck PC. Stress-induced neurogenic inflammation in murine skin skews dendritic cells towards maturation and migration: key role of intercellular adhesion molecule-1/leukocyte function-associated antigen interactions. *Am J Pathol.* 2008;173(5):1379–1388.

218. Viswanathan K, Daugherty C, Dhabhar FS. Stress as an endogenous adjuvant: augmentation of the immunization phase of cell-mediated immunity. *Int Immunol.* 2005;17(8):1059–1069.

219. Cross-Disorder Group of the Psychiatric Genomics Consortium. Identification of risk loci with shared effects on five major psychiatric disorders: a genome-wide analysis. *Lancet.* 2013;381(9875):1371–1379.

220. Wong ML, Dong C, Maestre-Mesa J, Licinio J. Polymorphisms in inflammation-related genes are associated with susceptibility to major depression and antidepressant response. *Mol Psychiatry.* 2008;13(8):800–812.

221. Cerri AP, Arosio B, Viazzoli C, Confalonieri R, Vergani C, Annoni G. The -308 (G/A) single nucleotide polymorphism in the TNF-alpha gene and the risk of major depression in the elderly. *Int J Geriatr Psychiatry.* 2010;25(3):219–223.

222. Clerici M, Arosio B, Mundo E, et al. Cytokine polymorphisms in the pathophysiology of mood disorders. *CNS Spectr.* 2009;14(8):419–425.

223. Jun TY, Pae CU, Hoon H, et al. Possible association between -G308A tumour necrosis factor-alpha gene polymorphism and major depressive disorder in the Korean population. *Psychiatr Genet.* 2003;13(3):179–181.

224. Pae CU, Lee KU, Han H, Serretti A, Jun TY. Tumor necrosis factor alpha gene-G308A polymorphism associated with bipolar I disorder in the Korean population. *Psychiatry Res.* 2004;125(1):65–68.

225. Bosker FJ, Hartman CA, Nolte IM, et al. Poor replication of candidate genes for major depressive disorder using genome-wide association data. *Mol Psychiatry.* 2011;16(5):516–532.

226. consortium C. Sparse whole-genome sequencing identifies two loci for major depressive disorder. *Nature.* 2015;523(7562):588–591.

227. Wheway J, Herzog H, Mackay F. NPY and receptors in immune and inflammatory diseases. *Curr Top Med Chem.* 2007;7(17):1743–1752.

228. Ferreira R, Xapelli S, Santos T, et al. Neuropeptide Y modulation of interleukin-1β (IL-1β)-induced nitric oxide production in microglia. *J Biol Chem.* 2010;285(53):41921–41934.

229. Wheway J, Herzog H, Mackay F. The Y1 receptor for NPY: a key modulator of the adaptive immune system. *Peptides.* 2007;28(2):453–458.

230. Heilig M, Zachrisson O, Thorsell A, et al. Decreased cerebrospinal fluid neuropeptide Y (NPY) in patients with treatment refractory unipolar major depression: preliminary evidence for association with preproNPY gene polymorphism. *J Psychiatr Res.* 2004;38(2):113–121.

231. Sjoholm LK, Melas PA, Forsell Y, Lavebratt C. PreproNPY Pro7 protects against depression despite exposure to environmental risk factors. *J Affect Disord.* 2009;118(1–3):124–130.

232. Mickey BJ, Zhou Z, Heitzeg MM, et al. Emotion processing, major depression, and functional genetic variation of neuropeptide Y. *Arch Gen Psychiatry.* 2011;68(2):158–166.

233. Morales-Medina JC, Dumont Y, Quirion R. A possible role of neuropeptide Y in depression and stress. *Brain Res.* 2010;1314:194–205.

234. Kallio J, Pesonen U, Kaipio K, et al. Altered intracellular processing and release of neuropeptide Y due to leucine 7 to proline 7 polymorphism in the signal peptide of preproneuropeptide Y in humans. *FASEB J.* 2001;15(7):1242–1244.

235. Wilson AG, di Giovine FS, Blakemore AI, Duff GW. Single base polymorphism in the human tumour necrosis factor alpha (TNF alpha) gene detectable by NcoI restriction of PCR product. *Hum Mol Genet.* 1992;1(5):353.

236. Lotrich FE, Ferrell RE, Rabinovitz M, Pollock BG. Labile anger during interferon alfa treatment is associated with a polymorphism in tumor necrosis factor alpha. *Clin Neuropharmacol.* 2010;33(4):191–197.

237. Correa PA, Gomez LM, Cadena J, Anaya JM. Autoimmunity and tuberculosis: opposite association with TNF polymorphism. *J Rheumatol.* 2005;32(2):219–224.

238. Kerr JR, McCoy M, Burke B, Mattey DL, Pravica V, Hutchinson IV. Cytokine gene polymorphisms associated with symptomatic parvovirus B19 infection. *J Clin Pathol.* 2003;56(10):725–727.

239. Chen DQ, Zeng Y, Zhou J, et al. Association of candidate susceptible loci with chronic infection with hepatitis B virus in a Chinese population. *J Med Virol.* 2010;82(3):371–378.

240. Surbatovic M, Grujic K, Cikota B, et al. Polymorphisms of genes encoding tumor necrosis factor-alpha, interleukin-10, cluster of differentiation-14 and interleukin-1ra in critically ill patients. *J Crit Care.* 2010;25(3):542 e541–e548.

241. Larcombe LA, Orr PH, Lodge AM, et al. Functional gene polymorphisms in canadian aboriginal populations with high rates of tuberculosis. *J Infect Dis.* 2008;198(8):1175–1179.

242. Masuda M, Senju S, Fujii Si S, et al. Identification and immunocytochemical analysis of DCNP1, a dendritic cell-associated nuclear protein. *Biochem Biophys Res Commun.* 2002;290(3):1022–1029.

243. Zhou T, Wang S, Ren H, et al. Dendritic cell nuclear protein-1, a novel depression-related protein, upregulates corticotropin-releasing hormone expression. *Brain.* 2010;133(10):3069–3079.

244. Kim Y, Park CS, Shin HD, et al. A promoter nucleotide variant of the dendritic cell-specific DCNP1 associates with serum IgE levels specific for dust mite allergens among the Korean asthmatics. *Genes Immun.* 2007;8(5):369–378.

245. Michan S, Sinclair D. Sirtuins in mammals: insights into their biological function. *Biochem J.* 2007;404(1):1–13.

246. Zhang Z, Lowry SF, Guarente L, Haimovich B. Roles of SIRT1 in the acute and restorative phases following induction of inflammation. *J Biol Chem.* 2010;285(53):41391–41401.

247. Vachharajani VT, Liu T, Wang X, Hoth JJ, Yoza BK, McCall CE. Sirtuins link inflammation and metabolism. *J Immunol Res.* 2016;2016:8167273.

248. Fernandez-Marcos PJ, Auwerx J. Regulation of PGC-1alpha, a nodal regulator of mitochondrial biogenesis. *Am J Clin Nutr.* 2011;93(4):884S–890S.

249. Liu TF, Brown CM, El Gazzar M, et al. Fueling the flame: bioenergy couples metabolism and inflammation. *J Leukoc Biol.* 2012;92(3):499–507.

250. Park SY, Lee SW, Kim HY, et al. SIRT1 inhibits differentiation of monocytes to macrophages: amelioration of synovial inflammation in rheumatoid arthritis. *J Mol Med (Berl).* 2016; 94(8):921–931.

251. Akimova T, Xiao H, Liu Y, et al. Targeting sirtuin-1 alleviates experimental autoimmune colitis by induction of Foxp3+ T-regulatory cells. *Mucosal Immunol.* 2014;7(5):1209–1220.

252. Ren JH, Tao Y, Zhang ZZ, et al. Sirtuin 1 regulates hepatitis B virus transcription and replication by targeting transcription factor AP-1. *J Virol.* 2014;88(5):2442–2451.

253. Lo Sasso G, Ryu D, Mouchiroud L, et al. Loss of Sirt1 function improves intestinal anti-bacterial defense and protects from colitis-induced colorectal cancer. *PLoS ONE.* 2014;9(7):e102495.

254. Annamanedi M, Kalle AM. Celecoxib sensitizes *Staphylococcus aureus* to antibiotics in macrophages by modulating SIRT1. *PLoS ONE.* 2014;9(6):e99285.

255. Zhang R, Chen HZ, Liu JJ, et al. SIRT1 suppresses activator protein-1 transcriptional activity and cyclooxygenase-2 expression in macrophages. *J Biol Chem.* 2010;285(10):7097–7110.

256. Owczarczyk AB, Schaller MA, Reed M, Rasky AJ, Lombard DB, Lukacs NW. Sirtuin 1 regulates dendritic cell activation and autophagy during respiratory syncytial virus-induced immune responses. *J Immunol.* 2015;195(4):1637–1646.

257. Tang HM, Gao WW, Chan CP, et al. SIRT1 suppresses human T-cell leukemia virus type 1 transcription. *J Virol.* 2015;89(16):8623–8631.

258. Lopez-Leon S, Janssens AC, Hofman A, et al. No association between the angiotensin-converting enzyme gene and major depression: a case-control study and meta-analysis. *Psychiatr Genet.* 2006;16(6):225–226.

259. Virchow S, Ansorge N, Rosskopf D, Rubben H, Siffert W. The G protein beta3 subunit splice variant Gbeta3-s causes enhanced chemotaxis of human neutrophils in response to interleukin-8. *Naunyn Schmiedebergs Arch Pharmacol.* 1999;360(1):27–32.

260. Lindemann M, Virchow S, Ramann F, et al. The G protein beta3 subunit 825T allele is a genetic marker for enhanced T cell response. *FEBS Lett.* 2001;495(1–2):82–86.

261. Romundstad S, Melien O, Holmen J. The G protein beta3 subunit C825T polymorphism is associated with microalbuminuria in hypertensive women and cardiovascular disease in hypertensive men. *Am J Hypertens.* 2010;23(10):1114–1120.

262. Holmen OL, Romundstad S, Melien O. Association between the G protein beta3 subunit C825T polymorphism and the occurrence of cardiovascular disease in hyperten-

sives: the Nord-Trondelag Health Study (HUNT). *Am J Hypertens.* 2010;23(10):1121–1127.

263. Hauge Opdal S, Melien O, Rootwelt H, Vege A, Arnestad M, Ole Rognum T. The G protein beta3 subunit 825C allele is associated with sudden infant death due to infection. *Acta Paediatr.* 2006;95(9):1129–1132.

264. Bagos PG, Elefsinioti AL, Nikolopoulos GK, Hamodrakas SJ. The GNB3 C825T polymorphism and essential hypertension: a meta-analysis of 34 studies including 14,094 cases and 17,760 controls. *J Hypertens.* 2007;25(3):487–500.

265. Ahlenstiel G, Nischalke HD, Bueren K, et al. The GNB3 C825T polymorphism affects response to HCV therapy with pegylated interferon in HCV/HIV co-infected but not in HCV mono-infected patients. *J Hepatol.* 2007;47(3):348–355.

266. Sarrazin C, Berg T, Weich V, et al. GNB3 C825T polymorphism and response to interferon-alfa/ribavirin treatment in patients with hepatitis C virus genotype 1 (HCV-1) infection. *J Hepatol.* 2005;43(3):388–393.

267. Brockmeyer NH, Potthoff A, Kasper A, Nabring C, Jockel KH, Siffert W. GNB3 C825T polymorphism and response to anti-retroviral combination therapy in HIV-1-infected patients—a pilot study. *Eur J Med Res.* 2005;10(11):489–494.

268. Lindemann M, Barsegian V, Siffert W, Ferencik S, Roggendorf M, Grosse-Wilde H. Role of G protein beta3 subunit C825T and HLA class II polymorphisms in the immune response after HBV vaccination. *Virology.* 2002;297(2):245–252.

269. Fodil-Cornu N, Kozij N, Wu Q, Rozen R, Vidal SM. Methylenetetrahydrofolate reductase (MTHFR) deficiency enhances resistance against cytomegalovirus infection. *Genes Immun.* 2009;10(7):662–666.

270. Imamura A, Murakami R, Takahashi R, et al. Low folate levels may be an atherogenic factor regardless of homocysteine levels in young healthy nonsmokers. *Metabolism.* 2010;59(5):728–733.

271. Fujimaki C, Hayashi H, Tsuboi S, et al. Plasma total homocysteine level and methylenetetrahydrofolate reductase 677C>T genetic polymorphism in Japanese patients with rheumatoid arthritis. *Biomarkers.* 2009;14(1):49–54.

272. Dedoussis GV, Panagiotakos DB, Pitsavos C, et al. An association between the methylenetetrahydrofolate reductase (MTHFR) C677T mutation and inflammation markers related to cardiovascular disease. *Int J Cardiol.* 2005;100(3):409–414.

273. Chen AR, Zhang HG, Wang ZP, et al. C-reactive protein, vitamin B12 and C677T polymorphism of N-5,10-methylenetetrahydrofolate reductase gene are related to insulin resistance and risk factors for metabolic syndrome in Chinese population. *Clin Invest Med.* 2010;33(5):E290–E297.

274. Hammons AL, Summers CM, Woodside JV, et al. Folate/homocysteine phenotypes and MTHFR 677C>T genotypes are associated with serum levels of monocyte chemoattractant protein-1. *Clin Immunol.* 2009;133(1):132–137.

275. Lu ZY, Morales M, Khartulyari S, et al. Genetic and biochemical determinants of serum concentrations of monocyte chemoattractant protein-1, a potential neural tube defect risk factor. *Birth Defects Res A Clin Mol Teratol.* 2008;82(10):736–741.

276. Bronowicki JP, Abdelmouttaleb I, Peyrin-Biroulet L, et al. Methylenetetrahydrofolate reductase 677 T allele protects against persistent HBV infection in West Africa. *J Hepatol.* 2008;48(4):532–539.

277. Simhan HN, Himes KP, Venkataramanan R, Bodnar LM. Maternal serum folate species in early pregnancy and lower genital tract inflammatory milieu. *Am J Obstet Gynecol.* 2011;205(1):61.e1–61.e7.

278. Chillemi R, Zappacosta B, Simpore J, Persichilli S, Musumeci M, Musumeci S. Hyperhomocysteinemia in acute *Plasmodium falciparum* malaria: an effect of host-parasite interaction. *Clin Chim Acta.* 2004;348(1–2):113–120.

279. Maeda M, Yamamoto I, Fukuda M, et al. MTHFR gene polymorphism is susceptible to diabetic retinopathy but not to diabetic nephropathy in Japanese type 2 diabetic patients. *J Diabetes Complic.* 2008;22(2):119–125.

280. Khandanpour N, Willis G, Meyer FJ, et al. Peripheral arterial disease and methylenetetrahydrofolate reductase (MTHFR) C677T mutations: a case-control study and meta-analysis. *J Vasc Surg.* 2009;49(3):711–718.

281. Ferrara F, Novo S, Grimaudo S, et al. Methylenetetrahydrofolate reductase mutation in subjects with abdominal aortic aneurysm subdivided for age. *Clin Hemorheol Microcirc.* 2006;34(3):421–426.

282. Pollex RL, Mamakeesick M, Zinman B, Harris SB, Hanley AJ, Hegele RA. Methylenetetrahydrofolate reductase polymorphism 677C>T is associated with peripheral arterial disease in type 2 diabetes. *Cardiovasc Diabetol.* 2005;4:17.

283. Chen J, Ma J, Stampfer MJ, Palomeque C, Selhub J, Hunter DJ. Linkage disequilibrium between the 677C>T and 1298A>C polymorphisms in human methylenetetrahydrofolate reductase gene and their contributions to risk of colorectal cancer. *Pharmacogenetics.* 2002;12(4):339–342.

284. Movva S, Alluri RV, Venkatasubramanian S, et al. Association of methylene tetrahydrofolate reductase C677T genotype with type 2 diabetes mellitus patients with and without renal complications. *Genet Test Mol Biomarkers.* 2011;15(4):257–261.

285. Reyes-Engel A, Munoz E, Gaitan MJ, et al. Implications on human fertility of the 677C→T and 1298A→C polymorphisms of the MTHFR gene: consequences of a possible genetic selection. *Mol Hum Reprod.* 2002;8(10):952–957.

286. Gerdes LU. The common polymorphism of apolipoprotein E: geographical aspects and new pathophysiological relations. *Clin Chem Lab Med.* 2003;41(5):628–631.

287. Urosevic N, Martins RN. Infection and Alzheimer's disease: the APOE epsilon4 connection and lipid metabolism. *J Alzheimers Dis.* 2008;13(4):421–435.

288. Mahley RW, Rall SC, Jr. Apolipoprotein E: far more than a lipid transport protein. *Annu Rev Genomics Hum Genet.* 2000;1:507–537.

289. Jofre-Monseny L, Minihane AM, Rimbach G. Impact of apoE genotype on oxidative stress, inflammation and disease risk. *Mol Nutr Food Res.* 2008;52(1):131–145.

290. Wozniak MA, Maude RJ, Innes JA, Hawkey PM, Itzhaki RF. Apolipoprotein E-epsilon2 confers risk of pulmonary tuberculosis in women from the Indian subcontinent—a preliminary study. *J Infect.* 2009;59(3):219–222.

291. Roy A, Karoum F, Pollack S. Marked reduction in indexes of dopamine metabolism among patients with depression who attempt suicide. *Arch Gen Psychiatry.* 1992;49(6):447–450.

292. Meyer JH, Kruger S, Wilson AA, et al. Lower dopamine transporter binding potential in striatum during depression. *Neuroreport.* 2001;12(18):4121–4125.

293. Lambert G, Johansson M, Agren H, Friberg P. Reduced brain norepinephrine and dopamine release in treatment-refractory depressive illness: evidence in support of the catecholamine hypothesis of mood disorders. *Arch Gen Psychiatry.* 2000;57(8):787–793.

294. Klimek V, Schenck JE, Han H, Stockmeier CA, Ordway GA. Dopaminergic abnormalities in amygdaloid nuclei in major depression: a postmortem study. *Biol Psychiatry.* 2002;52(7):740–748.

295. Kavelaars A, Cobelens PM, Teunis MA, Heijnen CJ. Changes in innate and acquired immune responses in mice with targeted deletion of the dopamine transporter gene. *J Neuroimmunol.* 2005;161(1–2):162–168.

296. Alaniz RC, Thomas SA, Perez-Melgosa M, et al. Dopamine beta-hydroxylase deficiency impairs cellular immunity. *Proc Natl Acad Sci U S A.* 1999;96(5):2274–2278.

297. Cobat A, Gallant CJ, Simkin L, et al. Two loci control tuberculin skin test reactivity in an area hyperendemic for tuberculosis. *J Exp Med.* 2009;206(12):2583–2591.

298. Stein CM, Zalwango S, Malone LL, et al. Genome scan of *M. tuberculosis* infection and disease in Ugandans. *PLoS One.* 2008;3(12):e4094.

299. Mill J, Asherson P, Browes C, D'Souza U, Craig I. Expression of the dopamine transporter gene is regulated by the 3′ UTR VNTR: evidence from brain and lymphocytes using quantitative RT-PCR. *Am J Med Genet.* 2002;114(8):975–979.

300. van de Giessen E, de Win MM, Tanck MW, van den Brink W, Baas F, Booij J. Striatal dopamine transporter availability associated with polymorphisms in the dopamine transporter gene SLC6A3. *J Nucl Med.* 2009;50(1):45–52.

301. Opdal SH, Vege A, Rognum TO. Serotonin transporter gene variation in sudden infant death syndrome. *Acta Paediatr.* 2008;97(7):861–865.

302. Narita N, Narita M, Takashima S, Nakayama M, Nagai T, Okado N. Serotonin transporter gene variation is a risk factor for sudden infant death syndrome in the Japanese population. *Pediatrics.* 2001;107(4):690–692.

303. Weese-Mayer DE, Berry-Kravis EM, Maher BS, Silvestri JM, Curran ME, Marazita ML. Sudden infant death syndrome: association with a promoter polymorphism of the serotonin transporter gene. *Am J Med Genet A.* 2003;117A(3):268–274.

304. Prandota J. Possible pathomechanisms of sudden infant death syndrome: key role of chronic hypoxia, infection/inflammation states, cytokine irregularities, and metabolic trauma in genetically predisposed infants. *Am J Ther.* 2004;11(6):517–546.

305. Fredericks CA, Drabant EM, Edge MD, et al. Healthy young women with serotonin transporter SS polymorphism show a pro-inflammatory bias under resting and stress conditions. *Brain Behav Immun.* 2010;24(3):350–357.

306. Su S, Zhao J, Bremner JD, et al. Serotonin transporter gene, depressive symptoms, and interleukin-6. *Circ Cardiovasc Genet.* 2009;2(6):614–620.

307. Murray DR, Schaller M. Historical prevalence of infectious diseases within 230 geopolitical regions: a tool for investigating origins of culture. *J Cross Cult Psychol.* 2010; 41(1):99–108.

308. Wray NR, Pergadia ML, Blackwood DH, et al. Genome-wide association study of major depressive disorder: new results, meta-analysis, and lessons learned. *Mol Psychiatry.* 2012;17(1):36–48.

309. Cattaneo M, Otsu M, Fagioli C, et al. SEL1L and HRD1 are involved in the degradation of unassembled secretory Ig-mu chains. *J Cell Physiol.* 2008;215(3):794–802.

310. Schelhaas M, Malmstrom J, Pelkmans L, et al. Simian virus 40 depends on ER protein folding and quality control factors for entry into host cells. *Cell.* 2007;131(3):516–529.

311. Oresic K, Ng CL, Tortorella D. TRAM1 participates in human cytomegalovirus US2- and US11-mediated dislocation of an endoplasmic reticulum membrane glycoprotein. *J Biol Chem.* 2009;284(9):5905–5914.

312. Ban Y, Taniyama M, Tozaki T, Yanagawa T, Tomita M. SEL1L microsatellite polymorphism in Japanese patients with autoimmune thyroid diseases. *Thyroid.* 2001;11(4): 335–338.

313. Song J, Duncan MJ, Li G, et al. A novel TLR4-mediated signaling pathway leading to IL-6 responses in human bladder epithelial cells. *PLoS Pathog.* 2007;3(4):e60.

314. Abera AB, Sales KJ, Catalano RD, Katz AA, Jabbour HN. EP2 receptor mediated cAMP release is augmented by PGF 2 alpha activation of the FP receptor via the calcium-calmodulin pathway. *Cell Signal.* 2010;22(1):71–79.

315. Klempan TA, Rujescu D, Merette C, et al. Profiling brain expression of the spermidine/spermine N1-acetyltransferase 1 (SAT1) gene in suicide. *Am J Med Genet B Neuropsychiatr Genet.* 2009;150B(7):934–943.

316. Tabeta K, Hoebe K, Janssen EM, et al. The Unc93b1 mutation 3d disrupts exogenous antigen presentation and signaling via Toll-like receptors 3, 7 and 9. *Nat Immunol.* 2006;7(2):156–164.

317. Koehn J, Huesken D, Jaritz M, et al. Assessing the function of human UNC-93B in Toll-like receptor signaling and major histocompatibility complex II response. *Hum Immunol.* 2007;68(11):871–878.

318. Pifer R, Benson A, Sturge CR, Yarovinsky F. UNC93B1 is essential for TLR11 activation and IL-12-dependent host resistance to *Toxoplasma gondii. J Biol Chem.* 2011;286(5):3307–3314.

319. Crozat K, Vivier E, Dalod M. Crosstalk between components of the innate immune system: promoting anti-microbial defenses and avoiding immunopathologies. *Immunol Rev.* 2009;227(1):129–149.

320. Lang R, Kofler B. The galanin peptide family in inflammation. *Neuropeptides.* 2011;45(1):1–8.

321. Matkowskyj KA, Danilkovich A, Marrero J, Savkovic SD, Hecht G, Benya RV. Galanin-1 receptor up-regulation mediates the excess colonic fluid production caused by infection with enteric pathogens. *Nat Med.* 2000;6(9):1048–1051.

322. McDonald AC, Schuijers JA, Gundlach AL, Grills BL. Galanin treatment offsets the inhibition of bone formation and downregulates the increase in mouse calvarial expression of TNFalpha and GalR2 mRNA induced by chronic daily injections of an injurious vehicle. *Bone.* 2007;40(4):895–903.

323. Su Y, Ganea D, Peng X, Jonakait GM. Galanin down-regulates microglial tumor necrosis factor-alpha production by a post-transcriptional mechanism. *J Neuroimmunol.* 2003;134(1–2):52–60.

324. Christiansen SH, Olesen MV, Wortwein G, Woldbye DP. Fluoxetine reverts chronic restraint stress-induced depression-like behaviour and increases neuropeptide Y and galanin expression in mice. *Behav Brain Res.* 2011;216(2):585–591.

325. Wardi Le Maitre T, Xia S, Le Maitre E, et al. Galanin receptor 2 overexpressing mice display an antidepressive-like phenotype: possible involvement of the subiculum. *Neuroscience.* 2011;190:270–288.

326. Davidson S, Lear M, Shanley L, et al. Differential activity by polymorphic variants of a remote enhancer that supports galanin expression in the hypothalamus and amygdala: implications for obesity, depression and alcoholism. *Neuropsychopharmacology.* 2011;36(11):2211–2221.

327. Rauch I, Lundstrom L, Hell M, Sperl W, Kofler B. Galanin message-associated peptide suppresses growth and the budded-to-hyphal-form transition of *Candida albicans. Antimicrob Agents Chemother.* 2007;51(11):4167–4170.

328. Ikegami K, Sato S, Nakamura K, Ostrowski LE, Setou M. Tubulin polyglutamylation is essential for airway ciliary function through the regulation of beating asymmetry. *Proc Natl Acad Sci U S A.* 2010;107(23):10490–10495.

329. Chen C, Han YH, Yang Z, Rodrigues AD. Effect of interferon-alpha2b on the expression of various drug-metabolizing enzymes and transporters in co-cultures of freshly prepared human primary hepatocytes. *Xenobiotica.* 2011;41(6):476–485.

330. Crossland H, Constantin-Teodosiu D, Greenhaff PL, Gardiner SM. Low-dose dexamethasone prevents endotoxaemia-induced muscle protein loss and impairment of carbohydrate oxidation in rat skeletal muscle. *J Physiol.* 2010;588(pt 8):1333–1347.

331. Palomer X, Alvarez-Guardia D, Rodriguez-Calvo R, et al. TNF-alpha reduces PGC-1alpha expression through NF-kappaB and p38 MAPK leading to increased glucose oxidation in a human cardiac cell model. *Cardiovasc Res.* 2009;81(4):703–712.

332. Zapata-Gonzalez F, Rueda F, Petriz J, et al. Human dendritic cell activities are modulated by the omega-3 fatty acid, docosahexaenoic acid, mainly through PPAR(gamma): RXR heterodimers: comparison with other polyunsaturated fatty acids. *J Leukoc Biol.* 2008;84(4):1172–1182.

333. Nawa Y, Kawahara K, Tancharoen S, et al. Nucleophosmin may act as an alarmin: implications for severe sepsis. *J Leukoc Biol.* 2009;86(3):645–653.

334. Sarek G, Jarviluoma A, Moore HM, et al. Nucleophosmin phosphorylation by v-cyclin-CDK6 controls KSHV latency. *PLoS Pathog.* 2010;6(3):e1000818.

335. Johnson JS, Samulski RJ. Enhancement of adeno-associated virus infection by mobilizing capsids into and out of the nucleolus. *J Virol.* 2009;83(6):2632–2644.

336. Lee JJ, Seah JB, Chow VT, Poh CL, Tan EL. Comparative proteome analyses of host protein expression in response to enterovirus 71 and coxsackievirus A16 infections. *J Proteomics.* 2011;74(10):2018–2024.

337. Zeng Y, Ye L, Zhu S, et al. The nucleocapsid protein of SARS-associated coronavirus inhibits B23 phosphorylation. *Biochem Biophys Res Commun.* 2008;369(2):287–291.

338. Fankhauser C, Izaurralde E, Adachi Y, Wingfield P, Laemmli UK. Specific complex of human immunodeficiency virus type 1 rev and nucleolar B23 proteins: dissociation by the Rev response element. *Mol Cell Biol.* 1991;11(5):2567–2575.

339. Lymberopoulos MH, Bourget A, Abdeljelil NB, Pearson A. Involvement of the UL24 protein in herpes simplex virus 1-induced dispersal of B23 and in nuclear egress. *Virology.* 2011;412(2):341–348.

340. Garcia MA, Meurs EF, Esteban M. The dsRNA protein kinase PKR: virus and cell control. *Biochimie.* 2007;89(6–7):799–811.

341. Burrows JF, McGrattan MJ, Johnston JA. The DUB/USP17 deubiquitinating enzymes, a multigene family within a tandemly repeated sequence. *Genomics.* 2005;85(4):524–529.

342. Burrows JF, McGrattan MJ, Rascle A, Humbert M, Baek KH, Johnston JA. DUB-3, a cytokine-inducible deubiquitinating enzyme that blocks proliferation. *J Biol Chem.* 2004;279(14):13993–14000.

343. Chen R, Zhang L, Zhong B, Tan B, Liu Y, Shu HB. The ubiquitin-specific protease 17 is involved in virus-triggered type I IFN signaling. *Cell Res.* 2010;20(7):802–811.

344. Detera-Wadleigh SD, Akula N. A systems approach to the biology of mood disorders through network analysis of candidate genes. *Pharmacopsychiatry.* 2011;44(suppl 1):S35–S42.

345. Liu Y, Blackwood DH, Caesar S, et al. Meta-analysis of genome-wide association data of bipolar disorder and major depressive disorder. *Mol Psychiatry.* 2011;16(1):2–4.

346. Green EK, Grozeva D, Jones I, et al. The bipolar disorder risk allele at CACNA1C also confers risk of recurrent major depression and of schizophrenia. *Mol Psychiatry.* 2010; 15(10):1016–1022.

347. Erk S, Meyer-Lindenberg A, Schnell K, et al. Brain function in carriers of a genome-wide supported bipolar disorder variant. *Arch Gen Psychiatry.* 2010;67(8):803–811.

348. Bigos KL, Mattay VS, Callicott JH, et al. Genetic variation in CACNA1C affects brain circuitries related to mental illness. *Arch Gen Psychiatry.* 2010;67(9):939–945.

349. Perrier E, Pompei F, Ruberto G, Vassos E, Collier D, Frangou S. Initial evidence for the role of CACNA1C on subcortical brain morphology in patients with bipolar disorder. *Eur Psychiatry.* 2011;26(3):135–137.

350. Suzuki Y, Inoue T, Ra C. L-type Ca2+ channels: a new player in the regulation of Ca2+ signaling, cell activation and cell survival in immune cells. *Mol Immunol.* 2010;47(4): 640–648.

351. Badou A, Jha MK, Matza D, et al. Critical role for the beta regulatory subunits of Cav channels in T lymphocyte function. *Proc Natl Acad Sci U S A.* 2006;103(42):15529–15534.

352. Matza D, Badou A, Kobayashi KS, et al. A scaffold protein, AHNAK1, is required for calcium signaling during T cell activation. *Immunity.* 2008;28(1):64–74.

353. Gupta S, Salam N, Srivastava V, et al. Voltage gated calcium channels negatively regulate protective immunity to *Mycobacterium tuberculosis. PLoS ONE.* 2009;4(4): e5305.

354. Radermacher AN, Crabtree GR. Monster protein controls calcium entry and fights infection. *Immunity.* 2008;28(1):13–14.

355. Suzuki Y, Yoshimaru T, Inoue T, Ra C. Ca v 1.2 L-type Ca2+ channel protects mast cells against activation-induced cell death by preventing mitochondrial integrity disruption. *Mol Immunol.* 2009;46(11–12):2370–2380.

356. Das R, Burke T, Van Wagoner DR, Plow EF. L-type calcium channel blockers exert an antiinflammatory effect by suppressing expression of plasminogen receptors on macrophages. *Circ Res.* 2009;105(2):167–175.

357. Matza D, Badou A, Jha MK, et al. Requirement for AHNAK1-mediated calcium signaling during T lymphocyte cytolysis. *Proc Natl Acad Sci U S A.* 2009;106(24):9785–9790.

358. Liao P, Soong TW. CaV1.2 channelopathies: from arrhythmias to autism, bipolar disorder, and immunodeficiency. *Pflugers Arch.* 2010;460(2):353–359.

359. Das R, Plow EF. A new function for old drugs. *Cell Cycle.* 2010;9(4):638–639.

360. Balog Z, Kiss I, Keri S. CACNA1C risk allele for psychotic disorders is related to the activation of the AKT-pathway. *Am J Psychiatry.* 2010;167(10):1276–1277.

361. Li XQ, Cao W, Li T, et al. Amlodipine inhibits TNF-alpha production and attenuates cardiac dysfunction induced by lipopolysaccharide involving PI3K/Akt pathway. *Int Immunopharmacol.* 2009;9(9):1032–1041.

362. Splawski I, Timothy KW, Sharpe LM, et al. Ca(V)1.2 calcium channel dysfunction causes a multisystem disorder including arrhythmia and autism. *Cell.* 2004;119(1): 19–31.

363. Okazaki R, Iwasaki YK, Miyauchi Y, et al. lipopolysaccharide induces atrial arrhythmogenesis via down-regulation of L-type Ca2+ channel genes in rats. *Int Heart J.* 2009;50(3):353–363.

364. Azenabor AA, Chaudhry AU. Effective macrophage redox defense against *Chlamydia pneumoniae* depends on L-type Ca2+ channel activation. *Med Microbiol Immunol.* 2003;192(2):99–106.

365. Wieland H, Hechtel N, Faigle M, Neumeister B. Efficient intracellular multiplication of *Legionella pneumophil*a in human monocytes requires functional host cell L-type calcium channels. *FEMS Immunol Med Microbiol.* 2006;47(2):296–301.

366. Hanff TC, Furst SJ, Minor TR. Biochemical and anatomical substrates of depression and sickness behavior. *Isr J Psychiatry Relat Sci.* 2010;47(1):64–71.

367. Hart BL. Biological basis of the behavior of sick animals. *Neurosci Biobehav Rev.* 1988;12(2):123–137.

368. Hart BL. Behavioral adaptations to pathogens and parasites: five strategies. *Neurosci Biobehav Rev.* 1990;14(3):273–294.

369. Kluger MJ. Phylogeny of fever. *Fed Proc.* 1979;38(1):30–34.

370. Kluger MJ, Kozak W, Conn CA, Leon LR, Soszynski D. Role of fever in disease. *Ann N Y Acad Sci.* 1998;856:224–233.

371. Sweet C, Cavanagh D, Collie MH, Smith H. Sensitivity to pyrexial temperatures: a factor contributing to virulence differences between two clones of influenza virus. *Br J Exp Pathol.* 1978;59(4):373–380.

372. Dixon G, Booth C, Price E, Westran R, Turner M, Klein N. Fever as nature's engine: part of beneficial host response? *BMJ.* 2010;340:c450.

373. Tyrrell D, Barrow I, Arthur J. Local hyperthermia benefits natural and experimental common colds. *BMJ.* 1989;298(6683):1280–1283.

374. Ostberg JR, Taylor SL, Baumann H, Repasky EA. Regulatory effects of fever-range whole-body hyperthermia on the LPS-induced acute inflammatory response. *J Leukoc Biol.* 2000;68(6):815–820.

375. Jiang Q, Detolla L, Singh IS, et al. Exposure to febrile temperature upregulates expression of pyrogenic cytokines in endotoxin-challenged mice. *Am J Physiol.* 1999;276(6 pt 2):R1653–R1660.

376. Ostberg JR, Dayanc BE, Yuan M, Oflazoglu E, Repasky EA. Enhancement of natural killer (NK) cell cytotoxicity by fever-range thermal stress is dependent on NKG2D function and is associated with plasma membrane NKG2D clustering and increased expression of MICA on target cells. *J Leukoc Biol.* 2007;82(5):1322–1331.

377. Ostberg JR, Repasky EA. Emerging evidence indicates that physiologically relevant thermal stress regulates dendritic cell function. *Cancer Immunol Immunother.* 2006; 55(3):292–298.

378. Evans SS, Wang WC, Bain MD, Burd R, Ostberg JR, Repasky EA. Fever-range hyperthermia dynamically regulates lymphocyte delivery to high endothelial venules. *Blood.* 2001;97(9):2727–2733.

379. Swenson BR, Hedrick TL, Popovsky K, Pruett TL, Sawyer RG. Is fever protective in surgical patients with bloodstream infection? *J Am Coll Surg.* 2007;204(5):815–823.

380. Mizushima Y, Ueno M, Idoguchi K, Ishikawa K, Matsuoka T. Fever in trauma patients: friend or foe? *J Trauma.* 2009;67(5):1062–1065.

381. Ohsugi Y. Recent advances in immunopathophysiology of interleukin-6: an innovative therapeutic drug, tocilizumab (recombinant humanized anti-human interleukin-6 receptor antibody), unveils the mysterious etiology of immune-mediated inflammatory diseases. *Biol Pharm Bull.* 2007;30(11):2001–2006.

382. Kung'u JK, Wright VJ, Haji HJ, et al. Adjusting for the acute phase response is essential to interpret iron status indicators among young Zanzibari children prone to chronic malaria and helminth infections. *J Nutr.* 2009;139(11):2124–2131.

383. Cartwright GE, Lauritsen MA, et al. The anemia of infection; hypoferremia, hypercupremia, and alterations in porphyrin metabolism in patients. *J Clin Invest.* 1946;25: 65–80.

384. Kochan I, Wagner SK, Wasynczuk J. Effect of iron on antibacterial immunity in vaccinated mice. *Infect Immun.* 1984;43(2):543–548.

385. Weinberg ED. Survival advantage of the hemochromatosis C282Y mutation. *Perspect Biol Med.* 2008;51(1):98–102.

386. Foster SL, Richardson SH, Failla ML. Elevated iron status increases bacterial invasion and survival and alters cytokine/chemokine mRNA expression in Caco-2 human intestinal cells. *J Nutr.* 2001;131(5):1452–1458.

387. Wander K, Shell-Duncan B, McDade TW. Evaluation of iron deficiency as a nutritional adaptation to infectious disease: an evolutionary medicine perspective. *Am J Hum Biol.* 2009;21(2):172–179.

388. Mitra AK, Akramuzzaman SM, Fuchs GJ, Rahman MM, Mahalanabis D. Long-term oral supplementation with iron is not harmful for young children in a poor community of Bangladesh. *J Nutr.* 1997;127(8):1451–1455.

389. Smith AW, Hendrickse RG, Harrison C, Hayes RJ, Greenwood BM. The effects on malaria of treatment of iron-deficiency anaemia with oral iron in Gambian children. *Ann Trop Paediatr.* 1989;9(1):17–23.

390. van den Hombergh J, Dalderop E, Smit Y. Does iron therapy benefit children with severe malaria-associated anaemia? A clinical trial with 12 weeks supplementation of oral iron in young children from the Turiani Division, Tanzania. *J Trop Pediatr.* 1996; 42(4):220–227.

391. Tielsch JM, Khatry SK, Stoltzfus RJ, et al. Effect of routine prophylactic supplementation with iron and folic acid on preschool child mortality in southern Nepal: community-based, cluster-randomised, placebo-controlled trial. *Lancet.* 2006;367(9505): 144–152.

392. Sazawal S, Black RE, Ramsan M, et al. Effects of routine prophylactic supplementation with iron and folic acid on admission to hospital and mortality in preschool children in a high malaria transmission setting: community-based, randomised, placebo-controlled trial. *Lancet.* 2006;367(9505):133–143.

393. Kluger MJ, O'Reilly B, Shope TR, Vander AJ. Further evidence that stress hyperthermia is a fever. *Physiol Behav.* 1987;39(6):763–766.

394. Oka T, Oka K, Hori T. Mechanisms and mediators of psychological stress-induced rise in core temperature. *Psychosom Med.* 2001;63(3):476–486.

395. Hayashida S, Oka T, Mera T, Tsuji S. Repeated social defeat stress induces chronic hyperthermia in rats. *Physiol Behav.* 2010;101(1):124–131.

396. Vinkers CH, Groenink L, van Bogaert MJ, et al. Stress-induced hyperthermia and infection-induced fever: two of a kind? *Physiol Behav.* 2009;98(1–2):37–43.

397. Chen J, Shen H, Chen C, et al. The effect of psychological stress on iron absorption in rats. *BMC Gastroenterol.* 2009;9:83.

398. Wei C, Zhou J, Huang X, Li M. Effects of psychological stress on serum iron and erythropoiesis. *Int J Hematol.* 2008;88(1):52–56.

399. Zhao M, Chen J, Wang W, et al. Psychological stress induces hypoferremia through the IL-6-hepcidin axis in rats. *Biochem Biophys Res Commun.* 2008;373(1):90–93.

400. Teng WF, Sun WM, Shi LF, Hou DD, Liu H. Effects of restraint stress on iron, zinc, calcium, and magnesium whole blood levels in mice. *Biol Trace Elem Res.* 2008;121(3): 243–248.

401. Kaneda Y, Tsuji S, Oka T. Age distribution and gender differences in psychogenic fever patients. *Biopsychosoc Med.* 2009;3:6.

402. Oka T, Oka K. Age and gender differences of psychogenic fever: a review of the Japanese literature. *Biopsychosoc Med.* 2007;1:11.

403. Singh A, Smoak BL, Patterson KY, LeMay LG, Veillon C, Deuster PA. Biochemical indices of selected trace minerals in men: effect of stress. *Am J Clin Nutr.* 1991;53(1): 126–131.

404. Dantzer R, O'Connor JC, Freund GG, Johnson RW, Kelley KW. From inflammation to sickness and depression: when the immune system subjugates the brain. *Nat Rev Neurosci.* 2008;9(1):46–56.

405. McEnany GW, Lee KA. Effects of light therapy on sleep, mood, and temperature in

women with nonseasonal major depression. *Issues Ment Health Nurs.* 2005;26(7): 781–794.

406. Rausch JL, Johnson ME, Corley KM, et al. Depressed patients have higher body temperature: 5-HT transporter long promoter region effects. *Neuropsychobiology.* 2003; 47(3):120–127.

407. Szuba MP, Guze BH, Baxter LR Jr. Electroconvulsive therapy increases circadian amplitude and lowers core body temperature in depressed subjects. *Biol Psychiat.* 1997;42(12):1130–1137.

408. Daimon K, Yamada N, Tsujimoto T, Takahashi S. Circadian rhythm abnormalities of deep body temperature in depressive disorders. *J Affect Disord.* 1992;26(3):191–198.

409. Avery DH, Shah SH, Eder DN, Wildschiodtz G. Nocturnal sweating and temperature in depression. *Acta Psychiatr Scand.* 1999;100(4):295–301.

410. Avery DH, Wildschiodtz G, Smallwood RG, Martin D, Rafaelsen OJ. REM latency and core temperature relationships in primary depression. *Acta Psychiatr Scand.* 1986; 74(3):269–280.

411. Avery DH, Wildschiodtz G, Rafaelsen OJ. Nocturnal temperature in affective disorder. *J Affect Disord.* 1982;4(1):61–71.

412. Sugahara H, Akamine M, Kondo T, et al. Somatic symptoms most often associated with depression in an urban hospital medical setting in Japan. *Psychiatry Res.* 2004; 128(3):305–311.

413. Rangan AM, Blight GD, Binns CW. Iron status and non-specific symptoms of female students. *J Am Coll Nutr.* 1998;17(4):351–355.

414. Maes M, Van de Vyvere J, Vandoolaeghe E, et al. Alterations in iron metabolism and the erythron in major depression: further evidence for a chronic inflammatory process. *J Affect Disord.* 1996;40(1–2):23–33.

415. Maes M, Vandewoude M, Scharpe S, et al. Anthropometric and biochemical assessment of the nutritional state in depression: evidence for lower visceral protein plasma levels in depression. *J Affect Disord.* 1991;23(1):25–33.

416. Maes M, Scharpe S, Bosmans E, et al. Disturbances in acute phase plasma proteins during melancholia: additional evidence for the presence of an inflammatory process during that illness. *Prog Neurospychopharmacol Biol Psychiatry.* 1992;16(4):501–515.

417. Albacar G, Sans T, Martin-Santos R, et al. An association between plasma ferritin concentrations measured 48h after delivery and postpartum depression. *J Affect Disord.* 2011;131(1–3):136–142.

418. Majer M, Wellberg LAM, Capuron L, Pagnoni G, Raison CL, Miller AH. IFN-alpha-induced motor slowing is associated with increased depression and fatigue in patients with chronic hepatitis C. *Brain Behav Immun.* 2008;25(10):870–880.

419. Capuron L, Gumnick JF, Musselman DL, et al. Neurobehavioral effects of interferon-alpha in cancer patients: phenomenology and paroxetine responsiveness of symptom dimensions. *Neuropsychopharmacology.* 2002;26(5):643–652.

420. Krueger JM, Majde JA. Humoral links between sleep and the immune system: research issues. *Ann N Y Acad Sci.* 2003;992:9–20.

421. Krueger JM, Toth LA. Cytokines as regulators of sleep. *Ann N Y Acad Sci.* 1994;739: 299–310.

422. Krueger JM, Majde JA. Microbial products and cytokines in sleep and fever regulation. *Crit Rev Immunol.* 1994;14(3–4):355–379.

423. Opp MR. Cytokines and sleep: the first hundred years. *Brain Behav Immun.* 2004; 18(4):295–297.

424. Opp MR. Sleeping to fuel the immune system: mammalian sleep and resistance to parasites. *BMC Evol Biol.* 2009;9:8.

425. Engel GL, Schmale AH. Conservation-withdrawal: a primary regulatory process for organismic homeostasis. *Ciba Found Symp.* 1972;8:57–75.

426. Nguyen KB, Biron CA. Synergism for cytokine-mediated disease during concurrent endotoxin and viral challenges: roles for NK and T cell IFN-gamma production. *J Immunol.* 1999;162(9):5238–5246.

427. Jakab GJ, Dick EC. Synergistic effect in viral-bacterial infection: combined infection of the murine respiratory tract with Sendai virus and *Pasteurella pneumotropica. Infect Immun.* 1973;8(5):762–768.

428. Degre M, Glasgow LA. Synergistic effect in viral-bacterial infection. I. Combined infection of the respiratory tract in mice with parainfluenza virus and *Hemophilus influenza. J Infect Dis.* 1968;118(5):449–462.

429. Jones WT, Menna JH, Wennerstrom DE. Lethal synergism induced in mice by influenza type A virus and type Ia group B streptococci. *Infect Immun.* 1983;41(2):618–623.

430. Beadling C, Slifka MK. How do viral infections predispose patients to bacterial infections? *Curr Opin Infect Dis.* 2004;17(3):185–191.

431. Molyneux EM, Tembo M, Kayira K, et al. The effect of HIV infection on paediatric bacterial meningitis in Blantyre, Malawi. *Arch Dis Child.* 2003;88(12):1112–1118.

432. McCullers JA, McAuley JL, Browall S, Iverson AR, Boyd KL, Henriques Normark B. Influenza enhances susceptibility to natural acquisition of and disease due to *Streptococcus pneumoniae* in ferrets. *J Infect Dis.* 2010;202(8):1287–1295.

433. Thornhill R, Fincher CL, Aran D. Parasites, democratization, and the liberalization of values across contemporary countries. *Biol Rev Camb Philos Soc.* 2009;84(1):113–131.

434. American Psychiatric Association. *Diagnostic and Statistical Manual of Mental Disorders—4th Edition Text Revision: DSM-IV–4–TR.* Washington, DC: American Psychiatric Association; 2000.

435. Miller GE, Cohen S. Infectious disease and psychoneuroimmunology. In: Vedhara K, Irwin MR, eds. *Human Psychoneuroimmunology.* Oxford, UK: Oxford University Press; 2005:219–242.

436. Capuron L, Gumnick JF, Musselman DL, et al. Neurobehavioral effects of interferon-alpha in cancer patients: phenomenology and paroxetine responsiveness of symptom dimensions. *Neuropsychopharmacology.* 2002;26(5):643–652.

437. Constant A, Castera L, Dantzer R, et al. Mood alterations during interferon-alfa therapy in patients with chronic hepatitis C: evidence for an overlap between manic/hypomanic and depressive symptoms. *J Clin Psychiatry.* 2005;66(8):1050–1057.

438. Critchley HD, Mathias CJ, Josephs O, et al. Human cingulate cortex and autonomic control: converging neuroimaging and clinical evidence. *Brain.* 2003;126(pt 10):2139–2152.

439. Eisenberger NI, Lieberman MD, Williams KD. Does rejection hurt? An fMRI study of social exclusion. *Science.* 2003;302(5643):290–292.

440. Slavich GM, Way BM, Eisenberger NI, Taylor SE. Neural sensitivity to social rejection is associated with inflammatory responses to social stress. *Proc Natl Acad Sci U S A.* 2010;107(33):14817–14822.

441. Brydon L, Harrison NA, Walker C, Steptoe A, Critchley HD. Peripheral inflammation is associated with altered substantia nigra activity and psychomotor slowing in humans. *Biol Psychiatry.* 2008;63(11):1022–1029.

442. Capuron L, Pagnoni G, Demetrashvili MF, et al. Basal ganglia hypermetabolism and symptoms of fatigue during interferon-alpha therapy. *Neuropsychopharmacology.* 2007;32(11):2384–2392.

443. Harrison NA, Brydon L, Walker C, et al. Neural origins of human sickness in interoceptive responses to inflammation. *Biol Psychiatry.* 2009;66(5):415–422.

444. Straub RH. Concepts of evolutionary medicine and energy regulation contribute to the etiology of systemic chronic inflammatory diseases. *Brain Behav Immun.* 2011;25(1): 1–5.

445. Adamo SA, Fidler TL, Forestell CA. Illness-induced anorexia and its possible function in the caterpillar, *Manduca sexta. Brain Behav Immun.* 2007;21(3):292–300.

446. Smith DJ, Kyle S, Forty L, et al. Differences in depressive symptom profile between males and females. *J Affect Disord.* 2008;108(3):279–284.

447. Wing EJ, Barczynski LK, Boehmer SM. Effect of acute nutritional deprivation on immune function in mice. I. Macrophages. *Immunology.* 1983;48(3):543–550.

448. Murray MJ, Murray AB. Anorexia of infection as a mechanism of host defense. *Am J Clin Nutr.* 1979;32(3):593–596.

449. Heuer JG, Bailey DL, Sharma GR, et al. Cecal ligation and puncture with total parenteral nutrition: a clinically relevant model of the metabolic, hormonal, and inflammatory dysfunction associated with critical illness. *J Surg Res.* 2004;121(2):178–186.

450. Sena MJ, Utter GH, Cuschieri J, et al. Early supplemental parenteral nutrition is associated with increased infectious complications in critically ill trauma patients. *J Am Coll Surg.* 2008;207(4):459–467.

451. Heyland DK. Parenteral nutrition in the critically-ill patient: more harm than good? *Proc Nutr Soc.* 2000;59(3):457–466.

452. Aubert A, Goodall G, Dantzer R. Compared effects of cold ambient temperature and cytokines on macronutrient intake in rats. *Physiol Behav.* 1995;57(5):869–873.

453. Heyland DK, MacDonald S, Keefe L, Drover JW. Total parenteral nutrition in the critically ill patient: a meta-analysis. *JAMA.* 1998;280(23):2013–2019.

454. Roura-Mir C, Wang L, Cheng TY, et al. *Mycobacterium tuberculosis* regulates CD1 antigen presentation pathways through TLR-2. *J Immunol.* 2005;175(3):1758–1766.

455. Amprey JL, Spath GF, Porcelli SA. Inhibition of CD1 expression in human dendritic cells during intracellular infection with Leishmania donovani. *Infect Immun.* 2004; 72(1):589–592.

456. Beekman M, Nederstigt C, Suchiman HE, et al. Genome-wide association study (GWAS)-identified disease risk alleles do not compromise human longevity. *Proc Natl Acad Sci U S A.* 2010;107(42):18046–18049.

457. Eaton WW, Anthony JC, Gallo J, et al. Natural history of Diagnostic Interview Schedule/*DSM-IV* major depression: the Baltimore Epidemiologic Catchment Area followup. *Arch Gen Psychiatry.* 1997;54(11):993–999.

458. Patten SB, Wang JL, Williams JV, et al. Descriptive epidemiology of major depression in Canada. *Can J Psychiatry.* 2006;51(2):84–90.

459. Kessler RC, Birnbaum H, Bromet E, Hwang I, Sampson N, Shahly V. Age differences in major depression: results from the National Comorbidity Survey Replication (NCS-R). *Psychol Med.* 2010;40(2):225–237.

460. Van Bodegom D, May L, Meij HJ, Westendorp RG. Regulation of human life histories: the role of the inflammatory host response. *Ann N Y Acad Sci.* 2007;1100:84–97.

461. Drenos F, Westendorp RG, Kirkwood TB. Trade-off mediated effects on the genetics of human survival caused by increasingly benign living conditions. *Biogerontology.* 2006;7(4):287–295.

462. Thase ME. Atypical depression: useful concept, but it's time to revise the *DSM-IV* criteria. *Neuropsychopharmacology.* 2009;34(13):2633–2641.

463. Matza LS, Revicki DA, Davidson JR, Stewart JW. Depression with atypical features in the National Comorbidity Survey: classification, description, and consequences. *Arch Gen Psychiatry.* 2003;60(8):817–826.

464. Posternak MA, Zimmerman M. Symptoms of atypical depression. *Psychiatry Res.* 2001;104(2):175–181.

465. Carter JD, Joyce PR, Mulder RT, Luty SE, McKenzie J. Gender differences in the presentation of depressed outpatients: a comparison of descriptive variables. *J Affect Disord.* 2000;61(1–2):59–67.

466. Patel SR, Zhu X, Storfer-Isser A, et al. Sleep duration and biomarkers of inflammation. *Sleep.* 2009;32(2):200–204.

467. El-Sheikh M, Buckhalt JA, Granger DA, Erath SA, Acebo C. The association between children's sleep disruption and salivary interleukin-6. *J Sleep Res.* 2007;16(2): 188–197.

468. Kleinridders A, Schenten D, Konner AC, et al. MyD88 signaling in the CNS is required for development of fatty acid-induced leptin resistance and diet-induced obesity. *Cell Metab.* 2009;10(4):249–259.

469. Zhang X, Zhang G, Zhang H, Karin M, Bai H, Cai D. Hypothalamic IKKbeta/NF-kappaB and ER stress link overnutrition to energy imbalance and obesity. *Cell.* 2008;135(1): 61–73.

470. Posey KA, Clegg DJ, Printz RL, et al. Hypothalamic proinflammatory lipid accumulation, inflammation, and insulin resistance in rats fed a high-fat diet. *Am J Physiol Endocrinol Metab.* 2009;296(5):E1003–E1012.

471. Milanski M, Degasperi G, Coope A, et al. Saturated fatty acids produce an inflammatory response predominantly through the activation of TLR4 signaling in hypothalamus: implications for the pathogenesis of obesity. *J Neurosci.* 2009;29(2):359–370.

472. Dahlgren J, Nilsson C, Jennische E, et al. Prenatal cytokine exposure results in obesity and gender-specific programming. *Am J Physiol Endocrinol Metab.* 2001;281(2):E326–E334.

473. Avitsur R, Mays JW, Sheridan JF. Sex differences in the response to influenza virus infection: modulation by stress. *Horm Behav.* 2011;59(2):257–264.

474. Atkinson RL. Could viruses contribute to the worldwide epidemic of obesity? *Int J Pediatr Obes.* 2008;3(suppl 1):37–43.

475. Mitra AK, Clarke K. Viral obesity: fact or fiction? *Obes Rev.* 2010;11(4):289–296.

476. Chuang JC, Krishnan V, Yu HG, et al. A beta3-adrenergic-leptin-melanocortin circuit regulates behavioral and metabolic changes induced by chronic stress. *Biol Psychiatry.* 2010;67(11):1075–1082.

477. Bailey MT, Engler H, Powell ND, Padgett DA, Sheridan JF. Repeated social defeat increases the bactericidal activity of splenic macrophages through a Toll-like receptor-dependent pathway. *Am J Physiol Regul Integr Comp Physiol.* 2007;293(3):R1180–R1190.

478. Cizza G, Nguyen VT, Eskandari F, et al. Low 24-hour adiponectin and high nocturnal leptin concentrations in a case-control study of community-dwelling premenopausal women with major depressive disorder: the Premenopausal, Osteopenia/Osteoporosis, Women, Alendronate, Depression (POWER) study. *J Clin Psychiatry.* 2010;71(8):1079–1087.

479. Zeman M, Jirak R, Jachymova M, Vecka M, Tvrzicka E, Zak A. Leptin, adiponectin, leptin to adiponectin ratio and insulin resistance in depressive women. *Neuro Endocrinol Lett.* 2009;30(3):387–395.

480. Pasco JA, Jacka FN, Williams LJ, et al. Leptin in depressed women: cross-sectional and longitudinal data from an epidemiologic study. *J Affect Disord.* 2008;107(1–3):221–225.

481. Yang K, Xie G, Zhang Z, et al. Levels of serum interleukin (IL)-6, IL-1beta, tumour necrosis factor-alpha and leptin and their correlation in depression. *Aust N Z J Psychiatry.* 2007;41(3):266–273.

482. Rubin RT, Rhodes ME, Czambel RK. Sexual diergism of baseline plasma leptin and leptin suppression by arginine vasopressin in major depressives and matched controls. *Psychiatry Res.* 2002;113(3):255–268.

483. Gecici O, Kuloglu M, Atmaca M, et al. High serum leptin levels in depressive disorders with atypical features. *Psychiatry Clin Neurosci.* 2005;59(6):736–738.

484. Buyukoglan H, Gulmez I, Kelestimur F, et al. Leptin levels in various manifestations of pulmonary tuberculosis. *Mediators Inflamm.* 2007;2007:64859.

485. van Crevel R, Karyadi E, Netea MG, et al. Decreased plasma leptin concentrations in tuberculosis patients are associated with wasting and inflammation. *J Clin Endocrinol Metab.* 2002;87(2):758–763.

486. Pednekar MS, Hakama M, Hebert JR, Gupta PC. Association of body mass index with all-cause and cause-specific mortality: findings from a prospective cohort study in Mumbai (Bombay), India. *Int J Epidemiol.* 2008;37(3):524–535.

487. Wieland CW, Florquin S, Chan ED, et al. Pulmonary *Mycobacterium tuberculosis* infection in leptin-deficient ob/ob mice. *Int Immunol.* 2005;17(11):1399–1408.

488. Leung CC, Lam TH, Chan WM, et al. Lower risk of tuberculosis in obesity. *Arch Intern Med.* 2007;167(12):1297–1304.

489. Roth J. Evolutionary speculation about tuberculosis and the metabolic and inflammatory processes of obesity. *JAMA.* 2009;301(24):2586–2588.

490. Raison CL, Lowry CA, Rook GA. Inflammation, sanitation, and consternation: loss of contact with coevolved, tolerogenic microorganisms and the pathophysiology and treatment of major depression. *Arch Gen Psychiatry.* 2010;67(12):1211–1224.

CHAPTER 11

The Case of Mary

Using Sensory Pathways as Deep Brain Stimulators to Treat Depression

When the research assistants were done, they came to get me to review their work, and that's how I met Mary. She sat hunched over a bit in our little interview room, an overweight 26-year-old white female dabbing her eyes with a tissue. I knew from the scales collected by my colleagues that Mary was severely depressed, had been so for more than a year, and had been depressed in the past. I also knew that she believed antidepressants had not helped her "that much" in the past. Perhaps, I thought to myself, this explained why she would volunteer for a study examining whether intense heat, in the form of whole-body hyperthermia (WBH), might show promise as a new treatment for major depressive disorder (MDD). Because she had been referred to the study by a colleague at the university, I had a special interest in hearing her story.

I sat down across a small table from Mary and waited for a moment. The two research assistants tried to settle as discreetly as possible into two chairs in the corner of the room. "I'm sorry you're feeling so badly," I said. "It looks like you're going to qualify for the study, but let me ask a few more questions. When did all this start?"

Mary dabbed her eyes. "I think I've always been a little depressed," she said. "I had a very hard childhood. My mom has bipolar disorder and growing up you never knew what mood you were going to find her in. Sometimes she'd be so sad she couldn't get out of bed. Other days she'd be full of anger and would beat us for no reason. Other times she'd be singing and kissing us. But especially as we got older and she got sicker, it was mostly the angers and beating. My dad did what he could, and that helped, but it was still hell."

"He's still with her?" I asked, drifting a little off topic.

"No, once he knew the kids were out of the house, he left her."

I nodded. "So was it always the same for you in terms of your own mood, or did you have a real down-turn at some point?"

"Downturn big time. Probably the best I ever felt was my first year at college. I was out of the house—such a relief. I did pretty well in school and I had a steady boyfriend. Problem was that at the start of my sophomore year he dumped me for my roommate. It was so terrible, I can't tell you. I just barely managed not to flunk out."

"What kind of symptoms did you have?" I asked

"Well I felt so depressed I could barely move, for one thing. And so bad about myself I started avoiding people. I got into this pattern where I'd sleep most of the day and then be up half the night. And I gained like 40 pounds."

"Trouble thinking and concentrating?" I asked. "And what about exhausted, no pleasure in life, all that?"

She nodded.

"So what finally happened?" I asked

"I got so bad that I started wanting to kill myself. I told a friend, who hauled me down to the campus clinic. They thought about sending me to the psych hospital, but when I promised I wouldn't hurt myself they let me go home with a prescription for Prozac."

"Did it help?"

"Yes," she replied. "I never went back to feeling as good as I did that first year of college, but I got to where I could go back to living my life. I was probably always at 'minus 1' after that, if you know what I mean. I stayed on it for a long time. When I first met my husband and we were dating I felt happier and got off it for a while, but then I started slipping with all the stress of planning a big Catholic wedding, so I went back on it and stayed on it until I got pregnant with our daughter."

Like many women, Mary did not want to take an antidepressant while pregnant, so she stopped it. She tried to "take up the slack," as she said, by going to a yoga class and by going to church more often. But despite these efforts her mood gradually deteriorated.

"I was hanging in there until I gave birth to Lizzie," she continued. "And then I spun down. Within a couple of weeks I couldn't find a way to stop crying. I can't tell you how guilty I felt . . ."

At this she burst into tears. I handed her a tissue and waited.

"Sorry," she finally said. "This is still a terrible problem for me. This guilt that I'm a terrible mother. I can't bear the thought that I might do to my little girl what my mom did to me."

Mary went on to describe a classic postpartum depression, with symptoms similar to her first major episode in college but with a critical difference: this time the depression didn't respond to fluoxetine (Prozac). She took it for six weeks at 20 mg a day with minimal response. Her psychiatrist increased it to 40 mg a day without any noticeable effect.

"At that high dose I had no sex drive whatsoever," Mary continued. "So then I became terrified I'd lose my husband like I'd lost that college boyfriend. And it made the feelings of failure and guilt worse."

Her doctor stopped the fluoxetine and tried several other selective serotonin reuptake inhibitor (SSRI) antidepressants, all of which Mary took at therapeutic doses for at least two months. Although she got a few weeks of improvement with escitalopram, it faded. The psychiatrist tried adding bupropion, but four weeks later at a full dose of both medications Mary was no better. Next came a trial of serotonin-norepinephrine reuptake inhibitors. Duloxetine caused intolerable nausea, and six weeks of extended-release venlafaxine "helped a little." Because her psychiatrist felt that the venlafaxine had been the most effective agent tried, he kept her on it and added the second-generation antipsychotic arapiprazole (Abilify).

"I was like a walking medicine cabinet," Mary said, smiling for the first time in our interview. "But I never felt more than about a third better, I think. And I still didn't have any sex drive, and I was gaining weight, and one day I'd just had it. I stopped all the medicine at once—I know that's stupid, but I did it. I felt a little weird and sick for a week or so, but then I got over it. I think I felt more depressed off the medicines, but not that much more depressed, so I just spent the next year or so trying to suffer through everything. Thank God my husband is like my dad. He really picks up the slack."

"And that's how you came to us?" I asked.

"Yes, that's how I came to you. I saw a flier for your study saying you were looking for depressed people not on an antidepressant. That's me."

"OK, one more question" I said. "Never had a manic or even a hypomanic episode like your mom's had?"

"No, it never happened," she said. "Sometimes I wish I could have a little hypomania, though."

Sadly, Mary's story is typical for many patients. Had she come to see me as a patient instead of as a research subject I would have been faced with the distressing truth that, although she might have a "miracle" response to the next medication we tried, it is more likely that subsequent efforts would also lead to a suboptimal response. This gloomy perspective comes from multiple studies showing that the more antidepressants people fail, the less likely they are to respond to whichever one they try next.[1] Related to this is the fact that people are also less likely to respond to antidepressants when they have been depressed for an extended period. Mary's current episode had lasted for three years and had clearly inflicted significant collateral damage on Mary's self-esteem, relationships, and work history.

So how would the new mind-body science of depression suggest we treat Mary if she wasn't about to be enrolled in a study? First and foremost, although Mary has tried a number of medications, she has not engaged in two modalities with known antidepressant effects: psychotherapy and exercise. Much has been written about both, and we discuss psychotherapy in another case (see Chapter 12). The evidence that exercise has both acute mood-elevating and longer-lasting antidepressant effects is now quite compelling.[2] Both strength training and aerobic exercise have this effect, and the combination of both is almost certainly better than either alone.[3] The challenge is that, unlike general health, which benefits from even modest amounts of physical activity, the full antidepressant effect of exercise is realized only when people commit to a serious exercise regimen.[4,5]

Serious in this case means something like 30–45 minutes a day five days a week. More than this doesn't seem to enhance antidepressant efficacy, but less than this rapidly diminishes the benefit. Aerobic and strength training are both effective; if anything, strength training might be the more effective of the two. An evolutionary theorist might hypothesize that this results in part from the fact that across most of their evolutionary history hominids escaped to safety by hoisting themselves into trees using upper body strength. Building up that capacity, even today, may in some way reignite ancient programming associated with security and community (as hominids likely slept in trees prior to becoming exclusively land dwelling).

Whether these types of musings have any scientific merit is unknown, but the effect of strength training has been shown again and again. And it is likely that a mix of strength and aerobic training is the most effective antidepressant strategy of all. But exercise has its downsides. It can promote injuries that over the long term increase sedentary behavior. It takes time, and it takes discipline. And finally, its effects are transient. It appears that its antidepressant effects fade rapidly once an exercise regimen is abandoned.

But Mary had come not as a patient but as a research subject. She passed all her screening tests and so entered our study and was randomly assigned to receive either active or sham/placebo WBH. At this point you might be wondering: why would we study WBH for depression, and more specifically, why does Mary's participation in our study merit inclusion as a case study in this book? The answer to both questions hinges on the fact that our study of WBH challenges standard understandings of the pathophysiology of depression but derives directly from the mind-body perspective that is underscored in this book.

We noted in Chapter 5 that the National Institute of Mental Health is deeply committed to the concept that mental illnesses are brain disorders. On one level this is so obvious that it hardly bears repeating, if one believes, as we do, that our thoughts and feelings arise from the functional activity of the brain. Indeed, if this perspective is right, then patterns of brain activity must always be the final cause of all mental disorders. But a full mind-body perspective also reveals important ways in which the dogma that "mental disorders are brain disorders" is manifestly not true and is, in fact, likely to prematurely foreclose and limit our ability to identify and develop new biological treatments for MDD.

To understand how a mind-body perspective differs from the currently fashionable brain-centered view—and to see why this difference has important treatment implications—we must start by digging a little deeper into what it would moan for mental illnesses to be brain disorders. And this in turn requires an exploration of what we mean when we say that something causes a mental disorder like depression, because when people say that mental disorders are brain disorders, what they mean is that the cause of mental illness is located in the brain. An immediate implication of this is that, if the cause of depression is in the brain, optimal treatments will always directly target brain function. Again, we tend to see this as so obvious that few of us question the fact that current research into somatic treatments for MDD, from ketamine to deep brain stimulation, focuses exclusively on the brain.

Again in deference to the primacy of the brain in mental functioning, let us grant that patterns of brain functioning are the most immediate cause of depressive thoughts and feelings—no brain, no depression. But the key point that is almost always overlooked is that just because the brain causes depression in this sense does not mean that this causation reflects a primary abnormality in the brain. To see this more clearly, consider two extreme cases. The first is a woman who never had a depressed day in her life until she suffered a stroke in her left anterior prefrontal cortex. Within a few days of the stroke she developed a catastrophic depression for no apparent psychosocial reason. The second case is a teenager with MDD whose life is being made miserable by a depressed single mother, whose care and attention are erratic at best and absent at worst.

We would all likely agree that the first case of depression resulted from malfunctioning of the brain. The brain broke, and depression resulted. It is worth pausing for a moment to realize that this is really what is meant by the claim that mental disorders like depression are brain disorders: their occurrence results from the brain being damaged—perhaps not as obviously as occurs with a stroke, but damaged nonetheless. On the other hand, although the second case manifests symptoms very similar to the first, we have no evidence that the teenager's brain is damaged or that any type of damage accounts for the young person's depression. In fact, a remarkable study suggests that most often these types of adolescent depression do not result from abnormal brain functioning arising from malfunctioning of the brain itself. In this study, researchers examined the impact of maternal response to an SSRI antidepressant on the emotional and behavioral functioning of their teenage children. If the mother had no significant clinical response to the antidepressant, her child experienced worsening depression over the study period, whereas if the mother went into remission, her child's depressive symptoms also showed marked improvement—in fact, more improvement than experienced by the mother herself.[6]

Unless one entertains the possibility that somehow the antidepressant vaporized and passed through the air from mother to child, the obvious conclusion from this study is that the mother's depression was causing the child's depression, if by "cause" we mean that reversing the relevant factor reverses the relevant result. The child's brain may have been in a functional state that produced depressive thoughts and feelings. But if this state had been caused by some type of abnormality within the child's brain, fixing the mother would not have fixed the child. Rather, the most parsimonious explanation is that the mother's behavior induced, or caused, the child's brain to go into a depressogenic functional pattern that normalized when the maternal cause normalized.

This is just one example of many we might offer to show that depression can have causes outside the brain, and not in some abstract sense but in the most concrete and important sense possible, given that reversing these "outside causes" can end the depression. What many of us in the world of mental health research have failed to do is differentiate between the proximal cause of depression, which can be found in the brain, and what might be called the "initiating cause," which may or may not reside in the brain. Once this distinction is grasped, another possibility becomes immediately apparent: what looks like abnormal brain functioning may in fact be a normal evolved response to depressogenic signals coming from domains outside the central nervous system (CNS). And here is the key point: depressogenic brain patterns emerging from a broken brain would not look any different than depressogenic brain patterns arising as a normal response to one or another type of signal coming from the wider world.

This line of reasoning became apparent to us only as an accidental result of a study we conducted examining whether the powerful anticytokine agent infliximab would work as an antidepressant. Our initial idea was simple: if depression is associated with increased inflammation, then blocking inflammation should work as an antidepressant. We selected infliximab because, unlike aspirin or nonsteroidal anti-inflammatories that have all manner of biological effects, infliximab does only one thing: it blocks the activity of the key inflammatory cytokine tumor necrosis factor-alpha.

We randomized 60 medically healthy adults with treatment-resistant MDD to three infusions of either infliximab or a saltwater placebo and followed changes in their depressive symptoms for 12 weeks.[7] We wanted to test the hypotheses that (a) cytokine blockade with infliximab would lead to a larger drop in depressive symptoms than exposure to the saltwater placebo and (b) subjects with higher levels of peripheral inflammation prior to treatment would have a larger antidepressant response than subjects with lower levels of inflammation. It is a powerful testimony to the strength of all the factors that comprise placebo that we saw an approximate 50 percent response rate to saltwater in this group of supposedly treatment-resistant patients. Importantly, we saw no benefit for infliximab in the depressed group as a whole, suggesting that anti-inflammatory approaches probably do not hold promise as an "all-purpose" antidepressant strategy. On the other hand we saw a striking dose-response relationship between inflammation before treatment and therapeutic response: the higher the inflammation, the better the antidepressant response to infliximab, exactly as one would predict.

These findings reflect everything we thought about as we planned the study, but they are not the key point for our current discussion. The key point here is that, although we did not make anything of this when we started the study, infliximab is too large a molecule to cross the blood–brain barrier and enter the CNS to any appreciable degree.[8] Although we didn't have the foresight to do lumbar punctures in our study, this has been done by other researchers, and the results are consistent that the medication stays outside the brain. Think for a moment about what this means in terms of our study findings. If our subjects with depression had low levels of peripheral inflammation, blocking this inflammation in the body had no antidepressant effect and in fact, for reasons we don't fully understand, actually made subjects worse compared with placebo. In contrast, in depressed subjects with higher levels of peripheral inflammation, blocking this inflammation in the body produced an antidepressant effect without presumably having any direct effect on the CNS. We think the simplest explanation for these findings is that, however it started, inflammation in the body was signaling the brain in ways that changed its function to produce depression. When this depressogenic signal was blocked by infliximab, the brain "recovered," meaning in this case that its functioning reverted to a state that promoted euthymia. If, on the other hand, the primary cause of depression in subjects with elevated inflammation had been within the brain itself, how could have a purely peripheral intervention, infliximab, produced an antidepressant effect?

Another finding from inflammation research makes the same point in a different way. Our colleagues at Emory University showed a number of years ago that chronic treatment with the inflammatory cytokine interferon-alpha (IFN-α) increased activity in the dorsal anterior cingulate cortex (dACC).[9] This finding has been confirmed so many times that we can say beyond a shadow of a doubt that the dACC is a primary target of peripheral inflammation.[10] Remarkably, meta-analyses have demonstrated that hyperactivity of this brain area is also among the most replicable brain functional abnormalities seen in MDD.[11]

Now consider a thought experiment. Two individuals who meet criteria for

MDD receive a functional MRI scan, and both have hyperactivity of the dACC. Indeed, their scans are indistinguishable. However, one of the individuals has "regular" depression and the other is depressed because she has been taking IFN-α for the prior two months. So here is the question: although their brain scans are indistinguishable, would we say that their conditions are caused by the same thing? Almost certainly not. What if we wanted to target the most powerful cause for each individual? What would we do? The answer is not so clear for the individual with idiopathic MDD, but for the patient on IFN-α the answer is clear: if we want to stop her depression we should stop the IFN-α. And indeed, studies show that almost always when this is done, the cytokine-driven depression resolves.[12] Here is the important point: while the patient with idiopathic MDD may or may not have a primary causal problem in the brain, the patient on IFN-α most certainly does not. Her problem is coming from the infusion of inflammation into her body, which is in turn inducing brain changes that manifest as depression. Nonetheless, one could never tell the difference between these two conditions based on a brain scan. Brain scans cannot differentiate between depression arising from subtle abnormalities within the wiring of the brain and depression arising from brain functional changes that are normal evolved responses to external signals of danger (including in this case an immune signal suggesting the body is infected and thus at increased risk of experiencing organismal death).

So if factors outside the brain can cause depression in nontrivial ways, might these factors also be harnessed to develop new treatments for depression? We think the answer is yes, and this brings us back to Mary, the depressed subject entering our study of WBH, and back to the question of why we would consider WBH as a depression treatment. Our work with infliximab convinced us that bodily pathways might be manipulated to change brain function in ways that might produce antidepressant effects. This, in turn, made us wonder what other pathways might hold antidepressant potential.

One way to begin addressing this question is to ask what the inflammatory system really is. The answer is that it is many things: a defense system, a communication pathway between the host and the microbial world, a pathway for regulating metabolism. But it is also importantly a sensory organ that tells the brain that the body is in danger as a result of infection, tissue damage, or a neoplasm. And like all sensory organs, the immune system evolved to be a truth teller: across evolutionary time organisms with faulty senses didn't stand much chance of survival or reproduction. Indeed, it is only through the senses that the brain is able to accurately ascertain what its current survival and reproductive chances are. This almost certainly accounts for why it is so very difficult for our minds to argue with our senses—we can't help but believe what we see, hear, taste, touch, and smell. And anyone who has tried to do anything social or complicated in the throes of the flu knows the power of the inflammatory sensory organ to control the brain and mind.

We suspect that all sensory pathways may have promise for the treatment of MDD, based on the idea that they might be employed as "deep brain stimulators" based on the fact that they project to specific brain areas and induce species-typical emotional and behavioral reactions depending on the signals they are sending. However, several factors made us zero in first on the antidepressant potential of thermosensory pathways that run from the periphery of the body to the brain.

A first factor influencing this choice is the fact that patients with MDD show a number of thermosensory abnormalities—something that has been known, but we think underappreciated, for many years. For example the observation that depressed patients sweat less than others (as measured by skin conductance, which is an indirect measure of sweating) was first made in 1890.[13] Since then, many studies have confirmed this original observation. In fact, so reliable is the association between decreased sweating and depression that daytime resting skin conductance was proposed in the 1980s as a potentially sensitive and specific marker for depression.[14] This suggestion was based on repeated findings that mean basal skin conductance levels are lower in unmedicated or medicated depressed subjects than in controls and that low daytime resting skin conductance levels are highly predictive of MDD.[14–22] In addition, a number of studies have documented reduced skin conductance responses to auditory stimuli in depressed patients, particularly patients with psychotic depression. Moreover, studies have found that reduced sweating is particularly associated with a history of suicide attempts.[23,24] Indeed, based on a meta-analysis, the sensitivity and specificity of electrodermal hyporeactivity for suicide in depressed patients were 97 percent and 93 percent, respectively.[24]

In addition to these observations, reduced sweating, as measured by skin conductance, has also been found to correlate with changes in brain function that have been linked to depression. For example, one study showed that neural activity in the ventromedial prefrontal cortex, associated with the "default mode" of brain function that is altered in depressed patients, as well as in the orbitofrontal cortex, covaries with skin conductance level during biofeedback and relaxation tasks.[25] Other brain areas that have been associated with transient skin conductance responses include the striate and extrastriate cortices, anterior cingulate and insular cortices, and lateral regions of prefrontal cortex.[26] Highlighting the close association between thermoregulatory functioning and CNS abnormalities linked to depression is the fact that all these brain areas have been repeatedly associated with MDD.

There may be both state and trait aspects of low skin conductance levels in depressed patients. Suggesting that decreased sweating may be a trait that increases vulnerability to MDD is a study reporting that one and two years following recovery from a depressive episode subjects continued to demonstrate skin conductance levels in the low end of the normal range.[27,28] In agreement with these findings, two other studies found that skin conductance levels do not normalize in association with acute clinical recovery following treatment with antidepressants or electroconvulsive therapy.[17,29] However, other studies suggest that decreased skin conductance to at least some degree reflects the depressive state itself. For example, one study found a correlation between increased basal skin conductance levels following eight weeks of treatment with fluoxetine and percent improvement in Beck Depression Inventory scores,[30] while another found that palmar digital sweating increased in association with clinical recovery following electroconvulsive therapy.[31] The latter findings are consistent with clinical studies reporting excessive sweating (an important thermoregulatory cooling mechanism in humans) as a common side effect of treatment with most currently available antidepressant agents (e.g., tricyclic antidepressants, SSRIs, serotonin-norepinephrine reuptake inhibitors).[32] Nevertheless, the issue of whether basal skin conductance increases following successful clinical outcomes requires further study, as does the intriguing possibility that increased sweating in response to antidepressants may either portend or correlate with clinical response.

If depressed people sweat less, and if sweating is an important thermoregulatory cooling mechanism in humans, one might predict that depression would be associated with increased core body temperature. And indeed a number of studies report that individuals with affective disorders have elevated body temperature. Depressed patients have elevated temperatures compared with healthy controls during the night,[33] a time when thermoregulatory cooling responses are important for sleep onset and sleep quality.[34–36] Elevated nocturnal temperatures decrease following clinical recovery (e.g., following electroconvulsive therapy, antidepressant drug treatment, or spontaneous recovery).[33] Similarly, an increase in nocturnal temperature is also observed in the depressed phase of bipolar disorder and seasonal affective disorder.[37,38] Interestingly, despite the higher nocturnal temperature in depressed patients, there is no concomitant increase in nighttime sweating.[39] Individuals with MDD also have higher daytime (morning) temperature that is predictive of MDD.[40]

Patients with MDD have also been reported to demonstrate increased mean 24-hour core body temperature and reduced circadian temperature amplitude compared with normal controls.[41] Interestingly, when treated with electroconvulsive therapy, both absolute temperature and circadian temperature amplitude reverted to values observed in the control subjects. The short allele of the serotonin transporter polymorphism 5HTTLPR, which has been widely replicated as a risk factor for depression in response to psychosocial stress, has also been associated with increased oral body temperature in both depressed and nondepressed individuals.[40] These findings suggest that thermoregulatory cooling mechanisms are dysfunctional in depressed patients, consistent with the low basal skin conductance levels in depressed patients, but may be restored following clinical recovery. Moreover, genetic risk factors for MDD may promote hyperthermia independently of current depressive status, again pointing to the intimate relationship between thermoregulatory activity and biological mechanisms important to the pathogenesis of MDD.

The associations between MDD and thermoregulatory abnormalities suggest, at the least, that brain changes common in depression impact how well the body is able to manage its heat load. But they do not provide evidence that thermal signals arising from the body might themselves impact brain function in ways relevant to emotional health. However, studies provide many examples of just this type of "bottom up" phenomenon. Human research in embodied social cognition has explored the emotional and behavioral consequences of exposure to warm (vs. cold) objects and local ambient temperatures. This research examines the overlap between the processing of physical temperature information and any corresponding change in psychological states associated with temperature, such as metaphorical warmth or coldness (being a warm person),[42] loneliness and social exclusion,[43] and social closeness.[44,45] For example, in one study exposed participants to either a hot or iced cup of coffee and after a delay asked participants to rate an ambiguous person on traits metaphorically associated with warmth (e.g., generosity, sociability) as well as traits unrelated to warmth (e.g., strength, honesty).[42] The authors found that those exposed to the physically warm object saw more "warmth" in the ambiguously described person. Extending these findings, researchers have explored the downstream behavioral consequences of exposure to warm versus cold temperatures. Exposure to warmth led people to prefer a gift for a friend over a reward for themselves and was associated with more trusting behavior in an economic game.[42,46] In the consumption domain, researchers find that people prefer to watch romantic movies when they feel cold.[47]

Interestingly, the relationship between physical warmth and perceptions of social warmth appears to be bidirectional. Just as physical warmth promotes perceptions of social warmth, social perceptions are capable of impacting perceptions of environmental temperatures. For example, one study found that just as exposure to ambient warm temperatures led people to feel socially closer to strangers, people reported feeling physically warmer when they thought about the similarities between themselves and others (prompting social closeness).[44] Similarly, another study found that when people feel socially excluded, they feel physically colder, leading to lower estimates of ambient temperatures.[43]

Our understanding of the psychological effects of exposure to warm temperatures is bolstered by functional neuroimaging work examining the neural correlates of perceptions of physical and psychological warmth. Consistent with earlier studies, a study by Naomi Eisenberger and colleagues found that exposure to a physically warm pack (vs. a room temperature ball) led participants to report stronger feelings of social connection to close friends and family.[48] Conversely, reading positive messages from close friends and family (vs. neutral messages) led participants to report feeling physically warmer. Using functional MRI, these researchers observed that exposure to physical and social warmth cues independently activated overlapping regions of the middle insula and ventral striatum.[48] These regions have been shown to be involved with temperature perception and emotional processing.[49,50] Findings such as these, while preliminary, begin to bridge the gap between the emotional and behavioral consequences tied to physical warmth perceptions and the underlying neural mechanisms through which such consequences arise. Moreover, brain-mediated associations between psychological and physiological warmth, while metaphorical, build upon actual physiological connections between physical warmth early in life and thermoregulation. For example, a study demonstrates that skin-to-skin contact during the first 24 hours of postnatal life significantly reduces the development of hypothermia in newborns.[51]

Taken together, these findings suggest the types of bidirectional relationships between thermosensory pathways and the brain that might be utilized to develop a new treatment for MDD. However, although we were aware of these findings, our initial impetus to examine WBH as a treatment for depression came not primarily from the thermal abnormalities of MDD but, rather, from a seemingly unrelated study conducted by our friend and colleague in the hyperthermia work, Christopher Lowry, at the University of Colorado Boulder. In a highly influential paper,[52] his research group reported that injection of the saprophytic bacteria *Mycobacterium vaccae* into the skin of mice produced an antidepressant-like effect on the forced swim test (a standard method for testing potential antidepressant medications in animal models) while simultaneously activating the intrafasicular and lateroventriculuar regions of the serotonergic dorsal raphe nucleus in the midbrain. The regions activated by *M. vaccae* were already known to project strongly to the rodent analogs of brain areas most implicated in the pathogenesis of MDD, and, interestingly to brainstem and hypothalamic regions crucial for the regulation of body temperature. Lowry had multiple reasons for believing that hyperthermia should have a similar effect, so he commenced studies examining whether heating mice would produce the same type of antidepressant response and patterns of serotonergic brain nuclei activation as he had seen with *M. vaccae*. These studies confirmed his hunch: hyperthermia worked as an antidepressant on the forced swim test and demonstrated an almost exact match with *M. vaccae* in terms of its impact on serotonin pathways in the brain (M. Hale et al., unpublished observations).

Based on the theoretical considerations and animal data discussed so far, one might predict that WBH in humans would induce two testable outcomes: a reduction in depressive symptoms and a lowering of core body temperature. In addition, if WBH works, at least in part, via activation and/or sensitization of the circuit that runs from peripheral biosensors in the skin and other bodily tissues to the brain areas discussed above (via ascending thermosensory pathways) and then back to the periphery (via descending thermoregulatory cooling pathways), one might predict that depressed subjects with evidence of abnormalities in this skin-to-brain-to-skin (S2B2S) circuit might be more likely than other depressed individuals to respond clinically to WBH. Although multiple measures of S2B2S are possible based on its functional anatomy (i.e., changes in autonomic tone, sleep, immune activity), the most direct measure of its activity is likely body temperature. People with suboptimal S2B2S functioning would be expected to have impairments in thermoregulatory cooling and therefore to show elevations in core body temperature. Thus, following this line of reasoning, increased body temperature should, somewhat paradoxically, be associated with enhanced antidepressant responses to hyperthermia.

As an initial first test of these predictions, we conducted a small open trial examining the acute antidepressant effects of a single session of WBH in Switzerland with our colleagues Kay Hanusch and Clemens Janssen.[53] In 16 medically healthy adults with MDD severe enough to warrant inpatient hospitalization, we found that WBH induced a rapid, robust, and sustained reduction in depressive symptom scores, assessed with the German version of the Centers for Epidemiologic Studies Depression Scale (CES-D), based on scores dropping from a mean ± standard deviation of 29.9 ± 10.6 before treatment to 19.2 ± 12.3 five days after treatment. Thirteen of these subjects received no other pharmacological or psychotherapeutic intervention during this period. However, three subjects were on chronic treatment with an SSRI antidepressant (with no change in dosage during the study period), and when looked at separately, WBH appeared to have no effect in these three and in fact worsened depressive symptoms in one of them. This finding is consistent with preclinical data from our group showing the chronic SSRI pretreatment antagonizes the ability of hyperthermia to activate CNS serotonergic nuclei (i.e., the dorsal raphe intrafasicular and lateroventricluar regions; CA Lowry, unpublished observation). With the three subjects receiving SSRIs were removed from analysis, the effect size of WBH increased. Interestingly, the antidepressant response observed five days after treatment actually increased six weeks later in nine patients for whom longer-term follow-up data were available (CES-D mean score 13.9). Although these patients received additional treatment during this period, these findings, while preliminary, suggest that WBH may induce a rapid antidepressant response that can be solidified by longer-term modalities.

We were able to obtain 24-hour mean core body temperature at baseline and posttreatment day 5 for seven of our patients who received WBH. A single session of WBH significantly reduced mean circadian core body temperature five days after treatment (pretreatment, 37.3 ± 0.24°C; posttreatment, 37.0 ± 0.14°C), suggesting that WBH enhanced thermoregulatory cooling capability. Moreover, consistent with the possibility that the S2B2S circuit represents a functionally unified pathway, reductions in core body temperature from pretreatment to posttreatment day 5 showed a large effect size correlation with reductions in depressive symptoms over the same period. Finally as predicted, increased circadian mean core body temperature prior to treatment showed a large effect size correlation with improved CES-D depressive symptom responses five days following a single WBH session ($r[9] = 0.62$, $p = 0.043$). Although this is the first study, to our knowledge, to examine WBH specifically for MDD, our findings are consistent with reports that WBH improves mood in patients with cancer and improves quality-of-life scores in patients with type II diabetes.[54,55]

So with this background in place, let us return to Mary, our depressed research subject. It should now be more apparent why she might benefit from treatment with WBH, and why, in fact, we might be so actively pursuing the study of WBH at the University of Arizona. Unlike the study done in Switzerland, our larger-scale study includes a placebo condition, in this case a sham version of WBH that controls for everything but the intense heat. The comparison of WBH with a believable sham control was an essential next step in our work, given the very real possibility that just being placed in a strange box and heated might induce an antidepressant response based on placebo mechanisms alone. Remember our study of infliximab in "treatment-resistant" depression and our higher than 50 percent response rate? This finding forever impressed us with the fact that any novel and invasive treatment for MDD can be judged effective only when nonspecific effects have been adequately controlled for.

As it turned out, Mary was randomized to receive active WBH. Like the other female subjects in both study arms, she changed into a sports bra and gym shorts, but not before self-inserting a rectal probe so that we could monitor her core body temperature during the treatment. These preliminaries completed, we helped her settle on her back on a stretcher bed and closed the hyperthermia tent around her, so that only her head emerged. The treatment commenced, growing hotter and hotter with each passing minute. She spent approximately 90 minutes receiving active heat until her core body temperature reached 38.5°C, at which point the heat lights were turned off and she was left in the box to gradually cool down for an hour. During this hour period, her skin temperature and heart rate dropped rapidly, but, as with most subjects, her core body temperature continued to gradually rise before slowly subsiding.

Two-and-a-half hours after entering the hyperthermia device, Mary emerged slightly lightheaded and tired but with an improved mood. Over the next several days her self-reported mood continued to improve, and when our clinical raters saw her a week after her treatment she had dropped from the severely depressed range to only mild symptoms. This pattern of improvement continued gradually over the next few weeks, such that when we saw her at the end of the study her Hamilton Depression Rating Scale score had dropped just below the cut-off for clinical remission. At the time we didn't know which arm of the study she'd been randomized to, so we couldn't know for sure that it was a hyperthermia effect. But as it happened, we elected to conduct an interim analysis of our study and saw a very strong benefit for WBH compared with the sham condition.

Wanting to get more insight into the experience of our subjects who had completed the study, I met with Mary three months after she had received her WBH treatment. When I walked into the exam room I couldn't believe my eyes. She literally looked like a different human being than the one who had sobbed in the same room at the start of the study prior to receiving her treatment. She was smiling. Gone too was the slumped posture. Instead of crying in guilt over the little daughter who had been suffering through her depression, Mary had brought the little girl with her and was allowing her to color quietly on the floor. In our discussion Mary confirmed that despite having had to face ongoing life challenges she had yet to relapse back into depression. "This is the first thing that has ever really worked for me," she said. "Antidepressants helped some in the past, but not like this."

We offer all our study subjects the chance to get an active WBH treatment once they have completed the study, as a way of giving each of them the chance to receive what we increasingly think might be an active treatment modality. Almost all our subjects want this treatment and many that get it, whatever they got during the actual study, request repeat treatments. But Mary was different. When I offered her the open treatment she just smiled and said, "Thanks, but no thanks. I don't need it."

References

1. Rush AJ. STAR*D: What have we learned. *Am J Psychiatry*. 2007;164(2):201–204.
2. Cooney GM, Dwan K, Greig CA, et al. Exercise for depression. *Cochrane Datab Syst Rev*. 2013;9:CD004366.
3. Mead GE, Morley W, Campbell P, Greig CA, McMurdo M, Lawlor DA. Exercise for depression. *Cochrane Datab Syst Rev*. 2008:CD004366.
4. Dunn AL, Trivedi MH, Kampert JB, Clark CG, Chambliss HO. Exercise treatment for depression: efficacy and dose response. *Am J Prev Med*. 2005;28:1–8.
5. Rethorst CD, Wipfli BM, Landers DM. The antidepressive effects of exercise: a meta-analysis of randomized trials. *Sports Med*. 2009;39:491–511.
6. Weissman MM, Pilowsky DJ, Wickramaratne PJ, et al. Remissions in maternal depression and child psychopathology: a STAR*D-child report. *JAMA*. 2006;295:1389–1398.
7. Raison CL, Rutherford RE, Woolwine BJ, et al. A randomized controlled trial of the tumor necrosis factor antagonist infliximab for treatment-resistant depression: the role of baseline inflammatory biomarkers. *Arch Gen Psychiatry*. 2012:1–11.
8. Kikuchi H, Aramaki K, Hirohata S. Effect of infliximab in progressive neuro-Behcet's syndrome. *J Neurol Sci*. 2008;272:99–105.
9. Capuron L, Pagnoni G, Demetrashvili M, et al. Anterior cingulate activation and error processing during interferon-alpha treatment. *Biol Psychiatry*. 2005;58:190–196.
10. Haroon E, Raison CL, Miller AH. Psychoneuroimmunology meets neuropsychopharmacology: translational implications of the impact of inflammation on behavior. *Neuropsychopharmacology*. 2012;37:137–162.
11. Hamilton JP, Etkin A, Furman DJ, Lemus MG, Johnson RF, Gotlib IH. Functional neuro-

imaging of major depressive disorder: a meta-analysis and new integration of base line activation and neural response data. *Am J Psychiatry.* 2012;169:693–703.

12. Raison CL, Demetrashvili M, Capuron L, Miller AH. Neuropsychiatric adverse effects of interferon-alpha: recognition and management. *CNS Drugs.* 2005;19:105–123.

13. Vigouroux A. Étude sur la résistance électrique chez les mélancholiques [dissertation]. Paris: University of Paris; 1890.

14. Ward NG, Doerr HO, Storrie MC. Skin conductance: a potentially sensitive test for depression. *Psychiatry Res.* 1983;10:295–302.

15. Ward NG, Doerr HO. Skin conductance: a potentially sensitive and specific marker for depression. *J Nerv Ment Dis.* 1986;174:553–559.

16. Dawson ME, Schell AM, Braaten JR, Catania JJ. Diagnostic utility of autonomic measures for major depressive disorders. *Psychiatry Res.* 1985;15:261–270.

17. Dawson ME, Schell AM, Catania JJ. Autonomic correlates of depression and clinical improvement following electroconvulsive shock therapy. *Psychophysiology.* 1977;14:569–578.

18. Donat DC, McCullough JP. Psychophysiological discriminants of depression at rest and in response to stress. *J Clin Psychol.* 1983;39:315–320.

19. McCarron LT. Psychophysiological discriminants of reactive depression. *Psychophysiology.* 1973;10:223–230.

20. Williams KM, Iacono WG, Remick RA. Electrodermal activity among subtypes of depression. *Biol Psychiatry.* 1985;20:158–162.

21. Carney RM, Hong BA, Kulkarni S, Kapila A. A comparison of EMG and SCL in normal and depressed subjects. *Pavlovian J Biol Sci.* 1981;16:212–216.

22. Mirkin AM, Coppen A. Electrodermal activity in depression: clinical and biochemical correlates. *Br J Psychiatry.* 1980;137:93–97.

23. Edman G, Asberg M, Levander S, Schalling D. Skin conductance habituation and cerebrospinal fluid 5-hydroxyindoleacetic acid in suicidal patients. *Arch Gen Psychiatry.* 1986;43:586–592.

24. Thorell LH. Valid electrodermal hyporeactivity for depressive suicidal propensity offers links to cognitive theory. *Acta Psychiatr Scand.* 2009;119:338–349.

25. Nagai Y, Critchley HD, Featherstone E, Trimble MR, Dolan RJ. Activity in ventromedial prefrontal cortex covaries with sympathetic skin conductance level: a physiological account of a "default mode" of brain function. *Neuroimage.* 2004;22:243–251.

26. Raison CL, Hale MW, Williams LE, Wager TD, Lowry CA. Somatic influences on subjective well-being and affective disorders: the convergence of thermosensory and central serotonergic systems. *Front Cogn.* 2015;5:1580.

27. Iacono WG, Lykken DT, Haroian KP, Peloquin LJ, Valentine RH, Tuason VB. Electrodermal activity in euthymic patients with affective disorders: one-year retest stability and the effects of stimulus intensity and significance. *J Abnorm Psychol.* 1984;93:304–311.

28. Iacono WG, Lykken DT, Peloquin LJ, Lumry AE, Valentine RH, Tuason VB. Electrodermal activity in euthymic unipolar and bipolar affective disorders: a possible marker for depression. *Arch Gen Psychiatry.* 1983;40:557–565.

29. Storrie MC, Doerr HO, Johnson MH. Skin conductance characteristics of depressed subjects before and after therapeutic intervention. *J Nerv Ment Dis.* 1981;169:176–179.

30. Fraguas R Jr, Marci C, Fava M, et al. Autonomic reactivity to induced emotion as potential predictor of response to antidepressant treatment. *Psychiatry Res.* 2007;151:169–172.

31. Bagg CE, Crookes TG. Palmar digital sweating in women suffering from depression. *Br J Psychiatry.* 1966;112:1251–1255.

32. Marcy TR, Britton ML. Antidepressant-induced sweating. *Ann Pharmacother.* 2005;39: 748–752.

33. Avery DH, Wildschiodtz G, Rafaelsen OJ. Nocturnal temperature in affective disorder. *J Affect Disord.* 1982;4:61–71.

34. Raymann RJ, Swaab DF, Van Someren EJ. Cutaneous warming promotes sleep onset. *Am J Physiol Regul Integr Comp Physiol.* 2005;288:R1589–R1597.

35. Raymann RJ, Swaab DF, Van Someren EJ. Skin deep: enhanced sleep depth by cutaneous temperature manipulation. *Brain.* 2008;131:500–513.

36. Romeijn N, Raymann RJ, Most E, et al. Sleep, vigilance, and thermosensitivity. *Pflugers Arch.* 2012;463:169–176.

37. Souetre E, Salvati E, Wehr TA, Sack DA, Krebs B, Darcourt G. Twenty-four-hour profiles of body temperature and plasma TSH in bipolar patients during depression and during remission and in normal control subjects. *Am J Psychiatry.* 1988;145:1133–1137.

38. Schwartz PJ, Rosenthal NE, Turner EH, Drake CL, Liberty V, Wehr TA. Seasonal variation in core temperature regulation during sleep in patients with winter seasonal affective disorder. *Biol Psychiatry.* 1997;42:122–131.

39. Avery DH, Shah SH, Eder DN, Wildschiodtz G. Nocturnal sweating and temperature in depression. *Acta Psychiatr Scand.* 1999;100:295–301.

40. Rausch JL, Johnson ME, Corley KM, et al. Depressed patients have higher body temperature: 5-HT transporter long promoter region effects. *Neuropsychobiology.* 2003;47:120–127.

41. Szuba MP, Guze BH, Baxter LR Jr. Electroconvulsive therapy increases circadian amplitude and lowers core body temperature in depressed subjects. *Biol Psychiatry.* 1997;42: 1130–1137.

42. Williams LE, Bargh JA. Experiencing physical warmth promotes interpersonal warmth. *Science.* 2008;322:606–607.

43. Zhong CB, Leonardelli GJ. Cold and lonely: does social exclusion literally feel cold? *Psychol Sci.* 2008;19:838–842.

44. Ijzerman H, Semin GR. The thermometer of social relations: mapping social proximity on temperature. *Psychol Sci.* 2009;20:1214–1220.

45. Izjerman H, Semin GR. Temperature perceptions as a ground for social proximity. *J Exp Soc Psychol.* 2010;46:867–873.

46. Kang Y, Williams LE, Clark MS, Gray JR, Bargh JA. Physical temperature effects on trust behavior: the role of insula. *Soc Cogn Affect Neurosci.* 2011;6:507–515.

47. Hong J, Sun Y. Warm it up with love: the effect of physical coldness on liking of romantic movies. *J Consumer Res.* 2012;39:293–306.

48. Inagaki TK, Eisenberger NI. Shared neural mechanisms underlying social warmth and physical warmth. *Psychol Sci.* 2013;24:2272–2280.

49. Davis KD, Kwan CL, Crawley AP, Mikulis DJ. Functional MRI study of thalamic and cortical activations evoked by cutaneous heat, cold, and tactile stimuli. *J Neurophysiol.* 1998;80:1533–1546.

50. Craig AD. Pain mechanisms: labeled lines versus convergence in central processing. *Annu Rev Neurosci.* 2003;26:1–30.

51. Nimbalkar SM, Patel VK, Patel DV, Nimbalkar AS, Sethi A, Phatak A. Effect of early skin-to-skin contact following normal delivery on incidence of hypothermia in neonates more than 1800 g: randomized control trial. *J Perinatol.* 2014;34:364–368.

52. Lowry CA, Hollis JH, de Vries A, et al. Identification of an immune-responsive mesolimbocortical serotonergic system: potential role in regulation of emotional behavior. *Neuroscience.* 2007;146:756–772.

53. Hanusch KU, Janssen CH, Billheimer D, et al. Whole-body hyperthermia for the treatment of major depression: associations with thermoregulatory cooling. *Am J Psychiatry.* 2013;170:802–804.

54. Koltyn KF, Robins HI, Schmitt CL, Cohen JD, Morgan WP. Changes in mood state following whole-body hyperthermia. *Int J Hyperthermia.* 1992;8:305–307.

55. Beever R. The effects of repeated thermal therapy on quality of life in patients with type II diabetes mellitus. *J Altern Complement Med.* 2010;16:677–681.

CHAPTER 12

The Case of Anna

Mrs. Anna S. is a 43-year-old married female referred to our practice by a primary care colleague.

I was running a bit late the morning that I went to greet Mrs. S in the waiting area. She was casually browsing through one of the weekly news magazines when I addressed her and introduced myself.

After a short walk to my office, I invited Mrs. S to sit down and make herself comfortable. She quickly scanned the room before sitting down in an armchair in the corner. The autumn sky outside was overcast, and I offered to turn the lights on, but she replied that it was fine the way it was.

Mrs. S was wearing a light-colored blouse under a navy cardigan and a gray tweed skirt. She had very discrete makeup and wore no jewelry aside from small pearl earrings, visible under her shoulder-length hair, and a thin gold chain around her neck. Mrs. S was an attractive woman of medium build, maybe a few pounds over her ideal weight. Her posture was a bit stiff and tense.

"I like your artwork."

"Thank you, Mrs. S. How can I be of help to you?"

"Please call me Anna."

"How can I help you, Anna?"

"I'm not sure that you can. I don't know where to start. I have been seeing Dr. G, our family medicine doctor for a couple of years. He has been treating me for depression. I feel much better now, and I don't want to be a whiner, but it is still not right. Maybe I expect too much—maybe this is as good as it will ever be for me? I'm sorry, I don't want to waste your time. I'm sure there are some really sick people out there who are in a greater need of your services."

I reassured Anna that visiting a psychiatrist can be quite anxiety pro-voking, and that if she is here, she probably has a good reason.

Anna smiled and relaxed a bit. "I almost changed my mind this morn-ing. I felt so anxious that I got sick to my stomach."

"So you mentioned that you have been feeling depressed?"

"I don't know if I would call it depression at this point. I just feel distant. Even when I read to my kids at night or laugh at their goofy jokes, I feel like a phony."

"A phony?"

"Like I'm not fully there, like I'm faking it. I'm not fully emotionally engaged. When I wake up in the morning I don't really feel like going to work. I make myself, but my heart is not really in it."

"What kind of work do you do?"

"I'm an accountant. Fall is pretty busy for us—people are in to discuss their deductions and investments. The market has been all over the place lately, so everybody is nervous and panicky. Sometimes it is hard to be empathetic when my thoughts are elsewhere."

"Has it been difficult to concentrate? Do you find yourself getting dis-tracted?"

"I don't know if I would say it is difficult, but my mind does drift a bit, and I have to go over my work to make sure I don't make any mistakes. I have been more scattered and forgetful lately. Usually I'm much more on top of things."

"You mentioned that you were seeing Dr. G. Has he initiated antidepres-sant treatment? Are you seeing a therapist?"

"Yes, I'm taking an antidepressant." She mentioned a name of a fre-quently prescribed selective serotonin reuptake inhibitor (SSRI). "It has helped a lot. I no longer feel weepy, and I'm getting things done around the house. Last winter, when it was really bad, I had stacks of laundry lying everywhere. Even when it was done, I didn't really feel like folding it. For a while my husband and kids would just get their stuff off the pile and take it to their rooms. You must think that I'm a slob, but that is not how I usually am. I'm a very organized person. I don't like clutter in my home. I felt so guilty, like I was letting everyone down. At times, I even wondered if they would be better off without me. It sounds dumb, I know, and I have never seriously considered killing myself. I could never do that to my kids. Grow-ing up my family was screwed up, and I'm still not fully healed from it. The last thing I would want to do is burden my children with their mother's sui-cide. It would be so selfish.

"It was really bad, though. I stopped cooking for a while. I had no energy after work. When I came home, I headed straight for the bedroom. After a nap, we would go out for fast food or order take-out. Sometimes, my husband would just heat up frozen food. Neither the kids nor my husband seemed to mind terribly, but it did bother me. Once I overheard the kids asking my husband if I was all right, because before this I'd always tried to make sure that we all ate healthy."

She glanced at her waist and blushed with a bit of chagrin. "I used to have a nice figure. Over the last couple of years when I would get down, I ate more. It's not like I was really hungry—I just snacked to feel better. Of course, it never worked. I would just get more frustrated and tell myself that I was turning into a fat pig. In the morning when I was getting ready for work, I avoided looking at myself in the mirror. You must think that I'm a vain and self-centered woman."

I replied that many people have difficulty regulating their appetite when their mood is off.

"I know its silly, but on top of everything I feared that my husband was going to have an affair or something, that he was going to leave us. I know that sounds crazy, because he is the last guy on earth who would do something like that. He is a typical engineer type, not very 'touchy-feely,' but you can always rely on him.

"We have had some tensions in the last few months. Things have not been going so well in the bedroom lately. I have gained weight, so maybe I feel more self-conscious. I don't feel very attractive or confident. I don't think that my medications have helped, either. A friend of mine, who also takes antidepressants, told me that they totally killed her sex life."

I agreed that antidepressants of the type that she is taking have been known to cause sexual side effects. "What kind of difficulties are you having—do you have less interest, or is it harder to reach climax?"

"Well, you don't go beating around the bush!" Anna blushed a bit and looked uneasy, averting her gaze to the painting on the side wall before reestablishing eye contact. "I'm not comfortable discussing my private life with strangers, but you are a doctor I guess. Jim, my husband, and I have never been a best match. Let's just say that our timing has always been a bit off. It may be silly, but I felt that he was always more focused on the mechanics of what he was doing than on me. Anyway, I have just not been in the mood lately. I stay up watching stupid TV programs until he falls asleep. Then I check on the kids before going to the bedroom. Fortunately, most of the time he is already snoozing by the time I get in. I try not to wake him up. I'm really not up for having awkward conversations at the end of the day. He has not said anything so far, but I know it bothers him. He has been very grumpy and more withdrawn. We argue more, about trivial things that don't really matter to either one of us. We don't even touch anymore when we watch TV together. It is like we are becoming roommates." She became pensive. "I guess it is worse than I thought. Should we change my antidepressant?"

"We will definitely discuss some alternatives, but before that I would like to learn more about your experience of depression. You mentioned that your mind drifts a bit at work. Sometimes that can happen if you are preoccupied or you have not slept well?"

"I have not slept well ever since my teenage years even though I often feel tired during the day. Sometimes I wish I could take a nap at work. I have hard time falling asleep at night. My mind just keeps on going—it won't turn off. I try to figure out why I feel the way I do, why I'm depressed and tired, why I can't fall asleep. Other people face more severe problems in their lives—how come I'm depressed? Is it because of the things that have happened in the past, or is my brain just not working right? Once this merry-go-round starts, I cannot get off. In the past, whenever I was out of sorts, I would go to my 'happy memory place.' It would calm me and make me feel better. Lately, when I'm keyed up, I can no longer reach those happy memories. Sometimes reading works, and I'm able to fall asleep. At other times I have to take a sleeping pill." She named a commonly prescribed benzodiazepine receptor modulator, indicated for sleep induction. "Most of the time it works well and I sleep at least until 5:30 or 6 a.m. At other times I wake up at 3 a.m. and toss and turn. Occasionally it takes me half an hour before I can fall back asleep. Sometimes I even go downstairs and make myself a snack. When I wake up, I feel groggy until my first cup of coffee. Even the kids know better than to ask me anything before my first cup. I guess it's that obvious. After the shower, though, I'm usually ready to go."

Ruminations are one of the most prominent symptoms of depression. Although they do not figure prominently in the diagnostic criteria, ruminations may be in the center of the spider web of depressive pathophysiology. Depressive ruminations can be conceived of as passive and repetitive dwelling on the causes, meaning, and unrelenting nature of sadness and symptoms of distress.[1,2] Several authors differentiate among components of rumination; self-reflection, which may have a more adaptive aspect; and brooding, which may have a causal association with depression, especially in individuals who have experienced childhood abuse.[3,4] Passivity, feeling stuck, and fixation on problems, their causes, and accompanying feelings rather then active coping is an important feature of ruminations.[1]

Ruminations predict the onset, severity, and duration of depression. They also promote an attentional bias toward negative information and diminish memory for positive experiences and the ability to utilize positive distractors, while increasing the tendency to overgeneralize from autobiographical memories, which often diverts attention from tasks on hand and causes problems with occupational and academic functioning.[1,5–8] Self-criticism, pessimism, hopelessness, and even suicidality in depressed individuals are all related to ruminative tendencies.[1,3] Women are more likely to ruminate than men and to engage in binging behaviors and alcohol use as a way of coping with dysphoric ruminations.[9]

Furthermore, depressive ruminations may interfere with social relationships. Social anxiety and depression are associated with more rumination following a social gathering and more pronounced negative feelings related to small talk.[10] Rumination-prone individuals are also likely to provide the most pessimistic explanations for interpersonal problems and engage family and friends in ways that are counterproductive and likely to engender friction. A final consequence of disappointing social interactions may be the avoidance of social events and a tendency toward escapist behavior.[9,11] Women with a chronic ruminative style suffer greater distress in the face of general somatic symptoms and are less likely to be compliant with medication regimens.[9]

It may be warranted to distinguish ruminations that are mostly past/present oriented from worries that are mostly future oriented and focused on anticipation and preparation for an oncoming dangerous/threatening event.[9,12] Individuals with high levels of ruminative activity, compared with ones with little rumination, are more likely to experience low sleep efficiency, wakening after sleep onset, poor sleep quality, disturbances in the regulation of arousal, fatigue, and concentration problems.[12] Furthermore, research suggests that the degree of ruminations at baseline predicts impaired cognitive control for emotional information and depressive symptoms a year later.[13]

We believe that we have made a good case for ruminations as a central factor of Anna's depressive experience. Will imaging studies provide a deeper understanding of this phenomenon and provide some guidance for helping Anna? We review imaging and genetic findings in some detail in previous chapters, so here we quickly recapitulate information that may have some bearing on Anna's clinical management. Anna's genetic predisposition is unknown to us, but if she had at-risk brain-derived neurotrophic factor and serotonin (5HT) transporter 5HTTLPR alleles, her recent life stress (work and marital issues) would put her at a greater risk for developing ruminations.[14] Furthermore, a high propensity toward ruminations/brooding interacts with dyadic adjustment (currently problematic in Anna's life) to predict increased depression persistence and severity.[15]

Resting functional networks are discussed in some detail in Chapter 8, so we provide a quick refresher here. The salience network (SN) includes a number of subcortical limbic structures, including thalamus and parts of the basal ganglia. Its major hubs are the subgenual anterior cingulate cortex (sgACC) and insula. The main role of the SN is to collect information about relevant changes in the environment while integrating sensory and emotional flow and engaging the executive network (EN) when necessary to initiate an adaptive response. The main hubs of EN are the dorsolateral prefontal cortex (dlPFC) and posterior parietal cortex. Some authors also include the superior temporal gyrus. The primary purpose of the EN is to process relevant sensory/emotional information, allocate attentional resources, store information in working memory, mount an adaptive response, and monitor its execution. When we are not actively engaged in a problem-solving mode, the default-mode network (DMN) may become more active. Self-reflection, rumination, planning future activity, processing social information, creative thinking, and reminiscing about past autobiographical events are all in the domain of the DMN. Principal nodes of the DMN include the ventromedial PFC (vmPFC), dorsomedial PFC (dmPFC), and precuneus/posterior cingulate complex (PCC). Some authors also include mesotemporal structures, primarily the hippocampus, in the DMN.

In healthy circumstances an influx of important information from the SN engages the EN, interrupting DMN activity. However, that does not always happen in major depressive disorder (MDD). Stressful life events may generate maladaptive communication patterns between the SN and DMN, exemplified by aberrant connectivity between the sgACC and PCC, which precipitates brooding and ruminative preoccupation with negative emotional states.[16,17] Unfortunately, ruminations based on aberrant SN-DMN coupling may become a self-perpetuating process. This is borne out in imaging studies, which have provided evidence that the duration of depressive episodes correlates inversely with the degree of connection between sgACC (an SN structure) and DMN components.[18] This of course gives Anna's situation some urgency, since she has suffered for an extended period of time.

Unfortunately, this is not where the story ends. In depressed individuals the mediodorsal PFC acts as a "dorsal nexus," short-circuiting all three networks together.[19] A likely consequence of this "hot-wiring" among the DMN, EN, and SN is an excessive self-focus and a proclivity toward rumination, which interferes with attention to cognitive tasks, accompanied by emotional and autonomic dysregulation.[19] Anna's predicament bears a clear resemblance to this scenario. Additionally, a state of hyperarousal may be a major contributor to Anna's sleep problems. How can we utilize this neurobiologically based information to help her?

Imaging studies have uncovered evidence that a dopamine-regulated cortico-striato-pallido-thalamo-cortical circuit may be malfunctional in depression. Several components of this neural loop also belong to the SN. Researchers have suggested a two-stage model. Mutual excitatory connections between insula, amygdala, dorsal anterior cingulate cortex (dACC), and thalamic pulvinar may be overly active in depression, "trapping" and amplifying negatively valenced emotional information in this subsection of the SN. At the same time, low striatal dopamine activity hinders the transfer of salient information from the dorsal caudate to the dlPFC (a major hub of the EN).[20] Therefore, negative emotionality is no longer subject to critical scrutiny and EN-initiated corrective responses. Studies that have described decreased connectivity between the caudate and PCC (a DMN hub) and diminished intra-EN connectivity, accompanied by elevated intra-DMN connectivity, further support and extend the previous findings.[21,22]

If the goal is deactivation of excessive DMN activity, enhancement of EN function, and consequent improvement of SN modulation, can pharmacological intervention be helpful? If so, which agent would be most effective? What would be the role of psychotherapy? Preliminary evidence suggests that antidepressants may be beneficial as they increase the activity in dlPFC and ventrolateral PFC, key EN areas also involved in the "top-down" regulation of emotions, and at the same time decrease activity in the SN-related amygdala, insula, and sgACC.[23] Furthermore, imaging studies evaluating antidepressant effects have found evidence of therapeutic DMN suppression and normalized connectivity.[23,24]

There is insufficient evidence at this time to conclude which antidepressant would be optimal to address Anna's multiple concerns. A preliminary chart-review study has found some evidence that individuals with irritability and ruminations may respond better to an SSRI, while driven, exercise- and achievement-oriented persons may do better with bupropion, a norepinephrine–dopamine reuptake inhibitor (NDRI).[25] These findings need to be replicated in controlled prospective studies. In other words, neuroscience research has provided us with useful information about the neural underpinning of ruminations, but thus far neurobiological studies have provided little guidance for selecting the most appropriate antidepressant for any given patient. Is there any indication that psychotherapy may be more helpful? Can residual symptoms or side effects help us make more optimal treatment choices?

> "You mentioned that your mind keeps on going at night, that it won't turn off. Are your thoughts racing?"
>
> "No, not really. And I'm not bipolar, if that is what you mean. I already went over all that stuff with my family doctor, he even had me fill out a questionnaire. I think, it is just plain old depression—nothing too exotic about me."
>
> "Are there some recurring thoughts or worries that you have at night?"
>
> Anna became visibly uncomfortable and shifted in her chair, recrossing her legs. "Sometimes there are, but I would rather not talk about it, if that's OK with you. There is some garbage from my past. My family was very dysfunctional when my brother and I were growing up. I went through most of it with my therapist in college, and I would rather not drudge it up again, if it's OK with you. It would just make me feel even more miserable, and besides, I don't think it has anything to do with my depression right now."
>
> "OK, we can leave it for some other time, if you feel like talking about it later. Have you seen any changes in your energy levels, or enthusiasm, in the last few months?"

"What energy? I'm just kidding. It has been better since I have started this new antidepressant last spring. As I mentioned, last winter was awful. I could barely function—everything made me cry. It is still hard to motivate myself to do things, but it's much better compared to how it was. At least I can sit down with my kids again and go over their homework. Math is still frustrating, though. Our son is struggling with it. I let my husband deal with math—he's much more patient.

"I'm all over the place. Yes, you asked me about my energy and motivation?"

"And enthusiasm . . ."

"Right, as I said, everyday life is still a chore, but at least I'm getting things done. I don't have a whole lot of enthusiasm about socializing and going out. My husband is not exactly a social butterfly, so it is mostly up to me to keep up with the family and our friends. To be honest with you, I don't really look forward to Thanksgiving. It's our turn to drive to my in-laws. His sister and brother-in-law are also going to be there. They are all nice people, but I really don't feel like talking with them. Am I awful for saying that?"

"Sometimes if our mood is off, it is harder to socialize."

"Absolutely. It was never a blast, but we used to have a good time, once we would get there. My in-laws have a bit of land around their home, and the kids loved to go exploring down by the creek.

"It is not only family visits. We used to get a babysitter and take dancing classes together. My husband was never Fred Astaire, but we would laugh and have a good time. It is just too much of a hassle now. We've probably not gone dancing in over a year. You might not see it now by looking at me, but I used to exercise regularly. Now that I could really afford to lose a few pounds, I just can't make myself do it. If it wasn't for walking the dog in the neighborhood, I don't know if we would even get out of the house.

"I love to read mystery novels at night, it is one of my little guilty pleasures. Chocolate is the other." Anna giggled. "I have been reading the same book for two months, it just does not pull me in the way it used to. Even chocolate doesn't taste as good. What is the world coming to? My depression must be worse than I thought," Anna said with a wry smile.

"Please don't misunderstand me, I'm not hopeless or desperate. My emotions just feel flat. Nothing excites me anymore—even food has less flavor. I would like colors in my life to be a bit more vivid, if you know what I mean. Do you think that some of this 'flat' feeling, some of my indifference may be caused by my medicine? Even if it isn't, is there another antidepressant that would have fewer sexual side effects? I'm a bit hesitant to switch, because I don't want to go back to feeling the way I did last winter, but I would rather not feel like I do now, either."

In the next segment of the intake interview, I collected information about Mr. S's family, past psychiatric, and medical history. We also spoke about habits and her social history and conducted a mental status exam. Here is the most relevant information.

Anna grew up in a suburban middle class family. She was nine and her younger brother six years old when her parents divorced after years of a "dysfunctional" marriage. Anna remembers their screaming fights at night, which her parents often denied the next morning. They would tell Anna that she just had bad dreams. She knew that they were lying because she found fragments of dishes broken during the previous night's argument. Whenever a fight started, she would take her younger brother by the hand and lead him to her room. They would watch TV shows with the volume up to drown out the noise of the escalating argument.

Anna's father moved away soon after the divorce due to a new work assignment. Her mother remarried when Anna was in middle school. She described her stepfather as a kind, although a bit "milk-toasty" kind of man. She missed her father, whom she later saw only during holidays and summer vacations. They kept in touch regularly by phone until her father remarried, several years later. Phone conversations continued to be warm, although a bit less frequent.

Anna developed her first depressive episode during her freshman year in college. She had a hard time adjusting to the new setting and a roommate who liked to party a lot and left the sink messy. Anna missed home and did not have an easy time making friends. She was always a very good student in high school, so her first C in college came as a shock. She started doubting her abilities and felt isolated. Shortly after returning to school after Thanksgiving, Anna found herself worrying about her final exams. She feared that this was just the beginning of her downfall. Her father was showing less interest in her since starting a new family. Recent conversations were mostly about school and grades. She ruminated increasingly on the possibility that she might fail at college and disappoint everyone. Maybe she really was not as smart as she thought; maybe her teachers in middle school gave her a break because she came from a broken home. No one in the cafeteria seemed too eager to start a conversation with her, it felt so awkward.

These negative thoughts would haunt her. At times she almost didn't want to go to sleep, just to avoid these upsetting thoughts. She became even more withdrawn. When she attempted to start a conversation with other students from her class, they appeared to be disinterested and disengaged. Loneliness and insomnia were becoming too difficult to bear. No amount of coffee seemed to be helpful enough. She studied hard but retained very little. It got so bad that she had a hard time getting out of bed and started skipping showers. She wore the same jeans for several weeks. Anna's adviser suggested that she might want to see a therapist in the student mental health service. Anna said that therapy helped a lot, because there were many things she needed to get off her chest. With the help of psychotherapy her mood lifted toward the end of winter. Although her first semester grades were "not great," her school performance significantly improved in the spring semester.

Anna's second depressive episode occurred at the age of 27, after the birth of her son. She felt very sad and dejected. Anna found herself crying frequently, often without a reason. She felt tired all the time, although Anna initially attributed her fatigue to having to wake up during the night to nurse the baby. Her whole life felt like it "was shrouded in a dark cloud. It was supposed to be the happiest part of my life, and I couldn't even enjoy my baby." Anna started doubting if she was cut out to be a mother. Her husband did not seem to be as interested in her. He had not approached her sexually in months, not that she was in the mood anyway. Anna would look at herself in the mirror and wondered who could possibly want her if her husband left. Maybe he was having an affair? They had just moved to a new town because of her husband's work, so she had very few acquaintances and felt isolated. Whenever they went to her husband's company parties, all the wives and girlfriends seemed more interested in talking to each other than to her. Anna tried hard to be a good conversationalist and make friends, but even women to whom she listened for an hour would not remember her name on the next occasion. These dark brooding thoughts made her depression more profound.

She saw her Ob/Gyn, who prescribed a new antidepressant, an early selective 5HT-norepinephrine reuptake inhibitor (SNRI). "At first it made me sick, but my doctor adjusted the dose. Several weeks later, I was much better. Although my mind was still foggy, and I was not sleeping well, at least I could function." Anna continued to take medication for several more months before stopping it, because she "no longer benefited from it." Additionally, she had sexual side effects on the antidepressant and wanted to get her marriage "back on track" now that her mood was better.

The most recent depressive episode started in the fall of last year. It felt similar to the previous ones, so she wasted no time in seeing her family doctor. An SSRI trial was initiated, since Anna did not wish to retry the SNRI due to previously experienced side effects.

Anna's mother had suffered from multiple depressive episodes. She believes that her maternal aunt may have also suffered from depression, but she is not sure because her aunt moved to Australia decades ago, and they have had very little contact since. Anna thinks that her mother has been treated with antidepressants, but she does not know which ones. "We don't usually talk about that stuff." I suggested that it would be helpful to find out which antidepressants her mother was treated with and what her response was like to these medicines. Anna said that it would be no problem to ask, she was sure that her mother would be glad to help.

Anna denied past drug use, aside from a couple of occasions when she tried "pot" in college. She couldn't get high, so she never bothered trying again. Anna never smoked tobacco. She admitted to occasional alcohol use. After her husband goes to sleep, she will sometimes have a couple of glasses of wine to unwind after a rough day.

Her past medical history is unremarkable, aside from tonsillectomy when she was seven years old and ongoing treatment of dyslipidemia with one of the statins since last year. Anna was not aware of any medication allergies.

At this point we engaged in a discussion of treatment options. I mentioned that marital therapy focused on improving her relationship with her husband might also help her mood. Furthermore, individual therapy might help Anna feel more comfortable in social situations and address the source of her perseverative "dark thoughts," which seem to augment depressive feelings and interfere with her sleep.

Anna indicated that she was not quite willing to "open up that can of worms right now" and that she would rather explore a medication adjustment. She wondered if there was an antidepressant that would help with her low energy, lack of enthusiasm, and memory problems without causing any more weight gain or sexual side effects. Anna also expressed concern about discontinuing her current antidepressant, if there was no guarantee that the "new one would work any better. I really don't want to go back to feeling the way I did the last winter."

I shared with her that there is an antidepressant known for modulating norepinephrine and dopamine transmission that could be combined with her current medication. This medicine, called bupropion, has some evidence of added effectiveness in patients who have experienced low energy, diminished ability to enjoy life, and antidepressant induced sexual side effects. It is also unlikely to contribute to weight gain. Furthermore, exercise may be a helpful adjunct, as the evidence suggests that it may help increase her energy and ameliorate antidepressant-related sexual side effects.

Does it make sense to add another antidepressant, rather then switching to a different medication? And if so, which antidepressant might be a good choice for Anna? Common wisdom would suggest that if a patient has had a partial response, adding an antidepressant may be a better choice than switching agents. Although switching to a different antidepressant class may minimize some of the presumably SSRI-related adverse reactions such as apathy, cognitive difficulties, and sexual side effects, large-scale studies, such as the STAR*D (Sequenced Treatment Alterna-tives to Relieve Depression) and GSRD (European Group for the Study of Resistant Depression), have found either only minimal benefit of switching from an SSRI to another SSRI, SNRI, or NDRI, or even a detriment, since patients who remained on the original antidepressant in GSRD did better than individuals who were switched to a different agent.[26–31] Based on STAR*D, switching to a different class of antide-pressant was no more effective than choosing another medication within the same class.[30] So who would do better by augmenting an existing antidepressant than by switching to a new one? Study data tentatively suggest that patients who have had a partial response and have tolerated the initial antidepressant may have a greater benefit from augmentation versus switching to another agent.[32]

Would an augmentation with psychotherapy be more advantageous to the patient? Possibly. Anna has marital issues that need to be addressed; moreover, cognitive-behavioral therapy (CBT) has proven value in the treatment of insom-nia[33] and may reduce the long-term risk of relapse and recurrence compared with antidepressant alone.[34] Moreover, unlike adding a second antidepressant, CBT would not potentially increase the side-effect burden of her treatment. Unfortu-nately, 71 percent of participants in STAR*D did not accept cognitive therapy,[35] and patient preference significantly influences treatment outcome.[36] Moreover, pharmacological augmentation may be more rapidly effective than addition of cognitive therapy.[37]

Bupropion is an NDRI, with predominantly noradrenergic activity, most likely attributable to its active metabolite hydroxybupropion. Bupropion is also possibly a nicotinic receptor modulator.[38,39] In healthy volunteers prolonged use of bupropion had stimulant-like effects, based on its tendency to decrease asthenia-fatigue, elevate blood pressure and body temperature, impair sleep onset, and cause weight loss.[40] Bupropion appears to have an overall antidepressant efficacy comparable to SSRIs, even in anxious depressed patients, with fewer complaints of somnolence, asthenia, and sexual dysfunction.[41,42] Controlled studies indicate that bupropion may be more effective than SSRIs in ameliorating hypersomno-lence and fatigue in the context of MDD.[43]

Although combining bupropion (an NDRI)[44,45] with an SSRI to provide an overall amelioration of depressive symptomatology remains controversial, this strategy may have an advantage in specific symptom domains and side-effect profile. For example, an open-label retrospective study reported an increase in energy and motivation in depressed patients treated with a combination of bupro-pion and a 5HT reuptake inhibitor (SRI) compared with an SRI alone.[47] Other studies have also reported symptomatic benefits from augmenting SSRIs with bupropion, but this is not a consistent finding.[46] Furthermore, there is limited evidence, based mostly from open-label and a few controlled studies, that bupro-pion can reverse sexual side effects of SSRIs, and only anecdotal evidence that it can reduce weight gain caused by SSRIs.[48] Apathy and emotional detachment can both accompany SSRI treatment; unfortunately, little research has investigated potential benefits from adjunct bupropion in ameliorating these undesirable SSRI effects.[28,48]

Are there any neuroscience advancements that could help us with our treatment choice? Would pharmacological manipulation of norepinephrine and dopamine signaling be ameliorative based on what we know of the neurobiological underpinning of sexual function/dysfunction, memory processes, apathy and cognition? Neuroimaging studies indicate that anhedonia in depression may be associated with decreased activity in the ventral striatum/nucleus accumbens (NAcc), dmPFC, and putamen.[49,50] Trait anhedonia in healthy individuals was associated with diminished activity in some of the same areas, including the NAcc and the basal forebrain, which are linked to the dopaminergic ventral tegmental area via the medial forebrain bundle.[51] Furthermore, an MRI study noted substantially reduced dopaminergic function in the NAcc, caudate, putamen, and dorsal brainstem of depressed patients suffering from marked affective flattening, compared with healthy controls.[52] What's more, patients who had the greatest improvement in positive affect following two months of antidepressant treatment demonstrated the largest increases in NAcc activity and frontolimbic connectivity, as established by functional MRI.[53] In summary, neurobiological evidence points to reduced ventral striatum activity and excessive activation of the vmPFC/orbitofrontal PFC, most likely related to inadequate dopamine transmission, as the main culprits behind anhedonia in MDD.[54]

Preclinical evidence suggests that there is significant crosstalk between the dopamine, norepinephrine, and 5HT signaling systems. While activation of several 5HT receptors, such as 5HT1A/B, 5HT2A, 5HT3, and 5HT4, has a facilitatory influence on dopamine release, stimulation of 5HT2C receptors inhibits dopamine transmission.[55] This is of particular relevance because the 5HT2C receptor has high levels of constitutive activity and is therefore most likely to be affected by sustained 5HT elevation due to SSRI use.[55] Moreover, apathy related to SSRI use has also been attributed to decreased noradrenergic transmission due to 5HT2C overactivation.[28] Even patients who were deemed responders following three months of SSRI treatment had high rates of impairment due to apathy (32.5 percent), sleepiness (52.3 percent), fatigue (48.8 percent), inattentiveness (35.9 percent), and forgetfulness (53.1 percent).[56] Interestingly, PFC and limbic areas involved in cognitive/executive function, working memory, regulation of arousal, and processing rewards are heavily innervated by dopamine and norepinephrine fibers, which are also subject to 5HT regulation.[57–59] While SSRIs may ameliorate depressive and anxious symptoms by enhancing 5HT transmission in limbic and paralimbic cortical areas, they may at the same time persistently activate 5HT2A/C receptors, thereby dampening norepinephrine and dopamine activity, thus contributing to residual symptoms of fatigue and anhedonia so often noted even after an overall positive response to SSRIs.[59]

Brain reward circuitry, which includes the NAcc, medial PFC, hippocampus, and parts of the thalamus, is generously innervated by mesolimbic and mesocortical dopaminergic projections originating from the mesencephalic ventral tegmental area.[60] Imaging evidence indicates that dopaminergic inputs to the NAcc play an excitatory role in the regulation of sexual arousal. Both estrogen and testosterone upregulate basal and stimulated dopamine release in the NAcc.[60] Consistent reports from imaging studies have implicated the reward system in response to sexual stimuli. The hypothalamus, ventral striatum/NAcc, and ACC are all involved in response to sexual intensity. Both the ACC and the insula have been implicated in interactions between sexual intensity and emotional valence.[60,61] The degree of insula activation may reflect the quality of orgasm in women. Several of the same areas, including the amygdala, thalamus, orbitofrontal PFC, ACC, insula, ventral striatum, and hypothalamus, have a role in sexual desire and arousal.[62] Most of these areas are components of the SN, which has altered connectivity in MDD. Interestingly, aberrant connectivity and information processing in DMN- and SN-related areas has also been implicated in sexual dysfunction and rumination.[63,64] In conclusion, proper dopaminergic transmission in the limbic and paralimbic areas, including the NAcc, is of paramount relevance in regulating healthy sexual behavior.[60]

Chronic administration of an SSRI to healthy individuals was found to diminish neural responses to erotic stimulation in the ACC (including sgACC, pregenual ACC, and mid-cingulate) and ventral striatum/NAcc and mesencephalon compared with placebo-treated individuals. Conversely, bupropion dosing was associated with unchanged or increased activity, relative to placebo, in the mid-cingulate, portions of the thalamus, extended amygdala, and NAcc. While SSRI usage was associated with reported sexual dysfunction, bupropion-treated subjects experienced either no change or improvement in their subjective ratings compared with placebo-treated subjects.[65,66] Another crossover study reported that, compared with individuals receiving placebo, SSRI-treated individuals had diminished response in the ventral striatum, vmPFC, and orbitofrontal PFC.[67] One could speculate that SSRI-induced changes in components of reward circuitry following pleasurable/erotic stimulation may in part be responsible for the sexual side effects of these medications.

An additional factor that may contribute to SSRI-induced sexual dysfunction involves SSRI-induced prolactin release. Dopamine and 5HT have opposing influences on prolactin secretion from the pituitary gland. Dopaminergic activation of D2 receptors via tuberoinfundibilar dopamine neurons inhibits prolactin release, whereas 5HT facilitates prolactin release by interacting with 5HT2A/C receptors.[68] Several clinical studies have reported increased peripheral prolactin levels related to the use of SSRIs or tricyclics with powerful serotonergic activity.[69-72] One of these studies discovered that 22 percent of women treated with a 12-week course of fluoxetine developed hyperprolactinemia.[73]

Prolactin and dopamine may represent another yin-and-yang regulatory coupling of sexual behavior. While dopamine has an important role in stimulating sexual desire and mediating orgasmic experience, prolactin seems to provide feedback inhibition of sexual drive, at least in part by modulating mesolimbic dopaminergic activity.[74] Clinical research has established that female orgasm may be associated with a more pronounced pituitary response and prolactin release than is male ejaculation.[75] Furthermore, postorgasmic prolactin release following intercourse is greater than after masturbatory activity, possibly producing a greater state of satiety.[76] The degree of prolactin elevation, which appears necessary to suppress libido in association with SSRI use, has not been sufficiently explored. Unlike SSRIs, bupropion is not associated with prolactin elevation.[77]

With all this in mind, below we summarize scientific evidence that may help guide Anna's treatment decisions.

"Great—if my energy improves I may start exercising again," remarked Anna.

I agreed that exercise would be a very helpful component of her treatment, and it may even help her sleep. I again reiterated that medicines may not be the answer to all her difficulties and that she might want to give psychotherapy some additional consideration. Anna agreed, although she did not appear to be persuaded by my arguments. After reviewing the expected benefits and common adverse reactions associated with the new antidepressant, Anna left with a bupropion prescription and directions to take one tablet in the morning for four to five days; if she tolerated the medicine well, she was then to increase her dose to two tablets daily.

EXCERPTS FROM THE OFFICE NOTES

Anna S is a 43-year-old married female suffering from recurrent depression.

First episode: 18 years of age, treated with psychotherapy, spontaneously resolved.

Second episode: 27 years of age (postpartum), treated with an SNRI, effective, acute GI side effects, sexual side effects contributed to medication discontinuation.

Third episode: Fall last year until this spring, presented with sad mood, decreased motivation, diminished ability to enjoy life, difficulty concentrating, low energy, sleep disturbance, frequent crying, hopelessness, and passive suicidal ideation. Partially successful treatment with an SSRI. Side effects: decreased libido, possibly SSRI-induced psychasthenia, and weight gain.

Present symptoms: Mildly depressed; anxious; distracted; frequently ruminates; suboptimal energy, enthusiasm, and ability to enjoy life; low libido (possibly due to SSRI).

Perpetuating factors: Marital tension, work-related stress, possibly unresolved
  issues related to an earlier trauma?
Relevant family history: Likely depression in mother and maternal aunt.
Plan: Bupropion augmentation, continue the SSRI and as-needed hypnotic
  agent, encourage exercise, individual and family therapy

Second Session, Three Weeks Later
Anna called two days before her scheduled appointment to ask if she could
increase her sleeping medicine. While she was excited about the benefits
from the new antidepressant, her sleep had become more problematic, and
there were other issues that she wanted to discuss.

Anna's affect appeared much brighter. She wore a brighter-colored
blouse with a navy knit skirt and more distinct makeup than on her first
visit. However, Anna's tension was betrayed by short, rapid swinging of her
lower leg and circular motions of her foot.

"Would you like me to start with good news, or not so good news?"

"Wherever you would like."

"I have more energy, that's good news. I think that even my concentration has somewhat improved. I'm getting more things done in the office,
anyway. I was able to go to two exercise classes last week, so I guess my
motivation is also better. I'm no longer as 'sexually dead' as I was, but I'm
not sure that I'm ready to resume intimacy with my husband. That is a complicated story, I'm not sure that I want to get into it today.

"After feeling a bit dizzy and queasy the first week, the medicine has
not been bothering me. Here is what troubles me. My sleep is getting
worse. It takes me forever to fall asleep. Then I have these very vivid, life-
like, troubling dreams, which wake me up. Although my energy is better, if I
don't get some good sleep soon, I don't know how long I will be able to function."

"You mentioned previously that you have some bothersome thoughts
before going to sleep. Now, you also have disturbing dreams. Is this something that you feel comfortable talking about?"

"Not really. But I guess I will have to tell you about it sooner or later.
Otherwise you are just going to keep on asking about it anyway." Anna had
a hint of a weary smile.

I assured her that she did not need to talk about any subject until she felt
ready.

"I will never really be ready. I might as well tell you about it now. I was
sexually abused as a teenager. It happened a couple of years after my parent's divorce. I felt so lonely and lost that swimming became my refuge.
When I was in the pool, swimming countless laps, all my worries were
washed away. At the end of the practice I would feel completely exhausted

and totally relaxed. Our swimming team coach seemed to take a special interest in me. I enjoyed his compliments and words of encouragement. I was only 14 but was already developing as a woman. One evening after a late practice, I was in the shower. The last girl had left the dressing room fifteen minutes earlier. I was late since the coach was helping me with the butterfly technique. He came in, apologizing that the hot water was not working in the men's dressing room. I was speechless and paralyzed, peeking from behind the curtain. He took his trunks off and turned the water on in the shower stall next to mine. I think that you can guess what happened next.

"Anyway, we didn't have sex that first time around. He begged for me not to tell anyone. He said that he would be fired right away. I'm sure that he was right. I kept my silence. It was so terribly confusing. Later, I found out that he was married and had a young child. I cannot tell you how awful and guilty I felt. On one hand I knew that what was going on was wrong. On the other hand—I'm embarrassed to say this—it was also exciting and at times even pleasurable.

"The fact that I liked some of it made it so much worse. I could not sleep at night. I was throwing up almost every evening. In school I was distracted and could not focus on my homework. My mother wanted to take me to a doctor. I was so afraid that they would discover everything that I cried hysterically. In the end I saw a church counselor and stopped swimming so that I could focus on my grades. I tried very hard to forget what had happened, but I was never completely successful.

"When I'm depressed it gets worse. Along with all the daily stuff, I can't stop thinking about what happened years ago. My bad thoughts spread like ripples, conjuring memories of my parents' fights and all the embarrassing episodes from my past. I'm not going crazy, am I? Sometimes I feel like I deserve all the bad things that have happened to me, that depression is a fair punishment for all the despicable things that I did.

"Toward the end of my senior year, another girl spoke up. There was a huge scandal. The swimming coach was fired. His court hearing made the local news. Every day I dreaded the news, fearing that my name was going to come out. I felt responsible for all the other girls. Had I spoken up it might not have happened to them. I felt so dirty. When he was sentenced, I was already in college. It would serve me right if it contributed to my depression." At this point Anna was in tears and sobbing.

"When I have come this far, I might as well come clean." She said drying her eyes with a tissue and discretely blowing her nose.

"I have been drinking more than I told you. Sometimes, it is more than a glass or two. If I have a rough day at work and my mind cannot find peace from these haunting thoughts, I will polish off a bottle of wine. I cannot bear the thought of my husband touching me when I'm in this frame of mind. I also don't want him to smell alcohol on my breath. I guess every-thing is not as hunky-dory as I have made it out to be."

Anna and I discussed how these brooding, ruminative thoughts may worsen her depression and make its recurrence more likely when she is dis-tressed. Anna was quite surprised to hear that ruminations may also inter-fere with her sleep and make it harder for her to stay focused at work. I strongly suggested that she see a local therapist skilled in rumination-focused CBT (RFCBT). I also asked for her permission to communicate her increased alcohol use to her future therapist. Moreover, I suggested that see-ing a couples' therapist may also help improve her home situation, which may additionally ameliorate her mood.

"I thought that medicines would take care of all of this. I guess I was wrong. Now that cat is out of the bag, I might as well go ahead with therapy. Can your office help me make an appointment? I would rather not get my husband involved for the time being, if it's OK with you. He doesn't know about the high school episode, and I'm really not in the mood to explain.

"I'm not questioning your recommendations. I'm sure that you mean well, but is there any hope that psychotherapy will work even after all the antidepressants haven't? I just don't want to get my hopes up and be disap-pointed again. It might send me right back to depression."

"While it would not be wise to guarantee success," I told her, "this form of cognitive therapy does have a good track record, even in patients who have not had a great success with antidepressant medication. Please don't forget this is only one component of our treatment plan. I'm still asking you to continue with medications and to cut down on alcohol. Furthermore, I would like to see you increase the exercise classes to at least three to four times a week, and to try to manage stress in your office as best as you can."

Several new developments have cast doubt on the utility of the further pursuit of antidepressant treatment for Anna and point to potential benefits of psychother-apy. Anna has not been fully successful in achieving symptom relief after trying several antidepressants. Research data indicate that a greater number of unsuc-cessful antidepressant trials translates into diminishing returns. Remission rates dropped from 36.8 percent to 30.6 percent to 13.7 percent and finally to 13 percent in the four consecutive treatment steps of STAR*D, and the likelihood of relapse in the follow-up period increased with each subsequent step.[78]

Furthermore, Anna has revealed that she has been abused in her early teen-age years and has had a very unsettled and disturbing early family life. A history of early-life adversity (ELA) has been associated with lesser response and remis-sion rates in antidepressant trials and greater benefits from psychotherapy.[79–81] Dyadic discord has also been associated with lower remission rates in response to pharmacotherapy while clearly benefiting from adjunct psychotherapy.[82] As a reminder, Anna has made several references to marital difficulties; they may also have contributed to her reported sexual dysfunction. Additionally, work-related and psychosocial stress can diminish the efficacy of antidepressants, resulting in approximately 50 percent lower remission rates.[83] In other words, while antidepressants may be a moderately effective treatment for depression, they are fairly ineffectual remedy for life's other vicissitudes.

The presence of any residual symptoms, even at the subthreshold level, especially anxiety and sleep disturbance, substantially increases the risk of future relapse.[84–86] Evidence from STAR*D suggests that the greater the number of residual symptoms. the more likely a person is to relapse, even while remaining on an antidepressant.[87] We have already established that prominent ruminative tendencies also represent a greater liability for relapse in stressful circumstances. A greater number of relapses appear to be associated with more pronounced cognitive dysfunction,[88] which like other residual symptoms substantially interferes with social and occupational functioning.[89,90] We have already heard from Anna that her cognitive difficulties at work are a major source of frustration and stress. Is there a way out of this vicious cycle?

Ample evidence supports the efficacy of cognitive therapy, both as an adjunct to antidepressants in treatment-resistant depression and in long-term relapse prevention.[91–93] Unlike antidepressant medications, which appear to have questionable relapse-preventing ability once they are discontinued, CBT has a very substantial carry-over relapse-preventing benefit, enduring for years after its completion.[93] However, how CBT and antidepressants compare in terms of relapse prevention during the maintenance phase of treatment remains an open question. While some studies showed superior relapse prevention associated with CBT,[93] others have failed to demonstrate a difference compared with an SSRI maintenance arm.[92]

Several elements in Anna's story bode well for the success of psychotherapy. First, Anna has made a decision to initiate psychotherapy on her own. In one of the studies patients who chose psychotherapy had more than double the remission rate (50 percent) compared with patients who preferred medications (22.2 percent) but ended in psychotherapy arm due to randomization.[36] Moreover, psychotherapy has established efficacy for two of the residual symptoms reported by Anna, sleep disturbance and anxiety.[33,94] In fact, CBT could help address potential posttraumatic issues (although Anna claims to have already worked through the consequences of trauma), as well as social anxiety.[94]

Anna has brought up a painful, traumatic episode from her past. Are there any neurobiological sequelae of ELA that are relevant for Anna's predicament? Imaging studies have reported that ELA can be associated with decreased gray and white matter volume of the hippocampus and reduced PFC volume, both of which are independent predictors of a severe course of illness.[95,96] Furthermore, reduced hippocampal volume in MDD has been associated with executive dysfunction.[97] Even individuals with family risk for depression who have suffered ELA have reduced volumes of dlPFC, ACC, and medial PFC, although they themselves have never experienced a depressive episode.[98] In other words, ELA is associated with structural and functional changes in the same limbic and cortical areas that are associated with the stress response, emotional regulation, and executive function. Moreover, repeated stress in individuals with ELA has a demonstrated association with reduced vmPFC perfusion and inadequate ability to modulate an amygdala response in stressful situations.[99] Early traumatic events may thus precipitate aberrant autonomic and endocrine regulation, which in turn may produce ongoing hyperarousal and sleep disturbance.[100–104] Cumulatively, research into the impact of ELA supports the two-strike model, whereby early adversity, in part mediated by epigenetic changes, generates functional and structural alterations in the key limbic and cortical areas involved in emotional regulation. The combined immune, autonomic, and endocrine disturbance that ensue set the stage for adult-life stressful events to act as activating agents of a future depressive episode.

Is there any scientific way to determine if one is more likely to benefit from psychotherapy or antidepressants? Are there any forms of psychotherapy that are more likely to be helpful to Anna and is there any evidence that they may reverse the brain changes underpinning depression? Very exciting preliminary evidence stemming from a positron emission tomography imaging study in a group of depressed patients suggests that one can predict remission in response to escitalopram versus CBT. Individuals with a higher baseline level of right insula activity responded better to escitalopram, whereas baseline insula hypometabolism was a positive predictor of remission following a 12-week course of CBT. Previous evidence of insula involvement in MDD, its principal role in translating sensory and visceral information into emotion, and its participation in the neural processes that result in self-awareness gives face validity to these findings.[105] If replicated, these findings may offer a very useful way to utilize a neuroscience discovery to guide effective clinical treatment.

People with a history of childhood abuse and subsequent adult stress are especially likely to experience a persistent course of depression. The presence of ruminations and depression severity also have a known association with lower remission rates in response to CBT.[105,106] Given these realities, is there a specific form of psychotherapy that is more likely to be effective for Anna? Although we are not aware of direct comparisons with other forms of psychotherapy, or specific studies in depressed patients who have experienced ELA, RFCBT has been associated with impressive efficacy in the treatment of MDD patients.

RFCBT was designed to specifically ameliorate unconstructive ruminations/brooding thoughts by replacing them with constructive ruminations/self-reflection based on functional analysis, experiential/imagery exercises, and behavioral experiments.[107] Compared with a previous study where CBT combined with pharmacotherapy resulted in a modest 25 percent remission rate, compared with 13 percent in the treatment-as-usual group, a combination of RFCBT and antidepressants (mostly SSRIs) was substantially more effective, generating a 62 percent remission rate compared with 21 percent in the treatment-as-usual group.[107] The treatment effect size in the RFCBT group relative to treatment as usual was 0.94–1.1, dwarfing the 0.34 effect size for antidepressants versus placebo.[107,108] Effect size is an average difference between the treatment and placebo divided by standard deviation. An effect size of 1 means that the average difference between treatment and placebo is about 1 S.D. Although, to some degree we are comparing apples to oranges, if RFCBT findings are replicated it may be an effective adjunct treatment for a great number of depressed patients still suffering from residual symptoms.

Are there other psychotherapies that may be helpful for depressed patients experiencing prominent ruminations like Anna? Systematic reviews and meta-analyses have suggested that mindfulness-based and cognitive-behavioral approaches may be beneficial interventions aimed at reduction of rumination and worries, whether delivered face to face or via the Internet.[109] A global review of mindfulness-based treatment approaches for a number of medical and psychiatric conditions concluded that they just as effective as pharmacotherapy, CBT, and other behavioral treatments.[110] Mindfulness-based approaches seem to be a particularly effective fit for rumination-prone depressed patients. Instead of engaging in circuitous elaboration of negative emotional experiences, beset with unanswerable "why" questions, patients are encouraged to practice reappraisal of emotion-eliciting experience in a nonevaluative and nonjudgmental manner. In some ways mindfulness is an existential antidote to ruminations: the focus shifts from fixation on past failures to the enriching experience of here and now.[111]

Metacognitive therapy may also be an effective modality for individuals with treatment-resistant depression accompanied by prominent ruminations. The theoretical underpinning of metacognitive therapy posits that vulnerable individuals engage in a cognitive attentional syndrome manifesting as "threat monitoring" in the form of rumination and worry, which paradoxically extends negative experience, induces a sense of helplessness, and reduces attentional flexibility. Interestingly, in metacognitive therapy ruminations and worries are not seen as part of a problem; rather, they are conceived of as coping methods. The primary goal of treatment is to reframe ruminations and worries as maladaptive and depression-enhancing activities. The patient is helped to realize that ruminations are not uncontrollable. Attention training is implemented to engender a belief that one has control over one's own thought processes. All the participants in one of the trials had failed both an appropriate course of antidepressant treatment and a prior psychological treatment. The metacognitive therapy intervention consisted of eight weekly sessions lasting 40–60 minutes. Patients were asked to continue the antidepressant on which they were stable for the previous six months. At the 6- and 12-month follow-up 75 percent of the original cohort achieved remission (defined as Hamilton Depression Rating Scale 17-item version [HAMD$_{17}$] score ≤ 7).[112] However, this truly remarkable outcome would need to be reproduced in a larger cohort with an appropriate control group to definitively establish this type of effectiveness.

Now that we have reviewed the clinical aspects of various psychotherapeutic approaches, let us focus on their neural correlates. Imaging literature evaluating the effect of mindfulness practices does not have the most consistent outcomes due to methodological differences and the utilization of diverse mindfulness techniques. Nevertheless, one can glean certain underlying commonalities. In general, mindfulness produces a shift from evaluative cognitive practices involving coupling of limbic SN and midline DMN-related brain areas to a heightened present-moment awareness, which couples sensory-related limbic areas, such as the thalamus and insula, with EN-related lateral PFC, dACC, and parietal areas.[113,114] Typically, overall activity and connectivity between DMN-related structures, such as the PCC, precuneus, dmPFC, and sgACC, is decreased.[115–118] Moreover, mindfulness-based practices may be associated with increase in gray matter volume of the hippocampus and PCC,[119] brain regions whose structure is often altered in the context of MDD. It is striking how the pattern of brain activity induced by mindfulness practices contrasts with the aberrant connectivity between the DMN and SN, which presumably underpins depressive ruminations, and abnormal DMN-EN coactivation, which is hypothetically associated with cognitive and attentional deficits in MDD.

Many imaging studies have investigated the effects of CBT and cognitive therapy on brain function. One of these studies comparing MDD patients with healthy controls found normalization of amygdala activity following 12 weeks of cognitive therapy and normalization of dlPFC activity during performance of a cognitive task, compared with brain activity in the same areas and during the same tasks prior to psychotherapy.[120] A higher degree of amygdala and sgACC activity prior to initiation of CBT predicted a more robust response and a greater reduction in depressive symptomatology. Interestingly, in the same study, greater amygdala activity was also associated with more ruminations.[121] Furthermore, a subsequent study by the same group reported that the patients who exhibited the lowest sgACC reactivity to negative emotional stimuli experienced the greatest posttreatment improvement. Pretreatment sgACC reactivity correctly classified 75 percent of future CBT responders and 70 percent of remitters. A different group of investigators expanded these findings by discovering that, compared with pretreatment, post-CBT medial PFC/sgACC activity in response to negative self-referential stimuli diminished, while the activity in the same brain areas increased in response to positive stimuli.[122] Clinical improvement of depressive symptoms correlated with reduction in sgACC activity in response to negative self-referential stimuli.[122] Another study found a relationship between baseline dACC activity in depressed patients and subsequent response to CBT.[123]

Preliminary imaging evidence suggests that long-term psychodynamic psychotherapy also influences brain activity. Depressed patients who initially exhibited increased activity in the hippocampus/amygdala, sgACC, and medial PFC showed a significant reduction in activation in the same brain regions following 15 months of psychodynamic therapy.[124] Furthermore, diffusion tensor imaging has provided evidence of microstructural improvements in the frontal lobe white matter tracts in depressed patients following a four-week course of guided imagery psychotherapy.[125]

In summary, imaging studies provide evidence that psychotherapeutic interventions produce changes in brain activity that are consistent with our understanding of the neurobiological underpinnings of depression. Psychotherapy is associated with uncoupling of the "dorsal nexus," whereby abnormal connection between the EN and DMN is severed. Adaptive connections between SN- and EN-related areas appear to be strengthened by psychotherapy. Excessive reactivity to negative emotional stimuli in limbic areas is reduced following successful psychotherapy, while the executive-cognitive lateral PFC and parietal areas involved in "top-down" emotional regulation manifest greater activation.

"Anything else? Do you want to help my kids with homework while I do all this? I will be glad to drop them off at your office.

"You don't have to answer that. I can already see that my life is going to be a blast in the next few months." Anna chuckled as she was leaving the office.

Excerpts from the second visit office notes
Anna has benefited from the combination of an SSRI and bupropion.
Energy, motivation, and libido have all improved.
SE: Anna has felt dizzy initially, sleep is worse.
Anna reported sexual abuse in her early teenage years. She has still not worked through some of the abuse related issues. Autonomic hyperarousal may be a consequence of the past trauma, and may contribute to the sleep disorder.
Alcohol use is more frequent and substantial (more than two glasses) than initially reported. It may have a negative impact on Anna's sleep and antidepressant response.
Plan: Specialized rumination-focused cognitive-behavioral therapy, family therapy; excessive alcohol use needs to be addressed in individual therapy. Will continue to encourage exercise.

Fifth Visit, Three Months After the Second Session

"Well, I think that psychotherapy may have finally paid dividends. I'm not sure if this is related to medicine or therapy, but I'm more comfortable in social situations. I'm able to get out of my brain and actually talk to people."

"What do you mean?"

"In the past I would focus on their expression, especially their eyes. Are they making as much eye contact with me as with other people in the group? Are they smiling? Why does Mary have that cynical expression? I would be so focused on faces that I would sometimes lose the thread of conversation. Are they going to pay attention to me if I say something, or am I just going to blend into the background noise? Sometimes, social gatherings would be such a pain that I would try to leave as soon as I could, without appearing rude. My husband would ask me what was the matter. I would just say that I was not feeling well rather than having to explain all this. He would probably think that I'm cuckoo anyway."

"You said that things are different now?"

"Well, yes. I'm more relaxed. It is easier to focus on the conversation without worrying how other people see me or if they approve of me. I have actually started enjoying some of the conversations, and people seem to genuinely like me."

"How about your sleep difficulties? Any improvement since last time?"

"Yes, it is easier to fall asleep. I don't allow the brooding thoughts to get out of control anymore. If there is an issue, I try to find a solution. All the catastrophizing serves no purpose—it just makes me miserable. I can now soothe myself with happy memories and drift off to sleep. Some nights it's not so easy. I still take my sleeping pills several times a week. Maybe it's because I'm sleeping better, but my work performance has also improved. I don't get distracted nearly as much."

"Any side effects from medications?"

"No, not really. I think that we can continue with treatment just the way it is."

"Do you plan to continue with psychotherapy?"

"Yes, there are some trust issues that I need to work on. Who knows, one of these days I may even drag in my husband."

In conclusion, advances in science have helped us gain a deeper understanding into some of the biochemical and imaging commonalities of MDD, despite the fact that it is clearly a neurobiologically diverse condition. While research has helped us understand the relationship between the mechanism of antidepressant action and some of the side effects of medication, it has done little to help us choose the most effective psychopharmacological intervention for a given patient. Nonetheless, there is some suggestion that cognitive difficulties, hypersomnolance, and fatigue may favor the norepinephrine- and dopamine-modulating agents over SSRIs.

There is preliminary evidence suggesting that imaging studies may help us predict which patients are more likely to benefit from psychotherapy versus pharmacotherapy. Furthermore, pretreatment activity in the limbic and paralimbic areas may also predict which depressed patients will respond and remit following psychotherapy.

References

1. Nolen-Hoeksema S, Wisco BE, Lyubomirsky S. Rethinking rumination. *Perspect Psychol Sci.* 2008;3:400–424.

2. Raes F, Hermans D, Williams JMG, Bijttebier P, Eelen P. A "triple W"-model of rumination on sadness: why am I feeling sad, what's the meaning of my sadness, and wish I could stop thinking about my sadness (but I can't!). *Cogn Ther Res.* 2008;32:526–541.

3. Miranda R, Nolen-Hoeksema S. Brooding and reflection: rumination predicts suicidal ideation at 1-year follow-up in a community sample. *Behav Res Ther.* 2007;45:3088–3095.

4. Raes F, Hermans D. On the mediating role of subtypes of rumination in the relationship between childhood emotional abuse and depressed mood: brooding versus reflection. *Depress Anxiety.* 2008;25:1067–1070.

5. Young KD, Erickson K, Drevets WC. Differential effects of emotionally versus neutrally cued autobiographical memories on performance of a subsequent cognitive task: effects of task difficulty. *Front Psychol.* 2012;3:299.

6. Young KD, Erickson K, Drevets WC. Match between cue and memory valence during autobiographical memory recall in depression. *Psychol Rep.* 2012;111:129–148.

7. Donaldson C, Lam D, Mathews A. Rumination and attention in major depression. *Behav Res Ther.* 2007;45:2664–2678.

8. Wilkinson PO, Croudace TJ, Goodyer IM. Rumination, anxiety, depressive symptoms and subsequent depression in adolescents at risk for psychopathology: a longitudinal cohort study. *BMC Psychiatry.* 2013;13:250.

9. Nolen-Hoeksema S. Emotion regulation and psychopathology: the role of gender. *Annu Rev Clin Psychol.* 2012;8:161–187.

10. Kashdan TB, Roberts JE. Social anxiety, depressive symptoms, and post-event rumination: affective consequences and social contextual influences. *J Anxiety Disord.* 2007;21:284–301.

11. Lyubomirsky S, Nolen-Hoeksema S. Effects of self-focused rumination on negative thinking and interpersonal problem solving. *J Pers Soc Psychol.* 1995;69:176–190.

12. Carney CE, Harris AL, Moss TG, Edinger JD. Distinguishing rumination from worry in clinical insomnia. *Behav Res Ther.* 2010;48:540–546.

13. Demeyer I, De Lissnyder E, Koster EH, De Raedt R. Rumination mediates the relationship between impaired cognitive control for emotional information and depressive symptoms: a prospective study in remitted depressed adults. *Behav Res Ther.* 2012;50:292–297.

14. Clasen PC, Wells TT, Knopik VS, McGeary JE, Beevers CG. 5-HTTLPR and BDNF Val-66Met polymorphisms moderate effects of stress on rumination. *Genes Brain Behav.* 2011;10:740–746.

15. Denton EG, Rieckmann N, Davidson KW, Chaplin WF. Psychosocial vulnerabilities to depression after acute coronary syndrome: the pivotal role of rumination in predicting and maintaining depression. *Front Psychol.* 2012;3:288.

16. Berman MG, Peltier S, Nee DE, Kross E, Deldin PJ, Jonides J. Depression, rumination and the default network. *Soc Cogn Affect Neurosci.* 2011;6:548–555.

17. Hamilton JP, Furman DJ, Chang C, Thomason ME, Dennis E, Gotlib IH. Default-mode and task-positive network activity in major depressive disorder: implications for adaptive and maladaptive rumination. *Biol Psychiatry.* 2011;70:327–333.

18. Greicius MD, Flores BH, Menon V, et al. Resting-state functional connectivity in major depression: abnormally increased contributions from subgenual cingulate cortex and thalamus. *Biol Psychiatry.* 2007;62:429–437.

19. Sheline YI, Price JL, Yan Z, Mintun MA. Resting-state functional MRI in depression unmasks increased connectivity between networks via the dorsal nexus. *Proc Natl Acad Sci U S A.* 2010;107:11020–11025.

20. Hamilton JP, Etkin A, Furman DJ, Lemus MG, Johnson RF, Gotlib IH. Functional neuroimaging of major depressive disorder: a meta-analysis and new integration of base line activation and neural response data. *Am J Psychiatry.* 2012;169:693–703.

21. Bluhm R, Williamson P, Lanius R, et al. Resting state default-mode network connectivity in early depression using a seed region-of-interest analysis: decreased connectivity with caudate nucleus. *Psychiatry Clin Neurosci.* 2009;63:754–761.

22. Alexopoulos GS, Hoptman MJ, Kanellopoulos D, Murphy CF, Lim KO, Gunning FM. Functional connectivity in the cognitive control network and the default mode network in late-life depression. *J Affect Disord.* 2012;139:56–65.

23. Delaveau P, Jabourian M, Lemogne C, Guionnet S, Bergouignan L, Fossati P. Brain effects of antidepressants in major depression: a meta-analysis of emotional processing studies. *J Affect Disord.* 2011;130:66–74.

24. Posner J, Hellerstein DJ, Gat I, et al. Antidepressants normalize the default mode network in patients with dysthymia. *JAMA Psychiatry.* 2013;70:373–382.

25. Bell DS, Shipman WM, Cleves MA, Siegelman J. Which drug for which patient? Is there a fluoxetine responding versus a bupropion responding personality profile? Clinical practice and epidemiology in mental health. *Clin Pract Epidemiol Ment Health.* 2013;9: 142–147.

26. Rothschild AJ, Raskin J, Wang CN, Marangell LB, Fava M. The relationship between change in apathy and changes in cognition and functional outcomes in currently nondepressed SSRI-treated patients with major depressive disorder. *Compr Psychiatry.* 2014;55:1–10.

27. Herrera-Guzman I, Gudayol-Ferre E, Herrera-Guzman D, Guardia-Olmos J, Hinojosa-Calvo E, Herrera-Abarca JE. Effects of selective serotonin reuptake and dual serotonergic-noradrenergic reuptake treatments on memory and mental processing speed in patients with major depressive disorder. *J Psychiatr Res.* 2009;43:855–863.

28. Raskin J, George T, Granger RE, Hussain N, Zhao GW, Marangell LB. Apathy in currently nondepressed patients treated with a SSRI for a major depressive episode: outcomes following randomized switch to either duloxetine or escitalopram. *J Psychiatr Res.* 2012;46:667–674.

29. Serretti A, Chiesa A. Treatment-emergent sexual dysfunction related to antidepressants: a meta-analysis. *J Clin Psychopharmacol.* 2009;29:259–266.

30. Rush AJ, Trivedi MH, Wisniewski SR, et al. Bupropion-SR, sertraline, or venlafaxine-XR after failure of SSRIs for depression. *N Engl J Med.* 2006;354:1231–1242.

31. Schosser A, Serretti A, Souery D, et al. European Group for the Study of Resistant Depression (GSRD)—where have we gone so far: review of clinical and genetic findings. *Eur Neuropsychopharmacol.* 2012;22:453–468.

32. Gaynes BN, Dusetzina SB, Ellis AR, et al. Treating depression after initial treatment failure: directly comparing switch and augmenting strategies in STAR*D. *J Clin Psychopharmacol.* 2012;32:114–119.

33. Carney CE, Segal ZV, Edinger JD, Krystal AD. A comparison of rates of residual insomnia symptoms following pharmacotherapy or cognitive-behavioral therapy for major depressive disorder. *J Clin Psychiatry.* 2007;68:254–260.

34. Shelton RC, Hollon SD. The long-term management of major depressive disorders. *Focus.* 2012;10:434–441.

35. Wisniewski SR, Fava M, Trivedi MH, et al. Acceptability of second-step treatments to depressed outpatients: a STAR*D report. *Am J Psychiatry.* 2007;164:753–760.

36. Kocsis JH, Leon AC, Markowitz JC, et al. Patient preference as a moderator of outcome for chronic forms of major depressive disorder treated with nefazodone, cognitive behavioral analysis system of psychotherapy, or their combination. *J Clin Psychiatry.* 2009;70: 354–361.

37. Thase ME, Friedman ES, Biggs MM, et al. Cognitive therapy versus medication in augmentation and switch strategies as second-step treatments: a STAR*D report. *Am J Psychiatry.* 2007;164:739–752.

38. Cadeddu R, Ibba M, Sadile A, Carboni E. Antidepressants share the ability to increase catecholamine output in the bed nucleus of stria terminalis: a possible role in antidepressant therapy? *Psychopharmacology (Berl).* 2014;231(9):1925–1933.

39. Dell'Osso B, Palazzo MC, Oldani L, Altamura AC. The noradrenergic action in antidepressant treatments: pharmacological and clinical aspects. *CNS Neurosci Ther.* 2011;17:7 23–732.

40. Chevassus H, Farret A, Gagnol JP, et al. Psychological and physiological effects of bupropion compared to methylphenidate after prolonged administration in healthy volunteers (NCT00285155). *Eur J Clin Pharmacol.* 2013;69:779–787.

41. Nieuwstraten CE, Dolovich LR. Bupropion versus selective serotonin-reuptake inhibitors for treatment of depression. *Ann Pharmacother.* 2001;35:1608–1613.

42. Papakostas GI, Trivedi MH, Alpert JE, et al. Efficacy of bupropion and the selective serotonin reuptake inhibitors in the treatment of anxiety symptoms in major depressive disorder: a meta-analysis of individual patient data from 10 double-blind, randomized clinical trials. *J Psychiatr Res.* 2008;42:134–140.

43. Papakostas GI, Nutt DJ, Hallett LA, Tucker VL, Krishen A, Fava M. Resolution of sleepiness and fatigue in major depressive disorder: a comparison of bupropion and the selective serotonin reuptake inhibitors. *Biol Psychiatry.* 2006;60:1350–1355.

44. Blier P, Ward HE, Tremblay P, Laberge L, Hebert C, Bergeron R. Combination of antidepressant medications from treatment initiation for major depressive disorder: a double-blind randomized study. *Am J Psychiatry.* 2010;167:281–288.

45. DeBattista C, Solvason HB, Poirier J, Kendrick E, Schatzberg AF. A prospective trial of bupropion SR augmentation of partial and non-responders to serotonergic antidepressants. *J Clin Psychopharmacol.* 2003;23:27–30.

46. Rush AJ, Trivedi MH, Stewart JW, et al. Combining medications to enhance depression outcomes (CO-MED): acute and long-term outcomes of a single-blind randomized study. *Am J Psychiatry.* 2011;168:689–701.

47. Bodkin JA, Lasser RA, Wines JD Jr, Gardner DM, Baldessarini RJ. Combining serotonin

reuptake inhibitors and bupropion in partial responders to antidepressant monotherapy. *J Clin Psychiatry.* 1997;58:137–145.

48. Demyttenaere K, Jaspers L. Review: bupropion and SSRI-induced side effects. *J Psychopharmacol.* 2008;22:792–804.

49. Epstein J, Pan H, Kocsis JH, et al. Lack of ventral striatal response to positive stimuli in depressed versus normal subjects. *Am J Psychiatry.* 2006;163:1784–1790.

50. Pizzagalli DA, Holmes AJ, Dillon DG, et al. Reduced caudate and nucleus accumbens response to rewards in unmedicated individuals with major depressive disorder. *Am J Psychiatry.* 2009;166:702–710.

51. Keller J, Young CB, Kelley E, Prater K, Levitin DJ, Menon V. Trait anhedonia is associated with reduced reactivity and connectivity of mesolimbic and paralimbic reward pathways. *J Psychiatr Res.* 2013;47:1319–1328.

52. Bragulat V, Paillere-Martinot ML, Artiges E, Frouin V, Poline JB, Martinot JL. Dopaminergic function in depressed patients with affective flattening or with impulsivity: [18F]fluoro-L-dopa positron emission tomography study with voxel-based analysis. *Psychiatry Res.* 2007;154:115–124.

53. Heller AS, Johnstone T, Light SN, et al. Relationships between changes in sustained fronto-striatal connectivity and positive affect in major depression resulting from antidepressant treatment. *Am J Psychiatry.* 2013;170:197–206.

54. Gorwood P. Neurobiological mechanisms of anhedonia. *Dialogues Clin Neurosci.* 2008;10:291–299.

55. Alex KD, Pehek EA. Pharmacologic mechanisms of serotonergic regulation of dopamine neurotransmission. *Pharmacol Ther.* 2007;113:296–320.

56. Fava M, Graves LM, Benazzi F, et al. A cross-sectional study of the prevalence of cognitive and physical symptoms during long-term antidepressant treatment. *J Clin Psychiatry.* 2006;67:1754–1759.

57. Drevets WC, Price JL, Furey ML. Brain structural and functional abnormalities in mood disorders: implications for neurocircuitry models of depression. *Brain Struct Funct.* 2008;213:93–118.

58. Chamberlain SR, Muller U, Robbins TW, Sahakian BJ. Neuropharmacological modulation of cognition. *Curr Opin Neurol.* 2006;19:607–612.

59. Blier P, Briley M. The noradrenergic symptom cluster: clinical expression and neuropharmacology. *Neuropsychiatr Dis Treat.* 2011;7:15–20.

60. Brom M, Both S, Laan E, Everaerd W, Spinhoven P. The role of conditioning, learning and dopamine in sexual behavior: a narrative review of animal and human studies. *Neurosci Biobehav Rev.* 2013;38C:38–59.

61. Ortigue S, Grafton ST, Bianchi-Demicheli F. Correlation between insula activation and self-reported quality of orgasm in women. *Neuroimage.* 2007;37:551–560.

62. Fonteille V, Stoleru S. The cerebral correlates of sexual desire: functional neuroimaging approach. *Sexologies.* 2011;20:142–148.

63. Motofei IG, Rowland DL. The ventral-hypothalamic input route: a common neural network for abstract cognition and sexuality. *BJU Int.* 2014;113(2):296–303.

64. Berman MG, Nee DE, Casement M, et al. Neural and behavioral effects of interference resolution in depression and rumination. *Cogn Affect Behav Neurosci.* 2011;11:85–96.

65. Abler B, Seeringer A, Hartmann A, et al. Neural correlates of antidepressant-related sexual dysfunction: a placebo-controlled fMRI study on healthy males under subchronic paroxetine and bupropion. *Neuropsychopharmacology.* 2011;36:1837–1847.

66. Abler B, Gron G, Hartmann A, Metzger C, Walter M. Modulation of frontostriatal inter-

action aligns with reduced primary reward processing under serotonergic drugs. *J Neurosci.* 2012;32:1329–1335.

67. McCabe C, Mishor Z, Cowen PJ, Harmer CJ. Diminished neural processing of aversive and rewarding stimuli during selective serotonin reuptake inhibitor treatment. *Biol Psychiatry.* 2010;67:439–445.

68. Mondal S, Saha I, Das S, Ganguly A, Das D, Tripathi SK. A new logical insight and putative mechanism behind fluoxetine-induced amenorrhea, hyperprolactinemia and galactorrhea in a case series. *Ther Adv Psychopharmacol.* 2013;3:322–334.

69. Hawken ER, Owen JA, Hudson RW, Delva NJ. Specific effects of escitalopram on neuroendocrine response. *Psychopharmacology (Berl).* 2009;207:27–34.

70. Lykouras L, Markianos M, Hatzimanolis Y. Prolactin and cortisol responses to acute intravenous clomipramine challenge in patients with mania, depression and healthy controls: evidence for reduced serotonergic responsivity. *Neuropsychobiology.* 2011;63: 77–81.

71. Cordes J, Kahl KG, Werner C, et al. Clomipramine-induced serum prolactin as a marker for serotonin and dopamine turnover: results of an open label study. *Eur Arch Psychiatry Clin Neurosci.* 2011;261:567–573.

72. Kim S, Park YM. Serum prolactin and macroprolactin levels among outpatients with major depressive disorder following the administration of selective serotonin-reuptake inhibitors: a cross-sectional pilot study. *PLoS ONE.* 2013;8:e82749.

73. Papakostas GI, Miller KK, Petersen T, et al. Serum prolactin levels among outpatients with major depressive disorder during the acute phase of treatment with fluoxetine. *J Clin Psychiatry.* 2006;67:952–957.

74. Kruger TH, Haake P, Hartmann U, Schedlowski M, Exton MS. Orgasm-induced prolactin secretion: feedback control of sexual drive? *Neurosci Biobehav Rev.* 2002;26:31–44.

75. Huynh HK, Willemsen AT, Holstege G. Female orgasm but not male ejaculation activates the pituitary: a PET-neuro-imaging study. *Neuroimage.* 2013;76:178–182.

76. Brody S, Kruger TH. The post-orgasmic prolactin increase following intercourse is greater than following masturbation and suggests greater satiety. *Biol Psychol.* 2006;71: 312–315.

77. Whiteman PD, Peck AW, Fowle AS, Smith P. Bupropion fails to affect plasma prolactin and growth hormone in normal subjects. *Br J Clin Pharmacol.* 1982;13:743–745.

78. Rush AJ, Trivedi MH, Wisniewski SR, et al. Acute and longer-term outcomes in depressed outpatients requiring one or several treatment steps: a STAR*D report. *Am J Psychiatry.* 2006;163:1905–1917.

79. Nanni V, Uher R, Danese A. Childhood maltreatment predicts unfavorable course of illness and treatment outcome in depression: a meta-analysis. *Am J Psychiatry.* 2012;169: 141–151.

80. Klein DN, Arnow BA, Barkin JL, et al. Early adversity in chronic depression: clinical correlates and response to pharmacotherapy. *Depress Anxiety.* 2009;26:701–710.

81. Nemeroff CB, Heim CM, Thase ME, et al. Differential responses to psychotherapy versus pharmacotherapy in patients with chronic forms of major depression and childhood trauma. *Proc Natl Acad Sci U S A.* 2003;100:14293–14296.

82. Denton WH, Carmody TJ, Rush AJ, et al. Dyadic discord at baseline is associated with lack of remission in the acute treatment of chronic depression. *Psychol Med.* 2010;40: 415–424.

83. Brown GW, Harris TO, Kendrick T, et al. Antidepressants, social adversity and outcome of depression in general practice. *J Affect Disord.* 2010;121:239–246.

84. Judd LL AH, Maser JD, et al. Major depressive disorder: a prospective study of residual subthreshold depressive symptoms as predictor of rapid relapse. *J Affect Disord.* 1998; 50:97–108.

85. Dombrovski AY, Mulsant BH, Houck PR, et al. Residual symptoms and recurrence during maintenance treatment of late-life depression. *J Affect Disord.* 2007;103:77–82.

86. Cho HJ, Lavretsky H, Olmstead R, Levin MJ, Oxman MN, Irwin MR. Sleep disturbance and depression recurrence in community-dwelling older adults: a prospective study. *Am J Psychiatry.* 2008;165:1543–1550.

87. Nierenberg AA, Husain MM, Trivedi MH, et al. Residual symptoms after remission of major depressive disorder with citalopram and risk of relapse: a STAR*D report. *Psychol Med.* 2010;40:41–50.

88. Gorwood P, Corruble E, Falissard B, Goodwin GM. Toxic effects of depression on brain function: impairment of delayed recall and the cumulative length of depressive disorder in a large sample of depressed outpatients. *Am J Psychiatry.* 2008;165:731–739.

89. Ormel J, Vonkorff M, Oldehinkel AJ, Simon G, Tiemens BG, Ustun TB. Onset of disability in depressed and non-depressed primary care patients. *Psychol Med.* 1999;29:847–853.

90. Jaeger J, Berns S, Uzelac S, Davis-Conway S. Neurocognitive deficits and disability in major depressive disorder. *Psychiatry Res.* 2006;145:39–48.

91. Wiles N, Thomas L, Abel A, et al. Cognitive behavioural therapy as an adjunct to pharmacotherapy for primary care based patients with treatment resistant depression: results of the CoBalT randomised controlled trial. *Lancet.* 2013;381:375–384.

92. Jarrett RB, Minhajuddin A, Gershenfeld H, Friedman ES, Thase ME. Preventing depressive relapse and recurrence in higher-risk cognitive therapy responders: a randomized trial of continuation phase cognitive therapy, fluoxetine, or matched pill placebo. *JAMA Psychiatry.* 2013;70:1152–1160.

93. Dobson KS, Hollon SD, Dimidjian S, et al. Randomized trial of behavioral activation, cognitive therapy, and antidepressant medication in the prevention of relapse and recurrence in major depression. *J Consult Clin Psychol.* 2008;76:468–477.

94. Otte C. Cognitive behavioral therapy in anxiety disorders: current state of the evidence. *Dialogues Clin Neurosci.* 2011;13:413–421.

95. Rao U, Chen LA, Bidesi AS, Shad MU, Thomas MA, Hammen CL. Hippocampal changes associated with early-life adversity and vulnerability to depression. *Biol Psychiatry.* 2010;67:357–364.

96. Frodl T, Reinhold E, Koutsouleris N, Reiser M, Meisenzahl EM. Interaction of childhood stress with hippocampus and prefrontal cortex volume reduction in major depression. *J Psychiatr Res.* 2010;44:799–807.

97. Frodl T, Schaub A, Banac S, et al. Reduced hippocampal volume correlates with executive dysfunctioning in major depression. *J Psychiatry Neurosci.* 2006;31:316–323.

98. Carballedo A, Lisiecka D, Fagan A, et al. Early life adversity is associated with brain changes in subjects at family risk for depression. *World J Biol Psychiatry.* 2012;13: 569–578.

99. Wang L, Paul N, Stanton SJ, Greeson JM, Smoski MJ. Loss of sustained activity in the ventromedial prefrontal cortex in response to repeated stress in individuals with early-life emotional abuse: implications for depression vulnerability. *Front Psychol.* 2013;4:320.

100. McEwen BS. Brain on stress: how the social environment gets under the skin. *Proc Natl Acad Sci U S A.* 2012;109(suppl 2):17180–17185.

101. McGowan PO. Epigenomic mechanisms of early adversity and HPA dysfunction: considerations for PTSD research. *Front Psychiatry.* 2013;4:110.

102. Struber N, Struber D, Roth G. Impact of early adversity on glucocorticoid regulation and later mental disorders. *Neurosci Biobehav Rev.* 2013;38C:17–37.

103. Espana RA, Scammell TE. Sleep neurobiology from a clinical perspective. *Sleep.* 2011;34:845–858.

104. Tsang AH, Barclay JL, Oster H. Interactions between endocrine and circadian systems. *J Mol Endocrinol.* 2014;52:R1–R16.

105. McGrath CL, Kelley ME, Holtzheimer PE, et al. Toward a neuroimaging treatment selection biomarker for major depressive disorder. *JAMA Psychiatry.* 2013;70:821–829.

106. Barnhofer T, Brennan K, Crane C, Duggan D, Williams JM. A comparison of vulnerability factors in patients with persistent and remitting lifetime symptom course of depression. *J Affect Disord.* 2014;152–154:155–161.

107. Watkins ER, Mullan E, Wingrove J, et al. Rumination-focused cognitive-behavioural therapy for residual depression: phase II randomised controlled trial. *Br J Psychiatry.* 2011;199:317–322.

108. Fountoulakis KN, Veroniki AA, Siamouli M, Moller HJ. No role for initial severity on the efficacy of antidepressants: results of a multi-meta-analysis. *Ann Gen Psychiatry.* 2013;12:26.

109. Querstret D, Cropley M. Assessing treatments used to reduce rumination and/or worry: a systematic review. *Clin Psychol Rev.* 2013;33:990–1009.

110. Khoury B, Lecomto T, Fortin G, et al. Mindfulness-based therapy: a comprehensive meta-analysis. *Clin Psychol Rev.* 2013;33:763–771.

111. Desrosiers A, Vine V, Klemanski DH, Nolen-Hoeksema S. Mindfulness and emotion regulation in depression and anxiety: common and distinct mechanisms of action. *Depress Anxiety.* 2013;30:654–661.

112. Wells A, Fisher P, Myers S, Wheatley J, Patel T, Brewin CR. Metacognitive therapy in treatment-resistant depression: a platform trial. *Behav Res Ther.* 2012;50:367–373.

113. Farb NA, Anderson AK, Segal ZV. The mindful brain and emotion regulation in mood disorders. *Can J Psychiatry.* 2012;57:70–77.

114. Dickenson J, Berkman ET, Arch J, Lieberman MD. Neural correlates of focused attention during a brief mindfulness induction. *Soc Cogn Affect Neurosci.* 2013;8:40–47.

115. Ives-Deliperi VL, Solms M, Meintjes EM. The neural substrates of mindfulness: an fMRI investigation. *Soc Neurosci.* 2011;6:231–242.

116. Taylor VA, Daneault V, Grant J, et al. Impact of meditation training on the default mode network during a restful state. *Soc Cogn Affect Neurosci.* 2013;8:4–14.

117. Brewer JA, Garrison KA. The posterior cingulate cortex as a plausible mechanistic target of meditation: findings from neuroimaging. *Ann N Y Acad Sci.* 2014;1307:19–27.

118. Farb NA, Segal ZV, Anderson AK. Mindfulness meditation training alters cortical representations of interoceptive attention. *Soc Cogn Affect Neurosci.* 2013;8:15–26.

119. Holzel BK, Carmody J, Vangel M, et al. Mindfulness practice leads to increases in regional brain gray matter density. *Psychiatry Res.* 2011;191:36–43.

120. DeRubeis RJ, Siegle GJ, Hollon SD. Cognitive therapy versus medication for depression: treatment outcomes and neural mechanisms. *Nat Rev Neurosci.* 2008;9:788–796.

121. Siegle GJ, Carter CS, Thase ME. Use of FMRI to predict recovery from unipolar depression with cognitive behavior therapy. *Am J Psychiatry.* 2006;163:735–738.

122. Yoshimura S, Okamoto Y, Onoda K, et al. Cognitive behavioral therapy for depression

changes medial prefrontal and ventral anterior cingulate cortex activity associated with self-referential processing. *Soc Cogn Affect Neurosci.* 2013.

123. Fu CH, Williams SC, Cleare AJ, et al. Neural responses to sad facial expressions in major depression following cognitive behavioral therapy. *Biol Psychiatry.* 2008;64:505–512.

124. Buchheim A, Viviani R, Kessler H, et al. Changes in prefrontal-limbic function in major depression after 15 months of long-term psychotherapy. *PLoS ONE.* 2012;7:e33745.

125. Wang T, Huang X, Huang P, et al. Early-stage psychotherapy produces elevated frontal white matter integrity in adult major depressive disorder. *PLoS ONE.* 2013;8:e63081.

CHAPTER 13

The Case of Thomas

Mr. Thomas W is a 57-year-old married male referred to the university mood disorder clinic by his community psychiatrist.

Mr. W was leafing through a magazine impassively as I greeted him in the waiting area. After shaking hands, we walked in silence toward my office. Once seated in a comfortable office, Mr. W glanced at me expectantly.

"How may I be of help to you, Mr. W?"

"Please call me Tom. I'm not sure if you can help me. You certainly come highly recommended. Dr. D and I have been working together for the last six years—it was his idea that I should see you. "

Tom's reply was dry, slow, and deliberate. It was a hot, humid summer day, and Tom had dark sweat stains around his armpits and in the front of his white shirt. His red tie was loosened up. Tom was an overweight man, approximately six feet tall. His scalp was glistening under his thinning and graying hair, neatly parted to the side.

"Can you tell me how you have been feeling?"

"I've been feeling like s***. Sorry, I'm a bit frustrated. We have tried so many medicines, nothing has worked. In the last few weeks I've been losing my temper at work. It's not a good time for that. Our insurance company is downsizing. If I don't get a grip soon, I may be out of a job. That would make my already lousy home life even worse."

"Is that new, losing your temper at work like that?"

"Why does it matter?" He cast a reproachful look at me. "I'm sorry, it's not your fault. I've been getting easily frustrated. I've been loosing my temper at home also. My youngest son, who's home from college, will hardly speak to me. I can't blame him. His mother and I are going through some rough times. We're in counseling. She was threatening to leave me this spring unless things got better."

Unfortunately, emerging evidence suggests that treatment with selective serotonin reuptake inhibitor (SSRI) antidepressants may have a negative impact on feelings of attachment and love in otherwise well-functioning marriages.[1] Tom may be caught in a vicious cycle, as his perceived distancing and anger may contribute to more negative marital interactions. The negative health implications of this cycle is highlighted by a study that found evidence that negative marital interactions may lead to an increase in carotid artery intima-media thickness, even after adjustment for other cardiovascular risk factors.[2] Marital counseling not only may help the family situation but also can potentially reduce Tom's risk for stroke.

> "I've not always been like this. Actually I'm kind of a laid-back guy when I feel well. It's just that I've been depressed for years. I can hardly remember what it feels like to be normal."
>
> "Can you describe for me what depression has been like for you?"
>
> "I feel tired and grumpy all the time. My concentration is off in the office. Last week I almost forgot a meeting with an important client. You can't do that in my line of work. I'm an actuary—do you know what that is?"
>
> I nodded.
>
> "My boss called me into his office last week. He wanted to know if I was OK. He has been very patient and understanding with me—he knows about our home situation. Whenever I get stressed out by work or have arguments at home, it stays with me. I keep on chewing on that stuff. Dwelling on things just makes me more distracted at work."

In this book we have highlighted that ruminations are one of the central symptoms of depression. Ruminations can increase negative affect and diminish positive affect. Furthermore, ruminations are associated with insomnia, impaired cognition, suicidality, and a greater likelihood of depressive recurrence in the face of stress (see Chapter 12 for more detail on these negative consequences of rumination). In Tom's case we are additionally concerned that ruminations may act as an "amplifier" of the biological correlates of stress. Studies have shown that rumination following stressful events may lead to extended cortisol response and sustained inflammation as measured by C-reactive protein (CRP) levels.[3] Both of these phenomena are likely to have a negative impact on Tom's cardiometabolic status.

> "But things can't go on like this much longer. We are a small company, and if I don't get my sh** together, they will have to let me go." Tom hesitated. "I apologize—I usually don't speak like this with other professionals. If I lose

my job, we will no longer be able to afford my son's tuition, and I'm sure that my wife will leave me. I might as well kill myself then."

Irritability is a common manifestation of major depressive disorder (MDD). Up to 40–50 percent of depressed patients report irritability as one of their presenting symptoms, making a good case for its inclusion as one of the core symptoms of MDD.[4,5] The presence of irritability is associated with more severe symptoms of depression, greater suicidality, less treatment response, longer depressive episodes, a tendency toward chronicity, and more pronounced psychosocial dysfunction.[4-6] Moreover, depressed irritable patients also frequently report fatigue, reversed vegetative signs manifesting as somnolence and weight gain, loss of interest, morbid thoughts of death, self-reproach, anxiety, psychomotor retardation, sympathetic overarousal, and anhedonia.[4,7,8] Although one would not be surprised by the link between irritability, anxiety, and sympathetic overarousal in MDD, it may be counterintuitive to associate elevated sympathetic tone with fatigue, somnolence, and psychomotor retardation. We discuss this point further below.

Depressed patients who have irritability and anger attacks tend to be female and tend to have an earlier onset of depression, comorbid impulse control disorders, substance use, anxiety disorders (including posttraumatic stress disorder), social anxiety, generalized anxiety disorder and panic attacks, and cardio- and cerebrovascular morbidity, but not bipolar spectrum features.[4-7] Antidepressants used in treatment of bipolar spectrum disorders can frequently precipitate irritable dysphoria.[9] It is important to acknowledge that irritability, even combined with psychotic-like symptoms, may occur in the context of MDD, without any relation to bipolarity.[6]

Irritability in the context of MDD may have specific neurobiological correlates. A positron emission tomography (PET) imaging study uncovered that depressed individuals exposed to angry as opposed to neutral autobiographical scripts manifested a positive correlation between increased blood flow in the ventromedial prefrontal cortex (vmPFC) and amygdala. There was no such association between amygdala and ventrolateral prefrontal cortex (vlPFC) activity in depressed patients with no history of anger attacks. In healthy individuals there was an inverse relationship between amygdala and vlPFC activation during the anger induction paradigm. This discovery suggests aberrant corticolimbic regulation in response to anger in this subset of depressed patients.[10] Further extending this finding, an MRI study has reported a higher density and severity of subcortical white matter hyperintensities in MDD patients with anger attacks, relative to individuals suffering from atypical or melancholy depression.[11]

Depressed patients with anger attacks may have an anomaly of central serotonergic transmission as manifested by a significantly blunted prolactin response to fenfluramine (a serotonergic agent) compared with healthy controls.[12] Treatment with SSRIs and serotonergic tricyclic antidepressants often suppresses anger attacks and mitigates the perception of stress in depressed patients.[13]

"Have you been thinking about suicide?" I asked.

"Sometimes when I get down. I wish that everything would just stop. I wouldn't care if I didn't wake up the next day." Tom noticed my concern. "I'm not going to do anything stupid, if that's what you were going to ask me. That's the last thing I want to put my kid through, after all that he has had to deal with. My uncle committed suicide—I saw what it did to his family.

"Tammy, my wife, had me get all the guns out of the house a few months ago. I used to go hunting with my friends. It's been a while. Nothing interests me anymore. I can't even sit through TV shows anymore. Most of them are just a mind-rot anyway.

"I wish that I could loose some weight." He looked at his gut disparagingly. "You wouldn't think it, but I was a football player in high school. All this weight came on when Dr. D added that medicine to my Cymbalta (duloxetine). He said that although it is an antipsychotic, it could help with my depression. All it did was make me gain weight and fall asleep at work. We stopped it after a month. I've been more on edge ever since."

"Has your energy and motivation improved?" I asked.

"Not really. I never feel rested. I feel tired the whole day. You would think that I could sleep well. But when I get to bed it's tossing and turning. Most nights I will take my sleep aid."

"Does that help?"

"Kind of. I sleep until 2 a.m. then I wake up to go to the bathroom. I rarely sleep well after that. My wife tells me that I snore loudly. Sometimes she kicks me so I'll turn over. Even on the weekends when I sleep in, it's still a struggle to get out of bed in the morning. Then I have to face my ugly mug in the mirror while I'm shaving. Can there be a better way to start a day?" asked Tom with a wry smile. "I stopped playing golf with my friends months ago—it is too much of a chore. I'm not in a very conversational mood lately. Silence would be awkward, and I'm not up to answering questions about what's wrong with me. My game's been lousy—not much of a loss."

"You mentioned previously that you have been losing your temper. How long has that been going on, and when do you remember first getting depressed?"

"I think that I may have been depressed in high school. I'm not sure—nobody called it depression back then. My father had just lost his job because of an argument at work. He started hitting the bottle too often. My sister was staying out late at night. The screaming arguments at home went on around the clock. On one occasion I got into my father's face because he was screaming at my Mom, something about the dinner. Bad move—he cleaned my clock."

"Was he abusive?"

"Not really, just old school. Parents didn't use to apologize a lot. You knew what to expect if you got out of line."

"You said that you became depressed?"

"I stopped caring about my grades. I was reading comic books under my desk in class. I wore the same pair of jeans and sweatshirt to school for weeks. Finally my Mom noticed. I also wasn't eating that well. I had a chip on my shoulder all the time. She spoke to the vice-principal, and they sent me to counseling. I straightened my act a few weeks later and pulled up my grades."

Relevant Psychiatric History

Tom first saw a therapist when he was twenty. He came home after sophomore year of college feeling "depleted." He was emotionally "flat and indifferent." At times he could not fall asleep until the early morning hours. On other occasions he slept 12–13 hours a day. Nothing in his life felt enjoyable, and everything "got on his nerves." He was completely withdrawn. Tom ate his meals in his room and did not return his friends' phone calls. When his parents approached him, wondering what was wrong, he said he wished that he had never been born. Alarmed, his parents took him to see their family doctor. After speaking to Tom, the doctor referred him to a local psychiatrist. Imipramine treatment and psychotherapy were initiated. By the time he returned to college for his junior year, Tom felt much better. He continued medicine until the end of the fall semester and then stopped it because it was giving him "cotton mouth" and causing constipation. Tom was depression-free for several years.

From age 25 to the present, Tom has had six more depressive episodes. In general the presentation of these episodes was similar to the initial one, except that problems with concentration and memory became more prominent. Tom was also becoming more despondent, dejected, and indignant. His anger on occasion turned into rage, which caused problems in his marriage and at work. After he lost his temper, Tom would be truthfully regretful and apologize profusely. He and his wife have been in marital therapy on two occasions, for several months each time. Additionally, Tom has sought individual therapy to help him cope with anger. Relationships in the family have improved some but still become tense and distant at times.

Tom has several significant risk factors predicting the recurrence of his illness. Several studies have identified a relationship between an increased number of previous episodes and the risk of future recurrence.[14–18] Typically one considers depression as recurrent if a patient has experienced four or more episodes,[14] which unfortunately is the case for Tom. As many as two-thirds of depressed patients suffer from a recurrent form of the disease. Furthermore, each successive episode may increase the risk of future occurrence by as much as 16 percent.[17] Although more than three previous episodes may substantially increase the odds of early relapse (odds ratio [OR] = 1.64), it is overshadowed by the ominous risk associated with residual symptoms (OR = 3.68).[14] The odds ratio is a measure of association between an exposure and an outcome. A more recent study has uncovered that residual symptoms are a common occurrence. Indeed, approximately 90 percent of remitted depressed patients had at least one residual symptom, with median number of three; the most common are weight increase (71.3 percent) and midnocturnal insomnia (54.9 percent).[19] Moreover, a greater number of residual symptom domains predicted a more substantial risk of disease recurrence.[19] Other studies have noted a high frequency of cognitive problems, fatigue, and sleep disturbance among residual symptoms.[20–23] These three symptoms not only dominated the course of depression but also were present 85–94 percent of the time; moreover, they occurred during 39–44 percent of the time in remission.[22]

Unfortunately, patients often fail to spontaneously mention indecisiveness, distractability, inattentiveness, and forgetfulness as part of their depressive experience, and clinicians omit asking about them. Furthermore, it is often difficult to ascertain if fatigue and cognitive problems are due to depression or are side effects of antidepressant therapy.[18,24] Additionally, cognitive symptoms and fatigue tend not to respond very well to treatment.[25] Some researchers have described the impact of repeated depressive episodes on declining cognitive function as "toxic."[26] Stimulants, noradrenergic antidepressants, and modafinil have been used with variable success in the treatment of depression-related fatigue.[27] In Tom's case these agents (possibly aside from modafinil) carry a risk of worsening his irritability, anger, anxiety, and sleep disturbance.

> After two courses of imipramine treatment, Tom was treated with fluoxetine. Initial response was favorable. Tom's anger subsided, and he enjoyed a year of good mood. Toward the end of that year, Tom developed sexual problems. He could no longer maintain an erection, which worsened his already difficult marital situation. Tom was next tried on sustained-release bupropion. Eventually, the dose was adjusted to 300 mg daily. Tom benefited from treatment: his mood improved, he had more enthusiasm and energy, he was less distracted, and he performed better at work. Unfortunately, Tom started having difficulty falling asleep and was becoming increasingly short-tempered.

Although bupropion, either as monotherapy or as an adjunct, tends to benefit depressed patients complaining of low energy, lack of enthusiasm, difficulty concentrating, and psychomotor retardation—most likely related to its ability to modulate dopamine (DA) and norepinephrine (NE)—it is not without its downside.[28,29] Insomnia, agitation, headache, constipation, and dizziness are all common side effects.[29,30]

At this point, we may wish to speculate about the hypothetical pathophysiological underpinning of Tom's depression. He is depressed, irritable, rumination prone, tired, and unenthusiastic. Tom has obvious cognitive difficulties and a chronic sleep disturbance. Many of the presenting symptoms point to central overarousal/hypervigilance, but is that explanation consistent with excessive daytime sleepiness, fatigue, and lack of enthusiasm/motivation? Apparently yes. Based on emerging evidence, it is increasingly clear that depression is a heterogeneous condition and may manifest simultaneously in a hypo- and hyperaroused form. Depression with low arousal/unstable vigilance may be associated with lower hypothalamic-pituitary-adrenal (HPA) function (as we discussed in the context of atypical depression), and lower NE turnover and locus ceruleus (LC) firing rate.[31–33] Clinically it would be associated with fatigue, low motivation, lack of interest in pleasurable activities, hypersomnolence, and difficulty sustaining focus. NE/DA-stimulating antidepressants, stimulants, and modafinil and armodafinil may be useful pharmacological interventions for these symptoms.[31–33] Vigilance Algorithm Leipzig (VIGALL) is a validated instrument that can be used to asses vigilance level in MDD patients.[32]

In contradistinction to hypoarousal, many if not most MDD patients suffer from the hyperaroused/hyperstable vigilant form of depression. The hyperaroused form of MDD is characterized by elevated and sustained LC firing, manifesting as increased NE turnover, associated with higher levels of its metabolite 3-methoxy-4-hydroxyphenylglycol (MHPG), and elevated corticotropin-releasing factor and HPA axis activity.[32–34] The clinical manifestations of hyperaroused depression include inner tension, irritability, prolonged sleep latency, fragmented sleep, fatigue, exhaustion, anhedonia, and not lack of drive but, rather, drive inhibition and psychomotor retardation.[32,33] Presumably, rapid burst firing of LC neurons results in an elevated release of galanin (see Chapter 9), which is colocalized in the NE vesicles. Galanin, along with excessive activation of postsynaptic adrenergic receptors, contributes to behavioral inhibition and suppression of ventral tegmental area (VTA) dopaminergic neuron activity. Reduced DA mesolimbic and mesocortical transmission may induce anhedonia, suppression of motivation, and concentration difficulties.[32,33] Furthermore, excessive LC activity in stressful circumstances, associated with deregulated stimulation of alpha-1 adrenergic receptors located on cortical pyramidal neurons, has been linked with a decline in executive function and working memory.[35]

Most antidepressants, including SSRIs, tricyclics, and serotonin-NE reuptake inhibitors (SNRIs), as well as electroconvulsive therapy (ECT) produce a sustained suppression of LC firing with an accompanying increase in dopaminergic activity. Some studies suggest that serotonin/NE-elevating agents may have an advantage over SSRIs in their ability to restore normative LC function.[34] Notable exceptions are bupropion, which is associated with only transient suppression of the LC activity, and a monoamine oxidase inhibitor, phenelzine, which does not activate VTA dopaminergic neurons.[33] Overaroused depressed patients are not likely to benefit from stimulant augmentation.

Tom is most likely, based on his clinical presentation, history, and comorbidities, suffering from the hyperaroused form of depression, sometimes referred to by psychiatrists as the "wired and tired" syndrome. Is there a relationship between Tom's depression and his chronic and disabling sleep disturbance? Since NE has an important role in the regulation of sleep and wakefulness, it is plausible that hyperarousal associated with excessive LC activity in the context of depression or stress interferes with sleep architecture. Especially vulnerable to increased LC activity is non-rapid eye-movement (non-REM), slow-wave sleep, also recognized as the most restorative sleep phase.[36] Both alpha-1 adrenergic antagonists and alpha-2 agonists (inhibitors of LC activity) have a demonstrated ability to suppress non-REM sleep.[36]

Etiological theories have placed overarousal center stage as an explanation for the origins of insomnia. Insomnia has been defined as a psychobiological phenomenon, characterized not only by difficulty falling asleep and maintaining sleep but also by a lack of refreshing sleep quality and an ensuing impairment in daytime functioning.[37] Physiological and cognitive hyperarousal is associated with myriad biological changes, including functional and structural brain changes, neuroimmune dysfunction, altered HPA axis regulation, and aberrant autonomic system function.[37–42] Moreover, primary insomnia is also associated with a profound disturbance of circadian and homeostatic drives, leading to a state "physiological confusion," whereby both sleep and arousal systems can be active simultaneously.[42] In this context, imaging studies demonstrate a sleep-related deactivation failure of frontoparietal system subserving executive function, attention, and self-awareness.[39]

Given the shared pathophysiological features of primary insomnia and MDD, such as autonomic, endocrine, and immune disturbance and functional and structural brain changes, including reduction in the orbitofrontal and hippocampal gray matter volumes, how can one draw a line separating the two conditions?[39–41,43,44] Adding to this challenge is the fact that primary insomnia and depression have many common clinical features, such as reduced positive affect and exaggerated negative affect, increased emotional reactions to adverse circumstances, fatigue, daytime somnolence, and attentional, executive, and memory deficits (also possibly related to hippocampal structural damage in both conditions).[40,45,46] Increased inflammation, which is often observed in both MDD and primary insomnia, may also contribute to cognitive clouding, irritability, fatigue, body aches, appetite, and sleep/wakefulness disturbance.[47,48] Insomnia and MDD also share common medical comorbidities, such as hypertension, heart disease, type 2 diabetes, cerebrovascular disease, respiratory and gastrointestinal ailments, and chronic pain disorders.[42,48,49]

This brings up the ubiquitous chicken-and-egg question: does the presence of insomnia precipitate depression, or is it the other way around? The answer is yes to both—there appears to be a bidirectional relationship between these two conditions. A meta-analysis has estimated that insomnia doubles the likelihood of developing depression over a five- to six-year observation period.[46] Moreover, insomnia is more likely to precipitate depression than the other way around; in contrast, anxiety is more predictive of insomnia than vice versa.[50] The relationship between these three diagnostic entities, insomnia, depression, and anxiety, is most likely mediated by emotional reactivity, cognitive, cortical, and autonomic hyperarousal.[45] Insomnia and depression additionally share circadian rhythm disturbances.[51]

What kind of advice can we provide for Tom based on this understanding of the overlap between, hyperarousal, insomnia, and depression? Good sleep hygiene, stable daily routines, improved dietary habits, insomnia-focused cognitive-behavioral therapy (CBT), and appropriate pharmacological management of insomnia would all go a long way toward improving depression treatment outcomes and Tom's functioning.

At his psychiatrist's suggestion, Tom agreed to a trial of lithium augmentation. Extended-release lithium carbonate, 300 mg, one in the morning and two at night, was utilized for several months. He did quite well. His mood was stable, and his irritability and sleep disturbance abated. Regrettably, however, Tom developed hypothyroidism and EKG changes, which were thought to be related to lithium therapy. Lithium was discontinued. As some of the side effects related to bupropion resurfaced, Tom and his psychiatrist initiated a cross-taper switch from bupropion to duloxetine. After a partial response to 60 mg duloxetine, his dose was adjusted to 90 mg a day.

Tom was overall feeling, and functioning better, yet sleep disturbance, irritability and a lack of enthusiasm continued to be an issue. His previous psychiatrist suggested olanzapine augmentation. Tom was concerned that olanzapine was classified as an antipsychotic. However, following a lengthy discussion, he decided to initiate an augmentation regimen. After his olanzapine dose was adjusted to 10 mg nightly, Tom experienced substantial relief. His sleep improved, and he "completely mellowed out." The combination of duloxetine at 90 mg a day and olanzapine at 10 mg a day was used for over a year.

However, as he worried would happen, Tom gained substantial weight (16 pounds) over this period. Since Tom had already been diagnosed with type 2 diabetes, hypertension, and dyslipidemia, he was justifiably concerned about this recent weight gain. Due to work demands and a busy family schedule, Tom's efforts to start exercising were not fruitful. He had also tried, albeit inconsistently, to change his diet.

Somewhat equivocal evidence points to a bidirectional relationship between depression and obesity, as well as between depression and metabolic syndrome.[52–55] Moreover, it appears that body mass index may mediate the association between depression and elevated peripheral inflammation, as well as the relationship between mood and anxiety disorders and metabolic syndrome.[56,57] Unfortunately, cardiometabolic, musculoskeletal, and psychiatric comorbidities have been shown to hasten the recurrence of depression and associated work disabilities.[58]

Tom reported considerable family- and work-related stress. Stress is an established precipitant of depressive episodes. Is it also likely to shape the relationship among depression, obesity, and metabolic abnormalities? Chronic stress, combined with a high-fat/high-sugar diet, is associated with more intense sympathetic signaling and elevated release of neuropeptide Y (NPY), an NE cotransmitter.[59] NPY, directly released into adipose tissue, interacts with NPY Y2 receptors, thereby initiating preadipocyte proliferation and lipid filling, as well as angiogenesis. In preclinical models, chronic stress precipitated release of NPY and upregulated Y2 receptor expression in adipose tissue, increasing its growth by 50 percent within a two-week period.[59] Another preclinical study uncovered stress-related activation of toll-like receptor-4 and an ensuing PFC upregulation of nuclear factor kappa-beta, a principal transcription factor mediating synthesis of proinflammatory molecules.[60] Furthermore, stress induced neuroinflammation in the PFC and local oxidative and nitrosative cellular damage.[60] These two preclinical studies elucidate physiological mechanisms that may explain the role of stress in the development of obesity, neuroinflammation, and oxidative/nitrosative cellular damage, all possibly contributing to the link between depression and metabolic derangement. Human studies have also shown that stress and depression interact, causing an altered metabolic response to high-fat meals, conducive to the development of obesity.[61] Moreover, as in preclinical studies, chronic stress in humans increases the vulnerability to diet-related abdominal obesity, oxidative stress, and metabolic abnormalities.[62]

Of course, from Tom's perspective it would be important to know if diet and exercise can mitigate the impact of depression and obesity on cardiometabolic disorder. There is some encouraging news stemming from research. In related studies, a six-month hypocaloric diet in individuals suffering from metabolic syndrome produced weight loss, elevation in peripheral blood DA and serotonin levels, and a reduction in anxiety.[63] Furthermore, a hypocaloric diet combined with increased folate consumption resulted in weight loss, an improvement in depressive symptomatology, and a reduction in markers of oxidative stress.[64] In another study, reduced depression, as measured by the Beck Depression Inventory, was correlated with decreased body fat mass, leptin, and CRP (an inflammatory marker).[65] The combination of sedentary lifestyle and high caloric intake may contribute to impaired glycemic control, decreased hepatic insulin, elevated cholesterol and low-density lipoproteins, and cognitive/attentional dysfunction. Normal physical activity (10,000 steps/day or more) was sufficient to abolish the detrimental metabolic effects of high-calorie food intake.[66] Robust scientific evidence supports the need for dietary counseling and the encouragement of exercise as standard treatment components for all obese depressed patients.

Currently Tom's psychiatric medication regimen includes duloxetine at 90 mg daily, 10 mg zolpidem as needed for insomnia, and 1 mg alprazolam every 8 hours as needed for anxiety. As we have learned, his current medications have not addressed Tom's depressive symptoms adequately. Reported side effects include constipation, which he manages with high-fiber diet, as well as a mild decrease in libido and a dry mouth.

Tom denied symptoms consistent with hypomania/mania such as elevated mood, excessive energy, racing thoughts, grandiosity, delusions, and hallucinations. Records from his previous psychiatrists offered no indication that lithium or atypical antipsychotics were utilized due to suspicion regarding bipolar disorder.

Social History

Tom is one of four children raised in a blue-collar family. After some minor difficulties in high school he graduated from collage and became an accountant. He had a brief seven-month marriage in his early twenties, which ended after his wife had an affair because "she was too bored." A few years later Tom met his current wife, Tammy. Following a short engagement they got married and had three children. His oldest daughter has graduated from nursing school and is married. She has two children and lives out of state. His middle daughter has just graduated from college and is working part-time. She is living with a roommate in the same town as Tom and Tammy. Their youngest son has just finished his sophomore year of college. Tom has worked for the same insurance company over twenty years.

Substance Use History

Tom admitted to occasional binge drinking during college. He also experimented with marijuana in his twenties but stopped using it because "it didn't do anything for me. I didn't even get high." Since then he usually has two to three beers with dinner and while he watches baseball games, several times a week. Tom smoked one to two packs a day for over two decades until he was diagnosed with hypertension and type 2 diabetes seven years ago.

Since then he has stopped smoking for the most part. On a few occasions he has relapsed: "Smoking helps me concentrate—it calms my nerves when the work gets too stressful."

Past Medical History

Tom fractured two ribs while playing high school football. Approximately twenty years ago he had an appendectomy. Seven years ago Tom was diagnosed with hypertension and type 2 diabetes. They are now well controlled with a calcium channel blocker, an ACE inhibitor, and a sulfonylurea agent. Initially Tom tried to adhere to a Mediterranean-type diet but has had a great deal of difficulty because he is "at heart a meat and potatoes kind a guy." Three years ago, due to his worsening dyslipidemia, Tom was started on a statin. Most of his metabolic indicators are now under control, although his high-sensitivity CRP level is still high at 3.4 mg/L. "My doctor told me that if I don't stop smoking and lose some weight, I might have a heart attack."

Eight years ago, after several months of lithium augmentation therapy, Tom developed hypothyroidism. It has been treated for several years with levothyroxine, but Tom has stopped it about three years ago. "I was on too many medicines as it is, and I didn't think I needed it anymore."

Family Psychiatric History

Tom mentioned that his father probably suffered from depression, although he was never treated for it. He also described his father as a "working alcoholic." Tom's father drank mostly during the weekends and occasionally during the weeknights but never went to work inebriated. His oldest sister has been treated for postpartum depression. He is not sure if she has had subsequent episodes. Tom's paternal uncle committed suicide. Based on family stories he had heard, Tom would not be surprised if his uncle suffered from depression. He described his mother as a "nervous Nelly." She tended to worry a lot and was overprotective as he was growing up. A few of the maternal family members have suffered from anxiety disorders and possible alcohol use disorders.

Relevant Mental Status Examination Findings

Tom is a 57-year-old married Caucasian male appearing slightly older than his stated age. His affect is dejected and at times morose. Tom reports feeling depressed and irritable. His range of affect is somewhat constricted. There is no evidence of a formal thought disorder. Tom denied hallucinations and delusions. On occasion he seemed distracted. Because Tom complained of memory problems, his recall was formally evaluated. His immediate recall was 4/4 words, and his delayed recall was 3/4. Tom endorsed transient hopeless feelings and indicated that at times he "wouldn't care if I never woke up in the morning" but denied any active suicidal thoughts, plans, or intent. His insight and judgment were intact.

Diagnostic Impression

Major depressive disorder, recurrent; history of hypertension, type 2 diabetes, dyslipidemia, hypothyroidism related to prior lithium use.

Treatment Plan

"I believe that you can benefit from adding aripiprazole to the duloxetine you are already taking. It may help with your mood overall but also address irritability."

"What kind of medicine is that?"

"It is classified as an atypical antipsychotic, just like olanzapine, but it is less likely to contribute to weight gain and metabolic issues."

"I don't know how I feel about that."

"There are other alternatives—would you like to hear about them?"

"Not really, not now—you're the expert. If you believe that it is the right medicine for me, let's try it. I guess I can always change my mind if it starts giving me problems."

Usage of atypical antipsychotics as augmenting agents in depressed patients who have not responded to antidepressants has become a common clinical practice. Studies suggest that approximately 30 percent of adult depression-related visits include an atypical antipsychotic agent (also often referred to as a second-generation antipsychotic [SGA]), less so if the sessions included psychotherapy.[67] Only three atypical antipsychotics have been approved by the U.S. FDA as adjunct treatments in antidepressant-unresponsive depression: quetiapine, aripiprazole, and the combination of olanzapine and fluoxetine.[67–69] A meta-analysis provides consistent evidence that SGAs provide significantly greater response (OR = 1.69; 95 percent confidence interval = 1.46–1.95, $p < 0.00001$) and remission rates (OR = 2.00, 95 percent confidence interval = 1.69–2.37, $p < 0.00001$) compared with placebo in patients suffering from nonpsychotic depression that has previously been unresponsive to antidepressant treatment.[69] Another meta-analysis quoted response and remission rates with adjunct atypical agents at 57.2 percent and 47.4 percent, respectively, compared with 35.4 percent and 22.3 percent for placebo.[70]

Not everything favors atypical antipsychotics, however. Discontinuation rates due to adverse reactions are consistently much higher with adjunct antipsychotics than with placebo. Furthermore, we still lack data to help us differentiate between the individual atypical antipsychotic augmenting agents based on their efficacy and to tailor our treatment to specific patient needs.[69] Few direct comparisons between augmenting strategies and a paucity of information about the relative efficacy of switch versus augmentation strategies make clinical decision making less obvious than it should be.[71–73] Nonetheless, it appears that the clinical community may be making its decisions based on perceived differences in side effect profiles.

Here we provide a rudimentary summary regarding the balance between the efficacy and safety of individual SGAs. While the olanzapine-fluoxetine combination clearly separates from placebo in treatment-resistant depressed (TRD) patients, its separation from antidepressant alone is less impressive and consistent. Weight gain, metabolic deregulation (manifesting as glucose, triglyceride, and cholesterol elevation), and ensuing cardiovascular risk have all been of concern.[68] Quetiapine augmentation has also had variable success in separating from antidepressant alone and has been associated with sedation, somnolence, and weight gain. Aripiprazole has established efficacy in TRD patients. However, its utilization has been hampered somewhat by relatively frequent complaints of akathisia, restlessness, headache, and sleep disturbance. Risperidone has not demonstrated consistent efficacy as an augmenting agent in TRD patients. Furthermore, reports of prolactin elevation, extrapyramidal side effects, and weight gain have all hindered its utilization. Clozapine and ziprasidone have inadequately been studied as augmenting strategies in MDD. Additionally, their use can be associated with serious adverse reactions.[68] More frequent use of SGAs may also be constrained by the dearth of studies evaluating their long-term efficacy and safety.

What should we suggest to Tom? Tom has voiced clear concerns about the risk of gaining weight and the cardiometabolic impact of a new medication. A randomized study evaluated change in metabolic parameters following a switch from olanzapine, quetiapine, or risperidone to aripiprazole. Non-high-density cholesterol levels, triglycerides, and body weight were reduced more in the patients who switched to aripiprazole for 24 weeks compared with the ones who remained on the previous treatment.[74] Moreover, the risk of acute major cardiovascular events in younger and middle-aged adults appears to be similar in the three frequently prescribed SGAs. The crude rate for any major cardiovascular event was 5.3 per 1,000 person-years for olanzapine, 3.4 for quetiapine, and 5.2 for risperidone users.

Both olanzapine and aripiprazole were found to induce insulin resistance compared with placebo. Unlike olanzapine, aripiprazole use was not associated with significant elevation of postprandial insulin and glucagon. However, it is important to emphasize that metabolic changes occurred even in absence of increased hunger, weight gain, or a change in psychiatric symptoms.[75] A study that specifically investigated the metabolic impact of adjunct aripiprazole in the treatment of resistant MDD discovered no change in waist circumference, total cholesterol, triglycerides, fasting plasma glucose, or hemoglobin A1C compared with placebo-treated patients. A greater number of aripiprazole-treated patients had significant weight gain (≥7 percent of body mass) relative to placebo.[76]

Several blinded, placebo-controlled, and open label studies have established the efficacy of aripiprazole in the treatment of depressed patients who have failed a previous antidepressant or suffer from chronic or recurrent form of illness, regardless of depression severity.[77–79] Adjunct aripiprazole was effective for core symptoms of depression, such as depressed mood, guilt, and psychic anxiety, but also helped with insomnia and drive.[80] Even depressed patients who had no response or got worse on a previous antidepressant benefited from aripiprazole augmentation. Patients who got worse in response to a prior antidepressant achieved a 25.4 percent remission rate with adjunct aripiprazole compared with only 12.4 percent on placebo.[81] Although aripiprazole augmentation was overall well tolerated, some of the patients experienced akathisia, restlessness, insomnia, headache, and constipation.[77,78,81,82]

Adjunctive aripiprazole has been compared with adjunctive bupropion in a retrospective chart review.[83] In this retrospective study, augmentation with aripiprazole was more effective than augmentation with bupropion, resulting in a 50 percent remission rate following five patient visits, as opposed to a 33 percent remission rate observed with bupropion.[83] Significantly, aripiprazole use was associated with a reduced score on the item measuring death and suicide. A prospective 52-week open label study evaluated aripiprazole safety when combined with bupropion, SSRIs, and SNRIs.[84] There were no unexpected adverse events, and symptomatic improvement was comparable in all the study arms.[84]

Therefore, we can with reasonable confidence suggest to Tom that the combination of duloxetine with aripiprazole may be a relatively metabolically safe and therapeutically feasible option. However, we should remember that past augmentation of an SSRI with bupropion led to increased irritability and agitation in Tom's case. Furthermore, Tom is complaining of difficulty regulating his temper and angry outbursts. Is aripiprazole a suitable choice in this respect? Although we are not aware of any published studies of adjunct aripiprazole benefits in depression with anger attacks, there are a few reports of its use in borderline patients who suffered from both depression and anger and in agitated/aggressive schizophrenic and developmentally disordered individuals.[85–88] All reports indicated that aripiprazole ameliorated both depressive symptoms and anger in subjects suffering from borderline personality disorder; one study noted that aripiprazole had a much larger effect size than other antipsychotics.[87] One can speculate that aripiprazole-mediated alpha-1 adrenergic antagonism, as well as modulation of serotonergic 5HT1A and dopaminergic D2 receptors, may have mitigated some of the effects of sympathetic overarousal and serotonergic dysfunction in these individuals, including anger and anxiety.[88] As Tom is also manifesting symptoms consistent with elevated sympathetic tone, this medication may be a good choice for him.

A daily dose of 5 mg aripiprazole was initiated. Tom was going to give me a call in a couple of weeks and let me know how he was doing. Additionally, we ordered his old medical records and several laboratory studies to reevaluate his metabolic status and thyroid function. We also ordered electrolytes, a complete blood count, B12, folate, high-sensitivity CRP, and homocysteine levels.

I encouraged Tom to make his best effort to exercise at least 30–40 minutes three to four times a week. Going for hikes with his family on weekends would be a particularly good idea, because it might also improve relationships in the family, and exercising in the natural environment might provide additional benefits. He agreed to try harder to adhere to his weight loss diet and cut down on alcohol.

Tom declined individual or family therapy but did agree to have a consultation with a sleep specialist.

Tom called the office about two weeks after starting aripiprazole as augmentation therapy. He reported minor improvement. His irritability and anger had subsided, but he was still feeling tired, had little enthusiasm, and experienced significant difficulty maintaining focus at work. He agreed to increase aripiprazole to 7.5 mg daily. As sleep continued to be a problem, Tom scheduled an appointment with the sleep specialist I had previously recommended.

Second Office Visit, Four Weeks Later

"Well, Doc, I have some good news and some bad news. Where would you like me to start?"

"Let's start with good news."

"OK, 7.5 mg of the new medicine really helped with irritability and anger. Even my wife noticed a difference and asked me if I was taking some new medication. Since it really helped with my short temper and I was still feeling tired and a bit tense, I decided on my own to increase the dose to 10 mg last week. I hope that you don't mind."

"Has it helped?"

"It's hard to say. My mood is better—I was looking forward to mountain biking with my son. On the other hand, I feel more fidgety and restless. At night I am nervous and have a harder time falling sleep. Could this be a side effect of the new medicine? Maybe I should have given you a call before increasing the dose."

As he was answering my question, Tom appeared restless: he was shifting in the chair and tapping his foot against the floor. "It may be a side effect of the new medication," I responded. "Sometimes medicines in this class will cause people to feel restless, like they need to move all the time. Some patients also describe it as inner tension or even anxiety. It is a side effect called akathisia."

"Sounds exactly like what I have. Is there anything that we can do about it? I like how this medicine is working for me, otherwise. I would like to keep it if I could."

"We can try to go back to 7.5 mg and see how it works. Maybe if you gave it a bit more time it will be able to help with the rest of the depressive symptoms."

"I guess we can try that." Tom did not look entirely convinced.

"How did your appointment with the sleep specialist go?"

"I really liked him. He did a sleep study ten days ago. It is one of those where I had to spend a night at the sleep center. Actually, the room was pretty nice and quiet. I'm used to softer pillows, and all those wires made it harder to sleep. I saw Dr. W again three days ago. He gave me a report to bring to you. I guess I have moderate sleep apnea. They are going to fit me for a mask. He recommended a CPAP (continuous positive airway pressure) machine. Do you have any other patients who use those?"

"Yes, several. Quite a few people have both mood disorders and obstructive sleep apnea. May I see the report that Dr. W has sent with you?"

There is robust evidence supporting an association between obstructive sleep apnea/hypopnea syndrome (OSAH) and MDD. Approximately half of OSAH patients also suffer from depression, and about one-third to a half experience anxiety.[89–91] In fact, OSAH patients are as likely to present to physicians with complaints of depression and anxiety as they are with more typical symptoms of this condition.[91] A prospective study uncovered that individuals with OSAH had twice the risk of developing depression within a year of follow-up compared with individuals without this condition.[92] Although in Tom's case depression most likely predated OSAH, it is conceivable that OSAH may have contributed to some of the symptoms that have aggravated Tom's depression or possibly made it more treatment resistant.

Pathophysiological mechanisms associated with sleep apnea may cause both functional and structural damage to key brain areas involved in regulation of mood, cognition, the stress response, neuroendocrine function, and autonomic regulation.[90] Furthermore, injury to the brainstem in OSAH may be associated with disturbance in DA, NE, and serotonin transmission, as well as autonomic regulation, leading to elevation of sympathetic tone.[90] Damage to the insula, anterior cingulate cortex (ACC), and thalamus may contribute to compromised emotional regulation and stress responsivity.[90,93] Magnetic resonance spectroscopy studies have found evidence of a correlation between insular metabolites and depression, anxiety, and sleep disturbance measures on standardized scales.[93] Cortical, hippocampal, and mammillary body structural abnormalities may be linked to deficits in concentration, executive function, and memory, all of which are included among Tom's complaints.[90,94]

Although the apnea/hypopnea index, an indirect measure of OSAH severity, does not appear to be directly linked with cognitive dysfunction, mean oxygen saturation in OSAH patients does correlate with measures of executive function and memory.[95] Moreover, OSAH has been identified as a risk factor for mild cognitive impairment and dementia.[96] Excessive daytime sleepiness and insomnia, both cardinal symptoms of OSAH, are also common features of MDD.[94,97,98] Excessive sleepiness in patients who are utilizing a CPAP machine is linked with more slow-wave sleep disturbance and fatigue.[96]

Sleepiness and fatigue can in part be explained by the fact that both MDD and OSAH are proinflammatory conditions.[43,96] Furthermore, OSAH and MDD are associated with a number of shared comorbidities where inflammation may be an etiological factor, such as cardio- and cerebrovascular disease, obesity, hypertension, and metabolic disorders, including type 2 diabetes.[43,96,97,99,100] Obesity is, of course, a risk factor for dysregulated inflammation, MDD, and OSAH.[96,101] The relationship between OSAH and endocrine/metabolic disorder may additionally be based on a derangement of hypothalamic function in OSAH, as manifested by aberrant thyroid, orexin, and leptin signaling.[90]

Given all this, untreated OSAH may have been involved in shaping the presentation of Tom's depression and its lack of treatment response but also various medical comorbidities from which he suffers. Proper OSAH treatment, a healthy diet, and exercise will be key components of Tom's future treatment.

The sleep study indicated that Tom had an apnea/hypopnea index of 17 (meaning 17 episodes of interrupted breathing per hour, classified as moderately severe OSAH). Additionally, Tom had 89 episodes of arousal per hour, wake-after-sleep onset time of 43 minutes, REM sleep of 2 percent, and no non-REM sleep.

"You seem concerned, Doc? Is something wrong?"

"Your sleep study is quite a bit off. Did Dr. W discuss the findings in detail?"

"He told me about the apnea and CPAP. He also mentioned a medication that we ought to consider. Dr. W also said that there is often a connection between apnea and the high blood pressure. Does that mean that if we are successful, I can get off my blood pressure medications?"

"Not necessarily. Dr. W suggested that we consider adding clonidine. It is a blood pressure medication and may replace some of the other medicines that you are taking or at least reduce their doses. Your sleep study shows that you have quite a few arousal episodes. They may be related to sleep apnea but may also be influenced by antidepressants that you are taking. Unfortunately, there is often a trade-off. While antidepressants, which boost norepinephrine and serotonin, help your mood, they may also interfere with your sleep. Your sleep architecture is also changed. It seems like you are getting very little REM and slow-wave sleep."

"Is that a problem?"

"It can be. Having frequent arousals during the night, which will interfere with REM and slow-wave sleep, may translate not only into frequent wake-ups but also feeling tired, unrefreshed, and foggy during the day. It may also interfere with your focus at work. Sleep disturbance of this sort is also a risk factor for your depression coming back. In other words, we need to do something about it."

"I'm not really keen about taking another medication, but if you think that it will help my sleep . . . "

"I think that it's worth trying. I will communicate with Dr. H, your family doctor, to let him know what we are doing. He might want to adjust some of the blood pressure medications that he is prescribing. Another thing that we need to focus on is diet and exercise. Would you consider seeing a nutritionist?"

"OK, Doc, but what are we going to do about my depression? Is this as good as it is going to get?"

"I'm not sure, but I hope that if we succeed in getting your sleep properly regulated, you might be feeling a bit better. After CPAP many patients report improvement in energy, wakefulness, and concentration. It is realistic to expect that even your motivation and enthusiasm may get better. Also, let's see what aripiprazole 7.5 mg will do for you with everything else in place. Have you been able to exercise more?"

"Not really. I feel so drained after work that I can hardly get off the couch. I've gone out a couple of times on the weekends. I mentioned that my son and I went mountain biking. My wife has been trying to get me to play some tennis with her. I guess I'll give it a shot. I'll be very rusty, I haven't picked up the racquet in years . . . Let's say all these things, aripiprazole, clonidine, CPAP, and exercise don't work well enough. What is our next step, is there one?"

"There can be. We can consider so called neuromodulatory treatments like electroconvulsive therapy, vagal nerve stimulation and transcranial magnetic stimulation."

"Sounds pretty sci-fi to me. I don't think that I'm interested in electroshock treatments. Even if you tell me that it is not as bad as the 'cuckoo's nest' movie, I would rather move on to the next option."

"Let's cross that bridge when we get to it. In the meantime, I've checked all your labs. Everything looks OK except for the high-sensitivity CRP—it's still elevated, at 3.14. I will write you a prescription for clonidine 0.1 mg. You can take up to two of these every night once you have had a chance to consult your family doctor. Let's plan on meeting again in three to four weeks. Will that work?"

"Sure, Doc."

Third Office Visit, a Month Later

"Well, Tom how's it been going?"

"I wish that I could give you a better report. The lower dose of aripiprazole has been helpful but not like 10 mg. It still helps with my anger and irritability, and I think that we should keep it, but my mood is not really that much better. Clonidine and CPAP have helped some. I now wake up only once or twice a night. My wife says that the machine humming bothers her sleep, so she has moved out to the guest bedroom. It doesn't really bother me much, but sleeping with the mask and the air blown into my lungs under pressure is not so fun. I had a follow-up appointment with Dr. W and mentioned to him what bothered me. He checked on the current machine settings and made some adjustments. It seems like there is some new model coming out, BiPAP or something like that. Dr. W thinks that I could be more comfortable. Hopefully, I will be able to persuade my wife to come back."

"You mentioned that your mood is not great?"

"No, not really. I still feel tired sleepy and foggy. My concentration is a bit better, but with reorganization in the company, I can hardly keep up. I'm doing a better job exercising on the weekend, though. We even played tennis a couple of times. There is less tension at home—everybody appreciates this change. Still I wish we did more together as a family. At least we have been better about eating dinner together, but that's about it."

"Speaking about food, have you made plans to visit a nutritionist, Tom?"

"Not yet, it sounds like I'm making excuses, but I've just been too busy . . . So, Doc, what's the next step? You mentioned that there are some other things that we can consider. I just don't want electroshock."

ECT is arguably the most effective antidepressant intervention. However, despite response rates as high as 79 percent and remission rates of 75 percent, ECT has been mostly relegated to the third line of treatment. Response rates in TRD patients are somewhat more modest, between 50 percent and 70 percent.[102] Other studies have confirmed that ECT is about five times more likely to produce response than placebo and four times more likely to generate a response than antidepressants.[70] Furthermore, bilateral ECT appears to be more effective than unilateral in treatment of depression.[103] Moreover, ECT may have a greater efficacy than some of the other neuromodulatory treatments. Compared with repeated transcranial magnetic stimulation (rTMS), ECT produced a 64.4 percent versus 48.7 percent response rate and a 52.9 percent versus 33.6 percent remission rate in treatment of depressed patients. Most of the ECT superiority over rTMS originates from its benefit in patients suffering from psychotic depression; in nonpsychotic patients there was no significant difference in outcome between these two treatments.[104] Due to its proven efficacy, ECT can be considered as a first-line treatment in suicidal or catatonic depressed patients and in psychotic depression and TRD.[70,103]

While the short-term efficacy of ECT remains beyond doubt, maintenance of the initial therapeutic effect remains a challenge. Among patients who have had at least one antidepressant trial, 9.8 percent will relapse within the first week after attaining remission with ECT, and 31.4 percent of TRD patients will experience the same outcome.[102] Eventually, about a third of the non-medication-resistant MDD patients and half of nonpsychotic TRD patients will experience a relapse following an acute ECT course.[102] Nonetheless, substantial evidence supports the efficacy of combination pharmacotherapy or maintenance ECT in preventing relapse/recurrence after ECT treatment. For example, studies compared the relative efficacy of continuation antidepressant pharmacotherapy alone, or combined with add-on CBT or add-on of brief-pulse continuation ECT. At the completion of the acute ECT phase, 70 percent of depressed patients responded and 47 percent attained remission. During the 12-month follow-up, 65 percent of patients in the CBT arm, 28 percent in the continuation ECT group, and 33 percent in the antidepressant-alone arm were able to sustain their response. This finding further affirms the robust benefit of CBT in the maintenance phase of depression treatment.[105]

The therapeutic effect of ECT may in part be mediated by stimulation of neurotrophic factors. A four-week prospective study found that a combination of 12 sessions of ECT and citalopram (an SSRI) was more effective in elevating plasma brain-derived neurotrophic factor (BDNF) than antidepressant alone.[106] Moreover, the same group evaluated the benefits of augmenting ECT and an SSRI with aerobic exercise and found that the addition of exercise resulted in a greater improvement in depressive symptoms, as measured by a standardized scale, than either ECT or aerobic exercise training alone.[107] Both interventions were also associated with an increase in peripheral BDNF levels, although surprisingly, ECT alone elevated BDNF significantly more than when combined with exercise.[107] In further support of favorable neuroplastic effects of ECT, an MRI study evaluated the volume of the amygdala and hippocampus a week prior and a week after the conclusion of ECT and found a significant volume increase in these two structures.[108]

The greatest detraction from more frequent utilization of ECT in the treatment of depression stems from its cognitive side effects. Confusion and anterograde amnesia are common and typically time-limited sequelae of the individual ECT treatments. Unfortunately, retrograde amnesia has been found to persist even beyond six months on occasion.[109] Lower premorbid intellectual functioning, lower education, and greater patient age are all associated with greater risk of cognitive impairment. There are reports that some of the psychotropics, such as lithium and venlafaxine, may aggravate ECT-related cognitive deficits, while others, like nortriptyline, may ameliorate them.[109] Although Tom might be an appropriate candidate for ECT, his reluctance and current cognitive difficulties are plausible reasons to pursue other treatment alternatives.

> "There is a relatively simple thing that we can do to help your sleepiness and maybe fatigue. Armodafinil is a medication that is approved for people who suffer from sleep apnea and still feel sleepy despite adjusted CPAP."
>
> Tom was frowning. "Do we really need to be adding another medicine. Didn't you say that there are some other, novel techniques that we could try? Can you tell me about those?"
>
> "Well, there is vagal nerve stimulation, or VNS; there's repetitive transcranial magnetic stimulation, or rTMS, and a procedure that is still not approved by the FDA, called deep brain stimulation. VNS involves a minor surgery to implant a pacemaker-like device. It then sends the signals along one of the branches of the vagal nerve to the brain. This stimulation hypothetically causes an increase in brain activity and improves neurotransmission in some of the brain areas affected by depression. There are a couple of problems with this for you. First, VNS may changes your voice and produce hoarseness, throat inflammation, and pain. Also, there is some risk that it may negatively influence your obstructive sleep apnea."

VNS was approved by the FDA in 2005 as an adjunctive treatment for chronic or recurrent TRD. It is intended as a long-term intervention for depressed individuals who have failed to respond to four or more adequate antidepressant trials, including different classes of antidepressants, combinations of agents, and augmentation attempts.[110]

A small pacemaker-like pulse generator is surgically implanted under the clavicle on the left side of the chest.[103,110] It intermittently delivers electrical pulses to the left vagus nerve via an electrode wrapped around its ascending fibers, in the midcervical section.[110] Electrical signals are initially delivered to the nucleus of the solitary tract and from there to the serotonergic nuclei raphae, noradrenergic LC, amygdala, hippocampus, hypothalamus, parahippocampus, thalamus, orbitofrontal cortex, and insula.[102,103,109,111] In addition to causing metabolic changes in the aforementioned limbic and paralimbic cortical formations, VNS activation is associated with changes in monoamine, glutamate, gamma-aminobutyric acid (GABA), and neurotrophic factor signaling.[112] Furthermore, imaging studies have reported that VNS treatment has been associated with suppressed vmPFC and subgenual anterior cingulate cortex (sgACC) resting-state activity, similar to findings linked with improvement following antidepressant, ECT, CBT, and deep brain stimulation (DBS) treatment.[113]

Three-month response rates in the acute open-label VNS studies have been approximately 30–35 percent; remission rates in the same time frame have been approximately 15 percent. Both response and remission rates considerably improved during a 12-month follow-up period and reached 45–55 percent and 20–30 percent, respectively.[111] In a comparative study of non-VNS-treated TRD patients, remission rates were 5.8 percent and 1.7 percent, respectively, at the 3-month time point and rose to 11.6 percent and 3.6 percent at 12 months.[111] Clearly, VNS appears to have an advantage over TRD treatment as usual. Furthermore, VNS benefits at 3 months have largely been sustained at 9 and 12 months (~70 percent of TRD patients). This was not the case with the non-VNS group, where only 4.6 percent of TRD patients maintained their 3-month response at the 9- and 12-month time points.[111] The number needed to treat (NNT—a statistical measure indicating an average number of patients needed to be treated in order to achieve a desired outcome which would otherwise not be present) for VNS ranges from 4 to 10.[111] However, the only randomized controlled 12-week trial failed to show a difference on the primary outcome measure (24-item HAMD), although it did show a difference on the secondary self-reported measure, the Inventory of Depressive Symptoms.[111] It is possible that the controlled study was not long enough to fully capture the benefits of VNS, since one of the studies reported average time to first response of 48.1 ± 31.7 days among eventual VNS responders.[114] Patients who respond best to VNS tend to be the ones with low to moderate resistance to antidepressants. Moreover, patients who have never received ECT are four times more likely to respond to VNS than those who have received it. Additionally, none of the patients who failed more than seven antidepressant trials responded to VNS.[112]

The use of VNS has been associated with improvement in several cognitive domains, such as executive function and psychomotor speed.[114] Moreover, some findings indicate that VNS can help improve sleep and food craving.[112,114] There would be good reasons for Tom to consider this treatment option, were it not for his obstructive sleep apnea and need for prompt symptom relief. Overall, VNS is quite well tolerated. Adverse events include incision pain (which usually resolves within a couple of weeks), sore throat, cough, hoarseness, dyspnea, headache, neck pain, jaw pain, nausea, rare worsening depression, anxiety, and the emergence of mania.[102,109,114]

In conclusion, VNS is best suited as an adjunct treatment for depressed patients with moderate resistance to previous antidepressant treatments, with persistent residual symptoms that do not require rapid relief, and where suppression of recurrences has been a challenge.[111]

"I think that I've heard enough. What's our next option?"

"Well, I think that we can consider rTMS. This procedure involves the application of a strong magnetic coil to your scalp in order to create weak electric currents in your brain."

"Is it like electroshock treatment? It sounds painful."

"No, not really. It is about the same strength of magnetic field as an MRI scan. Some patients report tingling, a sense of heat, or mild scalp irritation. Very rarely one can have a seizure. It is an outpatient procedure, so doctors who perform it have antiseizure medications in their office that can be given right away. There have also been reports of unintended changes in mood or thinking, but these are also fairly rare. Overall, it's a safe procedure, and you would be likely to experience relief within a matter of weeks. There is even some evidence that right-sided rTMS may improve your thinking."

"What are my chances of getting well with this treatment, and will my insurance company cover it?"

"About one in seven patients who have not responded to antidepressant treatments will be depression-free after this procedure based on the statistical analysis of the published studies. Some centers do report higher success rates. I'm not sure if your insurance company will cover this treatment. We can definitely check into it."

"How much would it cost if I had to pay out of the pocket?"

"It varies from center to center, but it is often between $20,000 and $30,000."

"You've got to be kidding me! There's no way that we can afford this, not with our kid in college. What's that last intervention that you mentioned?"

"Deep brain stimulation involves a minor neurosurgical procedure to implant a wire into the brain, which is later connected to a pacemaker device. If it's successful this treatment offers virtually instantaneous relief of depressive symptoms. Right now deep brain stimulation is approved for the treatment of Parkinson's disease but not yet for treatment of resistant depression."

DBS is an invasive procedure requiring stereotactical placement of a stimulation electrode in one of the target brain areas. This electrode is connected by a subcutaneously placed wire to a pulse generator, usually located under the skin in the subclavicular area.[109,112] Several target areas have been the most thoroughly studied in the context of TRD, including the sgACC (Brodmann area 25), anterior limb of the capsula interna, ventral capsule/ventral striatum (VC/VS) and adjacent nucleus accumbens (NAcc), and superolateral branch of the medial forebrain bundle (slMFB).[102,103,109,112,115–118]

DBS applied to the sgACC and adjacent white matter has probably been the most studied approach. Early reports suggested that treatment results are prompt and well maintained. Response rates were 40 percent at one week and 60 percent at six months, Remission rates over this time period reached 35 percent. At the end of a year response rates were 62.5 percent and remission rates were 18.8 percent, which declined somewhat after two years to 46.2 percent, with 15.4 percent remission rate. Interestingly, rates improved again at year 3, with 75 percent of patients showing response and 50 percent showing remission.[112,116]

Another group of DBS studies targeted the reward system, including the VC/VS and NAcc. All these brain areas are richly innervated with dopaminergic fibers. Electrical pulses were delivered via bilateral stimulating electrodes.[102,109,112] Response rates following VC/VS were surprisingly similar to sgACC stimulation: 53 percent at 3 months, 47 percent at 6 months, 53 percent at 12 months, and 71 percent at the last follow-up (ranging from 14 to 67 months). The corresponding remission rates were 35 percent, 29 percent, 41 percent, and 35 percent.[112] A study examining the therapeutic efficacy of DBS targeting NAcc reported a 50 percent response rate one year following treatment.[102] PET imaging studies found a decline of metabolic rate in several limbic areas associated with negative affect in depression, including the sgACC, orbitofrontal PFC, and amygdala.[102] Complementing these impressive clinical findings, preclinical studies discovered robust increases in serotonin, DA, and NE release in orbitofrontal and medial PFC areas as a result of the NAcc DBS intervention.[119] Furthermore, in addition to an increase in pleasurable activities, patients who underwent NAcc DBS also reported a decrease in anxiety.[112]

More recent DBS studies have focused on neural structures closely connected with the reward system, such as the anterior limb of the capsula interna and slMFB.[117] Stimulation of the slMFB appears particularly promising because this area has intimate functional and anatomical connections with the sgACC, NAcc, and anterior limb of the capsula interna. Hypothetically, DBS stimulation of the slMFB is likely to predominantly affect descending glutamatergic fibers, which would in turn activate dopaminergic VTA neurons. Increased signaling in the ascending VTA neurons would presumably ameliorate NAcc and PFC activity, thereby bringing about significant improvement of depressive symptoms.[117] Indeed, a pilot study reported that six of the seven TRD patients experienced a response at day 7, which persisted at the last observation (12–33 weeks). Four of the patients maintained remission until that time, also showing remarkable improvement in their social functioning.[120] These impressive results were achieved using a much milder electrical current, about one-third of the strength of the electrical impulses used in the sgACC and VC/VS studies.[120]

Unlike ECT, DBS is not associated with cognitive impairment. On the contrary, studies reported normalization of cognitive function,[118] including improved verbal memory, attention, executive function, processing speed, and motor speed, especially in patients who manifested pretreatment deficits in these cognitive domains.[109,117] The adverse effects associated with DBS were in general rare and transient. Wound infection, lead migration, one report of minor hemorrhage, erythema, anxiety, agitation, transient elevation in mood, and oculomotor side effects were generally relatively brief and resolved without sequelae.[117] Tom was not eager to undergo surgery, which is understandable given that some less invasive neuromodulatory interventions have not been exhausted.

"So they would have to drill a hole in my skull? That does not sound very appealing. I'm not really hearing any options that I would like pursue."

"If you are interested I can check with one of my colleagues doing research in rTMS. Maybe he can enroll you in one of his studies. It would be free of charge then. You might need to have MRIs done as part of the study, though."

"Well, if you wouldn't mind checking and letting me know. I will need some time to think about all this and to talk to my wife."

Fifth Office Visit, Two Months Later

"Thank you very much, Doc, for helping me get into that study. TMS worked like a charm! After a month I was feeling much better. As a matter of fact, I probably felt the best I can remember since high school. My sleep is fine with the new apnea machine. My mind feels much more clear when I wake up in the morning. I'm not quite sure what's doing it, if it's the magnet or medicines or exercise, maybe all of it, but even focus at work is noticeably improved. Energy is back—I'm getting a lot of chores done around the house. Tammy and I are doing much better. In fact, my interest in sex has returned. It's a bit awkward because we've had such a long hiatus, but with time it should be OK. Our son is now excited about going biking with me. I guess not yelling at him as much is making a difference."

rTMS is a noninvasive neuromodulatory treatment, approved by the FDA in 2008 as a treatment for adult patients suffering from MDD who have previously failed an adequate antidepressant trial.[102,121] Tom certainly meets that criterion. Transcranial magnetic stimulation is administered via an electromagnetic coil applied to the patient's scalp. The coil generates a powerful but brief magnetic field, which is converted into electrical energy as it passes through skin, muscle, and skull bone.[121] As the electromagnetic pulse comes into contact with neural tissue, it induces a flow of electrical current, thereby depolarizing neurons and/or modulating cortical excitability over a relatively small and circumscribed cortical area.[103,121,122]

Coil design and power level influence the depth of penetrance and focality of stimulation. Larger coils may provide a greater depth of stimulation while sacrificing the precision to target a specific neuroanatomical focus.[123,124] Coils and powers most often used in clinical rTMS research approximately penetrate 2–4 cm into brain tissue, leaving deeper limbic areas out of their direct reach.[123–125] rTMS is most often applied either as low-frequency (LF) stimulation (≤1 Hz) to the right dorsolateral PFC (dlPFC) or as high-frequency (HF) stimulation (usually 5–10 Hz) to the left dlPFC.[103,121,122] HF stimulation of the left dlPFC is believed to induce long-term potentiation of neuronal activity in this area, presumably correcting the hypofunction of this area observed in imaging studies.[103,121] In contrast, LF stimulation of the right dlPFC creates long-term depression, hypothetically addressing the hyperactivation of this brain area in MDD and the aberrant interhemispheric activity balance in this disease state.[103,121]

Scientific and clinical communities have still to reach a full consensus regarding the optimal, dose, time, type of coil and focus of magnetic stimulation. It would be more appropriate to consider rTMS as a class of treatments rather than as a singular entity. Here we provide a brief discussion of some of the most clinically important rTMS paradigms.[126] Arguably, HF (usually 10 Hz) stimulation of the left dlPFC is the modality most often utilized by practitioners. One of the meta-analyses of the randomized double-blind controlled trials examined the efficacy of HF-rTMS applied to the left dlPFC over 13 sessions and found 29.3 percent of the depressed patients were responders and 18.6 percent were remitters, compared with 10.4 percent response and 5 percent remission rates in sham-treated patients.[125,126] Furthermore, the pooled OR for both response and remission following HF-rTMS of the left dlPFC was 3.3, while NNT approached 6 and 8 for response and remission, respectively.[125] Moreover HF-rTMS efficacy in the treatment of more antidepressant-resistant depressed patients versus less resistant groups was virtually the same as measured by response and remission rates.[125] Additionally, no remarkable difference was noted between HF-rTMS as monotherapy and its use as an augmentation treatment.[125] While some of the meta-analyses dispute the significance of the clinical and functional benefits of HF-rTMS,[127] other authors point to methodological advances in localization of target brain areas, better study designs, longer treatment course, and individually tailored stimulation frequencies guided by functional imaging findings and larger clinical samples, resulting in more robust effect sizes for HF-rTMS (~0.75).[128,129] Overall, remission rates have doubled in rTMS studies published since 2010 compared with those published earlier.[128]

LF-rTMS administered over the right dlPFC has emerged as a valid alternative to HF-rTMS. LF-rTMS delivered as a total of 1,200 pulses or more over an average number of 13 sessions produces a response rate of 38.2 percent and remission rate of 34.6 percent, compared with 15.1 percent and 9.7 percent, respectively, in sham-treated patients.[130] NNT for both response and remission was 5. A meta-analysis suggested that the clinical benefits of LF-rTMS to the right dlPFC may be similar to those observed by the more often utilized HF-rTMS delivered to the left dlPFC and that it is at least as effective as second- or third-line pharmacotherapeutic alternatives.[126,130] Furthermore, smaller comparative studies suggest that HF-rTMS to the left dlPFC and LF-rTMS to the right dlPFC may have complementary therapeutic benefits: some of the HF-rTMS nonresponders may experience therapeutic benefit from LF-rTMS, and vice versa.[129] Moreover, emerging PET imaging evidence indicates that hypometabolism of the left dlPFC may be a positive marker of response to HF-rTMS.[128,129,131] Overall, relative response and remission risks for rTMS compared with sham were between 3.38 and 5.07, based on the most recent trials.[126]

Some studies have utilized bilateral rTMS consisting of a combination of LF-rTMS to the right dlPFC and HF-rTMS to the left dlPFC. An early six-week, randomized, sham-controlled trial evaluating the efficacy of this sequential approach found a robust 44 percent response rate relative to 8 percent of sham-treated patients, and a remission rate of 36 percent, compared with none in the placebo group.[132] The same group of researchers reported an impressive >50 percent response and 40 percent remission rates in a later large randomized trial involving TRD patients.[133] Moreover, bilateral rTMS was directly compared with unilateral LF-rTMS to the right dlPFC, utilizing a priming protocol, whereby LF stimulation is "primed" by a preceding brief HF stimulation of the same area. The study outcome demonstrated similar clinical benefits from the bilateral and unilateral "primed" LF-rTMS approaches.[133] Intriguingly, this particular study indicated that age, prior duration of disease, number of failed medication trials, and even history of nonresponse to ECT did not influence the response to rTMS.[133] A meta-analysis of seven randomized controlled trials of bilateral rTMS reported more modest outcomes.[134] A mean number of 13 bilateral rTMS sessions was associated with response rate of 24.7 percent versus 6.8 percent with sham treatment, and remission rate of 19 percent, compared with 2.6 percent rate with sham, ultimately translating into a clinically meaningful OR of 6.[134]

A few novel variations on the more common rTMS methods, such as intensive rTMS and low-field magnetic stimulation, have delivered very encouraging albeit preliminary results.[135,136] An intensive course, delivering 31,000 pulses of HF stimuli to the left dlPFC, in a total of 20 sessions over 4 days (five sessions a day), produced a 35 percent response rate in a group of TRD patients who had previously failed two SSRI/SNRI agents and a tricyclic antidepressant. Response was both robust and prompt (given that it was a four-day study). However, the longevity of this clinical benefit is difficult to predict without an adequate long-term follow-up. A shorter duration of the current episode was a positive predictor of response to rTMS, while poor response to prior ECT treatment predicted less treatment benefit.[135] A novel low-field magnetic stimulation induces a low-pulsed electrical field, insufficient to depolarize neurons but presumably adequate to influence dendritic function. This technique is hypothetically capable of affecting transmission in wide areas of the cerebral cortex. A small, sham-controlled study has reported a rapid and significant improvement in clinical symptoms of depression, measured by standard scales.[136] Larger-scale replication studies are needed before this method of magnetic stimulation becomes more widely clinically applicable.

Application of rTMS to sites other than the left and right dlPFC has also been explored. Although there is little room for questioning the efficacy of rTMS administered to the dlPFC, other accessible cortical sites, such as the ventromedial PFC (vmPFC), vlPFC, and dorsomedial PFC (dmPFC) are receiving more attention. Neuroimaging studies have provided consistent evidence of vmPFC, dmPFC, and vlPFC involvement in mood regulation via their crucial participation in cortico-limbic circuits.[128] In fact, the most consistent morphometric imaging evidence singles out the dmPFC and ACC as the primary areas altered in MDD.[128] Unlike the dlPFC, the dmPFC has much more pronounced functional connectivity with the amygdala, and due to its central role in coordination between major functional networks, and cognitive-emotional regulation, it has been dubbed the "dorsal nexus."[128,137] Response to HF-rTMS applied to the dmPFC was strongly influenced by lower connectivity in the reward circuit composed of the dopaminergic VTA, striatum, and vmPFC, clinically correlated with anhedonia. Response to rTMS was strongly bimodal. Higher baseline anhedonia and lower connectivity in reward circuitry predicted poor response to rTMS.[138]

The same group published a subsequent study demonstrating that higher dmPFC–sgACC and sgACC–dlPFC connectivity and lower corticolimbic connectivity predicted better treatment response to the bilateral HF-rTMS delivered to the dmPFC.[139] Therefore, strong connectivity between the principal hubs of major functional networks, sgACC–dmPFC (representing the salience network [SN] and default-mode network [DMN], respectively) and sgACC–dlPFC (SN and cognitive executive network [EN], respectively) may indicate more adaptive communication between principal networks involved in regulation of mood and cognition and better response to rTMS applied to the dmPFC. Furthermore, a different group of researchers reported that greater sgACC–dlPFC–mPFC connectivity predicted a good response to HF-rTMS delivered to the left dlPFC.[140] These authors found abnormally elevated DMN activity and diminished EN function in depressed patients, as well as aberrant connectivity between the EN and DMN in this group. Effective rTMS treatment had a normalizing influence on EN–DMN connectivity, as well as on DMN hyperconnectivity.[140] Yet other groups have linked a lower baseline cerebral blood flow ratio between the dlPFC and vmPFC in depressed patients to favorable HF-rTMS to the left dlPFC.[141] Moreover, certain EEG characteristics may also differentiate future responders from nonresponders to a combined rTMS/psychotherapy treatment.[142]

Several other practical issues may be relevant to Tom's predicament. How effective is rTMS as a maintenance treatment? How does rTMS compare with ECT? Are there cognitive sequelae associated with rTMS? What is the safety profile of rTMS? Only limited data are available about the long-term efficacy of rTMS. One small study estimated mean relapse time, following acute rTMS treatment, to be approximately 10 months.[103] Furthermore, maintenance treatment consisting of 20 sessions over a five-week period, combined with pharmacotherapy, may confer additional benefits compared with only acute treatment in combination with antidepressants. Twenty-week relapse rates in the nonmaintenance group was 81.8 percent, compared with only 37.8 percent in the rTMS maintenance cohort.[143] A long-term study followed up a small sample of unmedicated patients who had an initial response to rTMS treatment. If they relapsed, they were treated with rTMS once or twice a week. The authors reported a 26- to 43-month medication-free period and a 65 percent response retention rate. Preliminary evidence suggests a direct correlation between the number of sessions and the longevity of the rTMS-derived clinical benefits and an inverse relationship with depressed patient's age.[103,109]

Meta-analyses generally point to a greater clinical efficacy of ECT compared with either HF-rTMS or LF-rTMS, although one of the analyses found nonsignificant superiority of rTMS delivered at 20 Hz (HF) at a rate of ≥1,200 daily stimuli compared with ECT.[104,144,145] A meta-analysis reported a 52 percent after an average of 8.2 ECT sessions and a 33.6 percent remission rate after an average of 15.2 HF-rTMS sessions.[145] Another meta-analysis also found higher response (64.4 percent vs. 48.7 percent) and remission rates (52.9 percent vs. 33.6 percent) with ECT compared with HF-rTMS, although superiority of ECT over HF- and LF-rTMS was almost exclusively attributable to the greater ECT efficacy in patients suffering from psychotic depression.[104] However, ECT-treated patients suffered greater impairment in visual memory and verbal fluency.[104]

rTMS may provide additional benefits by suppressing anxiety in TRD patients,[146] improving sleep quality by reducing alpha activity during REM sleep in MDD patients (bilateral, sequential LF-rTMS over the right dlPFC, followed by HF-rTMS over the left dlPFC),[147] and improving visuospatial memory, working memory, verbal memory, and verbal fluency in some depressed patients.[148,149] Overall, rTMS is very well tolerated. The risk of seizures is very low, about 1 in 30,000 treatments, although it is possible that patients with neurological disorders and seizure-threshold-lowering medication may be at a greater risk.[121] Additionally, local scalp irritation, headaches, transient elevation of auditory threshold, facial pain due to muscular twitches, temporary attentional deficits, and dizziness are among the more commonly encountered side effects.[103,109,122]

While some meta-analyses cast doubt on the clinical relevance of rTMS benefits in MDD and TRD, despite statistical significance,[127] others remind us that more methodologically sound studies demonstrate substantially greater rTMS effects than is apparent in older research.[128] The preponderance of evidence supports the clinical usefulness of rTMS in the adjunctive treatment of depression. Issues of dose, application site, optimal duration, and coil type remain to be answered in future research.[121]

"These changes in your mood sound wonderful."

"Unfortunately, there is a flip side of the coin. My last TMS session was two weeks ago. Over the last week my mood has started slipping a bit. Especially in the afternoon, I feel a bit deflated. I try to get home from work as soon as I can. It's not like I'm in profoundly depressed. I still remember what real depression feels like. It is more of a glass half-empty kind of feeling."

It took me a minute to respond.

"You don't need to get gloomy on me, Doc. It's really not that bad. I just don't want to slide back into depression, not after the way I've been feeling the last month. Your friend, Dr. Z, who did the TMS said that some of the patients need 'booster' maintenance sessions. He's waiting to hear if his funding for the follow-up TMS will come through. In the worst-case scenario, I can mortgage the house and get some money out. He mentioned that he sometimes offers a discount for his established patients. Do you have some other ideas, Doc?"

"Well, I'm not sure about this one. Another member of our department is currently enrolling treatment-resistant depressed patients into a ketamine study. It's an anesthetic agent which can be given in a lower dose as an infusion. In some of the previous studies it has worked remarkably fast and well. Patients reported significant improvement in their depressive symptoms even during the first two hours after the start of the treatment."

"Wow! What are the side effects?"

"Well, the study that our department is doing is using repeated doses of ketamine. I'm not sure if it is every two or three days. Based on the past research experience, very few people experience any side effects. A few of the patients complained of 'feeling high' or 'weird,' drowsiness, confusion, and perceptual disturbances. To my knowledge, no one has had very serious or long-lasting side effects."

"If you were in my shoes, what would you do, Doc?"

"It's hard to say. You have had such a great response to TMS that it would make most sense to go with their maintenance study. On the other hand, no one really knows if and when the funding will come through. Paying for it out of pocket, even at the discounted rate, could be quite expensive."

"Let me talk to Dr. Z. Maybe he will have some good news for me. Either way I will let you know about ketamine in a couple of days. Would you have any articles about it that I can read and understand?"

"I will get some material together for you. The National Institute for Mental Health also has some information on its site that you might want to peruse. Please let me know if I can help you with the ketamine study."

"I definitely will. The last thing I want is to get depressed again. Not after experiencing a normal life for the last several weeks."

Ketamine has been defined as a noncompetitive, nonselective, high-affinity *N*-methyl-D-aspartate (NMDA) antagonist.[150,151] Based on preclinical research, perhaps paradoxically, because it is an NMDA glutamate receptor antagonist, ketamine enhances PFC glutamate efflux.[150–153] Most likely ketamine inhibits NMDA receptors located on GABA neurons as well as on other neural elements (including astrocytes and oligodendroglia).[150–154] By eliminating the glutamate-driven GABA-mediated tonic inhibition, ketamine effectively disinhibits glutamatergic neurons. Since postsynaptic NMDA receptors are occupied by ketamine, enhanced glutamate signaling is now "rerouted" to alpha-amino-3-hydroxy-5-methyl-4-isoxazole-propionic acid (AMPA) postsynaptic receptors. Increased activation of AMPA receptors has been associated with enhanced downstream synthesis of BDNF and elevated mTOR (mammalian target of rapamycin) signaling. Ketamine-driven synaptogenesis is believed to be primarily mediated by the BDNF–mTOR cascade.[150–154]

Some of the therapeutic actions of ketamine may also be related to its inhibition of glycogen synthase kinase-3, a proapoptotic intracellular signaling molecule also putatively involved in the mood-stabilizing effects of lithium and the antidepressant effect mediated by 5HT1A agonists.[152,155] It is uncertain if additional pharmacodynamic properties involving affinity for D2, 5HT2A, and opioid kappa and mu receptors and inhibition of inflammatory cytokines and peripheral monoamine uptake sites have any relevant role in ketamine's antidepressant action.[150–155] The robust change in levels of amino acid neurotransmitters (glutamate and GABA) following parenteral ketamine administration tends to dissipate rapidly, returning to baseline levels within an hour. Downstream effects of ketamine administration are also relatively short-lived. For example, BDNF elevation in the hippocampus lasts from 30 minutes to 24 hours after ketamine administration; mTOR increases, from 30 minutes to 2 hours; greater synaptic protein synthesis, from 2 to 72 hours; and increased neurotransmitter-induced postsynaptic currents, up to 24 hours.[153]

Ketamine is rapidly metabolized by liver CYP450 enzymes, mainly 2B6 and 3A4, which is reflected in a relatively short half-life of about 3 hours and low bioavailability of approximately 20 percent after oral dosing. Due to extensive first-pass metabolism, oral administration of ketamine in clinical trials has mostly been avoided. Parenteral administration, predominantly as a slow intravenous infusion, has been the preferred method of administration in clinical trials. A few studies were conducted using sublingual, inhaled, or intramuscular route.[150]

Most randomized controlled clinical trials of ketamine conducted to date have utilized the same route and similar methodology. Ketamine was administered in a subanesthetic dose as a 5 mg/kg intravenous infusion over 40 minutes.[150,151,153,155,156] Treatment effects were noticeable as early as 40–240 minutes after initiation.[150,151,153,155,157] Robust response and remission rates of approximately 77 percent and 43 percent were recorded between 4 and 72 hours after administration.[150] Although the typical duration of effect was estimated to be two to three days, some studies have noted a sustained treatment effect approximately two weeks after ketamine administration.[151,152,157] Another way of characterizing ketamine's efficacy in treatment of depressed patients is by calculating an NNT in order to achieve remission on ketamine versus a comparator (saline or midazolam). Ketamine intravenous infusion demonstrated robust remission rates compared with control, with NNT rates of 5 at 24 hours, 3 at 3 days, and 4 at 7 days after treatment initiation.[158] Ketamine often induces a mild and transient (usually ≤1 hour duration) but nevertheless distinct psychomimetic effect, which effectively "unblinds" it to both patients and researchers. A few studies utilized midazolam as a control to better preserve the blind. Midazolam infusion is associated with a change in mentation, which makes it more difficult to distinguish from ketamine, while it has no established antidepressant effect.[153,158]

Not enough is known about the efficacy and safety of repeated intravenous ketamine infusion. An augmentation study provided six ketamine 0.5 mg/kg infusions over a 40-minute period on a Monday-Wednesday-Friday schedule to TRD subjects previously on a stable antidepressant dose for two months.[159] An analysis of treatment completers indicated a 91.6 percent response and a 66.6 percent remission rate after the 12-day treatment period. The mean relapse time was 16 days over the course of a four-week follow-up period.[159] Ketamine infusion was also effective in augmenting ECT effect and suppressing suicidal ideation in depressed patients.[150,157,160]

There is only limited information regarding the efficacy and safety of ketamine administered via alternative routes. Sublingual ketamine achieves higher bioavailability than oral administration (~30 percent). In one study ketamine was dispensed every two to three days or weekly as a 10 mg dose from a 100 mg/ml solution, allowing for 5-minute sublingual absorption, and then swallowed. Remission was achieved by 77 percent of the patients, accompanied by significant improvements in mood, sleep, and cognition.[161] Furthermore, a randomized controlled trial compared the efficacy of two 50-mg ketamine intranasal treatments with saline administered in a similar fashion. Ketamine generated a treatment response in 44 percent of MDD patients compared with a 6 percent response rate on saline.[162] Ketamine has also been injected as a 0.2 mg/kg intravenous bolus to a group of suicidal patients, which produced a robust antidepressant effect four hours after administration that was largely sustained over the ensuing 10-day observation period.[150] Moreover, ketamine administered as a 50 mg intramuscular injection every three to four days, in an ongoing fashion, has proven to be exceptionally effective in producing enduring recovery. Patients stayed well for five to six months before experiencing a partial relapse.[150]

Imaging studies have attempted to establish neural correlates of ketamine response in depressed patients. A group of researchers utilized PET imaging to evaluate changes in brain metabolic rate associated with ketamine treatment. While whole-brain metabolism did not significantly change due to ketamine administration, there was a substantial reduction of regional metabolism in some of the key areas involved in mood regulation, working memory, and executive function, such as the insula, habenula, vlPFC, and dlPFC.[163] Furthermore, a placebo-controlled MRI study noted a significant reduction in signal emanating from the sgACC in MDD patients treated with ketamine infusion relative to the placebo-treated cohort.[164] Another magnetic resonance spectroscopy study evaluated a change in the ratio of glutamine plus glutamate (Glx) to glutamate, a proxy to change in glutamine, as a consequence of intravenous ketamine infusion.[154] Pretreatment Glx:glutamate ratio in the dmPFC and dorsal anterolateral PFC was negatively correlated with improvement in depressive symptomatology following ketamine infusion. Furthermore, Glx:glutamate ratio (proxy for glutamine) in the vmPFC was positively related with improvement in depression and anxiety scores 230 minutes after the ketamine treatment. A lower Glx:glutamate ratio is indicative of reduced glutamine and may reflect either impaired glia function or reduced glia density in these brain areas involved in cognition and emotional regulation.[154] Postmortem studies have established that reduction in astroglia and oligodendroglia density in the ACC, dlPFC, hippocampus, and amygdala represents the most pronounced cytopathological finding in MDD (see Chapter 7). Both astrocytes and oligodendroglia metabolize glutamine and possess glutamate receptors (including NMDA and AMPA). Moreover, a postmortem study established that glial reduction in the amygdala of deceased depressed patients was predominantly attributable to decreased oligodendrocyte density.[165]

How is all this relevant to Tom? Unfortunately, there are more open questions than there are answers. Tom has had only a partial response to monoamine-modulating agents. If we go out on the limb and assume that some of the key pathophysiological processes underpinning Tom's depression may have to do with inadequate glutamatergic transmission, compromised neuroplasticity, and/or astroglial/ologodendroglial dysfunction, monoamine-modulating interventions would be very indirect remedies. On the other hand, glutamate-modulating interventions, such as ketamine, may plausibly restore or improve glia function, glutamate transmission, and neuroplasticity, ushering in clinical improvement in clinical domains where previous treatments have fallen short. Indeed, ketamine treatment of previously TRD patients has been associated with improvement in visual and working memory[166] and slow-wave sleep.[153]

Do we have a way of prognosticating which depressed patient is a good candidate for ketamine treatment? Aside from the above-referenced pioneering imaging studies, others have noted that patients who had lower pregenual ACC activity during a working memory task, indicating more intact mood-regulating cortico-limbic circuitry, fared better 230 minutes after ketamine administration.[153] Furthermore, pretreatment connectivity between the pregenual ACC and amygdala during the working memory task negatively predicted response to ketamine four hours later. One can potentially interpret these findings as a suggestion that patients who have better-functioning corticolimbic circuitry, and therefore can suppress activity in limbic areas (e.g., the amygdala) during a cognitive task, tend to have a more robust ketamine response.[167] Additionally, patients who manifest greater disturbance of slow-wave sleep tend to have a more robust response to ketamine.[153] Consistent with purported role of BDNF modulation in mediation of the ketamine treatment effect, the Val66Met BDNF genetic polymorphism may influence clinical response to ketamine. Carriers of at least one copy of the less functional Met allele had substantially reduced antidepressant response to ketamine compared with individuals homozygous for the higher functioning Val allele. It is an interesting coincidence that the 30 percent nonresponse rate to ketamine matches approximately 30 percent prevalence of Met alleles.[151]

Finally, whenever we make a treatment decision, especially one involving an experimental agent, an extended and comprehensive discussion about the balance of potential benefits and risks is in order. Ketamine administration for the treatment of depression has been associated with transient adverse reactions, including psychotic-like symptoms, hallucination, dissociative experiences, manic-like experiences, elation, confusion, disinhibition, perceptual disturbances, and memory and concentration impairment. Neuropsychological disturbances related to ketamine administration are time-limited and tend to dissipate within two hours.[150,151] Physical side effects, such as headaches, drowsiness, dizziness, hypertension, tachycardia, light-headedness, and nausea, have also been reported. These adverse reactions appear to be dose-related and also transient, rarely lasting longer than 80 minutes.[150,151]

There are several unanswered questions regarding ketamine use in the treatment of previously resistant depression. What is the best route and frequency of administration? Is there a ketamine dose that offers an optimal efficacy-to-risk ratio? Are there biological markers predicting a favorable response to ketamine? Can ketamine be used for maintenance treatment? How can one combine ketamine with currently available medications and psychosocial interventions to achieve the best outcomes? Ongoing and future research will help answer some of these questions so that ketamine and other glutamatergic agents can be used to the greatest benefit of our depressed patients.

Visit Seven, Six Weeks Later

Because the rTMS maintenance study did not have a defined start date a week after our fifth appointment, Tom enrolled into the ketamine study.

"Well, Doc, I have no problems to report! After our last appointment my mood continued to slip, which ended up being good, since as you know, it qualified me for the ketamine study. It was just like you said: rapid and with no side effects! It wasn't even an injection—we used an inhaler. Two hours after the treatment, I was feeling perfectly well. My memory and concentration are better than they have been in a long time. We can keep this appointment short—I really have no concerns."

"Are you taking your other medications regularly?"

"Religiously. I heard from Dr. Z. His rTMS study finally got funded. They are starting next month. I'm not sure if I want to enroll, or even if they would accept me—I'm doing really well. For the first time since my treatment started, I'm feeling very hopeful!"

References

1. Marazziti D, Akiskal HS, Udo M, et al. Dimorphic changes of some features of loving relationships during long-term use of antidepressants in depressed outpatients. *J Affect Disord.* 2014;166C:151–155.

2. Joseph NT, Kamarck TW, Muldoon MF, Manuck SB. Daily marital interaction quality and carotid artery intima-medial thickness in healthy middle-aged adults. *Psychosom Med.* 2014;76:347–354.

3. Zoccola PM, Figueroa WS, Rabideau EM, Woody A, Benencia F. Differential effects of poststressor rumination and distraction on cortisol and C-reactive protein. *Health Psychol.* 2014;33(12):1606–1609.

4. Perlis RH, Fava M, Trivedi MH, et al. Irritability is associated with anxiety and greater severity, but not bipolar spectrum features, in major depressive disorder. *Acta Psychiatr Scand.* 2009;119:282–289.

5. Judd LL, Schettler PJ, Coryell W, Akiskal HS, Fiedorowicz JG. Overt irritability/anger in unipolar major depressive episodes: past and current characteristics and implications for long-term course. *JAMA Psychiatry.* 2013;70:1171–1180.

6. Perlis RH, Uher R, Ostacher M, et al. Association between bipolar spectrum features and treatment outcomes in outpatients with major depressive disorder. *Arch Gen Psychiatry.* 2011;68:351–360.

7. Fava M, Hwang I, Rush AJ, Sampson N, Walters EE, Kessler RC. The importance of irritability as a symptom of major depressive disorder: results from the National Comorbidity Survey Replication. *Mol Psychiatry.* 2010;15:856–867.

8. Pedrelli P, Nyer M, Holt D, et al. Correlates of irritability in college students with depressive symptoms. *J Nerv Ment Dis.* 2013;201:953–958.

9. El-Mallakh RS, Ghaemi SN, Sagduyu K, et al. Antidepressant-associated chronic irritable dysphoria (ACID) in STEP-BD patients. *J Affect Disord.* 2008;111:372–377.

10. Dougherty DD, Rauch SL, Deckersbach T, et al. Ventromedial prefrontal cortex and amygdala dysfunction during an anger induction positron emission tomography study in patients with major depressive disorder with anger attacks. *Arch Gen Psychiatry.* 2004;61:795–804.

11. Iosifescu DV, Renshaw PF, Dougherty DD, et al. Major depressive disorder with anger attacks and subcortical MRI white matter hyperintensities. *J Nerv Ment Dis.* 2007;195:175–178.

12. Fava M, Vuolo RD, Wright EC, Nierenberg AA, Alpert JE, Rosenbaum JF. Fenfluramine challenge in unipolar depression with and without anger attacks. *Psychiatry Res.* 2000;94:9–18.

13. Fava M, Rosenbaum JF. Anger attacks in depression. *Depress Anxiety.* 1998;8(suppl 1):59–63.

14. Judd LL, Akiskal HS, Maser JD, et al. Major depressive disorder: a prospective study of residual subthreshold depressive symptoms as predictor of rapid relapse. *J Affect Disord.* 1998;50:97–108.

15. Keller MB, Lavori PW, Lewis CE, Klerman GL. Predictors of relapse in major depressive disorder. *JAMA.* 1983;250:3299–3304.

16. Keller MB, Shapiro RW, Lavori PW, Wolfe N. Relapse in major depressive disorder: analysis with the life table. *Arch Gen Psychiatry.* 1982;39:911–915.

17. Solomon DA, Keller MB, Leon AC, et al. Multiple recurrences of major depressive disorder. *Am J Psychiatry*. 2000;157:229–233.

18. Zajecka J, Kornstein SG, Blier P. Residual symptoms in major depressive disorder: prevalence, effects, and management. *J Clin Psychiatry*. 2013;74:407–414.

19. Nierenberg AA, Husain MM, Trivedi MH, et al. Residual symptoms after remission of major depressive disorder with citalopram and risk of relapse: a STAR*D report. *Psychol Med*. 2010;40:41–50.

20. McClintock SM, Husain MM, Wisniewski SR, et al. Residual symptoms in depressed outpatients who respond by 50% but do not remit to antidepressant medication. *J Clin Psychopharmacol*. 2011;31:180–186.

21. McClintock SM, Husain MM, Greer TL, Cullum CM. Association between depression severity and neurocognitive function in major depressive disorder: a review and synthesis. *Neuropsychology*. 2010;24:9–34.

22. Conradi HJ, Ormel J, de Jonge P. Presence of individual (residual) symptoms during depressive episodes and periods of remission: a 3-year prospective study. *Psychol Med*. 2011;41:1165–1174.

23. Conradi HJ, Ormel J, de Jonge P. Symptom profiles of DSM-IV-defined remission, recovery, relapse, and recurrence of depression: the role of the core symptoms. *Depress Anxiety*. 2012;29:638–645.

24. Fava M, Graves LM, Benazzi F, et al. A cross-sectional study of the prevalence of cognitive and physical symptoms during long-term antidepressant treatment. *J Clin Psychiatry*. 2006;67:1754–1759.

25. Fava M. Symptoms of fatigue and cognitive/executive dysfunction in major depressive disorder before and after antidepressant treatment. *J Clin Psychiatry*. 2003;64(suppl 14):30–34.

26. Gorwood P, Corruble E, Falissard B, Goodwin GM. Toxic effects of depression on brain function: impairment of delayed recall and the cumulative length of depressive disorder in a large sample of depressed outpatients. *Am J Psychiatry*. 2008;165:731–739.

27. Fava M, Ball S, Nelson JC, et al. Clinical relevance of fatigue as a residual symptom in major depressive disorder. *Depress Anxiety*. 2014;31:250–257.

28. Cooper JA, Tucker VL, Papakostas GI. Resolution of sleepiness and fatigue: a comparison of bupropion and selective serotonin reuptake inhibitors in subjects with major depressive disorder achieving remission at doses approved in the European Union. *J Psychopharmacol*. 2014;28:118–124.

29. Fava M, Rush AJ, Thase ME, et al. Fifteen years of clinical experience with bupropion HCl: from bupropion to bupropion SR to bupropion XL. *Primary Care Companion J Clin Psychiatry*. 2005;7:106–113.

30. Papakostas GI, Worthington JJ 3rd, Iosifescu DV, et al. The combination of duloxetine and bupropion for treatment-resistant major depressive disorder. *Depress Anxiety*. 2006;23:178–181.

31. Lam RW, Malhi GS, McIntyre RS, et al. Fatigue and occupational functioning in major depressive disorder. *Aust N Z J Psychiatry*. 2013;47:989–991.

32. Hegerl U, Lam RW, Malhi GS, et al. Conceptualising the neurobiology of fatigue. *Aust N Z J Psychiatry*. 2013;47:312–316.

33. Hegerl U, Hensch T. The vigilance regulation model of affective disorders and ADHD. *Neurosci Biobehav Rev*. 2014;44:45–57.

34. Correa H, Duval F, Claude MM, et al. Noradrenergic dysfunction and antidepressant treatment response. *Eur Neuropsychopharmacol*. 2001;11:163–168.

35. Arnsten AF, Wang MJ, Paspalas CD. Neuromodulation of thought: flexibilities and vulnerabilities in prefrontal cortical network synapses. *Neuron*. 2012;76:223–239.

36. Espana RA, Scammell TE. Sleep neurobiology from a clinical perspective. *Sleep.* 2011; 34:845–858.

37. Riemann D, Spiegelhalder K, Feige B, et al. The hyperarousal model of insomnia: a review of the concept and its evidence. *Sleep Med Rev.* 2010;14:19–31.

38. Buysse DJ, Germain A, Hall M, Monk TH, Nofzinger EA. A neurobiological model of insomnia. *Drug Discov Today Dis Models.* 2011;8:129–137.

39. Corsi-Cabrera M, Figueredo-Rodriguez P, del Rio-Portilla Y, et al. Enhanced frontoparietal synchronized activation during the wake-sleep transition in patients with primary insomnia. *Sleep.* 2012;35:501–511.

40. Riemann D, Kloepfer C, Berger M. Functional and structural brain alterations in insomnia: implications for pathophysiology. *Eur J Neurosci.* 2009;29:1754–1760.

41. Altena E, Vrenken H, Van Der Werf YD, van den Heuvel OA, Van Someren EJ. Reduced orbitofrontal and parietal gray matter in chronic insomnia: a voxel-based morphometric study. *Biol Psychiatry.* 2010;67:182–185.

42. Bonnet MH, Arand DL. Hyperarousal and insomnia: state of the science. *Sleep Med Rev.* 2010;14:9–15.

43. Miller AH, Maletic V, Raison CL. Inflammation and its discontents: the role of cytokines in the pathophysiology of major depression. *Biol Psychiatry.* 2009;65:732–741.

44. Maletic V, Robinson M, Oakes T, Iyengar S, Ball SG, Russell J. Neurobiology of depression: an integrated view of key findings. *Int J Clin Pract.* 2007;61:2030–2040.

45. Baglioni C, Spiegelhalder K, Lombardo C, Riemann D. Sleep and emotions: a focus on insomnia. *Sleep Med Rev.* 2010;14:227–238.

46. Baglioni C, Spiegelhalder K, Nissen C, Riemann D. Clinical implications of the causal relationship between insomnia and depression: how individually tailored treatment of sleeping difficulties could prevent the onset of depression. *EPMA J.* 2011;2:287–293.

47. Lorton D, Lubahn CL, Estus C, et al. Bidirectional communication between the brain and the immune system: implications for physiological sleep and disorders with disrupted sleep. *Neuroimmunomodulation.* 2006;13:357–374.

48. Maletic V, Raison CL. Neurobiology of depression, fibromyalgia and neuropathic pain. *Front Biosci.* 2009;14:5291–5338.

49. Taylor DJ, Mallory LJ, Lichstein KL, Durrence HH, Riedel BW, Bush AJ. Comorbidity of chronic insomnia with medical problems. *Sleep.* 2007;30:213–218.

50. Jansson-Frojmark M, Lindblom K. A bidirectional relationship between anxiety and depression, and insomnia? A prospective study in the general population. *J Psychosom Res.* 2008;64:443–449.

51. Germain A, Kupfer DJ. Circadian rhythm disturbances in depression. *Hum Psychopharmacol.* 2008;23:571–585.

52. Pan A, Keum N, Okereke OI, et al. Bidirectional association between depression and metabolic syndrome: a systematic review and meta-analysis of epidemiological studies. *Diabetes Care.* 2012;35:1171–1180.

53. Pan A, Sun Q, Czernichow S, et al. Bidirectional association between depression and obesity in middle-aged and older women. *Int J Obes (Lond).* 2012;36:595–602.

54. Simon GE, Ludman EJ, Linde JA, et al. Association between obesity and depression in middle-aged women. *Gen Hosp Psychiatry.* 2008;30:32–39.

55. Sorberg A, Gunnell D, Falkstedt D, Allebeck P, Aberg M, Hemmingsson T. Body mass index in young adulthood and suicidal behavior up to age 59 in a cohort of Swedish men. *PLoS ONE.* 2014;9:e101213.

56. Hung CI, Liu CY, Hsiao MC, Yu NW, Chu CL. Metabolic syndrome among psychiatric outpatients with mood and anxiety disorders. *BMC Psychiatry.* 2014;14:185.

57. Liu Y, Al-Sayegh H, Jabrah R, Wang W, Yan F, Zhang J. Association between C-reactive protein and depression: modulated by gender and mediated by body weight. *Psychiatry Res.* 2014;219:103–108.

58. Ervasti J, Vahtera J, Pentti J, et al. The role of psychiatric, cardiometabolic, and musculoskeletal comorbidity in the recurrence of depression-related work disability. *Depress Anxiety.* 2014;31(9):796–803.

59. Kuo LE, Czarnecka M, Kitlinska JB, et al. Chronic stress, combined with a high-fat/high-sugar diet, shifts sympathetic signaling toward neuropeptide Y and leads to obesity and the metabolic syndrome. *Ann N Y Acad Sci.* 2008;1148:232–237.

60. Garate I, Garcia-Bueno B, Madrigal JL, et al. Stress-induced neuroinflammation: role of the Toll-like receptor-4 pathway. *Biol Psychiatry.* 2013;73:32–43.

61. Kiecolt-Glaser JK, Habash DL, Fagundes CP, et al. Daily stressors, past depression, and metabolic responses to high-fat meals: a novel path to obesity. *Biol Psychiatry.* 2015;77(7):653–660.

62. Aschbacher K, Kornfeld S, Picard M, et al. Chronic stress increases vulnerability to diet-related abdominal fat, oxidative stress, and metabolic risk. *Psychoneuroendocrinology.* 2014;46:14–22.

63. Perez-Cornago A, Ramirez MJ, Zulet MA, Martinez JA. Effect of dietary restriction on peripheral monoamines and anxiety symptoms in obese subjects with metabolic syndrome. *Psychoneuroendocrinology.* 2014;47:98–106.

64. Perez-Cornago A, Lopez-Legarrea P, de la Iglesia R, Lahortiga F, Martinez JA, Zulet MA. Longitudinal relationship of diet and oxidative stress with depressive symptoms in patients with metabolic syndrome after following a weight loss treatment: the RESMENA project. *Clin Nutr.* 2014;33(6):1061–1067.

65. Perez-Cornago A, de la Iglesia R, Lopez-Legarrea P, et al. A decline in inflammation is associated with less depressive symptoms after a dietary intervention in metabolic syndrome patients: a longitudinal study. *Nutrition J.* 2014;13:36.

66. Krogh-Madsen R, Pedersen M, Solomon TP, et al. Normal physical activity obliterates the deleterious effects of a high-caloric intake. *J Appl Physiol.* 2014;116:231–239.

67. Gerhard T, Akincigil A, Correll CU, Foglio NJ, Crystal S, Olfson M. National trends in second-generation antipsychotic augmentation for nonpsychotic depression. *J Clin Psychiatry.* 2014;75:490–497.

68. Wright BM, Eiland EH 3rd, Lorenz R. Augmentation with atypical antipsychotics for depression: a review of evidence-based support from the medical literature. *Pharmacotherapy.* 2013;33:344–359.

69. Nelson JC, Papakostas GI. Atypical antipsychotic augmentation in major depressive disorder: a meta-analysis of placebo-controlled randomized trials. *Am J Psychiatry.* 2009;166:980–991.

70. Mathys M, Mitchell BG. Targeting treatment-resistant depression. *J Pharm Pract.* 2011;24:520–533.

71. Pae CU, Patkar AA. Clinical issues in use of atypical antipsychotics for depressed patients. *CNS Drugs.* 2013;27(suppl 1):S39–S45.

72. Patkar AA, Pae CU. Atypical antipsychotic augmentation strategies in the context of guideline-based care for the treatment of major depressive disorder. *CNS Drugs.* 2013;27(suppl 1):S29–S37.

73. Vieta E, Colom F. Therapeutic options in treatment-resistant depression. *Ann Med.* 2011;43:512–530.

74. Stroup TS, McEvoy JP, Ring KD, et al. A randomized trial examining the effectiveness of switching from olanzapine, quetiapine, or risperidone to aripiprazole to reduce meta-

bolic risk: comparison of antipsychotics for metabolic problems (CAMP). *Am J Psychiatry.* 2011;168:947–956.

75. Teff KL, Rickels MR, Grudziak J, Fuller C, Nguyen HL, Rickels K. Antipsychotic-induced insulin resistance and postprandial hormonal dysregulation independent of weight gain or psychiatric disease. *Diabetes.* 2013;62:3232–3240.

76. Fava M, Wisniewski SR, Thase ME, et al. Metabolic assessment of aripiprazole as adjunctive therapy in major depressive disorder: a pooled analysis of 2 studies. *J Clin Psychopharmacol.* 2009;29:362–367.

77. Papakostas GI, Petersen TJ, Kinrys G, et al. Aripiprazole augmentation of selective serotonin reuptake inhibitors for treatment-resistant major depressive disorder. *J Clin Psychiatry.* 2005;66:1326–1330.

78. Pae CU, Jeon HJ, Lee BC, et al. Aripiprazole augmentation for treatment of patients with chronic or recurrent major depressive disorder: a 12-week prospective open-label multicentre study. *Int Clin Psychopharmacol.* 2013;28:322–329.

79. Stewart TD, Hatch A, Largay K, et al. Effect of symptom severity on efficacy and safety of aripiprazole adjunctive to antidepressant monotherapy in major depressive disorder: a pooled analysis. *J Affect Disord.* 2014;162:20–25.

80. Nelson JC, Mankoski R, Baker RA, et al. Effects of aripiprazole adjunctive to standard antidepressant treatment on the core symptoms of depression: a post-hoc, pooled analysis of two large, placebo-controlled studies. *J Affect Disord.* 2010;120:133–140.

81. Nelson JC, Rahman Z, Laubmeier KK, et al. Efficacy of adjunctive aripiprazole in patients with major depressive disorder whose symptoms worsened with antidepressant monotherapy. *CNS Spectr.* 2014;19(6):528–534.

82. Berman RM, Fava M, Thase ME, et al. Aripiprazole augmentation in major depressive disorder: a double-blind, placebo-controlled study in patients with inadequate response to antidepressants. *CNS Spectr.* 2009;14:197–206.

83. Nasr S, Wendt B, Popli A, Crayton J. Comparing outcomes of adjunctive treatment in depression: aripiprazole versus bupropion. *J Affect Disord.* 2014;162:50–54.

84. Clayton AH, Baker RA, Sheehan JJ, et al. Comparison of adjunctive use of aripiprazole with bupropion or selective serotonin reuptake inhibitors/serotonin-norepinephrine reuptake inhibitors: analysis of patients beginning adjunctive treatment in a 52-week, open-label study. *BMC Res Notes.* 2014;7:459.

85. Nickel MK, Loew TH, Pedrosa Gil F. Aripiprazole in treatment of borderline patients, part II: an 18-month follow-up. *Psychopharmacology (Berl).* 2007;191:1023–1026.

86. Nickel MK, Muehlbacher M, Nickel C, et al. Aripiprazole in the treatment of patients with borderline personality disorder: a double-blind, placebo-controlled study. *Am J Psychiatry.* 2006;163:833–838.

87. Mercer D, Douglass AB, Links PS. Meta-analyses of mood stabilizers, antidepressants and antipsychotics in the treatment of borderline personality disorder: effectiveness for depression and anger symptoms. *J Pers Disord.* 2009;23:156–174.

88. Comai S, Tau M, Pavlovic Z, Gobbi G. The psychopharmacology of aggressive behavior: a translational approach: part 2: clinical studies using atypical antipsychotics, anticonvulsants, and lithium. *J Clin Psychopharmacol.* 2012;32:237–260.

89. Douglas N, Young A, Roebuck T, et al. Prevalence of depression in patients referred with snoring and obstructive sleep apnoea. *Intern Med J.* 2013;43:630–634.

90. Harper RM, Kumar R, Ogren JA, Macey PM. Sleep-disordered breathing: effects on brain structure and function. *Respir Physiol Neurobiol.* 2013;188:383–391.

91. Rezaeitalab F, Moharrari F, Saberi S, Asadpour H, Rezaeetalab F. The correlation of

anxiety and depression with obstructive sleep apnea syndrome. *J Res Med Sci.* 2014;19: 205–210.

92. Chen YH, Keller JK, Kang JH, Hsieh HJ, Lin HC. Obstructive sleep apnea and the subsequent risk of depressive disorder: a population-based follow-up study. *J Clin Sleep Med.* 2013;9:417–423.

93. Yadav SK, Kumar R, Macey PM, Woo MA, Yan-Go FL, Harper RM. Insular cortex metabolite changes in obstructive sleep apnea. *Sleep.* 2014;37:951–958.

94. Vaessen TJ, Overeem S, Sitskoorn MM. Cognitive complaints in obstructive sleep apnea. *Sleep Med Rev.* 2015;19:51–58.

95. Borges JG, Ginani GE, Hachul H, Cintra FD, Tufik S, Pompeia S. Executive functioning in obstructive sleep apnea syndrome patients without comorbidities: focus on the fractionation of executive functions. *J Clin Exp Neuropsychol.* 2013;35:1094–1107.

96. Li Y, Veasey SC. Neurobiology and neuropathophysiology of obstructive sleep apnea. *Neuromol Med.* 2012;14:168–179.

97. Kendzerska T, Mollayeva T, Gershon AS, Leung RS, Hawker G, Tomlinson G. Untreated obstructive sleep apnea and the risk for serious long-term adverse outcomes: a systematic review. *Sleep Med Rev.* 2014;18:49–59.

98. Bjorvatn B, Pallesen S, Gronli J, Sivertsen B, Lehmann S. Prevalence and correlates of insomnia and excessive sleepiness in adults with obstructive sleep apnea symptoms. *Percept Motor Skills.* 2014;118:571–586.

99. Nicto FJ, Young TB, Lind BK, et al. Association of sleep-disordered breathing, sleep apnea, and hypertension in a large community-based study. Sleep Heart Health Study. *JAMA.* 2000;283:1829–1836.

100. Ösby U, Brandt L, Correia N, Ekbom A, Sparén P. Excess mortality in bipolar and unipolar disorder in Sweden. *Arch Gen Psychiatry.* 2001;58:844–850.

101. Shelton RC, Miller AH. Eating ourselves to death (and despair): the contribution of adiposity and inflammation to depression. *Prog Neurobiol.* 2010;91:275–299.

102. Al-Harbi KS, Qureshi NA. Neuromodulation therapies and treatment-resistant depression. *Med Devices.* 2012;5:53–65.

103. Brunoni AR, Teng CT, Correa C, et al. Neuromodulation approaches for the treatment of major depression: challenges and recommendations from a working group meeting. *Arq Neuropsiquiatr.* 2010;68:433–451.

104. Ren J, Li H, Palaniyappan L, et al. Repetitive transcranial magnetic stimulation versus electroconvulsive therapy for major depression: a systematic review and meta-analysis. *Prog Neuropsychopharmacol Biol Psychiatry.* 2014;51:181–189.

105. Brakemeier EL, Merkl A, Wilbertz G, et al. Cognitive-behavioral therapy as continuation treatment to sustain response after electroconvulsive therapy in depression: a randomized controlled trial. *Biol Psychiatry.* 2014;76:194–202.

106. Haghighi M, Salehi I, Erfani P, et al. Additional ECT increases BDNF-levels in patients suffering from major depressive disorders compared to patients treated with citalopram only. *J Psychiatr Res.* 2013;47:908–915.

107. Salehi I, Hosseini SM, Haghighi M, et al. Electroconvulsive therapy and aerobic exercise training increased BDNF and ameliorated depressive symptoms in patients suffering from treatment-resistant major depressive disorder. *J Psychiatr Res.* 2014.

108. Tendolkar I, van Beek M, van Oostrom I, et al. Electroconvulsive therapy increases hippocampal and amygdala volume in therapy refractory depression: a longitudinal pilot study. *Psychiatry Res.* 2013;214:197–203.

109. Moreines JL, McClintock SM, Holtzheimer PE. Neuropsychologic effects of neuromod-

ulation techniques for treatment-resistant depression: a review. *Brain Stimul.* 2011;4: 17–27.

110. Berry SM, Broglio K, Bunker M, Jayewardene A, Olin B, Rush AJ. A patient-level meta-analysis of studies evaluating vagus nerve stimulation therapy for treatment-resistant depression. *Med Devices.* 2013;6:17–35.

111. Rush AJ, Siefert SE. Clinical issues in considering vagus nerve stimulation for treatment-resistant depression. *Exp Neurol.* 2009;219:36–43.

112. Mohr P, Rodriguez M, Slavickova A, Hanka J. The application of vagus nerve stimulation and deep brain stimulation in depression. *Neuropsychobiology.* 2011;64:170–181.

113. Pardo JV, Sheikh SA, Schwindt GC, et al. Chronic vagus nerve stimulation for treatment-resistant depression decreases resting ventromedial prefrontal glucose metabolism. *Neuroimage.* 2008;42:879–889.

114. Daban C, Martinez-Aran A, Cruz N, Vieta E. Safety and efficacy of vagus nerve stimulation in treatment-resistant depression. A systematic review. *J Affect Disord.* 2008;110: 1–15.

115. Lozano AM, Giacobbe P, Hamani C, et al. A multicenter pilot study of subcallosal cingulate area deep brain stimulation for treatment-resistant depression. *J Neurosurg.* 2012;116:315–322.

116. Kennedy SH, Giacobbe P, Rizvi SJ, et al. Deep brain stimulation for treatment-resistant depression: follow-up after 3 to 6 years. *Am J Psychiatry.* 2011;168:502–510.

117. Schlaepfer TE, Bewernick BH, Kayser S, Hurlemann R, Coenen VA. Deep brain stimulation of the human reward system for major depression—rationale, outcomes and outlook. *Neuropsychopharmacology.* 2014;39:1303–1314.

118. McNeely HE, Mayberg HS, Lozano AM, Kennedy SH. Neuropsychological impact of Cg25 deep brain stimulation for treatment-resistant depression: preliminary results over 12 months. *J Nerv Ment Dis.* 2008;196:405–410.

119. van Dijk A, Klompmakers AA, Feenstra MG, Denys D. Deep brain stimulation of the accumbens increases dopamine, serotonin, and noradrenaline in the prefrontal cortex. *J Neurochem.* 2012;123:897–903.

120. Schlaepfer TE, Bewernick BH, Kayser S, Madler B, Coenen VA. Rapid effects of deep brain stimulation for treatment-resistant major depression. *Biol Psychiatry.* 2013;73: 1204–1212.

121. George MS, Taylor JJ, Short EB. The expanding evidence base for rTMS treatment of depression. *Curr Opin Psychiatry.* 2013;26:13–18.

122. Hovington CL, McGirr A, Lepage M, Berlim MT. Repetitive transcranial magnetic stimulation (rTMS) for treating major depression and schizophrenia: a systematic review of recent meta-analyses. *Ann Med.* 2013;45:308–321.

123. Deng ZD, Lisanby SH, Peterchev AV. Electric field depth-focality tradeoff in transcranial magnetic stimulation: simulation comparison of 50 coil designs. *Brain Stimul.* 2013;6:1–13.

124. Deng ZD, Lisanby SH, Peterchev AV. Coil design considerations for deep transcranial magnetic stimulation. *Clin Neurophysiol.* 2014;125:1202–1212.

125. Berlim MT, van den Eynde F, Tovar-Perdomo S, Daskalakis ZJ. Response, remission and drop-out rates following high-frequency repetitive transcranial magnetic stimulation (rTMS) for treating major depression: a systematic review and meta-analysis of randomized, double-blind and sham-controlled trials. *Psychol Med.* 2014;44:225–239.

126. Gaynes BN, Lloyd SW, Lux L, et al. Repetitive transcranial magnetic stimulation for treatment-resistant depression: a systematic review and meta-analysis. *J Clin Psychiatry.* 2014;75:477–489.

127. Lepping P, Schonfeldt-Lecuona C, Sambhi RS, et al. A systematic review of the clinical relevance of repetitive transcranial magnetic stimulation. *Acta Psychiatr Scand.* 2014; 130(5):326–341.

128. Downar J, Daskalakis ZJ. New targets for rTMS in depression: a review of convergent evidence. *Brain Stimul.* 2013;6:231–240.

129. Lefaucheur JP, Andre-Obadia N, Antal A, et al. Evidence-based guidelines on the therapeutic use of repetitive transcranial magnetic stimulation (rTMS). *Clin Neurophysiol.* 2014;125(11):2150–2206.

130. Berlim MT, Van den Eynde F, Daskalakis ZJ. Clinically meaningful efficacy and acceptability of low-frequency repetitive transcranial magnetic stimulation (rTMS) for treating primary major depression: a meta-analysis of randomized, double-blind and sham-controlled trials. *Neuropsychopharmacology.* 2013;36:543–551.

131. Speer AM, Benson BE, Kimbrell TK, et al. Opposite effects of high and low frequency rTMS on mood in depressed patients: relationship to baseline cerebral activity on PET. *J Affect Disord.* 2009;115:386–394.

132. Fitzgerald PB, Benitez J, de Castella A, Daskalakis ZJ, Brown TL, Kulkarni J. A randomized, controlled trial of sequential bilateral repetitive transcranial magnetic stimulation for treatment-resistant depression. *Am J Psychiatry.* 2006;163:88–94.

133. Fitzgerald PB, Hoy KE, Singh A, et al. Equivalent beneficial effects of unilateral and bilateral prefrontal cortex transcranial magnetic stimulation in a large randomized trial in treatment-resistant major depression. *Int J Neuropsychopharmacol.* 2013;16: 1975–1984.

134. Berlim MT, Van den Eynde F, Daskalakis ZJ. A systematic review and meta-analysis on the efficacy and acceptability of bilateral repetitive transcranial magnetic stimulation (rTMS) for treating major depression. *Psychol Med.* 2013;43:2245–2254.

135. Baeken C, Vanderhasselt MA, Remue J, et al. Intensive HF-rTMS treatment in refractory medication-resistant unipolar depressed patients. *J Affect Disord.* 2013;151:625–631.

136. Rohan ML, Yamamoto RT, Ravichandran CT, et al. Rapid mood-elevating effects of low field magnetic stimulation in depression. *Biol Psychiatry.* 2014;76:186–193.

137. Sheline YI, Price JL, Yan Z, Mintun MA. Resting-state functional MRI in depression unmasks increased connectivity between networks via the dorsal nexus. *Proc Natl Acad Sci U S A.* 2010;107:11020–11025.

138. Downar J, Geraci J, Salomons TV, et al. Anhedonia and reward-circuit connectivity distinguish nonresponders from responders to dorsomedial prefrontal repetitive transcranial magnetic stimulation in major depression. *Biol Psychiatry.* 2014;76:176–185.

139. Salomons TV, Dunlop K, Kennedy SH, et al. Resting-state cortico-thalamic-striatal connectivity predicts response to dorsomedial prefrontal rTMS in major depressive disorder. *Neuropsychopharmacology.* 2014;39:488–498.

140. Liston C, Chen AC, Zebley BD, et al. Default mode network mechanisms of transcranial magnetic stimulation in depression. *Biol Psychiatry.* 2014;76(7):517–526.

141. Kito S, Hasegawa T, Koga Y. Cerebral blood flow ratio of the dorsolateral prefrontal cortex to the ventromedial prefrontal cortex as a potential predictor of treatment response to transcranial magnetic stimulation in depression. *Brain Stimul.* 2012;5: 547–553.

142. Arns M, Drinkenburg WH, Fitzgerald PB, Kenemans JL. Neurophysiological predictors of non-response to rTMS in depression. *Brain Stimul.* 2012;5:569–576.

143. Richieri R, Guedj E, Michel P, et al. Maintenance transcranial magnetic stimulation reduces depression relapse: a propensity-adjusted analysis. *J Affect Disord.* 2013;151: 129–135.

144. Xie J, Chen J, Wei Q. Repetitive transcranial magnetic stimulation versus electroconvulsive therapy for major depression: a meta-analysis of stimulus parameter effects. *Neurol Res.* 2013;35:1084–1091.

145. Berlim MT, Van den Eynde F, Daskalakis ZJ. Efficacy and acceptability of high frequency repetitive transcranial magnetic stimulation (rTMS) versus electroconvulsive therapy (ECT) for major depression: a systematic review and meta-analysis of randomized trials. *Depress Anxiety.* 2013;30:614–623.

146. Diefenbach GJ, Bragdon L, Goethe JW. Treating anxious depression using repetitive transcranial magnetic stimulation. *J Affect Disord.* 2013;151:365–368.

147. Pellicciari MC, Cordone S, Marzano C, et al. Dorsolateral prefrontal transcranial magnetic stimulation in patients with major depression locally affects alpha power of REM sleep. *Front Hum Neurosci.* 2013;7:433.

148. Hoy KE, Segrave RA, Daskalakis ZJ, Fitzgerald PB. Investigating the relationship between cognitive change and antidepressant response following rTMS: a large scale retrospective study. *Brain Stimul.* 2012;5:539–546.

149. Nadeau SE, Bowers D, Jones TL, Wu SS, Triggs WJ, Heilman KM. Cognitive effects of treatment of depression with repetitive transcranial magnetic stimulation. *Cognit Behav Neurol.* 2014;27:77–87.

150. Katalinic N, Lai R, Somogyi A, Mitchell PB, Glue P, Loo CK. Ketamine as a new treatment for depression: a review of its efficacy and adverse effects. *Aust N Z J Psychiatry.* 2013;47:710–727.

151. Hasselmann HW. Ketamine as antidepressant? Current state and future perspectives. *Curr Neuropharmacol.* 2014;12:57–70.

152. Browne CA, Lucki I. Antidepressant effects of ketamine: mechanisms underlying fast-acting novel antidepressants. *Front Pharmacol.* 2013;4:161.

153. Salvadore G, Singh JB. Ketamine as a fast acting antidepressant: current knowledge and open questions. *CNS Neurosci Ther.* 2013;19:428–436.

154. Salvadore G, van der Veen JW, Zhang Y, et al. An investigation of amino-acid neurotransmitters as potential predictors of clinical improvement to ketamine in depression. *Int J Neuropsychopharmacol.* 2012;15:1063–1072.

155. Yang C, Zhou ZQ, Gao ZQ, Shi JY, Yang JJ. Acute increases in plasma mammalian target of rapamycin, glycogen synthase kinase-3beta, and eukaryotic elongation factor 2 phosphorylation after ketamine treatment in three depressed patients. *Biol Psychiatry.* 2013;73:e35–e36.

156. Ibrahim L, Diazgranados N, Franco-Chaves J, et al. Course of improvement in depressive symptoms to a single intravenous infusion of ketamine vs add-on riluzole: results from a 4-week, double-blind, placebo-controlled study. *Neuropsychopharmacology.* 2012;37:1526–1533.

157. Fond G, Loundou A, Rabu C, et al. Ketamine administration in depressive disorders: a systematic review and meta-analysis. *Psychopharmacology (Berl).* 2014.

158. McGirr A, Berlim MT, Bond DJ, Fleck MP, Yatham LN, Lam RW. A systematic review and meta-analysis of randomized, double-blind, placebo-controlled trials of ketamine in the rapid treatment of major depressive episodes. *Psychol Med.* 2015;45(4):693–704.

159. Shiroma PR, Johns B, Kuskowski M, et al. Augmentation of response and remission to serial intravenous subanesthetic ketamine in treatment resistant depression. *J Affect Disord.* 2014;155:123–129.
160. Zigman D, Blier P. Urgent ketamine infusion rapidly eliminated suicidal ideation for a patient with major depressive disorder: a case report. *J Clin Psychopharmacol.* 2013;33: 270–272.
161. Lara DR, Bisol LW, Munari LR. Antidepressant, mood stabilizing and procognitive effects of very low dose sublingual ketamine in refractory unipolar and bipolar depression. *Int J Neuropsychopharmacol.* 2013;16:2111–2117.
162. Lapidus KA, Levitch CF, Perez AM, et al. A randomized controlled trial of intranasal ketamine in major depressive disorder. *Biol Psychiatry.* 2014;76(12):970–976.
163. Carlson PJ, Diazgranados N, Nugent AC, et al. Neural correlates of rapid antidepressant response to ketamine in treatment-resistant unipolar depression: a preliminary positron emission tomography study. *Biol Psychiatry.* 2013;73:1213–1221.
164. Doyle OM, De Simoni S, Schwarz AJ, et al. Quantifying the attenuation of the ketamine pharmacological magnetic resonance imaging response in humans: a validation using antipsychotic and glutamatergic agents. *J Pharmacol Exp Ther.* 2013;345: 151–160.
165. Hamidi M, Drevets WC, Price JL. Glial reduction in amygdala in major depressive disorder is due to oligodendrocytes. *Biol Psychiatry.* 2004;55:563–569.
166. Shiroma PR, Albott CS, Johns B, Thuras P, Wels J, Lim KO. Neurocognitive performance and serial intravenous subanesthetic ketamine in treatment-resistant depression. *Int J Neuropsychopharmacol.* 2014;17(11):1805–1813.
167. Salvadore G, Cornwell BR, Sambataro F, et al. Anterior cingulate desynchronization and functional connectivity with the amygdala during a working memory task predict rapid antidepressant response to ketamine. *Neuropsychopharmacology.* 2010;35:1415–1422.

Index